The SAGES Manual of Evolving Techniques in Pancreatic Surgery

Eugene P. Ceppa • Kevin M. El-Hayek
Melissa E. Hogg • Nicolò Pecorelli
Editors

The SAGES Manual of Evolving Techniques in Pancreatic Surgery

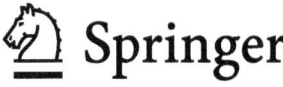 Springer

Editors
Eugene P. Ceppa
Department of Surgery
Indiana University School of Medicine
Indianapolis, IN, USA

Kevin M. El-Hayek
Division of General Surgery,
The MetroHealth System, Case Western
Reserve University School of Medicine
Cleveland, OH, USA

Melissa E. Hogg
NorthShore University HealthSystem
Evanston, IL, USA

Nicolò Pecorelli
Pancreas Translational & Clinical
Research Center
San Raffaele Scientific Institute, Vita-Salute
San Raffaele University
Milano, Italy

ISBN 978-3-031-78408-8   ISBN 978-3-031-78409-5   (eBook)
https://doi.org/10.1007/978-3-031-78409-5

This Springer imprint is published by the registered company Springer Nature Switzerland AG
The registered company address is: Gewerbestrasse 11, 6330 Cham, Switzerland

If disposing of this product, please recycle the paper.

Eugene P. Ceppa

I dedicate this to VXC, CLC, GDC, and DPC for their continued unwavering love, support, and patience. To IMC and PRC, I thank you for the love, guidance, and persistence to accomplish one's goals. I give thanks to my mentors along the way including Bertrand Garcia-Moreno, Gregory Bulkley, Keith Lillemoe, Ted Pappas, Paul Kuo, Kimberly Kirkwood, Bryan Clary, Rory Pryor, and Henry Pitt. With great admiration, I thank Kevin, Melissa, Nicolò, and Monia for their tireless effort, collegial collaboration, and making this experience feel more like a family and not just colleagues.

Kevin M. El-Hayek

To my mother and father, Annette and Salim El-Hayek for supporting my academic journey from day one. To my wife Raechel and my children, Keira, Alison, and Cameron for being supportive when my work extends into nights and weekends. I'd also like to dedicate this book to my mentors in hepato-pancreato-biliary surgery, namely,

R. Matthew Walsh, Sricharan Chalikonda, and J. Michael Henderson. Without your knowledge, experience, and willingness to share, I would not be the HPB surgeon I am today—I am eternally grateful. To the SAGES HPB leaders who supported my progress in the field of MIS HPB surgery, Horacio Asbun and Adnan Alseidi. And of course, this book would not be possible without the SAGES HPB/Solid Organ committee members (the BEST committee!) and the glue that keeps us together, Monia Ilunga.

Melissa E. Hogg

To young, old, current, and future pancreas surgeons as well as authors and editors of this manual. Continue to learn, evolve, and work hard to take care of sick patients.

Nicolò Pecorelli

To my mother Antonella, who was my number 1 supporter and would have loved to own a copy of this book. To my wife Ilaria and my kids Olivia, Arturo, and Lavinia— you are my everyday joy. To my father Sergio for inspiring my passion for research. Also, to my friend Jody for reminding me to stay hungry for science. I'd also like to dedicate this book to my first mentors in pancreatic surgery, Profs. Valerio Di Carlo, Marco Braga, and Gianpaolo Balzano, who taught me that surgery is not only a matter of hands, but also reason and soul. To my co-editors Melissa, Kevin, Eugene, and the SAGES HPB/Solid Organ committee friends who worked so hard to make this book happen.

Disclaimer

Disclaimer for Society of American Gastrointestinal and Endoscopic Surgeons (SAGES) Manual: The contents of this manual are intended exclusively for educational and informational purposes only, and nothing contained within constitutes medical advice. Neither this manual nor its contents have been subject to formal peer review. The information provided herein does not represent, nor should it be interpreted as, the official position, view, or endorsement of the Society of American Gastrointestinal and Endoscopic Surgeons (SAGES) or its governing body. This manual is not intended for use in diagnosing or treating any health problem, condition, or disease. Individuals seeking personal medical advice should consult an appropriate licensed professional.

Neither SAGES, nor its officers, directors, employees, members, nor any of the contributors to this manual make any representation or warranty, express or implied, regarding the accuracy, completeness, fitness for any intended purpose, or suitability of the information contained herein for any specific use or function. Neither access to nor use of this manual creates or implies any physician-patient relationship, and reliance on any information provided, contained, or implied herein is solely at the user's own risk.

Contents

Contributors

Martina Abati Division of Pancreatic Surgery, Pancreas Translational and Clinical Research Center, San Raffaele Scientific Institute, Milan, Italy
Nutrition Service, San Raffaele Scientific Institute, Milan, Italy

Gerard J. Abood Department of Surgery, Loyola University Medical Center, Maywood, IL, USA

Alexandra M. Adams Brooke Army Medical Center, Fort Sam Houston, TX, USA

Hemasat Alkhatib Division of General Surgery, MetroHealth System, Cleveland, OH, USA

Adnan Alseidi Department of Surgery, University of California, San Francisco, San Francisco, CA, USA

Osaid Alser Texas Tech University Health Sciences Center, Lubbock, TX, USA

Domenech Asbun Division of Hepatobiliary and Pancreas Surgery, Miami Cancer Institute, Miami, FL, USA

Horacio J. Asbun Division of Hepatobiliary and Pancreas Surgery, Miami Cancer Institute, Miami, FL, USA

Subhashini Ayloo Department of Surgery, Warren Alpert Medical School of Brown University, Providence, RI, USA

Elizabeth L. Barbera Brooke Army Medical Center, Fort Sam Houston, TX, USA

Jackson A. Baril Department of Surgery, Indiana University School of Medicine, Indianapolis, IN, USA

Jodie Adam Barkin Pancreas Center, Division of Gastroenterology, University of Miami Miller School of Medicine, Miami, FL, USA

Ricardo J. Bello Division of Surgical Oncology, Medical College of Wisconsin, Milwaukee, WI, USA

Marc G. Besselink Department of Surgery, Amsterdam UMC, Location University of Amsterdam, Amsterdam, The Netherlands
Amsterdam Gastroenterology Endocrinology Metabolism, Amsterdam, The Netherlands

Stefan A. W. Bouwense Department of Surgery, Maastricht University Medical Centre+, Maastricht, The Netherlands

Vincent Butano Digestive Health Institute at AdventHealth, Tampa, FL, USA

Nicholas Caminiti Department of Surgery, University of Louisville, Louisville, KY, USA

Mei Zhen Cao Department of General Surgery, The Brooklyn Hospital Center, Icahn School of Medicine at Mount Sinai, New York, NY, USA

Chelsea F. Cardell Department of Surgery, Loyola University Medical Center, Maywood, IL, USA

Fabio Casciani University of Verona, Verona, Italy
University of Pennsylvania Perelman School of Medicine, Philadelphia, PA, USA

Eugene P. Ceppa Department of Surgery, Indiana University School of Medicine, Indianapolis, IN, USA

Jenny Chang Department of General Surgery, Digestive Disease Institute, Cleveland Clinic, Cleveland, OH, USA

Zaim Chaudhary University of California, Berkeley, Berkeley, CA, USA

Ariana Chirban Department of Surgery, St. Elizabeth's Medical Center, Boston University School of Medicine, Boston, MA, USA
University of California, San Diego, School of Medicine, La Jolla, CA, USA

Edward Cho Department of Surgery, University of Oklahoma at Tulsa, Tulsa, OK, USA
Department of Surgery, University of Illinois Peoria, Peoria, IL, USA

Callisia N. Clarke Division of Surgical Oncology, Medical College of Wisconsin, Milwaukee, WI, USA

Claudius Conrad Department of Surgery, St. Elizabeth's Medical Center, Boston University School of Medicine, Boston, MA, USA
Carle Cancer Institute, Carle Illinois College of Medicine, Urbana, IL, USA

G. Corvino Department of General and Pancreatic Surgery, The Pancreas Institute Verona, University of Verona Hospital Trust, Verona, Italy

Kanak Das Texas Tech University Health Sciences Center, Lubbock, TX, USA

Jonathan C. DeLong Division of Surgical Oncology, University of Tennessee Medical Center Knoxville, Knoxville, TN, USA

Nicolas Demartines Department of Visceral Surgery, Lausanne University Hospital CHUV, University of Lausanne, Lausanne, Switzerland

Kevin M. El-Hayek Division of General Surgery, MetroHealth System, Cleveland, OH, USA
Case Western Reserve University School of Medicine, Cleveland, OH, USA
Northeast Ohio Medical University, Rootstown, OH, USA

Imad Elkhatib Advanced/Therapeutic Endoscopy, Advocate Christ Medical Center, Oak Lawn, IL, USA

Amir H. Fathi University of California San Francisco, Fresno MEP, Fresno, CA, USA

Ashley Faulx Division of Gastroenterology, University Hospitals of Cleveland, Case Western Reserve University School of Medicine, Cleveland, OH, USA

Alexandra Gangi Department of Surgical Oncology, Cedars-Sinai Medical Center, Los Angeles, CA, USA

Romulo Genato Department of General Surgery, The Brooklyn Hospital Center, Icahn School of Medicine at Mount Sinai, New York, NY, USA

Camilla Gomes Department of Surgery, University of California, San Francisco, San Francisco, CA, USA

Andrew Gumbs Department of General Surgery, The Brooklyn Hospital Center, Icahn School of Medicine at Mount Sinai, New York, NY, USA

Jessica Heard Department of Surgery, University of Oklahoma at Tulsa, Tulsa, OK, USA

Emily Hensler Department of Surgery, Warren Alpert Medical School of Brown University, Providence, RI, USA

Matthew Hernandez Department of Surgery, City of Hope National Medical Center, Duarte, CA, USA

Pamela J. Hodul Moffitt Cancer Center, Tampa, FL, USA

Melissa E. Hogg NorthShore University HealthSystem, Evanston, IL, USA

Carlos Theodore Huerta DeWitt Daughtry Family Department of Surgery, University of Miami Miller School of Medicine, Miami, FL, USA

Malynn Anne Ilanga Department of Surgery, University of Oklahoma at Tulsa, Tulsa, OK, USA

Harel Jacoby Advent Health Tampa Digestive Health Institute, Tampa, FL, USA
Sheba Medical Center, Tel-Aviv, Israel

Dhiresh Rohan Jeyarajah Department of Surgery, Methodist Health System, Dallas, TX, USA
Department of Surgery, TCU Burnett School of Medicine, Fort Worth, USA

Rachel C. Kim Department of Surgery, Indiana University School of Medicine, Indianapolis, IN, USA

Jörg Kleeff Department of Visceral, Vascular and Endocrine Surgery, University Hospital Halle (Saale), Martin-Luther-University Halle-Wittenberg, Halle (Saale), Germany

Johannes Klose Department of Visceral, Vascular and Endocrine Surgery, University Hospital Halle (Saale), Martin-Luther-University Halle-Wittenberg, Halle (Saale), Germany

Joshua P. Kronenfeld DeWitt Daughtry Department of Surgery, University of Miami Miller School of Medicine, Miami, FL, USA

Onur C. Kutlu DeWitt Daughtry Department of Surgery, University of Miami Miller School of Medicine, Miami, FL, USA

Jaewon Lee Department of Surgical Oncology, Cedars-Sinai Medical Center, Los Angeles, CA, USA

Chiara Limongi Vita-Salute San Raffaele University, Milan, Italy

Núria Lluís Division of Hepatobiliary and Pancreas Surgery, Miami Cancer Institute, Miami, FL, USA

Szu-Aun Long Department of Surgery, University of Cincinnati College of Medicine, Cincinnati, OH, USA

G. Marchegiani Hepatopancreatobiliary and Liver Transplant Surgery, Department of Surgery, Oncology and Gastroenterology (DiSCOG), University of Padua, Padua, Italy

David Martin Department of Visceral Surgery, Lausanne University Hospital CHUV, University of Lausanne, Lausanne, Switzerland

Robert Martin Department of Surgery, University of Louisville, Louisville, KY, USA

Heather E. Matheny Vascular Surgery, University of Washington, Seattle, WA, USA

Laleh Melstrom Department of Surgery, City of Hope National Medical Center, Duarte, CA, USA

Marc Mesleh Department of Surgery, University of Illinois Chicago (UIC), Chicago, IL, USA
Advocate Christ Medical Center, Oak Lawn, IL, USA

Luca Milone Division of Robotic Surgery, Department of General Surgery, The Brooklyn Hospital Center, Icahn School of Medicine at Mount Sinai, New York, NY, USA

David Caba Molina Loma Linda University, Loma Linda, CA, USA
Riverside University Health System/University of California-Riverside, Loma Linda, CA, USA

Ross Mudgway Loma Linda University, Loma Linda, CA, USA

Gilbert Murimwa Department of Surgery, University of Texas Southwestern Medical Center, Dallas, TX, USA

Anne Nagelhout Department of Surgery, Radboudumc, Nijmegen, The Netherlands
Department of Research and Development, St. Antonius Hospital, Nieuwegein, The Netherlands

Trang K. Nguyen Division of Surgical Oncology, Washington University in St. Louis, St. Louis, MO, USA

Daniel J. Oliveira Loma Linda University, Loma Linda, CA, USA

Edwin Onkendi Texas Tech University Health Sciences Center, Lubbock, TX, USA

Houssam G. Osman Department of Surgery, Methodist Health System, Dallas, TX, USA

Elena Panettieri Department of Surgery, St. Elizabeth's Medical Center, Boston University School of Medicine, Boston, MA, USA
Hepatobiliary Surgery, Fondazione "Policlinico Universitario A. Gemelli", IRCCS, Università Cattolica del Sacro Cuore, Rome, Italy

Nicolò Pecorelli Vita-Salute San Raffaele University, Milan, Italy
Division of Pancreatic Surgery, Pancreas Translational and Clinical Research Center, San Raffaele Scientific Institute, Milan, Italy
Pancreas Translational & Clinical Research Center, San Raffaele Scientific Institute, Vita-Salute San Raffaele University, Milan, Italy

G. Perri Hepatopancreatobiliary and Liver Transplant Surgery, Department of Surgery, Oncology and Gastroenterology (DiSCOG), University of Padua, Padua, Italy

Patricio M. Polanco Division of Surgical Oncology, Department of Surgery, University of Texas Southwestern Medical Center, Dallas, TX, USA

Ann Polcari University of Chicago, Chicago, IL, USA

Motaz Qadan Division of Surgical Oncology, Department of Surgery, Massachusetts General Hospital, Boston, MA, USA

Allen A. Razavi Department of Surgical Oncology, Cedars-Sinai Medical Center, Los Angeles, CA, USA

Aram Rojas NorthShore University HealthSystem, Evanston, IL, USA

Ulrich Ronellenfitsch Department of Visceral, Vascular and Endocrine Surgery, University Hospital Halle (Saale), Martin-Luther-University Halle-Wittenberg, Halle (Saale), Germany

Alexander Rosemurgy Department of Surgery, University of Central Florida, Orlando, FL, USA
Advent Health Tampal Digestive Health Institute, Tampa, FL, USA
Department of Surgery, Nova Southeastern University, Fort Lauderdale, FL, USA

Sharona Ross Department of Surgery, University of Central Florida, Orlando, FL, USA
Advent Health Tampal Digestive Health Institute, Tampa, FL, USA
Department of Surgery, Nova Southeastern University, Fort Lauderdale, FL, USA

Didier Roulin Department of Visceral Surgery, Lausanne University Hospital CHUV, University of Lausanne, Lausanne, Switzerland

R. Salvia Department of General and Pancreatic Surgery, The Pancreas Institute Verona, University of Verona Hospital Trust, Verona, Italy

Maximiliano Servin-Rojas Department of Surgery, Massachusetts General Hospital, Boston, MA, USA

Robert Simon Department of General Surgery, Digestive Disease Institute, Cleveland Clinic, Cleveland, OH, USA

Andrew J. Sinnamon Moffitt Cancer Center, Tampa, FL, USA

Rebecca A. Snyder Department of Surgical Oncology, The University of Texas MD Anderson Cancer Center, Houston, TX, USA

John Stauffer Department of Surgery, Mayo Clinic Florida, Jacksonville, FL, USA

Martijn W. J. Stommel Department of Surgery, Radboudumc, Nijmegen, The Netherlands

Iswanto Sucandy Department of Surgery, University of Central Florida, Orlando, FL, USA
Advent Health Tampal Digestive Health Institute, Tampa, FL, USA

Cameron Syblis University of South Florida Morsani College of Medicine, Tampa, FL, USA
Advent Health Tampal Digestive Health Institute, Tampa, FL, USA

Maxwell T. Trudeau University of Pennsylvania Perelman School of Medicine, Philadelphia, PA, USA
University of Connecticut School of Medicine, Farmington, CT, USA

Voranaddha Vacharathit Faculty of Medicine, Department of Surgery, Chulalongkorn University, Bangkok, Thailand

King Chulalongkorn Memorial Hospital, The Thai Red Cross Society, Bangkok, Thailand

Alessia Vallorani Vita-Salute San Raffaele University, Milan, Italy

Eduardo A. Vega Department of Surgery, St. Elizabeth's Medical Center, Boston University School of Medicine, Boston, MA, USA

Brendan C. Visser Division of Hepatobiliary and Pancreas Surgery, Stanford University, Stanford, CA, USA

Charles M. Vollmer University of Pennsylvania Perelman School of Medicine, Philadelphia, PA, USA

Catherine Vozzo Division of Gastroenterology, University Hospitals of Cleveland, Case Western Reserve University School of Medicine, Cleveland, OH, USA

Timothy J. Vreeland Brooke Army Medical Center, Fort Sam Houston, TX, USA

R. Matthew Walsh Department of General Surgery, Digestive Disease Institute, Cleveland Clinic, Cleveland, OH, USA

Jane Wang Department of Surgery, University of California, San Francisco, San Francisco, CA, USA

Paul Wong Department of Surgery, City of Hope National Medical Center, Duarte, CA, USA

Part I
Anatomy and Physiology

Chapter 1
Anatomy and Physiology

Jessica Heard, Malynn Anne Ilanga, and Edward Cho

Embryology

Rapid cell division of the blastula and subsequent gastrulation is completed by the end of the third embryonal week, giving the embryo the necessary endoderm, mesoderm, and ectoderm required for further development. Initially, these germ layers exist in a trilaminar disc which undergo craniocaudal and lateral folding as organogenesis begins in the fourth embryonal week. Ultimately, the endodermal cells will form the mucosal lining of the gastrointestinal tract in addition to the liver, pancreas, and gallbladder. The mesenteries and the muscular walls of the gastrointestinal organs develop from the splanchnic mesoderm. Finally, nerves, including the vagus nerve and the bowel wall plexuses, will develop from neural crest cell (ectoderm) origins.

Craniocaudal folding initiates the formation of the cranial and caudal portions of the primitive gut. In conjunction with craniocaudal folding, lateral folding completes the process of the primitive gut tube formation whereby the dorsal aspect of the yolk sac (endoderm) is slowly pinched off by the developing ventrolateral body walls (somatic mesoderm) in the formation of the midgut. During this process, splanchnic mesoderm is rolled with the endodermal cells resulting in an enveloping layer of mesoderm about the primitive gut tube. Migration of neural crest cells begins and will eventually provide innervation to the primitive gut [1].

J. Heard · M. A. Ilanga
Department of Surgery, University of Oklahoma at Tulsa, Tulsa, OK, USA
e-mail: MalynnAnne-Ilanga@ouhsc.edu

E. Cho (✉)
Department of Surgery, University of Oklahoma at Tulsa, Tulsa, OK, USA

Department of Surgery, University of Illinois Peoria, Peoria, IL, USA
e-mail: echo0818@uic.edu

© The Author(s), under exclusive license to Springer Nature Switzerland AG 2025
E. P. Ceppa et al. (eds.), *The SAGES Manual of Evolving Techniques in Pancreatic Surgery*, https://doi.org/10.1007/978-3-031-78409-5_1

The foregut will form gastrointestinal tissue from the oropharynx to the duodenum proximal to the major papilla in addition to the special digestive organs: the liver, gallbladder, and pancreas. The celiac artery is the primary vessel supplying the structures of the embryologic foregut. The midgut develops into the distal duodenum through the proximal transverse colon. The primary arterial supply of the midgut is derived from the superior mesenteric artery (SMA). Finally, the hindgut forms the distal transverse colon through the anus with its primary blood supply provided via the inferior mesenteric artery.

During the fifth embryonic week, proliferation of the primitive gut tube continues at a prolific rate resulting in occlusion of the lumen of the tube and the pancreatic buds first appear. These buds develop as direct outgrowths of the duodenal endoderm and as such, they too are covered on their ventral surface by splanchnic mesoderm. The dorsal pancreatic bud is relatively larger than the ventral pancreatic bud which is associated with the developing common bile duct, gallbladder, and liver.

By the end of the seventh embryonic week, the stomach completes a 90-degree clockwise rotation dragging with it the duodenum, the ventral pancreatic bud, and common bile duct. This rotation has several results, namely it creates the characteristic "C" of the duodenum, brings the pancreas and all but the most proximal duodenum into the retroperitoneum, and it puts the ventral pancreatic bud into contact with the posterior aspect of the dorsal pancreatic bud. The pancreatic buds, partially sandwiching the common bile duct, will then fuse by the end of week eight. The superior pancreatic head, neck, body, and tail originate from the dorsal pancreatic bud while the inferior pancreatic head and uncinate process are formed by the ventral bud. The main pancreatic duct (duct of Wirsung) is formed by fusion of the distal two thirds of the dorsal pancreatic duct with the entire ventral duct. The accessory pancreatic duct (duct of Santorini) is formed by the persistence of the proximal one third of the dorsal pancreatic duct, but the duct may completely regress in up to 40% of cases.

Prior to the arrival of week 10, the lumen of the gut is once again fully patent due to apoptosis of some endodermal cells. By the completion of week 10, acinar and primitive islet cells can be found within the pancreas of the embryo. Both exocrine and endocrine pancreatic cells form from endodermal buds. There is then an amplification of endocrine cells, particularly beta cells. By week 13, alpha, beta, and delta cells are present in the islets [2–4].

Normal Anatomy

Duodenal Anatomy

The duodenum is the first 20 to 25 cm of small bowel and connects the stomach to the jejunum. It is found in the upper abdomen, generally between lumbar vertebra one and three. Unlike the remainder of the small bowel, the duodenum does not have a mesentery. Its course forms a characteristic "C" shape which is divided into four parts: superior (D1), descending (D2), inferior (D3), and ascending (D4). D1 travels superiorly from the pylorus of the stomach. Approximately the first half of D1 is located intraperitoneally prior to transitioning to a retroperitoneal location. The hepatoduodenal ligament attaches D1 to the inferior aspect of the liver. D2 courses inferiorly, as the name implies, and curves around the head of the pancreas. It contains the major and minor duodenal papillae by which the liver and pancreas drain. D3 crosses from right to left, passing over the great vessels and behind the superior mesenteric vessels. Once the duodenum crosses over the aorta, it begins an anterosuperior ascension and is called D4. The most distal segment of D4 transitions into the intraperitoneal space and its terminal point is marked by a peritoneal fold, known as the ligament of Treitz (suspensory muscle of the duodenum). The ligament of Treitz creates a sharp anteroinferior turn known as the duodenojejunal flexure and signifies the start of the jejunum [2, 3, 5, 6].

Pancreatic Anatomy

Also located primarily in the retroperitoneum, the pancreas is positioned posterior to the stomach and mesentery of the transverse colon. It also is divided into four major sections: head, neck, body, and tail. The head is the most right-sided major division of the pancreas and can be found nestled within the C-loop of the duodenum, which overlies the inferior vena cava (IVC). The uncinate process, a subdivision of the head, extends inferiorly and medially to hook behind the superior mesenteric vein (SMV). The uncinate process generally terminates prior to the superior mesenteric artery (SMA). The neck is a short segment that connects the head and body of the pancreas and is located directly anterior to the SMV. The gastroduodenal artery (GDA) is located on the anterior surface of the pancreas and can be used to identify the border between the head and neck of the pancreas. The body then extends across the midline, crossing over the aorta and SMA. The tail lies anterior to the left kidney and can be intimately related to the splenic hilum and left colonic flexure. The splenic vein courses along the posterior surface of the body and tail, while the splenic artery runs along their superior surface [6–8].

Ductal Anatomy

The extrahepatic biliary ducts ultimately flow into the common bile duct, which travels in the hepatoduodenal ligament. The common bile duct passes posterior to D1, courses within a deep pancreatic groove on the posterior surface of the pancreatic head until eventually becoming intrapancreatic prior to its termination in the duodenum. The normal internal diameter of the common bile duct is less than 6 mm.

The main pancreatic duct is responsible for drainage of the entire length of the pancreas. It eventually joins the distal common bile duct to drain via the major duodenal papilla. The diameter of the main duct increases gradually as it travels from the tail to the pancreatic head with normal diameters of 1–2 mm in the tail, 2–3 mm in the body, and 3–4 mm in the head. The accessory duct drains the anterosuperior aspect of the pancreatic head. Approximately 60% of people have a bifid pancreatic duct configuration with the main and accessory pancreatic ducts both present although the main duct maintains the dominant role of drainage. The accessory pancreatic duct typically drains via the minor duodenal papilla, which is located within D2 proximal to the major duodenal papilla.

The ampulla of Vater (hepatopancreatic ampulla) contains the dilated fusion of the distal portion of the common bile and main pancreatic ducts. It is located within the wall of D2, in the most common configuration, producing a short common channel. The sphincter of Oddi (hepatopancreatic sphincter), a smooth muscle complex, is located within the ampulla of Vater and controls the flow of bile and pancreatic enzymes into the duodenum and prevents reflux into the common bile and main pancreatic ducts [2, 7, 9, 10].

Vasculature

The duodenum and head of the pancreas obtain their blood supply by a highly redundant arterial collateralization from branches of both the celiac trunk and SMA. The celiac trunk gives rise to the common hepatic artery. The common hepatic artery branches to form the gastroduodenal artery, which then gives off the anterior and posterior superior pancreaticoduodenal arteries. These supply D1 to the major duodenal papilla in D2. Meanwhile, the inferior pancreaticoduodenal artery, a branch of the SMA, bifurcates into the anterior and posterior inferior pancreaticoduodenal arteries. The paired inferior pancreaticoduodenal arteries provide for D2, distal to the major papilla, through D4. Together, the four pancreaticoduodenal arteries supply the head and uncinate process of the pancreas. The pancreatic neck, body, and tail all receive their arterial supply from branches of the splenic artery via the celiac trunk. The splenic artery produces several small branches along its length to supply the superior aspect. The inferior aspect of the neck, body, and tail are supplied by the dorsal (superior) and inferior (transverse) pancreatic arteries.

Venous drainage of the area generally mirrors that of the arterial system. All of the pancreaticoduodenal veins ultimately drain into the SMV. While the anterior and posterior inferior veins directly confluence with the SMV at the inferior border of the uncinate process, the posterior superior pancreaticoduodenal vein joins the SMV at the superior border of the pancreatic neck. The anterior superior flows into the right gastroepiploic vein prior to entering the SMV at the inferior border of the pancreas. Venous outflow of the pancreatic body and tail is via the branches of the splenic vein [2, 6].

Lymphatics

The body and tail of the pancreas directly drain to the pancreaticosplenic lymph nodes (stations 18, 10, 11), which subsequently go to the celiac lymph nodes (station 9). The head and neck of the pancreas primarily drain to the supra- and infra-pyloric lymph nodes (stations 5 and 6), anterior to the common hepatic artery (station 8a), around the cystic and common bile ducts (stations 12b1, 12b2, 12c), anterior and posterior to the head of the pancreas (stations 13a, 13b, 17a, 17b), and along the proximal SMA [14]. The duodenal lymphatics are located anterior and posterior to the head of the pancreas and around the SMA [11, 12].

Nerves

The vagus nerves provide parasympathetic innervation to the duodenum and pancreas. The left and right vagus nerves divide to form the anterior and posterior vagal trunks, respectively, which travel near the surface of the distal esophagus. The vagal trunks then pass through the celiac plexus before branching to innervate the submucosal layer of the duodenum and the pancreatic acinar and islet cells. Thoracic-level greater and lesser splanchnic nerves provide sympathetic innervation to both the duodenum and pancreas after passing through the sympathetic chain to the celiac and superior mesenteric plexuses [12, 13].

Clinically Relevant Anatomic Variations

Duodenum Inversum

In duodenum inversum, also known as inverted duodenum, the proximal duodenum travels posterosuperiorly so that the D3 curves over D2 ultimately terminating at a normally located ligament of Treitz. While the etiology is incompletely known, it is

Fig. 1.1 Abdominal radiograph demonstrating opacification of the stomach and duodenum. It is noted that the third part of the duodenum passes in a cranial direction over the second portion

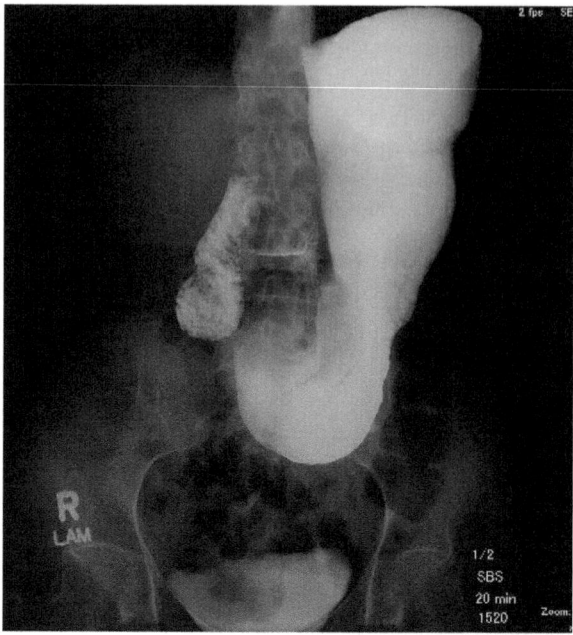

thought to result from a persistent pancreatic dorsal mesentery resulting in incomplete embryologic rotation. The reported prevalence is less than 1%, with the majority of these patients incidentally identified on imaging. Among the few who develop symptoms, nausea, vomiting, bloating, and epigastric pain are often seen. Notably, duodenum inversum is often reported in patients also found to have pancreas divisum [14] (Fig. 1.1).

Pancreas Divisum

Pancreas divisum is the most common pancreatic anatomic variant, occurring in up to 14% of the population. There are three primary variants, all of which result in a relative outflow obstruction through the minor papilla and may result in recurrent acute pancreatitis: type 1 (classical), type 2, and type 3 (incomplete). In type 1, there is a complete failure of fusion of the dorsal and ventral pancreatic buds resulting in the superior head, neck, body, and tail draining via the accessory duct and the minor papilla while the inferior head and uncinate process drain through the main pancreatic duct and the major duodenal papilla (Fig. 1.2). With type 2 pancreas divisum, there is an absence of the main pancreatic duct and pancreatic drainage is thus dependent upon the accessory duct alone. Type 3 is similar to type 1, except there is a diminutive communicating ductal branch between the main and accessory ducts [8, 10].

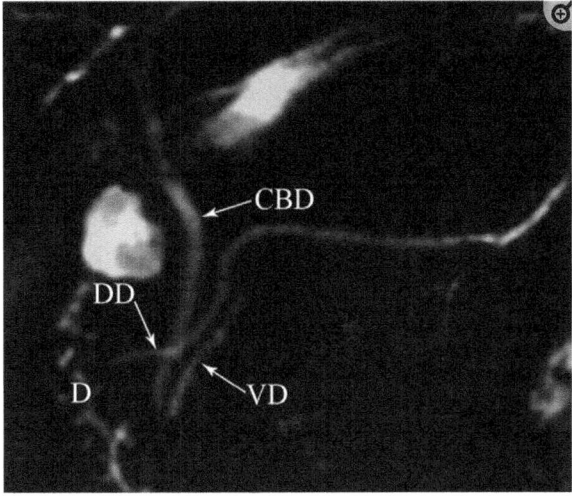

Fig. 1.2 An MRCP of classical pancreas divisum is shown. *CBD* common bile duct, *D* duodenum, *DD* dorsal duct, *VD* ventral duct

Annular Pancreas

The prevalence rate of annular pancreas is thought to be 0.01% and results from a failure of the ventral bud to properly rotate with the second portion of the duodenum during embryologic development. This results in complete, or partial, encasement of the duodenum by pancreatic tissue. There are two types: extramural and intramural. The most common type, extramural, occurs when the ventral pancreatic duct traverses posteriorly around the duodenum to join the main pancreatic duct in the usual fashion. When symptomatic, this often presents as a duodenal obstruction and has been associated with Down syndrome. The second type, intramural, results in many small ducts that drain directly into the duodenum from the ventral pancreatic bud and may cause duodenal ulcerations [7, 10].

Ectopic Pancreas

Ectopic pancreas occurs when normal pancreatic tissue exists without anatomic or vascular communication with the main pancreatic gland. Typically, these are identified in the submucosa of the gastric antrum (30%), duodenum (50%), or the remainder of the small bowel (20%). The embryologic origin for these islands of pancreatic tissue is thought to be residual primitive pancreatic cells that were not incorporated into the pancreatic buds. Ectopic pancreas is most often an incidental finding, but patients may develop abdominal pain, dyspepsia, or gastrointestinal bleeding. Although rare, there are reports of malignancy that develops within the ectopic pancreatic tissue which may be significant in patients with known pancreatic field defects [7, 8, 10].

Pancreatic Agenesis and Hypoplasia

Total pancreatic agenesis is considered incompatible with life, but partial agenesis, also known as hypoplasia, does occasionally occur as a result of a failure of the ventral or dorsal pancreatic buds to develop. Total dorsal pancreatic agenesis ("short pancreas") is extremely rare and has been associated with visceral heterotaxy. More commonly, partial dorsal agenesis occurs resulting in a variable degree of tail, body, neck, or anterior head absence. In partial dorsal agenesis, the accessory pancreatic duct and minor papilla are present, which differentiates it from total dorsal agenesis. Patients with dorsal agenesis are at elevated risk for diabetes as the islet cells are primarily located in the pancreatic tail [7, 8, 10].

Ansa Pancreatica

The rarest pancreatic duct anomaly, ansa pancreatica, is associated with the development of recurrent acute pancreatitis. In this anomaly, there is an obliteration of the accessory duct prior to joining the main pancreatic duct. This missing segment is replaced with a dilated branch of the main duct which takes an "S-shaped" or looping path to the remnant accessory duct allowing for drainage through the minor papilla [7, 15].

Pancreaticobiliary Maljunction

Pancreaticobiliary maljunction (anomalous pancreaticobiliary junction) occurs when the common bile duct and main pancreatic duct fuse prior to entering the duodenal wall which results in a long common channel (>15 mm) outside of the purview of the sphincter of Oddi. The estimated prevalence is near 3% worldwide although significantly higher rates are observed in Asia. In recent years, studies have associated pancreaticobiliary maljunction with development of biliary tract malignancies and pancreatitis, which are believed to result from bidirectional reflux of pancreatic juices and bile. While pancreaticobiliary maljunction is associated with a choledochal cyst (types A and C) in 70% of cases, it also occurs without dilation (type B) or as a product of annular pancreas, pancreas divisum, or other atypical duct configurations (type D) [16–18].

Duplication Anomalies

Duplication cysts are characterized by an epithelial mucosal lining, a smooth muscle layer, and an attachment, whether communicating or non-communicating, to the native alimentary tract. They may occur anywhere along the gastrointestinal tract and are named for their native-organ attachment from which they obtain their blood supply. Notably, up to 35% of duplication cysts contain ectopic tissue with gastric and pancreatic being common. Overall, the incidence of duplication cysts is 1 in 4500 births with duodenal duplication cysts accounting for 5% of those identified. Pancreatic duplication cysts are exceedingly uncommon with less than 75 reported cases in the literature.

Generally, duodenal duplication cysts are identified in early childhood as a result of abdominal pain, gastrointestinal bleeding, or intestinal obstruction although severe pancreatitis and cyst rupture do occur. Duodenal duplication cysts are typically located in the second or third portion of the duodenum and may communicate with the native duodenum, the pancreatic duct, or the common bile duct. Very little is known about pancreatic duplication cysts, but they are thought to have a connection with the native pancreatic duct [19–21].

Physiology

Duodenal Physiology

Mechanical Function

The migrating motor complex (MMC) is a recurring gastrointestinal pattern that occurs every 90 min in the fasted state. The MMC is thought to originate in the gastric antrum or duodenum and propagate a peristaltic contraction distally in order to propel residual material toward the colon. The MMC occurs in four phases with the third affecting the strongest contractions. Motilin, an active gastrointestinal peptide, is known to play a large role during phase III MMC contractions [22].

During the fed state, the duodenal motion serves two purposes: to mix the chyme deposited from the stomach and to increase the chyme's contact with the brush border of the intestines (segmentation contractions) and to propel the chyme forward through the intestinal tract (peristalsis) [23]. Peristalsis is increased by cholecystokinin, gastrin, serotonin, and insulin and decreased by glucagon and secretin [24].

Digestive and Absorptive Functions

The duodenum is a significant location for digestion of fats, carbohydrates, and proteins within the gastrointestinal tract and is primarily responsible for the absorption of starches, amino acids, vitamins, minerals, and water.

Oral and pancreatic amylase debranch almost all dietary starches (lactulose, sucrose, maltose) to maltose, saccharides, and dextrins prior to their passage into the jejunum. The more simplified starches then come into contact with the brush border of the intestines which completes the process of converting them primarily to glucose. SGLT1 transporters, present on the brush border in the upper one third of the small bowel, allow active transport of glucose and galactose from the digestive tract. GLUT5 allows for the facilitated diffusion of fructose across the brush border of the small intestines.

Denatured proteins, present in chyme, are further broken down by secreted pancreatic enzymes that are activated by the duodenal brush border in a cascade-like manner. Trypsin, activated from the secreted enzyme trypsinogen, then activates other proteolytic enzymes such as chymotrypsin, elastase, and carboxypeptidase. Together these enzymes complete the digestion of proteins to amino acids allowing for up to 90% of protein absorption by the end of the jejunum.

The duodenum is responsible for the uptake of several vitamins and minerals. Duodenal active transport of calcium is enhanced by the relatively acidic environment, vitamin D, and parathyroid hormone. Similarly, iron, in its ferrous form or as heme, is actively transported primarily in the duodenum by the transporter DMT1. Ferric iron is reduced to the ferrous form by brush border enzyme cytochrome b. DMT1 also transports zinc and copper within the duodenum. Finally, vitamin B12 (cobalamin), absorbed in the terminal ileum, requires pancreatic proteases in the duodenum to cleave intrinsic factor from B12 to allow for future absorption [25].

Endocrine Function

The second portion of the duodenum is the entry point for both stomach contents and pancreatic fluid into the small bowel. The duodenum plays an important role in hormone secretion in several negative feedback loops. G cells, primarily located in the gastric antrum, can be found in the duodenum. G cells are stimulated to release gastrin in response to vagal stimulation and gastrin-releasing peptide (bombesin) due to protein ingestion, gastric distention, and an elevated gastric pH. Gastrin stimulates gastric parietal cells to acidify the stomach, stimulates gastrointestinal mucosal growth, and increases gastric motility [26].

Cholecystokinin (CCK) is produced by I-cells in the duodenum, but also the jejunum, in response to the release of fats and digested proteins deposited from the stomach. CCK's primary functions are known to aid in digestion. It stimulates the gallbladder to contract, relaxes the sphincter of Oddi, inhibits further stomach contraction, and plays a role in inducing satiety. Additionally, CCK stimulates pancreatic release of bicarbonate rich fluid although to a much lesser extent than that of secretin [27].

Passage of gastric chyme into the duodenum and jejunum also stimulates the S cells to produce secretin. Specifically, a pH less than 4.5, fatty acids, and bile salts have been shown to stimulate secretin production. Secretin limits further gastrin release in the stomach and induces the pancreas to produce a high-volume bicarbonate fluid to neutralize the acidic chyme and digestive enzymes to aid fat digestion.

Somatostatin (SST) is produced by D cells in the pancreas as well as in the gastric antrum, duodenum, and central nervous system. Within the gut, SST is secreted in the presence of acid, fat, proteins, glucose, and cholecystokinin and acts as an inhibitor of pancreatic, biliary, gastric, and colonic secretion. Additionally, it inhibits the release of vasoactive intestinal peptide (VIP) [28].

Gastric inhibitory peptide (GIP) is produced primarily by the K cells of the duodenum and proximal jejunum, yet can be found throughout the small intestine. GIP is secreted in response to intraluminal glucose, high concentrations of amino acids, or long-chain fatty acids. The gastrointestinal related effects of GIP include stimulation of pancreatic islet cells to increase insulin levels and inhibition of G cell gastrin secretion [27, 29].

M cells, found in the duodenum, produce motilin which aids in propulsion of food through the gastrointestinal tract, increases gallbladder contractility, increases the lower esophageal sphincter tone, increases gastric pepsin release, and is thought to play a role in increasing hunger. Several factors increase motilin release including prolonged fasting and the presence of fat or acid in the duodenum [30, 31].

VIP, like SST, has a multitude of roles throughout the body. In the gastrointestinal tract, it is produced by the myenteric and submucosal plexus nerves in the intestinal walls and by the islet cells of the pancreas in response to vagal stimulation. Generally, VIP results in smooth muscle relaxation of the lower esophageal sphincter, stomach, gallbladder, small bowel, and blood vessels. Additionally, it causes secretion of water and electrolytes from the small bowel and bicarbonate rich fluid from the pancreas. Finally, in the stomach it reduces gastrin-related acid production [32].

Pancreatic Physiology

Exocrine Physiology

The exocrine structures of the pancreas make up about 80–90% of the pancreatic mass, and the endocrine structures contribute to about 2% of the pancreas. The rest of the pancreas is made up of the extracellular matrix, blood vessels, and ductal structures. The function of the exocrine pancreas is to aid in the digestion of carbohydrates, fats, and proteins.

There are two main components of the exocrine pancreas: the acinar cells and the ductal system. The pancreas secretes about 1 L of pancreatic fluid daily, containing the enzymes and zymogens that aid in digestion, as well as alkaline fluid, which are produced by the acinar cells and secreted into the ductal system. Initially, the acinar cells drain into intercalated ducts that come together to form interlobular ducts, which then join together to form secondary ducts that drain into the main pancreatic duct, and subsequently the duodenum at the ampulla of Vater.

The composition of pancreatic fluid varies depending on whether the body is in a fasting state or a stimulated phase. When fasting, pancreatic fluid has a bicarbonate concentration of 80 mEq/L and is rich in protein. However, when the pancreas is stimulated after a meal, the concentration of bicarbonate increases, and this alkaline fluid enters the duodenum. The fluid has a pH of 7.6–9.0 and acts to neutralize gastric acid while delivering digestive enzymes in their inactive state to the duodenum.

Vagal parasympathetic stimulation is largely responsible for the secretion of enzyme-rich fluid, while fluid and electrolyte secretion are more hormonally regulated. The main hormones involved are secretin and cholecystokinin. The presence of acid in the duodenum results in the release of secretin from the duodenal mucosa. Secretin subsequently stimulates the interlobular duct cells to release bicarbonate and water. As the bicarbonate concentration increases in the pancreatic fluid, chloride concentration decreases in order to maintain isotonicity. CCK, released in the presence of fat and protein, stimulates the pancreatic acinar cells to release proenzymes. Pancreatic secretion is also influenced by neuropeptides, which have an inhibitory effect [13].

Endocrine Physiology

The main endocrine function of the pancreas is regulation of carbohydrate metabolism and glucose homeostasis via insulin and glucagon secretion. While insulin functions to transport glucose into cells, stimulate protein synthesis, and inhibit glycogenolysis and fatty acid breakdown, glucagon stimulates glycogenolysis and gluconeogenesis, increasing blood glucose levels. Pancreatic islet cells of Langerhans comprise the endocrine structure of the pancreas and are of neural crest origin. Blood enters the islet cells via an afferent arteriole, which then enters into a capillary bed within the cell. Hormones secreted as part of the pancreatic endocrine system are secreted into this capillary bed, and blood then exits via an efferent collecting venule to the portal venous circulation.

The islets of Langerhans are composed of several types of cells, 70% of which are beta cells, which are mostly found in the core of the islet. These beta cells are surrounded by alpha cells, delta cells, and pancreatic polypeptide cells, which communicate with each other via extracellular spaces and gap junctions, allowing for cellular products secreted from one cell type to influence the function of another. The four main cell types—A (alpha), B (beta), D cells, and F cells—have varied distributions and secretory products. While B and D cells are found in the tail of the pancreas, F cells are primarily located in the head and uncinate process and A cells are evenly distributed throughout. B cells make up about 70% of the islet cell mass and are located centrally in the islet cell. The primary secretory product is insulin though amylin and cholecystokinin are also secreted by B cells.

Insulin is first produced as preproinsulin in the ribosomes of the rough endoplasmic reticulum before being cleaved into proinsulin and transported to the Golgi apparatus, where it is packaged into secretory granules. Proinsulin is then cleaved into insulin and C-peptide, and the secretory granules fuse with the cell membrane to secrete insulin. A cells are found more peripherally in the islet cells and comprise about 10% of islet cell mass. The main secretory product is glucagon. Also found peripherally within the islets are F cells, which make up 15% of islet cell mass. These cells secrete pancreatic polypeptide. D cells are distributed evenly within islet cells and make up 5% of their mass. D cells secrete somatostatin, while D2 cells secrete VIP.

Glucose is the main regulator of insulin secretion and is taken up by Beta cells through GLUT2 transporters. Glucokinase then phosphorylates glucose into glucose-6-phosphate and subsequently produces ATP in the process of glycolysis. When the pancreas is unstimulated, insulin is secreted at a basal rate. However, rapid increases in blood glucose result in a "first-phase" of insulin release that peaks within 5 min and decreases within 10 min. If the concentration of glucose in the blood remains high, a second phase is entered and insulin secretion is sustained by the release of both stored and newly synthesized insulin [2, 13].

References

1. Slack JM. Developmental biology of the pancreas. Development. 1995;121(6):1569–80.
2. Townsend CM, Beauchamp RD, Evers BM, Mattox KL, editors. Sabiston textbook of surgery: the biological basis of modern surgical practice. 20th ed. Elsevier; 2017.
3. Hurtado CW, Waasdorp C, Sferra T, Polk B. Embryology and anatomy of the gastrointestinal tract. 2023.
4. Dudek R. Embryology. In: High-yield embryology. 4th ed. Lippincott Williams & Wilkins. p. 1–55. 2009.
5. Jones O. The Small Intestine—Duodenum—Jejunum—Ileum—TeachMeAnatomy [Internet]. 2020 [cited 2022 Aug 18]. https://teachmeanatomy.info/abdomen/gi-tract/small-intestine/
6. Talathi SS, Zimmerman R, Young M. Anatomy, abdomen and pelvis, pancreas. In: StatPearls [Internet]. Treasure Island, FL: StatPearls Publishing; 2022. http://www.ncbi.nlm.nih.gov/books/NBK532912/.
7. Borghei P, Sokhandon F, Shirkhoda A, Morgan D. Anomalies, anatomic variants, and sources of diagnostic pitfalls in pancreatic imaging. Radiology. 2013;266(1):28–36. https://doi.org/10.1148/radiol.12112469.
8. Raichholz G, Giménez S, Dumoulin S, Sañudo JL. Segmental anatomy of the pancreas and its developmental variants. Imagenes. 2016;5:10.
9. Aljiffry M, Abbas M, Wazzan MAM, Abduljabbar AH, Aloufi S, Aljahdli E. Biliary anatomy and pancreatic duct variations: a cross-sectional study. Saudi J Gastroenterol. 2020;26(4):188–93.
10. Türkvatan A, Erden A, Türkoğlu MA, Yener Ö. Congenital variants and anomalies of the pancreas and pancreatic duct: imaging by magnetic resonance cholangiopancreaticography and multidetector computed tomography. Korean J Radiol. 2013;14(6):905–13.
11. Tol JAMG, Gouma DJ, Bassi C, Dervenis C, Montorsi M, Adham M, et al. Definition of a standard lymphadenectomy in surgery for pancreatic ductal adenocarcinoma: a consen-

sus statement by the international study group on pancreatic surgery (ISGPS). Surgery. 2014;156(3):591–600.

12. Japan Pancreas Society, editor. Classification of pancreatic carcinoma. 4th ed. Tokyo: Kanehara & Co., Ltd.; 2017. http://www.suizou.org/pdf/Classification_of_Pancreatic_Carcinoma_4th_Engl_ed.pdf

13. Mulholland MW, Lillemoe KD, Doherty GM, Upchurch GR Jr, Hasan HB, Pawlik TM. Chapter 52: pancreas anatomy and physiology. In: Greenfield's surgery scientific principles & practice. 6th ed. Philadelphia, PA: Wolters Kluwer Health/Lippincott Williams & Wilkins; 2017.

14. Yap CH, Coupland D, Au J, Raju S. Duodenum inversum: a rare cause of nausea and epigastric pain. BJR Case Rep. 2022;8(3):20210144.

15. Shaikh DH, Alemam A, von Ende J, Ghazanfar H, Dev A, Balar B. Ansa pancreatica, an uncommon cause of acute, recurrent pancreatitis. Case Rep Gastroenterol. 2021;15(2):587–93.

16. Ono Y, Kaneko K, Tainaka T, Sumida W, Ando H. Pancreaticobiliary maljunction without bile duct dilatation in children: distinction from choledochal cyst. J Pediatr Gastroenterol Nutr. 2008;46(5):555–60.

17. Urushihara N, Hamada Y, Kamisawa T, Fujii H, Koshinaga T, Morotomi Y, et al. Classification of pancreaticobiliary maljunction and clinical features in children. J Hepato-Biliary-Pancreat Sci. 2017;24(8):449–55.

18. Nagata E, Sakai K, Kinoshita H, Kobayashi Y. The relation between carcinoma of the gallbladder and an anomalous connection between the choledochus and the pancreatic duct. Ann Surg. 1985;202(2):182–90.

19. Chen JJ, Lee HC, Yeung CY, Chan WT, Jiang CB, Sheu JC. Meta-analysis: the clinical features of the duodenal duplication cyst. J Pediatr Surg. 2010;45(8):1598–606.

20. Macpherson RI. Gastrointestinal tract duplications: clinical, pathologic, etiologic, and radiologic considerations. Radiographics. 1993;13:1063–80. https://doi.org/10.1148/radiographics.13.5.8210590.

21. Cadili L, Cullen KL, Finn NJ, Singh A, Webber E, Hayashi AH. A rare case of a congenital pancreatic duplication cyst in an infant complicated by an upper GI bleed, pancreatitis, cyst infection and gastric outlet obstruction. J Surg Case Rep. 2022;2022(7):rjac326.

22. Deloose E, Janssen P, Depoortere I, Tack J. The migrating motor complex: control mechanisms and its role in health and disease. Nat Rev Gastroenterol Hepatol. 2012;9(5):271–85.

23. Bowen R. Small intestinal motility [Internet]. VIVO Pathophysiology. [cited 2022 Oct 29]. http://www.vivo.colostate.edu/hbooks/pathphys/digestion/smallgut/motility.html.

24. Kitazawa T, Kaiya H. Regulation of gastrointestinal motility by motilin and ghrelin in vertebrates. Front Endocrinol. 2019;10:278.

25. Kiela PR, Ghishan FK. Physiology of intestinal absorption and secretion. Best Pract Res Clin Gastroenterol. 2016;30(2):145–59.

26. Schubert ML. Gastric acid secretion. Curr Opin Gastroenterol. 2016;32(6):452–60.

27. Field BCT. Neuroendocrinology of obesity. Br Med Bull. 2014;109(1):73–82.

28. Cakir M, Dworakowska D, Grossman A. Somatostatin receptor biology in neuroendocrine and pituitary tumours: part 1—molecular pathways. J Cell Mol Med. 2010;14(11):2570–84.

29. Villar HV, Fender HR, Rayford PL, Bloom SR, Ramus NI, Thompson JC. Suppression of gastrin release and gastric secretion by gastric inhibitory polypeptide (GIP) and vasoactive intestinal polypeptide (VIP). Ann Surg. 1976;184(1):97–102.

30. Modlin IM, Mitznegg P, Bloom SR. Motilin release in the pig. Gut. 1978;19(5):399–402.

31. Korimilli A, Parkman HP. Effect of Atilmotin, a motilin receptor agonist, on esophageal, lower esophageal sphincter, and gastric pressures. Dig Dis Sci. 2010;55(2):300–6.

32. Iwasaki M, Akiba Y, Kaunitz JD. Recent advances in vasoactive intestinal peptide physiology and pathophysiology: focus on the gastrointestinal system. F1000Res. 2019;8:F1000 Fac Rev-1629. https://www.ncbi.nlm.nih.gov/pmc/articles/PMC6743256/.

Part II
Acute Pancreatitis

Chapter 2
Diagnosis and Medical Management of Acute Pancreatitis

Carlos Theodore Huerta, Jodie Adam Barkin, and Onur C. Kutlu

Etiology

Acute pancreatitis is a major source of economic burden with an estimated cost of AP-related hospitalizations exceeding 2 billion dollars to the US healthcare system. [1, 2] The incidence of AP has been reported ranging between 15 and 45 cases per 100,000 patients in the United States and 5 and 73 cases per 100,000 patients globally, with an increase observed in recent years [3]. However, the two most frequent etiologies in the US patient population include gallstones and excess alcohol consumption, which are estimated to occur between 40–70% and 25–35% of cases, respectively [4–6]. Given the importance of early diagnosis and recognition of the etiology of AP to prevent future recurrent episodes, abdominal ultrasound should be used to screen for the presence of cholelithiasis in all patients with AP [7, 8, 9]. Should the presence of cholelithiasis be confirmed in the setting of AP, these patients should be referred for consideration of interval cholecystectomy to prevent future episodes of disease.

Regarding pancreatitis secondary to alcohol consumption, symptoms can manifest along the entire disease spectrum ranging from individual, acute episodes to recurrent, chronic pancreatic dysfunction. Although multifactorial in nature due to other sensitizing factors such as smoking and genetic factors, patients with

C. T. Huerta
DeWitt Daughtry Family Department of Surgery, University of Miami Miller School of Medicine, Miami, FL, USA

J. A. Barkin
Pancreas Center, Division of Gastroenterology, University of Miami Miller School of Medicine, Miami, FL, USA

O. C. Kutlu (✉)
DeWitt Daughtry Department of Surgery, University of Miami Miller School of Medicine, Miami, FL, USA
e-mail: okutlu@med.miami.edu

© The Author(s), under exclusive license to Springer Nature Switzerland AG 2025
E. P. Ceppa et al. (eds.), *The SAGES Manual of Evolving Techniques in Pancreatic Surgery*, https://doi.org/10.1007/978-3-031-78409-5_2

alcohol-induced AP may have a history of excess alcohol intake more than 50 g per day for more than 5 years [6, 9–14].

Although alcohol and cholelithiasis-related AP predominate as the most commonly encountered cases in patients, the remaining differential includes a broad list of potential etiologies that should be carefully evaluated. While only estimated to constitute less than 4% of cases, hypertriglyceridemia is a well-studied cause of AP. Serum levels of triglycerides are often >1000 mg/dL in patients with either primary or secondary hypertriglyceridemia-induced pancreatitis, and a fasting serum triglyceride taken 30 days after discharge is often recommended in this population to confirm the diagnosis [15–18]. Electrolyte disturbances including hypercalcemia in isolation, or as a result of another medical cause such as hyperparathyroidism, have been documented as a causative factor in some patients. Pharmacologic insults from drugs known to cause AP such as azathioprine and 6-mercaptopurine are capable of eliciting disease episodes [6, 19]. Although uncommon, polymicrobial infections and toxins have also been shown to induce AP.

Anatomic causes resulting in hepatobiliary obstruction can similarly result in AP. Both benign and malignant masses of the hepatobiliary and pancreatic system as well as the duodenum that impact the main pancreatic duct have been recognized as less common causes of AP. Previous series have identified up to 14% of patients with idiopathic AP (IAP) may have underlying pancreatic or biliary malignancies [20–22]. Given the increasing incidence of pancreatic malignancy, a high degree of clinical suspicion for neoplastic etiologies associated with AP should be maintained particularly in younger patients and those with recurrent or prolonged episodes with no clearly identified etiology on routine workup [23–25]. Focused cross-sectional imaging of the pancreas through abdominal contrast-enhanced CT or MRI/MRCP as well as endoscopic ultrasound (EUS) can be considered in these patients [6, 26, 27].

Aberrant pancreatic anatomy and function can further predispose patients to develop AP. Congenital anomalies such as pancreas divisum can result in ampullary stenosis or obstruction impeding outflow of the main pancreatic duct [28, 29]. Physiologic outflow obstruction secondary to functional biliary dysfunction syndrome is also a rare physiologic cause of AP [30]. Instrumentation procedures of the ampulla such as endoscopic radiographic cholangiopancreatography (ERCP) for these and other conditions can further precipitate AP episodes [31]. Newer genetic targets including mutations and polymorphisms in genes such as SPINK1, CFTR, and PRSS1 have been implicated in the development AP, and the role of testing for these allelic defects in patients with a significant family history of AP and pancreatic disease is still to be fully determined in future work [28, 32]. Patients with more than one family member with pancreatic disease may benefit from formal genetic counseling. Together, these native genetic defects can further worsen the risk of disease in patients with the aforementioned anatomic and environmental factors contributing to a tissue milieu highly predisposed to inflammation.

IAP occurs in patients without these aforementioned risk factors and in whom no clear etiology is elucidated on diagnostic laboratory workup and imaging tests [33, 34]. In these patients without a structural cause identified on abdominal cross-sectional imaging, EUS may be considered to interrogate for the presence of microlithiasis.

Etiology of Acute Pancreatitis

A	Alcohol, autoimmune
B	Biliary, including gallstones, microlithiasis, and sludge
C	Congenital—Pancreas divisum associated with genetic abnormality and pancreas, Crohn's disease via inflammation, ampulla, or duodenal obstruction
D	Drugs, toxins (including, smoking, tobacco, and marijuana use)
E	Post-ERCP pancreatitis, eosinophilic pancreatitis
F	Formations—Primary cancers (pancreatic ductal adenocarcinoma, especially in patients >50 years, lymphomas, carcinoids, metastatic cancers, small cell of lungs, renal, melanoma
G	Genetic mutations and polymorphisms—cystic fibrosis, transmembrane conductance regulator [CFTR], cationic trypsinogen (PRSS1), serine protease inhibitor Kayal type 1 (SPINK1) and claudin-2 (CTRC)
H	Hypertriglyceridemia, hypercalcemia, hypertriglyceridemia may be associated with metabolic pancreatitis, i.e., elevated glucose, obesity, hypercalcemia associated with hyperparathyroidism or iatrogenic infusion
I	Infection—Including viruses, CMV, mumps and EBV (Forsmark NEJM), ascariasis and Clonorchis sinensis, bacteria tuberculosis
J	Juxta ampullary diverticula—Likely mechanism obstruction
K	Kinetic injury and other trauma, including seat belt injuries

Ref. Barkin JS, Barkin JA

Pathophysiology

The pathophysiology of AP is incompletely understood. However, the clinical and pathologic features appear similar regardless of the etiology. Inciting physiologic insults from the aforementioned etiological factors are thought to result in the loss of intracellular and extracellular compartmentalization and lead to aberrant activation of pancreatic enzymes within the pancreatic acinar cells [6–9]. This may subsequently result in autodigestive injury to the pancreas. Under normal conditions, the exocrine pancreas synthesizes and secretes several inactive digestive enzymes that are released into the duodenum via the pancreatic ducts and activated by trypsin. Under physiologic conditions, small amounts of these zymogens are activated spontaneously within the pancreas but are offset by natural inhibitory factors including pancreatic secretory trypsin inhibitor (PSTI or SPINK1), mesotrypsin, and enzyme Y which inactivate and lyse trypsin [10, 11, 35]. Nonspecific antiproteases in the pancreatic parenchyma such as alpha-1-antitrypsin and alpha-2-macroglobulin also help to prevent damage from inappropriate trypsin activation [10, 11]. During AP episodes, an overabundant pool of trypsin is activated within the pancreas and overwhelms these native defenses. Pathologic autodigestion develops from the colocalization of lysosomal enzymes including cathepsin B and trypsinogen in the acinar cells as well as subsequent activation of trypsinogen and other glandular enzymes such as chymotrypsin, phospholipase A, and elastase within the pancreas [10, 13]. Elastase overactivity may result in the breakdown of the elastic fibers within the vasculature wall and lead to hemorrhage. Phospholipase A among other factors has been implicated in fat necrosis observed in AP [14, 27]. This cascade of pathological enzymatic-induced degradation spreads throughout the pancreatic gland propagating further intrapancreatic enzyme activation and cell damage in a positive loop. The resultant activation of the systemic inflammatory response syndrome (SIRS) is responsible for driving systemic complications including extra-pancreatic end organ damage and failure [36].

Although most patients typically experience minimum to mild organ dysfunction as a result of pancreatitis, approximately 10–20% develop SIRS [36–38]. This is defined by the presence of at least two of the following features: temperature below 36 °C or above 38 °C; heart rate above 90 beats per minute; respiratory rate above 20 breaths per minute or $PaCO_2$ below 32 torr; white blood cell count above 12,000 cells/mm^3, below 4000 cells/mm^3, or above 10% immature cells (bands) [12]. Pancreatic inflammation can trigger SIRS via the activation of an inflammatory cascade mediated by cytokines, immunologic cells, and the complement system. These inflammatory cytokines cause dispersion and trafficking of macrophages and migration distant from the pancreas such as the lungs and kidneys. SIRS can lead to a fulminant course with multiorgan failure in addition to the development of local or systemic complications [3, 15, 31].

Diagnosis

The diagnosis of AP is established by the presence of two or more of the three following criteria: (i) abdominal pain consistent with the disease (acute onset of a persistent, severe, epigastric pain often radiating to the back), (ii) serum amylase and/or lipase greater than three times the upper limit of normal, and/or (iii) characteristic findings from abdominal imaging [39].

Clinical Presentation

Physical exam findings in AP vary based on the severity of disease presentation. As a result, the nonspecific nature of AP symptomatology may lead to misdiagnosis based on physical examination alone. Patients with mild AP may present only with minimal tenderness to palpation in the epigastrium, while those with severe pancreatitis may have significant tenderness diffusely throughout the abdomen and associated fever, tachypnea, hypoxemia, and hypotension [40, 41].

The most common presentation is significant abdominal pain, which may be so severe that the patient is reluctant to initiate deep respiratory efforts. This may subsequently result in hypoventilation and contribute to the increased incidence of respiratory complications observed in these patients, such as atelectasis and pulmonary consolidation [42, 43]. Given these patients' abdominal pain and associated nausea and/or emesis, they may present with profound dehydration resulting in tachycardia, orthostatic hypotension, and even shock physiology. Sequestration of fluid outside of the intravascular space in the retroperitoneum and other anatomic compartments due to inflammatory mediators can further compound extra-pancreatic organ system failure such as in the renal system [36, 41].

Abdominal distention precipitated by the extravasation of fluid into the retroperitoneum is common. Fulminant peritonitis may evolve as a rare, late finding associated with severe AP and is associated with a worse prognosis [44, 45]. Although uncommon, palpation of abdominal masses in the epigastrium or upper abdomen may suggest the presence of a pancreatic pseudocyst. Cullen's sign (bruising of the periumbilical area) and Grey Turner's sign (bruising of the flank) are consistent with retroperitoneal bleeding that can manifest in severe AP. These signs are rare and are associated with increased mortality [44, 45]. Signs of hepatobiliary obstruction including jaundice may be present on exam and should raise concern for an obstructive process due to neoplastic lesions or anatomic causes.

This third-spacing of extracellular fluid may further precipitate hemoconcentration evidenced by elevated hematocrit and leukocytosis on serologic laboratory testing [42, 46]. Electrolyte abnormalities, elevated blood urea nitrogen, hypocalcemia, and hyperglycemia are also seen. Elevated bilirubin and alkaline phosphatase, with or without the presence of elevated aminotransferases, should raise the suspicion for biliary obstruction—a common presentation of biliary pancreatitis [42, 46].

Laboratory Tests

Serum amylase and lipase are the most common laboratory tests used to diagnose AP [47, 48]. Early during AP, there is blockage of pancreatic digestive enzymes secretion while synthesis continues. Digestive enzymes leak from acinar cells through the basolateral membrane and into the interstitial space eventually entering systemic circulation. Serum amylase levels may rise 6–12 h after the onset of symptoms and usually return to normal within 3–5 days in uncomplicated cases [49]. Serum amylase elevation is considered a nonspecific finding with sensitivity and specificity for the diagnosis of AP of 67–83% and 85–98%, respectively [48]. Serum amylase may be elevated in other conditions with an extra-pancreatic cause, such as diseases of the salivary glands, which also produce amylase. Patients with alcoholic pancreatitis may have an inability to produce sufficient amylase levels to meet criteria for pancreatitis in as high as 20% of cases and elevated triglyceride levels in hypertriglyceridemia-associated pancreatitis may interfere with accuracy of the amylase assay in up to 50% of patients [50, 51]. Furthermore, mild elevations in amylase or lipase in the setting of multiorgan failure and shock may be incidental findings of systemic hypoperfusion and not true acute pancreatitis. A threefold elevation of serum lipase level is more diagnostic, especially in patients seen several days after the acute attack, and serum lipase is elevated in both alcoholic and nonalcoholic pancreatitis [48]. Serum lipase has a sensitivity of 82–100% for the diagnosis of acute pancreatitis, often rising within 4–8 h after symptom onset and peaking at 24 h. Lipase levels remain elevated longer than amylase, generally returning to normal within 8–14 days after an episode of acute pancreatitis [48, 50, 51]. Trending of amylase and lipase levels in an acute episode is not indicated, and once a diagnosis of acute pancreatitis is made, management should be driven only by symptomatology. The only utility to repeating enzyme levels is when a patient has initially improved, then clinically declines with concern for complication such as a collection (necrotic or inflammatory) or recurrent episode of acute pancreatitis [39].

Imaging

At presentation, abdominal radiographs are useful in the exclusion of other causes of abdominal pain, such as bowel obstruction, ileus, or perforated bowel, but are not diagnostic for AP. Chest X-ray studies may show infiltrates, left lower lobe atelectasis, or effusion [52, 53]. Abdominal films may be unremarkable or show localized ileus of the small intestine, paucity of air in the distal colon to the splenic flexure due to functional spasm of the descending colon, or ground glass appearance indicating an acute peripancreatic fluid collection [52, 53].

On abdominal ultrasonography, the pancreas may appear diffusely enlarged and hypoechoic in AP [53]. Peripancreatic fluid collections can be seen as anechoic areas that may contain internal echoes if pancreatic necrosis is present. Sensitivity of abdominal ultrasonography is as high as 95% in diagnosing uncomplicated cholelithiasis though its sensitivity decreases in the setting of biliary pancreatitis due to concurrent bowel distention [52, 53]. Up to 25–35% of patients have a limited radiologic exam on abdominal ultrasonography due to ileus or bowel gas that precludes adequate visualization of the gland or the bile duct [54]. Nonetheless, abdominal ultrasonography is recommended to be performed in all patients with acute pancreatitis to evaluate for biliary etiologies and gallstones [53, 55]. Additional imaging should be used only when the diagnosis is not conclusive from the history, physical examination, and laboratory findings or when a complicated course is anticipated.

CT imaging is not routinely indicated as the diagnosis is obvious in many cases, and many patients may have a mild and uncomplicated course. Despite this, intravenous contrast-enhanced CT scanning is a useful imaging technique not only for diagnosis of acute pancreatitis but also for detection of local complications of pancreatitis. This should be delayed until the patient is rehydrated if there is uncertainty of diagnosis because impairment of pancreatic perfusion and signs of pancreatic necrosis, recognized by the lack of enhancement on contrast-enhanced CT, can take several days [52]. After this time contrasted CT has been demonstrated to reliably identify the presence and extent of necrosis as well as local complications. If a patient is not improving clinically after 72 h, CT with contrast preferably over magnetic resonance imaging (MRI) is recommended to assess for the presence of local complications [54, 56]. If the patient meets only clinical symptoms suggestive of pancreatitis or biochemical evidence, then a radiologic study CT imaging can also be considered to confirm the diagnosis.

MRI and magnetic resonance cholangiopancreatography (MRCP) are used in the diagnosis of acute pancreatitis and have higher sensitivity for diagnosis of early pancreatitis than contrasted CT imaging [44, 54, 56]. Focal or diffuse enlargement with blurring of the margins may be seen, failure of the pancreatic parenchyma to enhance on a contrasted study is indicative of necrosis. MRI is considered more useful in the effort to categorize acute fluid collections and assess main pancreatic duct anatomy and is more sensitive in diagnosis of milder forms of pancreatitis. MRCP is better able to delineate the pancreatic and bile ducts [52, 56]. The use of MRI may be limited due to longer scanning time, local expertise, and availability. While not routinely used in the diagnosis of acute pancreatitis, EUS is the most sensitive test for evaluation of small amounts of sludge or microlithiasis [57]. EUS may be able to discern pancreatic divisum or parenchymal abnormalities and can detect small masses that may be obscured via inflammation on cross-sectional imaging.

Patients with recurrent AP may benefit from EUS for further evaluation of the pancreatic parenchyma and ducts, or ERCP as a therapeutic modality to remove common bile duct stones or debris [54]. Patients with unexplained pancreatitis who are older than 40 years are at an increased risk of pancreatic malignancy and should have further imaging with CT or EUS. ERCP should be used only as a therapeutic modality for common bile duct stone removal because it can exacerbate biliary pancreatitis with manipulation of the pancreatic duct [39]. In cases of IAP, patients should be referred to centers of expertise.

American College of Gastroenterology Guidelines recommend:

1. Transabdominal ultrasound should be performed in all patients with acute pancreatitis.
2. In the absence of gallstones and/or significant history of alcohol use, a serum triglyceride should be obtained and considered the etiology if >1000 mg/dL.
3. In a patient older than 40 years, a pancreatic tumor should be considered as a possible cause of acute pancreatitis.
4. Endoscopic investigation in patients with acute idiopathic pancreatitis should be limited, as the risks and benefits of investigation in these patients are unclear.
5. Patients with idiopathic pancreatitis should be referred to centers of expertise.
6. Genetic testing may be considered in young patients (<30 years old) if no cause is evident and a family history of pancreatic disease is present.

Disease Severity and Classification

There have been multiple scoring systems used over time including Apache II criteria, Bedside Index of Severity in Acute Pancreatitis (BISAP), Ranson Criteria, etc. [58, 59]. All of these scoring systems have fallen out of favor and have been replaced by evaluating for the presence and persistence of organ failure with presence of SIRS criteria as a surrogate marker for this as predictors of increased morbidity and mortality.

Risk Stratification

Use of a severity index should allow prediction of the small group of patients who are going to develop severe disease, characterized by organ system failure, pancreatic necrosis ± infection and increased mortality. Overall mortality for AP is 2% and increases to 30% in those with severe acute pancreatitis [43, 52]. However, others found that the test characteristics and clinical utility if these AP severity scores remain uncertain [60]. Investigators did not find studies that directly assessed the influence of these models on patient management.

Predicting severity of AP should be simple and allow for prediction early in the patient's course. This is best accomplished by the BISAP or SIRS, which can predict severity within the first 24 h. The BISAP includes blood urea nitrogen of >25 mg/dL, impaired mental status (Glasgow Coma Scale score <15), SIRS score ≥2, age >60, and pleural effusion. One point is given for each and a score of more than three indicates an increased risk of death [58]. A follow-up evaluation by Singh on the BISAP score reported that a score ≥3 was associated with an increased risk of developing organ failure, persistent organ failure, and pancreatic necrosis [61].

The systemic inflammatory response syndrome is defined by the presence of two or more criteria. These consist of heart rate >90 beats/min, respiratory rate >20 breaths/min or partial pressure of carbon dioxide <32 mm/hg, body temperature <36 °C or >38 °C, and leukocyte count <4 or >12,000 per cubic mm. Its presence during the first 24 h of admission has high sensitivity for predicting severe disease (85%). Persistent SIRS predicted persistent organ failure in only a minority of patients [36].

On admission, hematocrit >44% and a rise in BUN at 24 h may be optional predictive tools. Reducing blood urea nitrogen and hematocrit should be used to guide fluid resuscitation over the first 12–24 h and are an accurate predictor of death [11, 62, 63]. Forsmark and Yadav noted that following serum BUN and hematocrit along with SIRS over the first 48 h are simple and an effective scoring system to predict severe AP (Table 2.1).

Table 2.1 Predictors of severe acute pancreatitis

- Patient: Age, obesity (BMI >30 kg/m^2), altered mental status, numerous and severe, comorbidities including coronary artery disease, CHF, COPD, diabetes mellitus, chronic liver disease, long history of alcohol abuse
- SIRS: Present and persists >48 h
- Laboratory:
  - Hematocrit >44% and no decrease with hydration,
  - Urea nitrogen >20 mg/dL (>7.1 mmol/L), rising and/or no decrease with hydration, and/ or elevated creatinine >1.8 deciliter −159 mmol/L
- Imaging: Pleural effusion or infiltrates

Modified from: Bell D, et al. Medicine 43;3:174–181
Forsmark C, et al. NEJM 2016;375:1972–1981

Table 2.2 Classification of severity of acute pancreatitis

	Mild	Moderate	Severe
Organ failure	None	Transient (resolves within 48 h)	Persistent organ failure (>48 h) of one or more organs
Local complications	None	Yes, without persistent organ failure	
Systemic complications	None	Yes, without persistent organ failure	

Banks PA, Bollen TL, Dervenis C, et al. GUT 2013;62:102–111

Classification of Severity

Important revisions introduced to the Atlanta classification originally devised in 1992 have added radiographic and clinical criteria to further stratify AP into mild, moderately severe, and severe categories [41]. Severe AP includes persistent organ failure per the modified Marshall score criteria more than 48 h compared to mild AP, which has no associated findings of organ failure or local or systemic complications. Moderate AP includes transient organ failure less than 48 h in the presence of local and systemic complications [41]. Moderately severe AP, as a new intermediary category, has been further added and defined as transient organ failure less than 48 h in the presence of complications. Although it may substantially worsen underlying comorbid diseases, moderately severe AP is associated with lower mortality compared to severe AP. Temporal phases of AP-associated complications have been described including the propagation of end organ failure or SIRS within 1 week (early phase) and local complications manifesting after 1 week (late phase). Local complications often include pancreatic fluid collections, pseudocysts, infected or sterile wall-off necrosis, and fulminant parenchymal necrosis of the pancreas. Necrotizing pancreatitis may include isolated peripancreatic tissue necrosis and is often associated with infection, severe systemic end organ damage, and even mortality [64, 65] (Table 2.2).

In mild AP, patients usually improve rapidly with supportive care (fluid resuscitation) and mortality is rare, unless other severe medical comorbidities are present

[42, 46]. Patients with acute, mild pancreatitis by definition do not have local complications or have a modified Marshall score >2 or more that defines the presence of organ failure (respiratory, renal, cardiovascular) [66].

Moderately severe AP is defined as the presence of transient organ system failure (less than 48 h) and/or local complications or systemic complications exacerbation of comorbid disease without persistent organ failure [66]. Severe AP is characterized by single or multiple organ system failure >48 h. These usually include respiratory, renal, and/or cardiovascular failure as measured by (systolic blood pressure mm/hg off inotropic support) as determined by modified Marshall scoring system. Patients with persistent SIRS >48 h or infected necrosis are usually in this category although infected necrosis can be present without organ failure.

Medical Management

Fluid Resuscitation

The cornerstone for therapy for patients with AP is judicious fluid, as one of the major sequelae of pancreatic inflammation is fluid sequestration. Goals of fluid therapy are to replenish lost circulatory fluids to maintain organ system perfusion and oxygenation. However, conflicting evidence has been reported in the literature with regard to the benefits of aggressive fluid resuscitation [46]. Sinha et al. reported factors that independently predicted increased fluid sequestration within the first 48 h after hospital admission [46] including younger age <40 years, alcohol etiology, hemoconcentration, and SIRS. Increasing volumes of fluid sequestration were associated with longer hospitalizations, persistent SIRS and persistent organ system failure [42]. Buxbaum et al. similarly reported a randomized trial of patients with non-severe AP to aggressive (20 mL/Kg Bolus followed by 3 mL/Kg/h vs. standard therapy (10 mL/Kg bolus followed by 1.5 mg/Kg/h) hydration with lactated Ringers solution [67]. A significantly higher proportion of patients treated with aggressive fluid therapy demonstrated clinical improvement compared to standard hydration. In addition to higher volumes of fluid, early fluid administration correlates with reduced morbidity among patients with AP. Gardner et al. reported that early resuscitation, defined as receipt of ≥1/3 of the total calculated 72 h fluid volume given within the first 24 h of presentation, was associated with decreased development of SIRS as well as reduced organ failure, lower rate of ICU admissions, and reduced length of hospitalization [68, 69]. The optimal fluid in this study was Ringer's lactate [68, 69]. Clinically relevant parameters followed during fluid replacement include heart rate, urine output, and blood pressure as well as laboratory markers such as BUN and hematocrit. Therefore, the volumes infused are based on the patient's hemodynamic status measured by vital signs, incorporating blood pressure, pulse and respiratory rates, age, cardiac and renal disease, laboratory values (BUN, creatinine, and HcT) and the presence of SIRS. This "goal-directed therapy" for fluid management is defined as titration of IV fluids to specific clinical and bio-chemical targets of perfusion [68].

Fluid therapy is most effective when given early in the course of AP. This was shown by an international, multicenter study, which found that early moderate fluid repletion (>500–1000 mL) compared to non-aggressive (<500) mL fluid volume administration in the ER, was associated with lower rates of local complications [70]. Furthermore, the aggressive fluid therapy groups who received >1000 mL in the ER, also had significantly lower need for intervention [70]. We utilize a combination of initial bolus and high-volume IV infusion (10 mL/kg bolus in case of hypovolemia, followed by 1.5 mL/kg/h) and assess our goal-directed therapy using patients' vital signs, urine output hourly and with laboratory values (BUN, creatinine and hematocrit every 6–8 h). When hemodynamic stability and laboratory values (BUN <20 and HcT <35) are reached, we decrease rates of infusion.

Analgesics

Abdominal pain in AP can be severe and is often the primary symptom of a flare. Moreover, failure to adequately control abdominal pain can worsen hemodynamic instability. However, pain management in pancreatitis has been poorly studied, leading to significant heterogeneity both between and within different clinical practices. Adequate pain control requires a multimodal approach which may rely on the use of intravenous opiates such as fentanyl, morphine, or hydromorphone in addition to non-opioid pain medications including acetaminophen, NSAIDs, and metamizole [44]. Epidural analgesia may also be an effective opiate sparing modality. Among opiates, fentanyl is favorable due to its safety profile particularly in patients with renal impairment. Although it has not been shown to incite or aggravate AP, morphine has been known to increase sphincter of Oddi pressure and is often avoided for this reason [44]. Historically, meperidine has been used with good efficacy; yet, it must be used cautiously due to the risk of neuromuscular irritation and seizures caused by accumulation of the metabolite normeperidine.

Prophylactic Antibiotics

Historically, the administration of prophylactic antibiotics in patients with AP in the past was to prevent infection and the development of necrotizing AP. Prophylactic antibiotics were similarly thought to help address the risk of extra-pancreatic infections such as bacteremia, pneumonia, and urinary tract infections that may be observed in up to 20% of patients with pancreatitis [65, 71]. The mortality in patients with necrosis is up to 20% vs. interstitial AP, whose associated mortality is 5% [45, 64]. Once infection complicates necrosis, mortality increases to 30–40% [64]. Therefore, prophylactic antibiotics would appear to be a reasonable therapeutic approach. However, it has been shown not to be effective in a recent Cochrane Database systematic review of antibiotic therapy for prophylaxis against infection of pancreatic necrosis in AP by Villatoro et al. They found that there was no benefit of antibiotics in preventing infection of pancreatic necrosis or decreasing mortality [71].

A subgroup analysis of patients in this study who received imipenem demonstrated a significant decrease in pancreatic infections in the absence of any reduction in mortality. Antibiotics should only be administered early in the course of patients with AP who have suspected biliary sepsis or have extra-pancreatic infection (urinary tract infection and/or positive blood cultures) [39, 71]. Additionally, antibiotic therapy should be reserved for suspected or diagnosed pancreatic or peripancreatic infections in the later phase (at least 1–2 weeks) after onset of disease [65]. The role of antibiotics in this phase is to allow the focal organization of parenchymal necrosis as well as to delay surgery, usually until 4 weeks, as this is associated with decreased mortality compared to earlier intervention [65]. Furthermore, the delay utilization of antibiotics may allow for application of less invasive drainage procedures. As Adler and Runzi reported, antibiotic therapy alone can also effectively treat a subgroup of patients with infected pancreatic necrosis [72, 73]. An initial report by Runzi et al. examining nonsurgical treatment of 16 patients with severe AP with infected pancreatic necrosis (IPN), utilized only with an antibiotic regimen tailored to bacteriology culture results and nonsurgical therapy, reported a 12% (2/16 patients) mortality rate [73]. Six recovered without further complications, and 10 patients developed single or multiple organ failure. This study challenged the dogma that all patients with IPN require immediate open pancreatic surgical drainage [73]. The currently accepted management of patients with IPN is that early in their course they can generally be managed nonsurgically with antibiotics in the initial stage and that antibiotics alone can also be definitive therapy. The second concept is that surgery can be delayed, which allows operative intervention to be performed electively for more chronic sequelae of AP and with less invasive interventions.

Nutrition

One of the goals in treating patients with AP is early enteral feeding. This should commence as soon as the patient is hungry and ideally once nausea, emesis, and abdominal pain are improving. Oral feeds help maintain small bowel integrity, thereby decreasing bacterial translocation. Early gastric feeds administered via nasogastric tube have not been shown to have significant benefits in reducing infection or death compared to oral feeding at 72 h [74]. In one randomized study, over two-thirds of patients tolerated an oral diet after its initiation at 72 h after presentation, which demonstrated that starting an oral diet at 72 h is not harmful to the patient [74]. In patients with moderate or severe AP, early oral feeding once patients demonstrate an appetite has been shown to be safe and may even shorten hospitalization compared to conventional oral feeding initiated after clinical and laboratory parameters resolve [75]. Vaughn et al. in a systematic review of early (<48 h) vs. delayed (>48 h) feeding in patients with AP, found that adverse events did not increase in patients with early feeds [76]. In patients with mild to moderate AP, early enteral feeds have been associated with a reduction in the length of hospital stay [76]. Their early nutrition group included oral as well as tube feeding.

Oral feeding intolerance (OFI), defined as relapse of symptoms following oral feeding, occurs in approximately one of six patients with AP [77]. Predictive factors for OFI include complicated or severe disease reflected by the presence of pleural effusion and/or peripancreatic collections. If patients have OFI, enteral nutrition (EN) can be initiated with either nasogastric or nasojejunal feedings, as they have similar safety profiles and efficacy in these patients [77]. This should be initiated early (<48 h) in the course of severe AP and occasionally delayed for up to 72 h in patients with mild-to-moderate AP to determine if they can tolerate oral feeding. Low rates of infusion possibly decrease bowel permeability, but the goal should aim to meet patients' caloric demands. Enteral nutrition should be started prior to 48 h in patients with severe pancreatitis, especially those who are intubated. Khaled et al. showed that benefits of early feeding were more evident in the sickest (treated with multiple vasopressors) ICU patients [77].

Bakker OJ reported a meta-analysis of 165 individuals from 8 randomized trials [78]. The cohort was divided into those who received EN within 24 h of admission vs. those who received EN after 24 h of admission. Those receiving EN within 24 h of admission had decreased organ failure, 42 vs. 16% (OR 0.42), and a reduction in the complications of infected pancreatic necrosis and/or organ failure. No difference in mortality was observed and earlier initiation of EN was deemed better for patients with severe AP. However, benefits of EN begun within 3 days could reduce the risk of secondary infection and improve the nutritional status of patients with AP [78].

Overall, enteral nutrition should be utilized over parenteral nutrition in patients with AP. Enteral nutrition has a multitude of advantages over parenteral nutrition including avoidance of complications of invasive central venous access procedures, catheter-related sepsis, lower cost, maintenance of enteral barrier function, and decreasing bacterial translocation, which is a critical factor in the evolution of infections in AP patients [79, 80]. Enteral vs. parenteral nutrition results in reduction in the risk of total and pancreatic infectious complications and risk of death [79, 80].

Complications

Most patients with AP experience acute interstitial edematous pancreatitis, which is mild in severity with resolution in 3–5 days without complications [45]. Twenty percent experience moderately severe or severe acute pancreatitis with local or systemic complications [45]. Local complications of AP include peripancreatic collections such as acute fluid collections, pseudocysts, acute necrotic collections, and walled-off necrosis [81]. Acute peripancreatic fluid collections and acute necrotic collections usually develop within 4 weeks of an episode of AP, while pseudocysts and walled-off necrosis usually occur after 4 weeks once there is maturation of a wall [81]. Necrotic collections have tissue debris as well as fluid contents, whereas acute fluid collections and pseudocysts only have fluid contents. Approximately 50% of patients with necrotizing AP will develop portosplenomesenteric thrombosis, which is uncommon in the absence of necrosis [82]. Contrast-enhanced CT scan to investigate for the presence of necrosis should be considered in patients who fail to respond to supportive management after 72 h [52]. Pancreatic necrosis should be managed conservatively with a step-up approach focusing on supportive care measures, followed by catheter drainage if there are ongoing symptoms or a need for drainage of infected necrosis. Interventions with EUS or a minimally invasive surgical approach should be considered for those patients with walled-off infected necrosis who are not clinically improving despite antibiotic treatment [55]. The advent of procedures such as EUS-guided placement of lumen apposing metal stents (LAMS) has enabled cyst-gastrostomy of fluid collections with immediate drainage, and endoscopic necrosectomy for walled-off necrosis [53]. Timing of the intervention is of utmost importance, and treatment should be delayed for at least 3–4 weeks after the initial episode of AP to allow for maturation of fluid collection walls and to enable delineation of tissue planes. Open necrosectomy should be reserved for severe refractory cases in which minimally invasive approaches fail, as this operation is associated with significant complications and an overall poor prognosis [45, 47].

Systemic complications of AP are defined according to the revised Atlanta classification as an exacerbation of an underlying comorbidity [41]. Such conditions may include coronary artery disease or chronic lung disease. Organ failure is a distinct entity related to activation of a cytokine cascade from acute pancreatic inflammation, which results in SIRS [36]. SIRS may lead to organ failure of one or more organ systems leading to renal failure, shock, and respiratory failure and is the major cause of death due to acute pancreatitis [36]. Patients may also develop complications of hypocalcemia and other metabolic abnormalities, blindness, pseudocysts, necrosis, hemorrhage, and multisystem organ failure. Long-term, if there is disruption with disconnection of the pancreatic duct due to an episode of acute pancreatitis, this may lead to recurrent complications including fluid collections as well as exocrine pancreatic insufficiency [43].

Long-Term Sequelae of Acute Pancreatitis

Patients who have recovered from AP are at significant risk for recurrence if the initial cause has not been elucidated and corrected. The morbidity of a bout of AP persists in some patients after recovery of AP. An episode of AP increases a patient's risk of developing diabetes mellitus, progressing to chronic pancreatitis with exocrine pancreatic insufficiency and is associated with an increased risk of harboring or developing pancreatic cancer [32, 81]. Patients who had severe AP that required critical care were found to have a high risk for developing new onset of diabetes mellitus. Therefore, multidisciplinary management of these patients and ensuring follow-up with gastroenterology is crucial.

References

1. Peery AF, Dellon ES, Lund J, Crockett SD, McGowan CE, Bulsiewicz WJ, et al. Burden of gastrointestinal disease in the United States: 2012 update. Gastroenterology. 2012;143(5):1179–1187.e3.
2. Fagenholz PJ, Fernández-del Castillo C, Harris NS, Pelletier AJ, Camargo CA. Direct medical costs of acute pancreatitis hospitalizations in the United States. Pancreas. 2007;35(4):302–7.
3. Fagenholz PJ, del Castillo CF, Harris NS, Pelletier AJ, Camargo CA. Increasing United States hospital admissions for acute pancreatitis, 1988–2003. Ann Epidemiol. 2007;17(7):491–7.
4. Lankisch PG, Assmus C, Lehnick D, Maisonneuve P, Lowenfels AB. Acute pancreatitis: does gender matter? Dig Dis Sci. 2001;46(11):2470–4.
5. Gullo L, Migliori M, Oláh A, Farkas G, Levy P, Arvanitakis C, et al. Acute pancreatitis in five European countries: etiology and mortality. Pancreas. 2002;24(3):223–7.
6. Lowenfels AB, Maisonneuve P, Sullivan T. The changing character of acute pancreatitis: epidemiology, etiology, and prognosis. Curr Gastroenterol Rep. 2009;11(2):97–103.
7. Yadav D, Lowenfels AB. Trends in the epidemiology of the first attack of acute pancreatitis: a systematic review. Pancreas. 2006;33(4):323–30.
8. Johnson C, Lévy P. Detection of gallstones in acute pancreatitis: when and how? Pancreatology. 2010;10(1):27–32.
9. Moreau JA, Zinsmeister AR, Melton LJ, DiMagno EP. Gallstone pancreatitis and the effect of cholecystectomy: a population-based cohort study. Mayo Clin Proc. 1988;63(5):466–73.
10. Ammann RW. The natural history of alcoholic chronic pancreatitis. Intern Med. 2001;40(5):368–75.
11. Yadav D, O'Connell M, Papachristou GI. Natural history following the first attack of acute pancreatitis. Am J Gastroenterol. 2012;107(7):1096–103.
12. Whitcomb DC. Genetic polymorphisms in alcoholic pancreatitis. Dig Dis. 2005;23(3–4):247–54.
13. Steinberg W, Tenner S. Acute pancreatitis. N Engl J Med. 1994;330(17):1198–210.
14. Rebours V, Vullierme MP, Hentic O, Maire F, Hammel P, Ruszniewski P, et al. Smoking and the course of recurrent acute and chronic alcoholic pancreatitis: a dose-dependent relationship. Pancreas. 2012;41(8):1219–24.
15. Fortson MR, Freedman SN, Webster PD. Clinical assessment of hyperlipidemic pancreatitis. Am J Gastroenterol. 1995;90(12):2134–9.
16. Parenti DM, Steinberg W, Kang P. Infectious causes of acute pancreatitis. Pancreas. 1996;13(4):356–71.
17. Toskes PP. Hyperlipidemic pancreatitis. Gastroenterol Clin N Am. 1990;19(4):783–91.
18. Yadav D, Pitchumoni CS. Issues in hyperlipidemic pancreatitis. J Clin Gastroenterol. 2003;36(1):54–62.
19. Lippi G, Valentino M, Cervellin G. Laboratory diagnosis of acute pancreatitis: in search of the holy grail. Crit Rev Clin Lab Sci. 2012;49(1):18–31.
20. Simpson WF, Adams DB, Metcalf JS, Anderson MC. Nonfunctioning pancreatic neuroendocrine tumors presenting as pancreatitis: report of four cases. Pancreas. 1988;3(2):223–31.
21. Köhler H, Lankisch PG. Acute pancreatitis and hyperamylasaemia in pancreatic carcinoma. Pancreas. 1987;2(1):117–9.

22. Robertson JF, Imrie CW. Acute pancreatitis associated with carcinoma of the ampulla of Vater. Br J Surg. 1987;74(5):395–7.
23. Busquets J, Fabregat J, Pelaez N, Millan M, Secanella L, Garcia-Borobia F, et al. Factors influencing mortality in patients undergoing surgery for acute pancreatitis: importance of peripancreatic tissue and fluid infection. Pancreas. 2013;42(2):285–92.
24. Bollen TL, Singh VK, Maurer R, Repas K, van Es HW, Banks PA, et al. Comparative evaluation of the modified CT severity index and CT severity index in assessing severity of acute pancreatitis. AJR Am J Roentgenol. 2011;197(2):386–92.
25. Stimac D, Miletić D, Radić M, Krznarić I, Mazur-Grbac M, Perković D, et al. The role of nonenhanced magnetic resonance imaging in the early assessment of acute pancreatitis. Am J Gastroenterol. 2007;102(5):997–1004.
26. Bank S, Indaram A. Causes of acute and recurrent pancreatitis. Clinical considerations and clues to diagnosis. Gastroenterol Clin N Am. 1999;28(3):571–89. viii
27. Banks PA. Epidemiology, natural history, and predictors of disease outcome in acute and chronic pancreatitis. Gastrointest Endosc. 2002;56(6 Suppl):S226–30.
28. DiMagno MJ, Dimagno EP. Pancreas divisum does not cause pancreatitis, but associates with CFTR mutations. Am J Gastroenterol. 2012;107(2):318–20.
29. Al-Haddad M, Wallace MB. Diagnostic approach to patients with acute idiopathic and recurrent pancreatitis, what should be done? World J Gastroenterol. 2008;14(7):1007–10.
30. Neoptolemos JP, Carr-Locke DL, London NJ, Bailey IA, James D, Fossard DP. Controlled trial of urgent endoscopic retrograde cholangiopancreatography and endoscopic sphincterotomy versus conservative treatment for acute pancreatitis due to gallstones. Lancet. 1988;2(8618):979–83.
31. Badalov N, Tenner S, Baillie J. The prevention, recognition and treatment of post-ERCP pancreatitis. JOP. 2009;10(2):88–97.
32. Bakker OJ, van Santvoort H, Besselink MGH, Boermeester MA, van Eijck C, Dejong K, et al. Extrapancreatic necrosis without pancreatic parenchymal necrosis: a separate entity in necrotising pancreatitis? Gut. 2013;62(10):1475–80.
33. Tandon M, Topazian M. Endoscopic ultrasound in idiopathic acute pancreatitis. Am J Gastroenterol. 2001;96(3):705–9.
34. Steinberg WM, Chari ST, Forsmark CE, Sherman S, Reber HA, Bradley EL, et al. Controversies in clinical pancreatology: management of acute idiopathic recurrent pancreatitis. Pancreas. 2003;27(2):103–17.
35. Hasan A, Moscoso DI, Kastrinos F. The role of genetics in pancreatitis. Gastrointest Endosc Clin N Am. 2018;28(4):587–603.
36. Singh VK, Wu BU, Bollen TL, Repas K, Maurer R, Mortele KJ, et al. Early systemic inflammatory response syndrome is associated with severe acute pancreatitis. Clin Gastroenterol Hepatol. 2009;7(11):1247–51.
37. Tenner S. Initial management of acute pancreatitis: critical issues during the first 72 hours. Am J Gastroenterol. 2004;99(12):2489–94.
38. Banks PA, Freeman ML, Practice Parameters Committee of the American College of Gastroenterology. Practice guidelines in acute pancreatitis. Am J Gastroenterol. 2006;101(10):2379–400.
39. Tenner S, Baillie J, De Witt J, Vege SS, American College of Gastroenterology. American College of Gastroenterology guideline: management of acute pancreatitis. Am J Gastroenterol. 2013;108(9):1400–15, 1416
40. Talukdar R, Vege SS. Recent developments in acute pancreatitis. Clin Gastroenterol Hepatol. 2009;7(11 Suppl):S3–9.
41. Zaheer A, Singh VK, Qureshi RO, Fishman EK. The revised Atlanta classification for acute pancreatitis: updates in imaging terminology and guidelines. Abdom Imaging. 2013;38(1):125–36.

42. de Madaria E, Banks PA, Moya-Hoyo N, Wu BU, Rey-Riveiro M, Acevedo-Piedra NG, et al. Early factors associated with fluid sequestration and outcomes of patients with acute pancreatitis. Clin Gastroenterol Hepatol. 2014;12(6):997–1002.
43. Jang JW, Kim MH, Oh D, Cho DH, Song TJ, Park DH, et al. Factors and outcomes associated with pancreatic duct disruption in patients with acute necrotizing pancreatitis. Pancreatology. 2016;16(6):958–65.
44. Crockett SD, Wani S, Gardner TB, Falck-Ytter Y, Barkun AN, American Gastroenterological Association Institute Clinical Guidelines Committee. American Gastroenterological Association Institute Guideline on Initial Management of Acute Pancreatitis. Gastroenterology. 2018;154(4):1096–101.
45. Singh VK, Bollen TL, Wu BU, Repas K, Maurer R, Yu S, et al. An assessment of the severity of interstitial pancreatitis. Clin Gastroenterol Hepatol. 2011;9(12):1098–103.
46. Sinha A, Quesada-Vázquez N, Faghih M, Afghani E, Zaheer A, Khashab MA, et al. Early predictors of fluid sequestration in acute pancreatitis: a validation study. Pancreas. 2016;45(2):306–10.
47. Kiriyama S, Gabata T, Takada T, Hirata K, Yoshida M, Mayumi T, et al. New diagnostic criteria of acute pancreatitis. J Hepatobiliary Pancreat Sci. 2010;17(1):24–36.
48. Ismail OZ, Bhayana V. Lipase or amylase for the diagnosis of acute pancreatitis? Clin Biochem. 2017;50(18):1275–80.
49. Weiss FU, Hesselbarth N, Párniczky A, Mosztbacher D, Lämmerhirt F, Ruffert C, et al. Common variants in the CLDN2-MORC4 and PRSS1-PRSS2 loci confer susceptibility to acute pancreatitis. Pancreatology. 2018;18(5):477–81.
50. Garg R, Rustagi T. Management of Hypertriglyceridemia Induced Acute Pancreatitis. Biomed Res Int. 2018;2018:4721357.
51. Vipperla K, Somerville C, Furlan A, Koutroumpakis E, Saul M, Chennat J, et al. Clinical profile and natural course in a large cohort of patients with hypertriglyceridemia and pancreatitis. J Clin Gastroenterol. 2017;51(1):77–85.
52. Türkvatan A, Erden A, Türkoğlu MA, Seçil M, Yener Ö. Imaging of acute pancreatitis and its complications. Part 1: acute pancreatitis. Diagn Interv Imaging. 2015;96(2):151–60.
53. Kondo S, Isayama H, Akahane M, Toda N, Sasahira N, Nakai Y, et al. Detection of common bile duct stones: comparison between endoscopic ultrasonography, magnetic resonance cholangiography, and helical-computed-tomographic cholangiography. Eur J Radiol. 2005;54(2):271–5.
54. Wan J, Ouyang Y, Yu C, Yang X, Xia L, Lu N. Comparison of EUS with MRCP in idiopathic acute pancreatitis: a systematic review and meta-analysis. Gastrointest Endosc. 2018;87(5):1180–1188.e9.
55. De Lisi S, Leandro G, Buscarini E. Endoscopic ultrasonography versus endoscopic retrograde cholangiopancreatography in acute biliary pancreatitis: a systematic review. Eur J Gastroenterol Hepatol. 2011;23(5):367–74.
56. Makary MA, Duncan MD, Harmon JW, Freeswick PD, Bender JS, Bohlman M, et al. The role of magnetic resonance cholangiography in the management of patients with gallstone pancreatitis. Ann Surg. 2005;241(1):119–24.
57. Ardengh JC, Malheiros CA, Rahal F, Pereira V, Ganc AJ. Microlithiasis of the gallbladder: role of endoscopic ultrasonography in patients with idiopathic acute pancreatitis. Rev Assoc Med Bras (1992). 2010;56(1):27–31.
58. Papachristou GI, Muddana V, Yadav D, O'Connell M, Sanders MK, Slivka A, et al. Comparison of BISAP, Ranson's, APACHE-II, and CTSI scores in predicting organ failure, complications, and mortality in acute pancreatitis. Am J Gastroenterol. 2010;105(2):435–41. quiz 442
59. Ranson JH, Pasternack BS. Statistical methods for quantifying the severity of clinical acute pancreatitis. J Surg Res. 1977;22(2):79–91.
60. Di MY, Liu H, Yang ZY, Bonis PAL, Tang JL, Lau J. Prediction models of mortality in acute pancreatitis in adults: a systematic review. Ann Intern Med. 2016;165(7):482–90.

61. Singh VK, Wu BU, Bollen TL, Repas K, Maurer R, Johannes RS, et al. A prospective evaluation of the bedside index for severity in acute pancreatitis score in assessing mortality and intermediate markers of severity in acute pancreatitis. Am J Gastroenterol. 2009;104(4):966–71.
62. Forsmark CE, Yadav D. Predicting the prognosis of acute pancreatitis. Ann Intern Med. 2016;165(7):523–4.
63. Koutroumpakis E, Wu BU, Bakker OJ, Dudekula A, Singh VK, Besselink MG, et al. Admission hematocrit and rise in blood urea nitrogen at 24 h outperform other laboratory markers in predicting persistent organ failure and pancreatic necrosis in acute pancreatitis: a post hoc analysis of three large prospective databases. Am J Gastroenterol. 2015;110(12):1707–16.
64. Umapathy C, Raina A, Saligram S, Tang G, Papachristou GI, Rabinovitz M, et al. Natural history after acute necrotizing pancreatitis: a large US tertiary care experience. J Gastrointest Surg. 2016;20(11):1844–53.
65. Zavyalov T, Khotsyna Y, Tenner S. The role of antibiotics in the management of patients with acute necrotizing pancreatitis. Curr Infect Dis Rep. 2010;12(1):13–8.
66. Banks PA, Bollen TL, Dervenis C, Gooszen HG, Johnson CD, Sarr MG, et al. Classification of acute pancreatitis—2012: revision of the Atlanta classification and definitions by international consensus. Gut. 2013;62(1):102–11.
67. Buxbaum JL, Quezada M, Da B, Jani N, Lane C, Mwengela D, et al. Early aggressive hydration hastens clinical improvement in mild acute pancreatitis. Am J Gastroenterol. 2017;112(5):797–803.
68. Gardner TB, Vege SS, Pearson RK, Chari ST. Fluid resuscitation in acute pancreatitis. Clin Gastroenterol Hepatol. 2008;6(10):1070–6.
69. Gardner TB, Vege SS, Chari ST, Petersen BT, Topazian MD, Clain JE, et al. Faster rate of initial fluid resuscitation in severe acute pancreatitis diminishes in-hospital mortality. Pancreatology. 2009;9(6):770–6.
70. Singh VK, Gardner TB, Papachristou GI, Rey-Riveiro M, Faghih M, Koutroumpakis E, et al. An international multicenter study of early intravenous fluid administration and outcome in acute pancreatitis. United European Gastroenterol J. 2017;5(4):491–8.
71. Villatoro E, Mulla M, Larvin M. Antibiotic therapy for prophylaxis against infection of pancreatic necrosis in acute pancreatitis. Cochrane Database Syst Rev. 2010;2010(5):CD002941.
72. Adler DG, Chari ST, Dahl TJ, Farnell MB, Pearson RK. Conservative management of infected necrosis complicating severe acute pancreatitis. Am J Gastroenterol. 2003;98(1):98–103.
73. Runzi M, Niebel W, Goebell H, Gerken G, Layer P. Severe acute pancreatitis: nonsurgical treatment of infected necroses. Pancreas. 2005;30(3):195–9.
74. Bakker OJ, van Brunschot S, van Santvoort HC, Besselink MG, Bollen TL, Boermeester MA, et al. Early versus on-demand nasoenteric tube feeding in acute pancreatitis. N Engl J Med. 2014;371(21):1983–93.
75. Coté GA. Early enteral feeding does not improve outcomes in patients with predicted severe acute pancreatitis. Gastroenterology. 2015;148(7):1476–8.
76. Vaughn VM, Shuster D, Rogers MAM, Mann J, Conte ML, Saint S, et al. Early versus delayed feeding in patients with acute pancreatitis: a systematic review. Ann Intern Med. 2017;166(12):883–92.
77. Bevan MG, Asrani VM, Bharmal S, Wu LM, Windsor JA, Petrov MS. Incidence and predictors of oral feeding intolerance in acute pancreatitis: a systematic review, meta-analysis, and meta-regression. Clin Nutr. 2017;36(3):722–9.
78. Bakker OJ, van Brunschot S, Farre A, Johnson CD, Kalfarentzos F, Louie BE, et al. Timing of enteral nutrition in acute pancreatitis: meta-analysis of individuals using a single-arm of randomised trials. Pancreatology. 2014;14(5):340–6.
79. Jin M, Zhang H, Lu B, Li Y, Wu D, Qian J, et al. The optimal timing of enteral nutrition and its effect on the prognosis of acute pancreatitis: a propensity score matched cohort study. Pancreatology. 2017;17(5):651–7.
80. Petrov MS, van Santvoort HC, Besselink MGH, van der Heijden GJMG, Windsor JA, Gooszen HG. Enteral nutrition and the risk of mortality and infectious complications in

patients with severe acute pancreatitis: a meta-analysis of randomized trials. Arch Surg. 2008;143(11):1111–7.
81. Afghani E, Pandol SJ, Shimosegawa T, Sutton R, Wu BU, Vege SS, et al. Acute pancreatitis-progress and challenges: a report on an international symposium. Pancreas. 2015;44(8):1195–210.
82. Vege SS, DiMagno MJ, Forsmark CE, Martel M, Barkun AN. Initial medical treatment of acute pancreatitis: American Gastroenterological Association Institute Technical Review. Gastroenterology. 2018;154(4):1103–39.

Chapter 3
Acute Pancreatitis: Non-surgical Therapies Including Gallstone Management

Anne Nagelhout, Martijn W. J. Stommel, Stefan A. W. Bouwense, Marc G. Besselink, and for the Dutch Pancreatitis Study Group

Introduction

Acute pancreatitis has an increasing incidence worldwide and is one of the most common gastrointestinal disorders requiring acute hospitalization [1, 2]. The current incidence in the Western World is 34 per 100.000 person-years [3]. The clinical course and severity of acute pancreatitis varies a lot, ranging from a mild course with transient abdominal discomfort till a severe course with multiorgan failure and high mortality.

Approximately 80% of the patients present with mild acute pancreatitis, which is self-limiting, usually within 1 week [4, 5]. The other 20% of patients develop moderate to severe acute pancreatitis, with (multiple) organ failure and often (infected)

A. Nagelhout (✉)
Department of Surgery, Radboudumc, Nijmegen, The Netherlands

Department of Research and Development, St. Antonius Hospital, Nieuwegein, The Netherlands
e-mail: a.nagelhout@antoniusziekenhuis.nl

M. W. J. Stommel
Department of Surgery, Radboudumc, Nijmegen, The Netherlands
e-mail: martijn.stommel@radboudumc.nl

S. A. W. Bouwense
Department of Surgery, Maastricht University Medical Centre+, Maastricht, The Netherlands
e-mail: stefan.bouwense@mumc.nl

M. G. Besselink
Department of Surgery, Amsterdam UMC, Location University of Amsterdam, Amsterdam, The Netherlands

Amsterdam Gastroenterology Endocrinology Metabolism, Amsterdam, The Netherlands
e-mail: m.g.besselink@amsterdamumc.nl

© The Author(s), under exclusive license to Springer Nature Switzerland AG 2025
E. P. Ceppa et al. (eds.), *The SAGES Manual of Evolving Techniques in Pancreatic Surgery*, https://doi.org/10.1007/978-3-031-78409-5_3

necrosis of the pancreatic or peripancreatic tissue [4–6]. In these patients, the mortality rate is high (10–30%) in contrast to low mortality in mild pancreatitis (less than 1%) [5, 7, 8]. The treatment of pancreatitis patients is predominantly aimed at supporting the vital organ systems and providing comfort and nutrition when needed.

This chapter provides an overview of the non-surgical therapy of acute pancreatitis. First, initial therapies (i.e., fluid resuscitation, pain management, nutrition, and the role of antibiotics) will be discussed, followed by the specific treatment for biliary pancreatitis, including the role of endoscopic retrograde cholangiopancreatography (ERCP), magnetic resonance cholangiopancreatography (MRCP), and endoscopic ultrasound (EUS), the timing of cholecystectomy. The prevention of disease recurrence and recommendations for future research will also be discussed.

Early and Late Phase of Acute Pancreatitis

In case of mild pancreatitis, the disease is limited to the early phase. A mild systemic inflammatory reaction may take place and patients usually improve spontaneously after a few days. However, in case of a more severe inflammatory response, two overlapping phases of acute pancreatitis can be recognized: the early and the late phase. Due to excessive local pancreatic cell injury, the early phase is characterized by activation of large cytokine cascades which can cause the systemic inflammatory response syndrome (SIRS) [4]. As a result of persistent SIRS, the risk of infections and development of organ failure arises [4, 9]. (Multi)organ failure, including cardiovascular, respiratory, or renal failure, can develop early in acute pancreatitis and is the main reason for early mortality in patients with severe acute pancreatitis [4, 9, 10]. The late phase of acute pancreatitis is characterized by persistence of systemic signs of inflammation, generally caused by compensatory anti-inflammatory response syndrome (CARS) [5]. During this phase, patients are again susceptible to infections like pneumonia, sepsis, or secondary infection of (peri)pancreatic necrosis [5, 7].

Initial Treatment

The initial treatment of acute pancreatitis in the early phase consists of supportive measures and preventing/treating (multi)organ failure which comprises fluid resuscitation, pain management, and proper nutrition. For management of the disease, a multidisciplinary team (including a surgeon, gastroenterologist, radiologist, and dietitian) in hospitals is recommended.

Reducing Severity of Acute Pancreatitis

Until this date, the cornerstone of treatment in patients with severe acute pancreatitis is supportive care. Several studies have been conducted in the early phase of acute pancreatitis in order to prevent severe disease progression and reduce complications [11–14]. Unfortunately, these studies showed no improvement in clinical outcomes and the right treatment in the early phase of acute pancreatitis for reduction of organ failure and mortality is still lacking. An option for treatment may be modification of the immune response in the early phase of predicted severe acute pancreatitis through the administration of early intravenous omega-3 fatty acids in patients. Omega-3 fatty acids replace arachidonic acids (omega-6) in the inflammatory mediator production cascade [15]. In addition, omega-3 fatty acids provide increased production of resolvins which improve normalization of inflammatory tissue [16]. These actions of omega-3 fatty acids could potentially lead to an effective response of the immune system. A meta-analysis [17] was performed to investigate the safety and efficacy of omega-3 in patients with acute pancreatitis and sepsis. The meta-analysis demonstrated a lower incidence of mortality after omega-3 fatty acids infusion. Furthermore, a recent single-center randomized controlled trial [18] demonstrated decreased CRP levels and decreased onset of new organ failure in patients with predicted severe pancreatitis after administration of omega-3 fatty acids. To provide solid evidence on the true potential of omega-3 fatty acids, the PLANCTON multicenter randomized trial is currently in progress in the Netherlands in patients with predicted severe acute pancreatitis.

Fluid Resuscitation

Adequate fluid resuscitation is required during the first few days of acute pancreatitis to correct for possible intravascular hypovolemia, which is caused by local and systemic immune responses. Infusion with Ringer's lactate is recommended as it reduces the risk of developing SIRS when compared to normal saline infusion [1, 19–22]. In fact, such immune responses induce cell apoptosis and increase vascular permeability, resulting in extravasation of fluid in the third space, and could lead to hypoperfusion, (multiple) organ failure, and ultimately death [2, 23, 24]. On the other hand, aggressive and undirected fluid infusion contributes to higher morbidity and even higher mortality as was shown by two randomized trials [25, 26]. Therefore, careful monitoring of the vital signs during fluid resuscitation is necessary [1, 25, 26]. The preferred approach according to the current IAP/APA treatment guideline for acute pancreatitis focuses on resuscitation until certain goals are reached (heart rate less than 120 per minute, mean arterial pressure between 65 and 85 mmHg, and urinary output more than 0.5 till 1.0 mL/kg/h) [1].

The recent Waterfall trial [27] compared aggressive versus moderate fluid resuscitation in patients with acute pancreatitis. Aggressive fluid resuscitation consisted of 20 mL/kg Ringer's lactate over 2 h, followed by 3 mL/kg/h. Patients in the moderate-resuscitation group received 1.5 mL/kg/h and only a bolus of 10 mL/kg/2 h in patients with hypovolemia. This trial demonstrated that patients with aggressive fluid resuscitation had a higher risk of fluid overload compared to moderate resuscitation (20.5 vs. 6.3%). These findings underline the importance of carefully monitoring vital signs and achieving the resuscitation goals to prevent both hypovolemia and hypervolemia.

Pain Management

Severe, persistent upper abdominal pain is the predominant symptom in patients with acute pancreatitis, which remains dominant during the first few days of hospital admission. Therefore, adequate pain treatment according to the World Health Organization (WHO) analgesic ladder is required [28]. The use of opioids could reduce the number of patients that need supplementary analgesia [29]. One study suggested that epidural anesthesia prevents early tissue damage and improves the perfusion of the pancreas [30]. More recent, a multicenter retrospective study suggested that the use of epidural anesthesia was associated with reduced 30-day mortality in patients with severe acute pancreatitis compared to patients without epidural anesthesia (2 vs. 17%) [31]. Nevertheless, more prospective studies are needed on the use of epidural anesthesia before it can be recommended in the standard supportive care for acute pancreatitis.

Nutrition

Gut barrier dysfunction is present in most patients with acute pancreatitis [32]. Therefore, optimal enteral nutritional support is important to maintain the intestinal barrier integrity, but it also prevents bacterial overgrowth and decreases SIRS. [32, 33] According to the multicenter randomized PYTHON trial [11], early enteral tube feeding within 24 h after admission does not decrease rates of infection (25 vs. 26%) or mortality (11 vs. 7%) in comparison to on-demand feeding in patients with predicted severe acute pancreatitis. Oral feeding on-demand is recommended and can be started as early as a patient request. Enteral tube feeding should only be considered if an oral diet is not tolerated after 72 h form the time of presentation. Enteral feeding is strongly preferred over parenteral feeding because of the lower risks of complications such as (multi)organ failure, central venous catheter infections, and mortality [34, 35].

Preventing Infectious Complications

In acute pancreatitis, both early infections, especially bacteremia, and secondary infection of (peri)pancreatic necrosis in a later phase, may increase mortality [9]. Disruption of the normal gut barrier, which results in translocation of microorganisms, is believed to be the major cause of secondary infection of (peri)pancreatic necrosis [32, 36, 37]. Multiple studies have shown that prophylactic administration of antibiotics does not reduce the risk of infected (peri)pancreatic necrosis [38–41]. Moreover, the use of prophylactic antibiotics is associated with an increased incidence of fungal and multidrug-resistant bacterial infections [42, 43]. Administration of antibiotics in acute pancreatitis are therefore only advised as treatment for proven or clinically suspected infected necrosis [1, 44]. Another believed potential prophylactic strategy for the prevention of (secondary) infections by protecting the gut barrier was the use of probiotics. The multicenter randomized PROPATRIA trial [12] found a higher rate of mortality in patients with predicted severe acute pancreatitis who received probiotics compared to a placebo group. Therefore, the administration of probiotics for the treatment of acute pancreatitis is not recommended.

Nevertheless, the perfect strategy for protecting the gut barrier and eventually preventing infectious complications remains challenging. A possible strategy may be the use of the short-chain fatty acid "butyrate" which is produced by different types of bacteria in the gut. Butyrate has an anti-inflammatory and antimicrobial effect in the gut that improves the gut integrity and the mucosal immune system [45]. A recent study showed the positive effect of oral supplementation of butyrate in a mouse model of biliary necrotizing pancreatitis on the gut barrier [46]. Another possible beneficial effect on preventing bacterial translocation may be modulating the gut's microflora. The gut microbiome is believed to play a role in the development of sepsis and (multi)organ failure [47]. Future research should be conducted to investigate both possible strategies.

Management of Biliary Pancreatitis

Currently, the most frequent cause of acute pancreatitis in the Western world is gallstones (45%) [48]. Gallstones can induce acute biliary pancreatitis as a result of (transient) obstruction of the bile and pancreatic duct. Cholangitis, organ failure, and further potentially fatal consequences can occur in patients with biliary pancreatitis [4, 49, 50].

Role of ERCP

According to current guidelines, ERCP is not recommended for mild biliary pancreatitis without cholangitis or predicted severe biliary pancreatitis without cholangitis
and no presence of common bile duct obstruction [1, 51]. Urgent ERCP (within 24 h
of admission) might be favorable in patients with persistent cholestasis and is currently only indicated in patients with biliary pancreatitis and concurrent acute cholangitis [1, 52, 53]. It was hypothesized that ERCP combined with papillotomy
might also reduce the severity of biliary pancreatitis by reducing pressure in the
common bile duct [54]. The multicenter randomized APEC trial [55] demonstrated
that routine urgent ERCP with biliary papillotomy did not lower rates of mortality
or major complications in patients with predicted severe acute biliary pancreatitis
when compared to conservative treatment (38 vs. 44%). It therefore appears that
only patients with acute biliary pancreatitis and concurrent cholangitis benefit from
ERCP, especially in the first 24 h of admission.

Role of EUS and MRCP

Similar to ERCP, EUS and MRCP are not advised in patients with mild biliary pancreatitis without signs of common bile duct obstruction [1]. In case of uncertainty
regarding common bile duct obstruction in the absence of cholangitis, an EUS (or
MRCP) could detect gallstones in the common bile duct. A negative MRCP, however, does not reliably (sensitivity of 88%) rule out the presence of small stones (less
than 5 mm) in the common bile duct, which are known to cause acute biliary pancreatitis [56, 57]. If stones are visualized on EUS, an elective ERCP with papillotomy and stone extraction may be indicated to prevent new episodes of biliary
pancreatitis [58]. However, an ERCP with papillotomy does not prevent gallbladder
stones-related conditions such as cholecystitis and biliary colic [1, 59]. For that
reason, cholecystectomy after ERCP and papillotomy is recommended [1].

Timing of Cholecystectomy

In case of mild biliary pancreatitis, same-admission cholecystectomy is advised [1].
This advice emerged out of the multicenter randomized PONCHO trial [60], which
demonstrated that same-admission cholecystectomy safely reduces the risk of
recurrent gallstone-related complications and mortality when compared with a
delayed elective cholecystectomy (5 vs. 17%). In patients with necrotizing biliary
pancreatitis, cholecystectomy is advised if necrotic peripancreatic collections have
resolved or persist after 6 weeks [1, 61]. Before cholecystectomy, assessment of the
presence and location of peripancreatic collections should be performed [62].

Whether or not cholecystectomy can be performed safely obviously depends on the clinical condition of the patient, but also on the location of the persistent peripancreatic collections, which should be avoided in the surgical field of the cholecystectomy.

Prevention of Recurrence

Besides gallstones, alcohol and smoking are common risk factors for recurrence of acute pancreatitis [63]. Recurrence could be reduced by alcohol abstinence after the first episode of the acute alcoholic pancreatitis [64–66]. However, quitting excessive use of alcohol is widely known to be difficult. A single-center randomized trial from Finland reported that standardized follow-up with repeated intervention against alcohol consumption lowers the recurrence rate of acute alcoholic pancreatitis after 2 years compared to single standardized intervention alone during the initial hospitalization (8 vs. 21%) [66]. Currently, the multicenter randomized PANDA trial in the Netherlands is assessing the effect of an optimally timed personalized multidisciplinary alcohol cessation program on the recurrence rate in patients with acute alcoholic pancreatitis.

Approximately 20% of the etiology of acute pancreatitis in patients remains idiopathic [67, 68]. In these patients, it is advised to repeat the transabdominal ultrasound after discharge, as the accuracy of a second transabdominal ultrasound is higher than the first one [1, 69]. In 2015, a multicenter randomized trial from Finland reported that patients with idiopathic pancreatitis should undergo laparoscopic cholecystectomy [70]. However, in this study EUS was not used. The current advice is, in case of a negative repeat transabdominal ultrasound, to perform EUS to detect occult microlithiasis, as well as neoplasms and chronic pancreatitis [1, 71, 72]. If both transabdominal and EUS are negative, some experts advise (secretin-enhanced) MRCP to search for rare anatomical anomalies [1]. In case of recurrent attacks of idiopathic pancreatitis, genetic counseling should be considered [1]. The role of laparoscopic cholecystectomy in patients with "EUS-negative" idiopathic pancreatitis is currently unclear and being studied in the multicenter randomized PICUS-2 trial.

References

1. IAP/APA evidence-based guidelines for the management of acute pancreatitis. Pancreatology. 2013;13(4):e1–15.
2. Boxhoorn L, Voermans RP, Bouwense SA, Bruno MJ, Verdonk RC, Boermeester MA, et al. Acute pancreatitis. Lancet. 2020;396(10252):726–34.
3. Xiao AY, Tan MLY, Wu LM, Asrani VM, Windsor JA, Yadav D, et al. Global incidence and mortality of pancreatic diseases: a systematic review, meta-analysis, and meta-regression of population-based cohort studies. Lancet Gastroenterol Hepatol. 2016;1(1):45–55.

4. Banks PA, Bollen TL, Dervenis C, Gooszen HG, Johnson CD, Sarr MG, et al. Classification of acute pancreatitis—2012: revision of the Atlanta classification and definitions by international consensus. Gut. 2013;62(1):102–11.
5. Schepers NJ, Bakker OJ, Besselink MG, Ahmed Ali U, Bollen TL, Gooszen HG, et al. Impact of characteristics of organ failure and infected necrosis on mortality in necrotising pancreatitis. Gut. 2019;68(6):1044–51.
6. Bakker OJ, van Santvoort H, Besselink MGH, Boermeester MA, van Eijck C, Dejong K, et al. Extrapancreatic necrosis without pancreatic parenchymal necrosis: a separate entity in necrotising pancreatitis? Gut. 2013;62(10):1475–80.
7. van Santvoort HC, Bakker OJ, Bollen TL, Besselink MG, Ahmed Ali U, Schrijver AM, et al. A conservative and minimally invasive approach to necrotizing pancreatitis improves outcome. Gastroenterology. 2011;141(4):1254–63.
8. Petrov MS, Shanbhag S, Chakraborty M, Phillips ARJ, Windsor JA. Organ failure and infection of pancreatic necrosis as determinants of mortality in patients with acute pancreatitis. Gastroenterology. 2010;139(3):813–20.
9. Besselink MG, van Santvoort HC, Boermeester MA, Nieuweohuijs VB, van Goor H, Dejong CHC, et al. Timing and impact of infections in acute pancreatitis. Br J Surg. 2009;96(3):267–73.
10. Carnovale A, Rabitti P, Manes G, Esposito P, Pacelli L, Uomo G. Mortality in acute pancreatitis: is it an early or a late event. J Pancreas. 2005;6(5):438–44.
11. Bakker OJ, van Brunschot S, van Santvoort HC, Besselink MG, Bollen TL, Boermeester MA, et al. Early versus on-demand nasoenteric tube feeding in acute pancreatitis. N Engl J Med. 2014;371(21):1983–93.
12. Besselink MG, van Santvoort HC, Buskens E, Boermeester MA, van Goor H, Timmerman HM, et al. Probiotic prophylaxis in predicted severe acute pancreatitis: a randomised, double-blind, placebo-controlled trial. Lancet. 2008;371(9613):651–9.
13. de Vries AC, Besselink MGH, Buskens E, Ridwan BU, Schipper M, van Erpecum KJ, et al. Randomized controlled trials of antibiotic prophylaxis in severe acute pancreatitis: relationship between methodological quality and outcome. Pancreatology. 2007;7(5–6):531–8.
14. Moggia E, Koti R, Belgaumkar AP, Fazio F, Pereira SP, Davidson BR, et al. Pharmacological interventions for acute pancreatitis. Cochrane Database Syst Rev. 2017;2017(4).
15. Calder PC. n−3 Fatty acids, inflammation, and immunity— Relevance to postsurgical and critically III patients. Lipids. 2004;39(12):1147.
16. Calder PC. Marine omega-3 fatty acids and inflammatory processes: effects, mechanisms and clinical relevance. Biochim Biophys Acta. 2015;1851(4):469–84.
17. Wolbrink DRJ, Grundsell JR, Witteman B, van de Poll M, van Santvoort HC, Issa E, et al. Are omega-3 fatty acids safe and effective in acute pancreatitis or sepsis? A systematic review and meta-analysis. Clin Nutr. 2020;39(9):2686–94.
18. Al-Leswas D, Eltweri AM, Chung WY, Arshad A, Stephenson JA, Al-Taan O, et al. Intravenous omega-3 fatty acids are associated with better clinical outcome and less inflammation in patients with predicted severe acute pancreatitis: a randomised double blind controlled trial. Clin Nutr. 2020;39(9):2711–9.
19. Wu BU, Hwang JQ, Gardner TH, Repas K, Delee R, Yu S, et al. Lactated Ringer's solution reduces systemic inflammation compared with saline in patients with acute pancreatitis. Clin Gastroenterol Hepatol. 2011;9(8):710–717.e1.
20. de-Madaria E, Herrera-Marante I, González-Camacho V, Bonjoch L, Quesada-Vázquez N, Almenta-Saavedra I, et al. Fluid resuscitation with lactated Ringer's solution vs normal saline in acute pancreatitis: a triple-blind, randomized, controlled trial. United European Gastroenterol J. 2018;6(1):63.
21. Choosakul S, Harinwan K, Chirapongsathorn S, Opuchar K, Sanpajit T, Piyanirun W, et al. Comparison of normal saline versus Lactated Ringer's solution for fluid resuscitation in patients with mild acute pancreatitis, A randomized controlled trial. Pancreatology. 2018;18(5):507–12.

22. Iqbal U, Anwar H, Scribani M. Ringer's lactate versus normal saline in acute pancreatitis: a systematic review and meta-analysis. J Dig Dis. 2018;19(6):335–41.
23. Warndorf MG, Kurtzman JT, Bartel MJ, Cox M, Mackenzie T, Robinson S, et al. Early fluid resuscitation reduces morbidity among patients with acute pancreatitis. Clin Gastroenterol Hepatol. 2011;9(8):705–9.
24. Gukovsky I, Pandol SJ, Mareninova OA, Shalbueva N, Jia W, Gukovskaya AS. Impaired autophagy and organellar dysfunction in pancreatitis. J Gastroenterol Hepatol. 2012;27(Suppl 2):27.
25. Mao EQ, Fei J, Peng YB, Huang J, Tang YQ, Zhang SD. Rapid hemodilution is associated with increased sepsis and mortality among patients with severe acute pancreatitis. Chin Med J (Engl). 2010;123(13):1639–44.
26. Mao EQ, Tang YQ, Fei J, Qin S, Wu J, Li L, et al. Fluid therapy for severe acute pancreatitis in acute response stage. Chin Med J (Engl). 2009;122(2):169–73.
27. de-Madaria E, Buxbaum JL, Maisonneuve P, García García de Paredes A, Zapater P, Guilabert L, et al. Aggressive or moderate fluid resuscitation in acute pancreatitis. New Engl J Med. 2022;387(11):989–1000.
28. Jadad AR, Browman GP. The WHO analgesic ladder for cancer pain management: stepping up the quality of its evaluation. JAMA. 1995;274(23):1870–3.
29. Basurto Ona X, Rigau Comas D, Urrútia G. Opioids for acute pancreatitis pain. Cochrane Database Syst Rev. 2013;2013(7):CD009179.
30. Sadowski SM, Andres A, Morel P, Schiffer E, Frossard JL, Platon A, et al. Epidural anesthesia improves pancreatic perfusion and decreases the severity of acute pancreatitis. World J Gastroenterol. 2015;21(43):12448.
31. Jabaudon M, Belhadj-Tahar N, Rimmelé T, Joannes-Boyau O, Bulyez S, Lefrant JY, et al. Thoracic epidural analgesia and mortality in acute pancreatitis: a multicenter propensity analysis. Crit Care Med. 2018;46(3):E198–205.
32. Wu LM, Sankaran SJ, Plank LD, Windsor JA, Petrov MS. Meta-analysis of gut barrier dysfunction in patients with acute pancreatitis. Br J Surg. 2014;101(13):1644–56.
33. Capurso G, Zerboni G, Signoretti M, Valente R, Stigliano S, Piciucchi M, et al. Role of the gut barrier in acute pancreatitis. J Clin Gastroenterol. 2012;46(SUPPL. 1):S46–51.
34. Al-Omran M, AlBalawi ZH, Tashkandi MF, Al-Ansary LA. Enteral versus parenteral nutrition for acute pancreatitis. Cochrane Database Syst Rev. 2010;2010(1):CD002837.
35. Li W, Liu J, Zhao S, Li J. Safety and efficacy of total parenteral nutrition versus total enteral nutrition for patients with severe acute pancreatitis: a meta-analysis. J Int Med Res. 2018;46(9):3948.
36. Petrov MS, Td Correia I, Windsor JA. Nasogastric tube feeding in predicted severe acute pancreatitis. A systematic review of the literature to determine safety and tolerance. JOP. 2008;9(4):440–8.
37. Mowbray NG, Ben-Ismaeil B, Hammoda M, Shingler G, Al-Sarireh B. The microbiology of infected pancreatic necrosis. Hepatobiliary Pancreat Dis Int. 2018;17(5):456–60.
38. Wittau M, Mayer B, Scheele J, Henne-Bruns D, Dellinger EP, Isenmann R. Systematic review and meta-analysis of antibiotic prophylaxis in severe acute pancreatitis. Scand J Gastroenterol. 2011;46(3):261–70.
39. Lim CLL, Lee W, Liew YX, Tang SSL, Chlebicki MP, Kwa ALH. Role of antibiotic prophylaxis in necrotizing pancreatitis: a meta-analysis. J Gastrointest Surg. 2015;19(3):480–91.
40. Jiang K, Huang W, Yang XN, Xia Q. Present and future of prophylactic antibiotics for severe acute pancreatitis. World J Gastroenterol: WJG. 2012;18(3):279.
41. Villatoro E, Mulla M, Larvin M. Antibiotic therapy for prophylaxis against infection of pancreatic necrosis in acute pancreatitis. Cochrane Database Syst Rev. 2010;2010(5):CD002941.
42. Uchil RR, Kohli GS, Katekhaye VM, Swami OC. Strategies to combat antimicrobial resistance. J Clin Diagn Res. 2014;8(7):ME01.
43. Lee HS, Lee SK, Park DH, Lee SS, Seo DW, Kim MH, et al. Emergence of multidrug resistant infection in patients with severe acute pancreatitis. Pancreatology. 2014;14(6):450–3.

44. Baron TH, DiMaio CJ, Wang AY, Morgan KA. American gastroenterological asso-ciation clinical practice update: management of pancreatic necrosis. Gastroenterology. 2020;158(1):67–75.e1.
45. Tan J, McKenzie C, Potamitis M, Thorburn AN, Mackay CR, Macia L. The role of short-chain fatty acids in health and disease. Adv Immunol. 2014;121:91–119.
46. van den Berg FF, van Dalen D, Hyoju SK, van Santvoort HC, Besselink MG, Wiersinga WJ, et al. Western-type diet influences mortality from necrotising pancreatitis and demonstrates a central role for butyrate. Gut. 2021;70(5):915–27.
47. Haak BW, Wiersinga WJ. The role of the gut microbiota in sepsis. Lancet Gastroenterol Hepatol. 2017;2(2):135–43.
48. Roberts SE, Morrison-Rees S, John A, Williams JG, Brown TH, Samuel DG. The incidence and aetiology of acute pancreatitis across Europe. Pancreatology. 2017;17(2):155–65.
49. Tenner S, Baillie J, Dewitt J, Vege SS. American college of gastroenterology guideline: man-agement of acute pancreatitis. Am J Gastroenterol. 2013;108(9):1400–15.
50. Kimura Y, Takada T, Kawarada Y, Nimura Y, Hirata K, Sekimoto M, et al. Definitions, patho-physiology, and epidemiology of acute cholangitis and cholecystitis: Tokyo guidelines. J Hepatobiliary Pancreat Surg. 2007;14(1):15.
51. Tse F, Yuan Y. Early routine endoscopic retrograde cholangiopancreatography strategy versus early conservative management strategy in acute gallstone pancreatitis. Cochrane Database Syst Rev. 2012;(5):CD009779.
52. Arvanitakis M, Dumonceau JM, Albert J, Badaoui A, Bali MA, Barthet M, et al. Endoscopic management of acute necrotizing pancreatitis: European Society of Gastrointestinal Endoscopy (ESGE) evidence-based multidisciplinary guidelines. Endoscopy. 2018;50(5):524–46.
53. Fan ST, Lai E, Mok F, Lo CM, Zheng SS, Wong J. Early treatment of acute biliary pancreatitis by endoscopic papillotomy. New Engl J Med. 1993;328(4):228–32.
54. van Santvoort HC, Besselink MG, de Vries AC, Boermeester MA, Fischer K, Bollen TL, et al. Early endoscopic retrograde cholangiopancreatography in predicted severe acute biliary pan-creatitis: a prospective multicenter study. Ann Surg. 2009;250(1):68–75.
55. Schepers NJ, Hallensleben NDL, Besselink MG, Anten MPGF, Bollen TL, da Costa DW, et al. Urgent endoscopic retrograde cholangiopancreatography with sphincterotomy versus conservative treatment in predicted severe acute gallstone pancreatitis (APEC): a multicentre randomised controlled trial. Lancet. 2020;396(10245):167–76.
56. Kondo S, Isayama H, Akahane M, Toda N, Sasahira N, Nakai Y, et al. Detection of com-mon bile duct stones: comparison between endoscopic ultrasonography, magnetic reso-nance cholangiography, and helical-computed- tomographic cholangiography. Eur J Radiol. 2005;54(2):271–5.
57. Venneman N, Buskens E, Besselink M, Stads S, Go PM, Bosscha K, et al. Small gallstones are associated with increased risk of acute pancreatitis: potential benefits of prohylacctic cholecys-tectomy? Am J Gastroenterol. 2005;100(11):2540–50.
58. Bakker OJ, van Santvoort HC, Hagenaars JC, Besselink MG, Bollen TL, Gooszen HG, et al. Timing of cholecystectomy after mild biliary pancreatitis. Br J Surg. 2011;98(10):1446–54.
59. van Baal MC, Besselink MG, Bakker OJ, van Santvoort HC, Schaapherder AF, Nieuwenhuijs VB, et al. Timing of cholecystectomy after mild biliary pancreatitis: a systematic review. Ann Surg. 2012;255(5):860–6.
60. da Costa DW, Bouwense SA, Schepers NJ, Besselink MG, van Santvoort HC, van Brunschot S, et al. Same-admission versus interval cholecystectomy for mild gallstone pancreatitis (PONCHO): a multicentre randomised controlled trial. Lancet. 2015;386(10000):1261–8.
61. Nealon WH, Bawduniak J, Walser EM, Pitt HA, Behrns KE, Stain SC. Appropriate timing of cholecystectomy in patients who present with moderate to severe gallstone-associated acute pancreatitis with peripancreatic fluid collections. Ann Surg. 2004;239(6):741.
62. Hallensleben ND, Timmerhuis HC, Hollemans RA, Pocornie S, van Grinsven J, van Brunschot S, et al. Optimal timing of cholecystectomy after necrotising biliary pancreatitis. Gut. 2022;71(5):974–82.

63. Bertilsson S, Swärd P, Kalaitzakis E. Factors that affect disease progression after first attack of acute pancreatitis. Clin Gastroenterol Hepatol. 2015;13(9):1662–1669.e3.
64. Pelli H, Lappalainen-Lehto R, Piironen A, Sand J, Nordback I. Risk factors for recurrent acute alcohol-associated pancreatitis: a prospective analysis. Scand J Gastroenterol. 2009;43(5):614–21.
65. Nikkola J, Räty S, Laukkarinen J, Seppänen H, Lappalainen-Lehto R, Järvinen S, et al. Abstinence after first acute alcohol-associated pancreatitis protects against recurrent pancreatitis and minimizes the risk of pancreatic dysfunction. Alcohol Alcohol. 2013;48(4):483–6.
66. Nordback I, Pelli H, Lappalainen-Lehto R, Järvinen S, Räty S, Sand J. The recurrence of acute alcohol-associated pancreatitis can be reduced: a randomized controlled trial. Gastroenterology. 2009;136(3):848–55.
67. Párniczky A, Kui B, Szentesi A, Balázs A, Szűcs Á, Mosztbacher D, et al. Prospective, multicentre, nationwide clinical data from 600 cases of acute pancreatitis. PLoS One. 2016;11(10):e0165309.
68. Nesvaderani M, Eslick GD, Vagg D, Faraj S, Cox MR. Epidemiology, aetiology and outcomes of acute pancreatitis: a retrospective cohort study. Int J Surg. 2015;23:68–74.
69. Signoretti M, Baccini F, Piciucchi M, Iannicelli E, Valente R, Zerboni G, et al. Repeated transabdominal ultrasonography is a simple and accurate strategy to diagnose a biliary etiology of acute pancreatitis. Pancreas. 2014;43(7):1106–10.
70. Räty S, Pulkkinen J, Nordback I, Sand J, Victorzon M, Grönroos J, et al. Can laparoscopic cholecystectomy prevent recurrent idiopathic acute pancreatitis? Ann Surg. 2015;262(5):736–41.
71. Smith I, Ramesh J, Kyanam Kabir Baig KR, Mönkemüller K, Wilcox CM. Emerging role of endoscopic ultrasound in the diagnostic evaluation of idiopathic pancreatitis. Am J Med Sci. 2015;350(3):229–34.
72. Pereira R, Eslick G, Cox M. Endoscopic ultrasound for routine assessment in idiopathic acute pancreatitis. J Gastrointest Surg. 2019;23(8):1694–700.

Chapter 4
Acute Pancreatitis: Surgical Therapies

Osaid Alser, Kanak Das, and Edwin Onkendi

Introduction

According the 2012 Revised Atlanta Classification of Acute Pancreatitis (RACAP), acute pancreatitis is classified based on morphology and computed tomography findings, as interstitial edematous pancreatitis, where the pancreas shows localized or diffuse enlargement on computed tomography (CT) scans, and necrotizing pancreatitis where necrosis develops in the pancreatic parenchyma or in the peripancreatic tissues and appears as non-enhancement on contrast-enhanced CT scans. Acute pancreatitis is further classified based on severity as mild, moderately severe, and severe types [1]. These are:

(a) *Mild acute pancreatitis*, the most common form (estimated incidence is around 80%), has no associated organ failure, local or systemic complications, and usually resolves with no sequelae in the first week with medical management only [2, 3].
(b) *Moderately severe acute pancreatitis* (~15%) is defined as acute pancreatitis associated with the presence of transient organ failure, local complications or exacerbation of comorbid disease.
(c) *Severe acute pancreatitis* (SAP) (<5%) is defined as acute pancreatitis associated with persistent organ failure (>48 h).

Local complications as per the RACAP 2012 include the following four entities:

1. Acute peripancreatic fluid collection (APFC) occurring in the early phase of interstitial pancreatitis with no defined capsule (Fig. 4.1a).

O. Alser · K. Das · E. Onkendi (✉)
Texas Tech University Health Sciences Center, Lubbock, TX, USA
e-mail: Edwin.onkendi@ttuhsc.edu

© The Author(s), under exclusive license to Springer Nature Switzerland AG 2025
E. P. Ceppa et al. (eds.), *The SAGES Manual of Evolving Techniques in Pancreatic Surgery*, https://doi.org/10.1007/978-3-031-78409-5_4

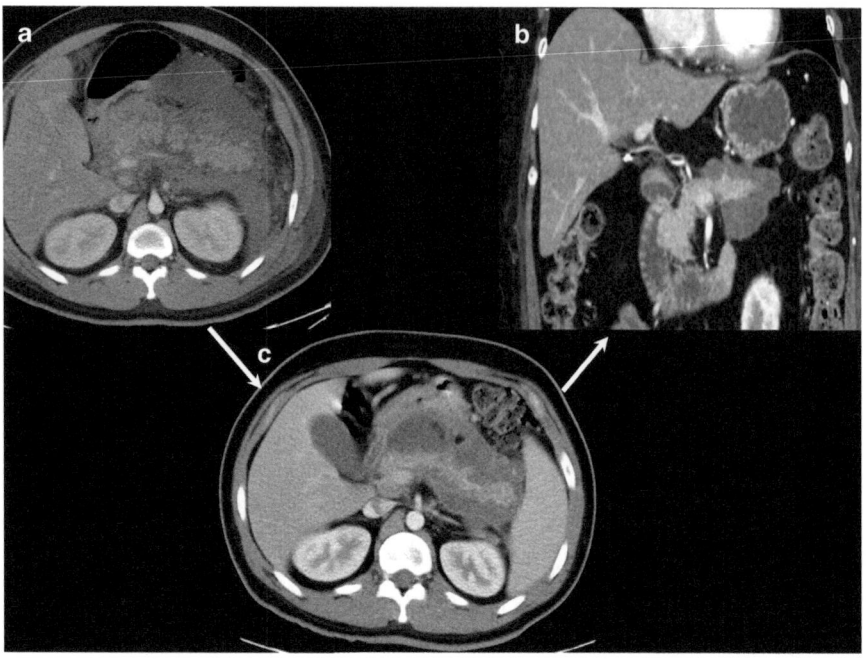

Fig. 4.1 Evolution of an acute peripancreatic fluid collection (APFC) with time. APFC appears as fluid that merges into surrounding peripancreatic, peritoneal, and retroperitoneal tissue plains without clear demarcation (**a**). The pancreas enhances with contrast suggesting maintained perfusion and viability. However, it is still difficult to rule out pancreatic necrosis until after the first week of onset of pancreatitis pain. The APFC evolves into a pseudocyst by developing a wall of granulation tissue 4 or more weeks later (**b**). Majority of APFCs and pseudocysts will resolve over time without intervention (**c**)

2. Pancreatic pseudocyst which is a chronic (usually 4 weeks or more) sequelae of APFC from interstitial pancreatitis that has developed encapsulation in the form of a well-defined wall formed from non-epithelialized granulation tissues (Figs. 4.1b, 4.1c, 4.2, and 4.3).
3. Acute necrotic collection (ANC) in the early phase before demarcation in necrotizing pancreatitis (Fig. 4.4a, b).
4. Walled-off pancreatic necrosis (WOPN), which represents a mature form of ANC where the necrosis is surrounded by a mature wall of granulation tissue between the necrosis and the surrounding tissues. This mature wall typically develops 4 weeks or more from the onset of pancreatitis (Fig. 4.4c, d) (Table 4.1) [4–6].

APFC and ANC are indistinguishable in the first week, usually appearing as homogenous enhancements on contrast-enhanced CT images [7]. Distinction between APFC and ANC becomes possible after the first week of onset once

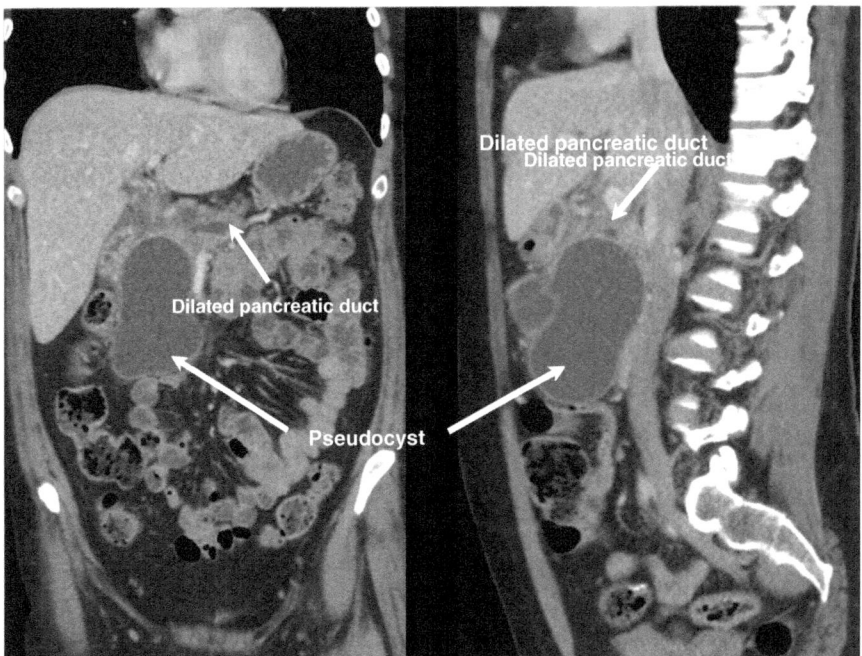

Fig. 4.2 Coronal and sagittal CT scan images showing a peripancreatic fluid collection 7 weeks after onset of pancreatitis. The fluid collection is extrapancreatic with pressure effects on the proximal pancreatic duct and the duodenum. The main pancreatic duct is dilated

necrosis becomes confluent and demarcated. The distinction between these two is important since APFC is usually self-limited, resolving spontaneously over time (Fig. 4.1), and therefore supportive measures alone usually sufficient [8, 9]. Since both pseudocyst and WOPN represent mature forms of acute pancreatitis complications, the distinction is usually easier than APFC and ANC. In contrast to a pseudocyst, WOPN contains necrotic pancreatic parenchyma or necrotic fat which appears as solid heterogeneous density within the walled-off cavity on imaging. The ability to differentiate between these pathologies is extremely important since it guides decision-making about their management. The majority of pancreatic fluid collections (acute and chronic) remains asymptomatic and resolve spontaneously over time, and therefore do not require any intervention. About 25% become symptomatic or infected, which necessitates intervention. Any of the above pancreatitis-related collections and complications can be sterile or secondarily infected (Fig. 4.5a–d). Collections that contain solid material are more likely to become infected (i.e., ANC and WOPN) [10]. Infection can be suggested by clinical criteria with signs and symptoms of sepsis as well as on contrast-enhanced CT images by the presence of gas bubbles, which are produced by gas-forming organisms, or from

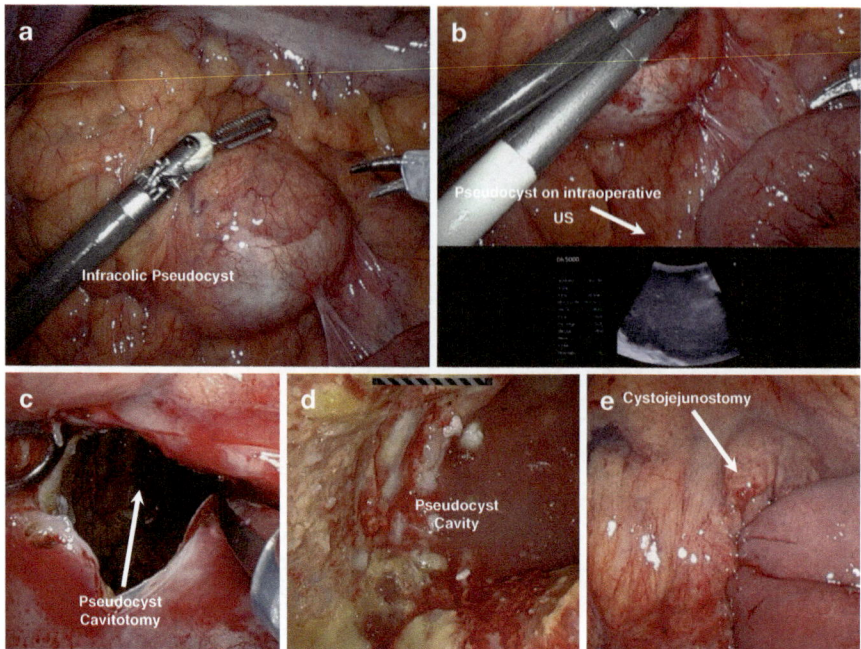

Fig. 4.3 Intraoperative photos showing the extrapancreatic infracolic pseudocyst (**a**). Intraoperative ultrasound shows no intracystic solid tissue (**b**), and this is confirmed by cystic drainage through a cavitotomy (**c**), with no solid debri found in the cyst cavity (**d**). A cystojejunostomy is then performed for internal drainage (**e**)

fistulization into the alimentary tract [11, 12]. Interestingly, SIRS can serve as an early predictor of acute pancreatitis severity and mortality. However, SIRS may result from the development of superimposed infection of pancreatic and/or peripancreatic collections [13, 14]. One must differentiate between pure pancreatitis-induced SIRS response and the development of superimposed infection on a pancreatic or peripancreatic collection, which can be difficult especially early in the course (the first 2 weeks from onset of pain) of acute pancreatitis. As we discuss below, the management of these complications requires a multidisciplinary team approach involving gastroenterologists, surgeons (including general surgeons and specialist acute care and hepatopancreatobiliary surgeons), interventional radiologists, infectious disease specialists, etc. The 2012 revised Atlanta classification is summarized in Table 4.1 below.

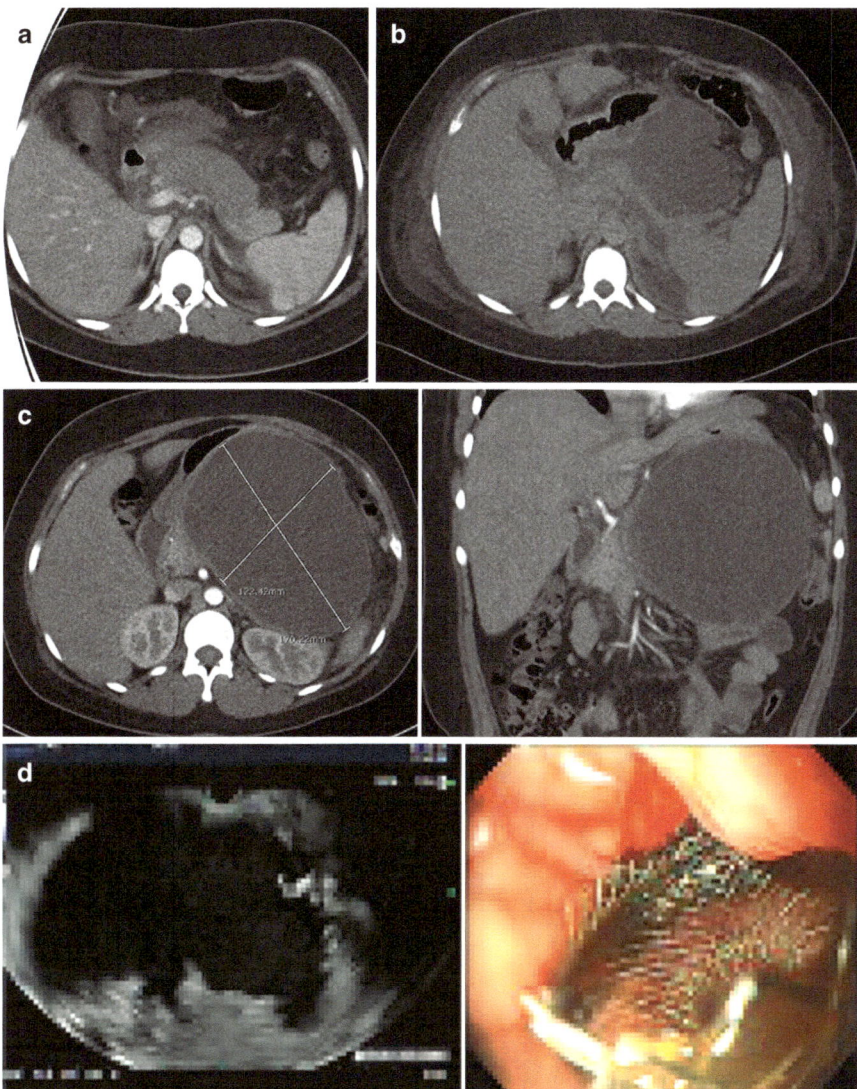

Fig. 4.4 (**a–d**) Evolution of pancreatic necrosis. Contrast-enhanced CT 2 weeks after onset of pancreatitis pain showing non-enhancement of the pancreatic body and tail due to confluent necrosis (**a**). This transforms into an acute necrotic collection 3 weeks after onset of pancreatitis pain (**b**). Patient was discharged asymptomatic. She returned 10 weeks after onset of pancreatitis pain, with abdominal pain, nausea, and emesis, and CT showed that the ANC had evolved into a predominantly intraabdominal, 17 cm walled-off pancreatic necrosis with local compressive features (**c**). This was misinterpreted as a pancreatic pseudocyst, and patient underwent endoscopic ultrasound (EUS)-guided cystogastrostomy (**d**). EUS, however, showed solid component (necrotic tissue) in the collection

Table 4.1 Types of acute pancreatitis and its complications. (Adapted from the 2012 Revised Atlanta Classification of Pancreatic and Peripancreatic Fluid Collections)

Types of acute pancreatitis	Acute peripancreatic collection (<4 weeks after onset of pain)	Chronic peripancreatic collection (≥4 weeks after onset of pain)
Interstitial edematous (85%)	**Acute peripancreatic fluid collection (APFC)** Homogenous fluid density No solid or necrotic tissue component Merges into the peripancreatic tissue planes with NO clear demarcated encapsulation No associated pancreatic necrosis No intra-pancreatic involvement	**Pancreatic pseudocyst** Homogenous fluid density A well-defined wall, pseudocapsule Fully encapsulated by a thick wall that demarcates it from surrounding tissue and structures Extra-pancreatic with no associated necrosis No solid tissue in the cavity
Necrotizing (10%)	**Acute necrotic collection (ANC)** Intra-pancreatic with pancreatic parenchymal necrosis and/or peripancreatic extension of necrosis Heterogeneous density, with solid component (necrosis) Not encapsulated yet and no demarcation from surrounding tissues and structures Can be sterile vs. infected	**Walled-off pancreatic necrosis (WOPN)** Intra-pancreatic with pancreatic parenchymal necrosis with/without peripancreatic extension of necrosis Heterogeneous density, with solid component (necrosis) A well-defined wall completely encapsulates the necrosis, separating it from the surrounding tissues and structures Can be sterile or infected

APFC acute peripancreatic fluid collection, *ANC* acute necrotic collection, *WON* walled-off necrosis

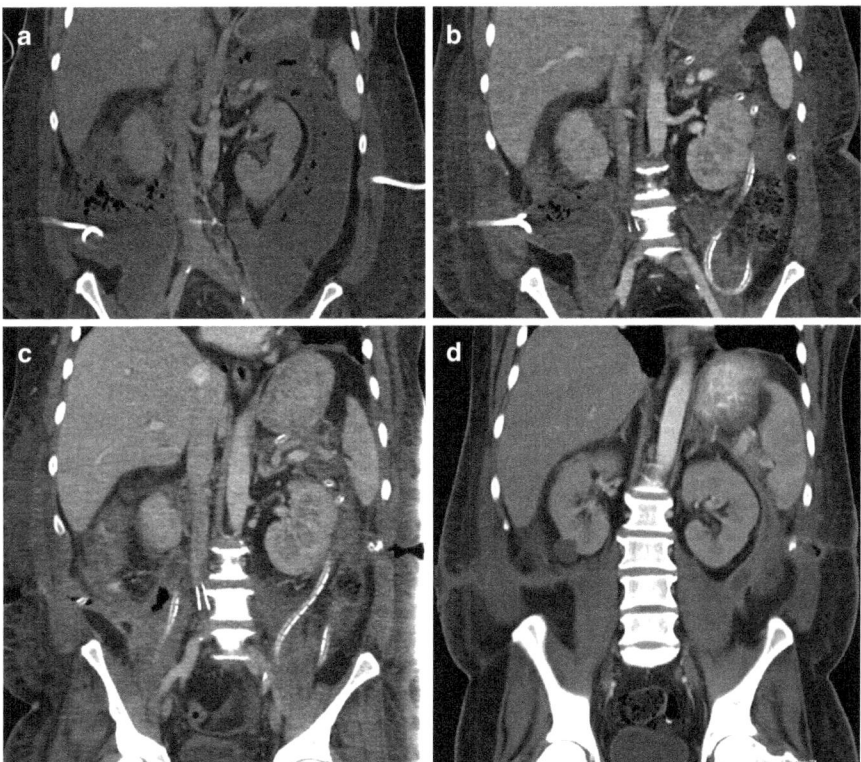

Fig. 4.5 (**a–d**) Coronal CT scan of the abdomen showing bilateral retroperitoneal walled-off necrosis 3 weeks after onset of pancreatitis, with associated fluid and air within the necrosis, suggesting infected necrosis (**a**). This patient had features of sepsis with recurrent fever, leukocytosis, and tachycardia. Bilateral retroperitoneal percutaneous drainage catheters were placed as part of a step-up approach to management. Patient was subsequently taken for a staged pneumoretroperitoneum-assisted VARD (PRA-VARD), starting with the left retroperitoneal infected necrosis as shown in image **b**. A surgical drain is indwelling post left PRA-VARD procedure (**b**). Following recovery from the left PRA-VARD procedure, the patient was taken back to the operating room for a right PRA-VARD procedure, and a surgical drain was placed (**c**). Patient was subsequently discharged 10 days later after drain removal. Follow-up 6 weeks postoperatively with CT showed complete resolution of the necrosis cavity (**d**)

Early Vs. Delayed Intervention for Acute Peripancreatic Collections

As mentioned above, 80% of patients with acute pancreatitis have mild acute pancreatitis that resolves within 1 week with basic supportive care [1, 15]. The remaining 20% develop moderately severe or SAP with associated organ dysfunction, SIRS, and associated pancreatic and peripancreatic fluid collections and necrosis. These patients with SAP are usually systemically ill due to the multi-system inflammatory response syndrome resulting from the severe pancreatitis [16, 17]. As a result, most of them are vulnerable to systemic decompensation from a second pathophysiologic insult that may come in the form of superimposed infection on pancreatic necrosis, acute bleeding from vascular erosion/pseudoaneurysm or operative intervention in the acute phase of SAP [16, 17].

As a result, a number of factors should be taken into account in managing these acutely ill patients in a multidisciplinary team approach to minimize or prevent patient deterioration [18]. Some of these factors include:

(a) The hemodynamic compromise and extent of organ and systemic compromise due to severe acute pancreatitis, if any
(b) Patient's associated comorbidities and suitability for general anesthesia
(c) Time since onset of acute pancreatitis pain
(d) Presence or absence of pancreatic necrosis
(e) Presence/absence of superimposed infection

The contribution of each of these factors to the decision-making on timing of intervention is described in more detail in the Table 4.2 below.

Table 4.2 The contribution of patient and pancreatitis factors to the decision-making on timing of intervention for the management of pancreatic and peripancreatic fluid collections and necrosis

Patient and pancreatitis factors	Description	Evaluation	Intervention timing recommendations
Type and age of pancreatic fluid collections associated with pancreatitis (from onset of pain)	Early (<2 weeks) PFCs are amorphous, poorly defined, and usually sterile. Patient ill with systemic and organ effects of acute pancreatitis Late (>4 weeks) in the course of pancreatitis, the patient has usually recovered for the SIRS response, any PFCs will have resolve, or walled-off and localize	CT with IV contrast, >1 week from onset of pain; look for associated necrosis CT with IV contrast. Delineates viable and non-viable pancreas and its relationship to PFCs. MRI with MRCP may be useful	Delay intervention to >4 weeks from onset of pain; allows patients to recover, and PFCs to spontaneously resolve or wall-off Most PFCs spontaneously resolve and/or are asymptomatic. Those that need intervention will have developed a mature wall for safer intervention

(continued)

Table 4.2 (continued)

Patient and pancreatitis factors	Description	Evaluation	Intervention timing recommendations
Pancreatic necrosis	Not usually detected in the first 7 days from the onset of pain Initially, necrosis is patchy. Necrosis evolves into demarcated confluent necrosis over time	CT with IV contrast: Initial patchy hypoattenuation in the early stages, then evolves into demarcated, confluent necrosis after the first week from onset of pain. Non-enhancement of the pancreas on contrast CT Pancreatic necrosis <40 Hounsfield units compared to normal pancreas (100–150 HU)	Early on, developing necrosis is patchy, amorphous, and sterile. Demarcates after the first 1–2 weeks from onset of pain Intervention if superimposed infection or local complications like pseudoaneurysm with bleeding, erosion of nearby structures with fistulization
Infection of pancreatic necrosis	A small proportion of pancreatic necrosis cases develop infected necrosis, >75% of infections occur >2 weeks from onset of pain; worse outcomes SIRS from sepsis difficult to distinguish in the first 2 weeks. Infection of necrosis must be confirmed before antibiotics treatment by positive blood culture or presence of gas on imaging After the first 14 days, clinical signs of infection suffice for diagnosing infected necrosis while having no other focus for infection	CT scan with/without contrast: Necrosis with pockets of air in it Air in necrosis can be due to gas-forming bacteria, fistulization to the alimentary tract, or instrumentation of the necrosis cavity Imaging with intraluminal contrast may help identify fistulization to alimentary tract Imaging guided aspiration of the necrosis cavity with cultures is the gold-standard to diagnosis of infected necrosis	Understanding the timing of development of necrosis is critical to decision-making on intervention. APFC, ANC, pseudocyst, and WOPN are often confused with each other, which is inappropriate management Review of imaging is necessary to differentiate these four and accurately diagnose each Intervention by drainage only for confirmed infection of necrosis; should follow the STEP-UP approach

(continued)

Table 4.2 (continued)

Patient and pancreatitis factors	Description	Evaluation	Intervention timing recommendations
Patient condition and comorbidities	Early in SAP, and due to severe pancreatitis, patients have profound SIRS sometimes with organ dysfunction Associated necrosis worsens the patient condition Superimposed infection causes further deterioration Patient's comorbidities can contribute to worse clinical outcomes Extent of hemodynamic, pulmonary, and organ compromise determines the prognosis	Early in the course of SAP, clinical presentation may be misinterpreted; profound SIRS response may cause high fevers, leukocytosis, and elevated inflammatory markers. Can be mistaken for infected necrosis when none is present Positive blood cultures will differentiate these two scenarios Organ specific work-up and invasive monitoring will guide management	Early intervention usually necessary in critically ill patients with infected pancreatic necrosis; STEP-UP approach protocol best Goal is to delay operative necrosectomy until at >4 weeks from onset of pain Use of empiric antibiotics without infected necrosis is discouraged

Sterile Pancreatic Necrosis

About 20–30% of acute pancreatitis cases develop pancreatic necrosis. This occurs as a result of several factors including pancreatic microcirculatory vasoconstriction, reduced microvascular inflow and outflow, microvascular stasis, and TNF-alpha-induced apoptosis and necrosis. All these initially lead to patchy areas of ischemia early in the course of pancreatitis. This patchy necrosis may subsequently progress to confluent pancreatic necrosis later on in the course of disease with clear demarcation between viable and necrotic tissue, which becomes apparent on imaging after the first week [19].

Pancreatic necrosis is often sterile, with no associated infection. However, a small subset of cases develops superimposed infection. Sterile pancreatic necrosis usually resolves spontaneously over time and rarely requires intervention. Sterile necrosis can, therefore, be followed without intervention once the patient recovers from acute pancreatitis and becomes asymptomatic.

Indications for intervention for sterile necrosis include persistent signs of systemic inflammatory response syndrome, persistent unresolving pain, obstructive/erosive complications involving the biliary or enteric tract by the necrosis, and general illness and unwellness after the acute pancreatitis (including inability to tolerate oral intake, nausea, emesis, generalized fatigue, persistent fevers, etc.). These patients' symptoms often recover once the necrosis is debrided and cleared.

Infected Pancreatic Necrosis and STEP-UP Approach to Management

Superimposed infection on pancreatic necrosis is associated with a 30–50% mortality rate and is virtually always an indication for intervention [18]. The diagnosis of infected necrosis depends on the timing since the onset of acute pancreatitis. This is because, in the first 14 days after onset of pain due to severe acute pancreatitis, it is difficult to distinguish SIRS response from sepsis [20, 21]. Therefore, in patients with suspected infection based on clinical signs of infection in the first 14 days but without gas in the necrotic collection in contrast-enhanced CT scan, proof of infection usually by positive blood culture or presence of gas on contrast-enhanced computed tomography imaging is needed. The presence of gas in the pancreatic/extra-pancreatic necrotic collection is an indicator of infection of the necrosis, irrespective of the source of the gas. This is because the gas in the necrotic collection is present either from gas-forming bacterial infection or loss of integrity of the bacteria-laden gastrointestinal tract that leads to bacterial contamination of the necrosis [20].

Based on the PANTER trial, after the first 14 days from onset of acute pancreatitis, clinical signs alone are much more reliable at diagnosis of infection of necrosis. Clinical criteria alone had a 91% accuracy in the diagnosis of infected necrosis. The clinical criteria include persistent organ failure in patients admitted to the intensive care unit or the persistence of two inflammatory variables (temperature $> 38.5\,^\circ$C or elevated C-reactive protein levels or leukocyte counts) during three consecutive days in patients in a regular hospital room [20, 21].

Historically, intervention for infected pancreatic necrosis involved open necrosectomy via a bilateral subcostal or midline incision, with debridement of the infected pancreatic necrosis, drainage of purulence, and placement of large bore drains for postoperative continuous lavage of the cavity. Feeding tube access is considered as well at the completion of the procedure. This was associated with high morbidity and mortality [20].

The optimal management strategies of infected pancreatic necrosis have evolved in the past two decades. The PANTER trial by van Santvoort et al. compared patients with infected pancreatic necrosis, who were randomized for open necrosectomy, or a minimally invasive step-up approach, which consisted of percutaneous drainage followed, if necessary, by minimally invasive retroperitoneal necrosectomy. The step-up approach had a reduced rate of the composite end point of major complications (new onset multi-organ failure or multiple systemic complications, perforation of viscus or enterocutaneous fistula or bleeding) of 40 vs. 69% (risk ratio with the step-up approach, 0.57; 95% confidence interval, 0.38–0.87; $P = 0.006$). However, the mortality rate did not differ significantly (19 vs. 16%, $P = 0.70$) [20]. This landmark study created a paradigm shift in the management of infected pancreatic necrosis (Fig. 4.7).

The key benefits of using this step-up approach include the following:

(a) **Necrosectomy may be avoided:** Percutaneous drainage may be all that is needed in some patients to address the infected necrosis. From the PANTER trial, 35% of patients were successfully managed by percutaneous catheter or endoscopic drainage alone, without need for necrosectomy. This is hypothesized to be due to the drainage of the liquid portion (pus) of the infected contents, which is pus-under-pressure, and therefore decreasing and resolving the pressurized translocation of the infected fluid and bacteria into the systemic circulation. Once the infected fluid is drained and pressure relieved, the semisolid and solid necrosis tissue can be left in situ to resolve over time in 35% of patients managed this way.

(b) **Avoid "second-hit" on vulnerable patients:** Percutaneous drainage allows for postponement of major operative necrosectomy to a later time in the course of disease. Therefore, a "second-hit" of pro-inflammatory systemic reaction is avoided on patients who are already critically ill and vulnerable earlier on in the course of severe acute pancreatitis, often with significant systemic effects from SAP, infected necrosis and associated organ dysfunction and failure. Use of a minimally invasive intervention decreases intervention-associated trauma and stirring of additional systemic inflammatory response. Based on the results of the PANTER trial, this is therefore associated with lower morbidity and mortality.

(c) **Viable-pancreas-parenchymal-sparing treatment:** Step-up approach allows for a viable-pancreas-parenchymal-sparing treatment at a time when clear demarcation of necrotic devitalized pancreatic tissue may not be complete early in the course of SAP, and some of the presumably necrotic pancreatic parenchyma may potentially recover. Allowing for preservation of the potentially recoverable pancreatic parenchyma likely explains the lower rates (7–17%) of long-term new onset of pancreatic insufficiency in patients managed by step-up approach in the PANTER trial. Conversely, early maximal necrosectomy leads to debridement and removal of potentially recoverable and viable pancreatic tissue and therefore is associated with higher rates (33–38%) of new onset of pancreatic insufficiency.

(d) **Minimize injury risk to critical structures:** Early in the course of pancreatic necrosis, the critical structures (splenic and mesenteric vessels, the alimentary tract and retroperitoneal structures are intermixed with, and "bathing" in the pancreatic necrosis collection, and the associated inflammation, with no demarcation between these critical structures and the pathological tissue. Intervention at this time risks injury to these structures with a higher morbidity and mortality. The postponement of operative necrosectomy to a later time (usually >4 weeks since onset of demarcated necrosis) allows for a mature thick wall to develop around the necrosis, forming a protective interface between the necrosis cavity contents and the critical structures outside of the cavity including major vessels, bowel and retroperitoneal structures (Fig. 4.6a, b). The clear demarcation by the mature thick wall allows for a safer debridement of the cavity with significantly decreased risk of injury to the surrounding structures.

Fig. 4.6 Intraoperative photos of the PRA-VARD procedure for patient in Fig. 4.5. The Alexis® wound retractor is inserted through the incision into the necrosis cavity (**a**), and a GelPort® laparoscopic system is used to achieve wide insufflation of the necrosis cavity and provides excellent visualization of the necrosis cavity (**b**) and allows for a technically easier and potentially safer necrosectomy

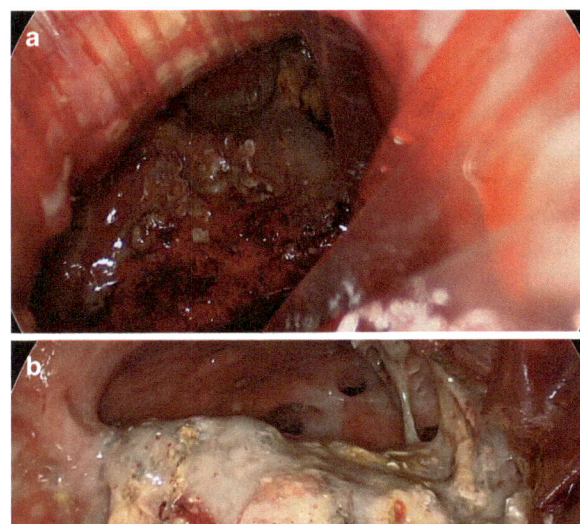

(e) **Allow for technically easier intervention later:** Delay in intervention allows the necrotic tissues to be organized into a localized walled-off cavity (as opposed to a widespread amorphous necrosis merging to nearby tissues), therefore allowing for a technically easier and safer necrosectomy.

Of the remaining 65% of patients who did not recover by percutaneous drainage alone in the PANTER trial, even if they required necrosectomy after percutaneous drainage, almost all (92%) of these patients were able to undergo a minimally invasive video-assisted retroperitoneal debridement (VARD) procedure. This indicates that step-up approach allows a minimally invasive intervention for the majority of patients with infected necrosis, and this represents a paradigm shift from the previous decade where open maximal necrosectomy was the standard approach [20].

The PENGUIN trial in 2012 by Bakker et al. soon followed PANTER trial to directly compare surgical necrosectomy with endoscopic trans-gastric necrosectomy, a form of natural orifice transluminal endoscopic surgery (NOTES), in 20 randomized patients. Endoscopic necrosectomy comprised of trans-gastric puncture, balloon dilatation, retroperitoneal drainage, and necrosectomy while surgical necrosectomy comprised of video-assisted retroperitoneal debridement (VARD) or, if not feasible, laparotomy. Post-processing pro-inflammatory response as measured by serum interleukin 6 (IL-6) levels was the primary end point while the composite end point of major complications as defined in PANTER trial or death was the secondary end point. When compared with surgical necrosectomy, endoscopic necrosectomy reduced post procedural IL-6 level ($p = 0.004$) and the composite clinical end point of death or major complications happened less frequently with endoscopic necrosectomy (20 vs. 80%, $p = 0.03$) [22].

In another study, van Brunschot et al. in 2017 conducted a multicenter randomized superiority trial (TENSION) in 98 patients with infected necrotizing pancreatitis comparing the endoscopic step-up approach with surgical step-up approach. The endoscopic approach comprised of endoscopic ultrasound-guided transluminal drainage followed, if needed, by endoscopic necrosectomy while the surgical step-up approach consisted of percutaneous catheter drainage followed, if necessary, by video-assisted retroperitoneal debridement. The primary end point was a composite of major complications as defined before or death during 6-month follow-up. The study showed that the endoscopic step-up approach was not superior to the surgical step-up approach as far as the primary end point was concerned ($p = 0.88$), but the rate of pancreatic fistulae formation and length of hospital stay were lower in the endoscopy group [23].

Based on information from the studies above, the current standard approach for infected pancreatic necrosis is the step-up approach defined by catheter drainage, followed, when necessary, by minimally invasive necrosectomy. In this approach, catheter drainage is typically postponed till 4 weeks following the onset of acute pancreatitis with necrosis to allow for the development of WOPN. Controversies exist whether earlier intervention for such patients could benefit the current step-up approach.

In the step-up approach, percutaneous drainage is often postponed until the infected necrosis cavity becomes encapsulated by a "mature" wall of granulation tissue (walled-off pancreatic necrosis, WOPN), a process that usually takes 4 weeks from onset of disease to complete. During this wait period, patients with infected necrosis are usually managed with intravenous antibiotics, while waiting for WOPN to develop. This may, in rare cases, lead to resolution of symptoms or reduce systemic illness, with the rationale being the postponement of invasive intervention until the WOPN stage allows for lower morbidity and mortality. In theory, there are a few downsides to this approach of delaying intervention until the WOPN stage, including prolonged hospital stay, early and prolonged use of empiric antibiotics contributes to the development of antibiotic resistance with increase in fungal infections, and increased healthcare costs. Furthermore, delaying intervention may be associated with clinical deterioration of the patient, and mortality. The recently published POINTER trial investigated if immediate (<24 h) catheter drainage in patients with acutely infected pancreatic necrosis is superior to the current standard of step-up approach. Boxhoom et al. in 2021 published the data on a total of 104 randomly assigned patients, indicating non-superiority of immediate drainage over postponed drainage (comprehensive complication index: $p = 0.90$; death: relative risk 1.25, 95% CI—0.42–3.68) while patients assigned to the postponed-drainage strategy needed fewer invasive interventions (catheter drainage and necrosectomy) with a mean number interventions of 4.4 vs. 2.6 [21, 24]. In summary, the key findings of the POINTER trial were:

(a) Patients in the postponed-drainage group required fewer interventions for infected necrosis.
(b) Antibiotic therapy was successful in 35% of patients in the postponed-drainage group, these patients were successfully treated conservatively with antibiotics only.
(c) There was no difference in complications and mortality between the immediate catheter drainage and postponed catheter drainage. As a result, immediate catheter drainage remains an option for patients who clinically deteriorate while on conservative treatment with antibiotics only.

Therefore, postponed catheter drainage is still the ideal option if the patient can tolerate delaying drainage intervention until the walled-off necrosis stage. However, if a patient clinically deteriorates despite appropriate antibiotic treatment during the waiting period, early catheter drainage can still be performed at any time.

The TENSION trial group published the 5–7 years follow-up data from the same trial (ex-TENSION) with similar end points. The trial revealed no difference in achieving the primary end point ($p = 0.688$) but fewer pancreatico-cutaneous fistulae occurred in patients assigned to endoscopy group (8 vs. 34%) and fewer re-interventions took place for endoscopy group than surgery group (7 vs. 24%) [25].

Typical indications for intervention (radiological, endoscopic, or surgical) in acute necrotizing pancreatitis include proven infected pancreatic and/or peripancreatic necrosis (IPN) [15, 26]. It may be indicated in clinically suspected IPN without any documented IPN but with ongoing organ failure or failure to thrive for several weeks after the onset of pancreatitis despite adequate medical management. A retrospective study on 164 such patients identified IPN in 42% of cases [26, 27]. Interventions in ANP may even be indicated in patients with organ compression including gastric outlet obstruction, biliary or intestinal obstruction, and pain relative to the mass effect from the large WON though secondary infection remains a major concern [26, 28, 29]. A less common scenario when intervention of ANP is needed is abdominal compartment syndrome which may require radiological or surgical decompression without exploration of lesser sac and performance of the necrosectomy at the same session to avoid bleeding and microbial inoculation into sterile necrosis [26, 30, 31].

Detailed Management of Infected Necrosis

Antibiotic Therapy

- For clinically suspected or documented infection as defined above, appropriate targeted antibiotics must be initiated. According to the POINTER trial, up to 35% of these patients may recover with intravenous antibiotics alone. Patients who clinically respond need no further intervention as long as they proceed to recover. For non-responders or patients with infected necrosis who clinically deteriorate while on antibiotics, management should follow the step-up approach with the next step being catheter drainage. With the latest advancement in minimally invasive techniques, open necrosectomy is no longer the first-line approach to management of infected pancreatic necrosis. Minimally invasive techniques include image-guided catheter drainage, endoscopic ultrasound-guided transgastric/transduodenal drainage and necrosectomy, and laparoscopic/robotic drainage and debridement [18].

Catheter Drainage

- Percutaneous or endoscopic catheter drainage is a key modality in the step-up approach to management of patients with infected necrosis, and in up to 35%, it is the only intervention needed and averts the need for subsequent necrosectomy. Furthermore, catheter drainage may be useful in stabilizing infected necrosis patients during the waiting period prior to the WOPN stage when they will then undergo operative necrosectomy. The step-up approach is summarized in Fig. 4.7a below and Fig. 4.5a–d [20].

Although the POINTER trial did not show superiority of immediate catheter drainage over postponed catheter drainage, there was no difference in complication rates or mortality between these two approaches. Therefore, immediate catheter drainage is a good option for patients with infected necrosis in case of acute deterioration at any time during the wait period to WOPN.

Catheter drainage is usually performed percutaneously under image-guidance (ultrasound or CT) by interventional radiology team, and sometimes by the surgical team. Catheter drainage is considered successful when there is full patient recovery after catheter drainage of the "pus under pressure" while the solid necrosis tissue is left in situ. In these cases, the solid infected necrosis does not need to be subsequently removed in at least 35% of infected necrosis cases.

According to the PANTER trial protocol, additional drainage catheters can be placed or existing drain(s) repositioned/re-adjusted if needed in the first 3–6 days after initial catheter placement, to achieve optimal and complete drainage of the "pus under pressure" (Fig. 4.7b). In patients managed by this protocol in the PANTER trial, sepsis was able to be resolved in 62–84% of cases, therefore allowing for postponement of definitive necrosectomy until mature walled-off necrosis stage when a safer and technically easier necrosectomy could be performed.

In the remaining 65% of cases of infected necrosis with unsuccessful catheter drainage, percutaneous catheter drainage serves as a bridge during the wait period to subsequent definitive operative necrosectomy at the WOPN stage.

Pre-procedure Preparation Pearls for Catheter Drainage
- A thorough review of the patient's preoperative imaging is critical to inform the intervention, including the anatomy around the infected necrosis cavity. Percutaneous catheter drainage relies on availability of a safe "window" devoid

of critical structures along the path of the catheter from the skin puncture site to the necrosis cavity. At a minimum, CT scan with intravenous contrast is needed to provide detailed information of the necrosis cavity and its relationship to surrounding structures.

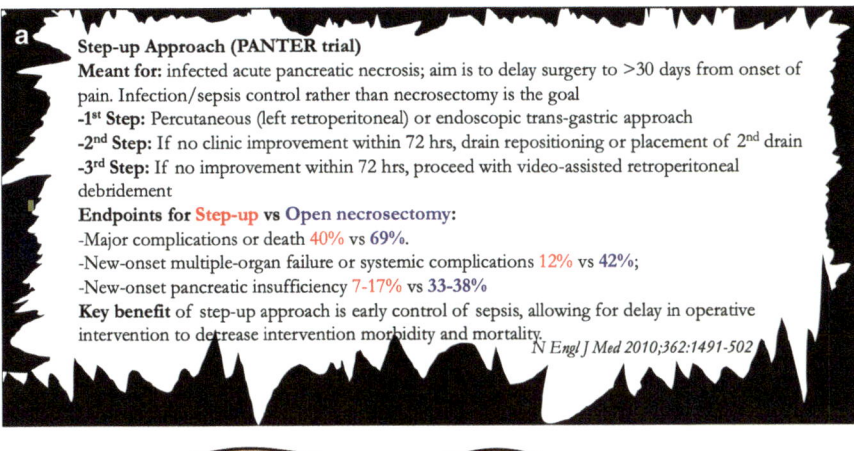

a   Step-up Approach (PANTER trial)
Meant for: infected acute pancreatic necrosis; aim is to delay surgery to >30 days from onset of pain. Infection/sepsis control rather than necrosectomy is the goal
-1st Step: Percutaneous (left retroperitoneal) or endoscopic trans-gastric approach
-2nd Step: If no clinic improvement within 72 hrs, drain repositioning or placement of 2nd drain
-3rd Step: If no improvement within 72 hrs, proceed with video-assisted retroperitoneal debridement
Endpoints for Step-up vs Open necrosectomy:
-Major complications or death 40% vs 69%.
-New-onset multiple-organ failure or systemic complications 12% vs 42%;
-New-onset pancreatic insufficiency 7-17% vs 33-38%
Key benefit of step-up approach is early control of sepsis, allowing for delay in operative intervention to decrease intervention morbidity and mortality.
N Engl J Med 2010;362:1491-502

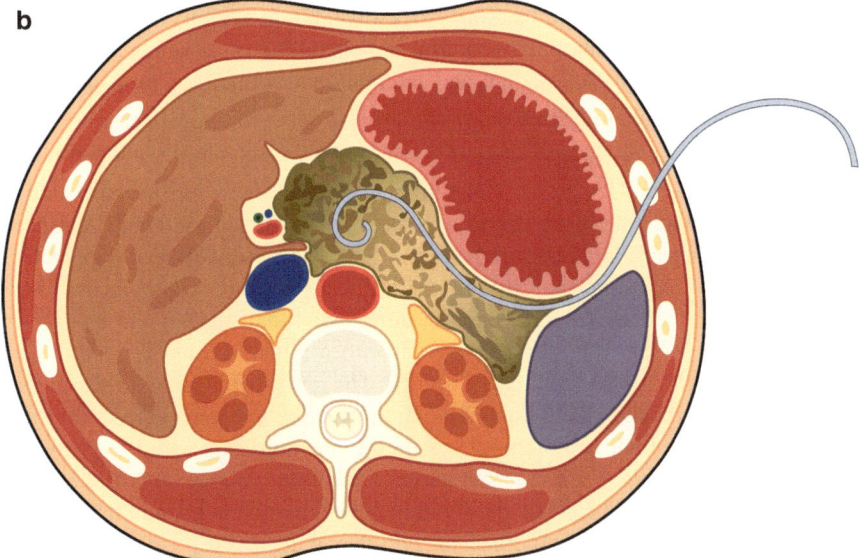

Fig. 4.7 (**a**) Summary of the step-up approach (PANTER trial) for management of infected acute pancreatic necrosis. (**b**) Axial abdominal schematic showing a large, retroperitoneal peripancreatic walled-off cavity filled with necrotic debris. A percutaneous drain is placed in this retroperitoneal cavity. (**c**) Pneumoretroperitoneum-assisted VARD (PRA-VARD) procedure: (*A*) An incision is made around the percutaneous drain leading into the necrotic peripancreatic cavity. (*B*) A gel port is placed into this incision with two 5 mm trocars and one 12 mm trocar. (*C*) The cavity is insufflated and a laparoscope, a grasper, and a suction irrigator are used to clear the necrotic debris

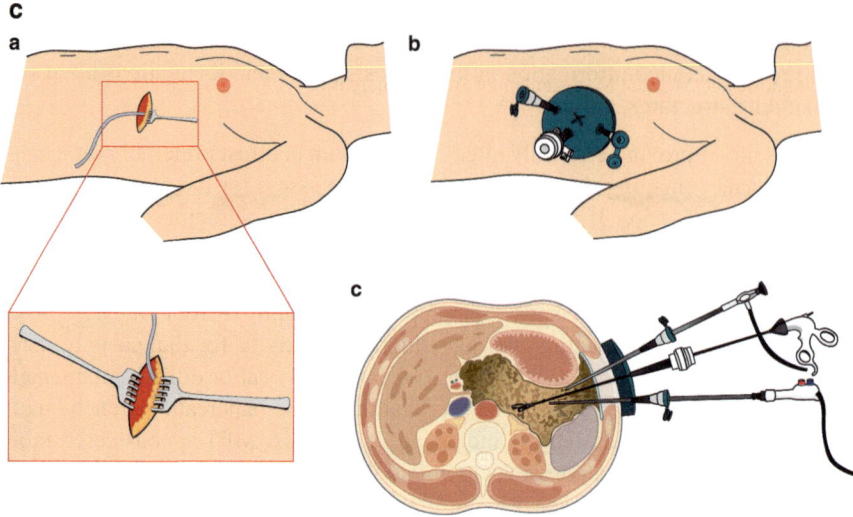

Fig. 4.7 (continued)

- If feasible, anticoagulation should be held prior to the procedure to allow for sufficient time for anticoagulation effects to resolve. If urgent intervention is needed, reversal of anticoagulation may be utilized depending on the anticoagulation in question. Patient's platelet count and international normalized ratio should be checked prior to the procedure.

Catheter Drainage Procedure Steps
- Following imaging review, a choice of the route of approach to the cavity is made. Almost all pancreatic necrosis collections can be accessed via a retroperitoneal or transperitoneal approach (Fig. 4.7b). The retroperitoneal approach is preferred and recommended (usually the left retroperitoneal route) due to lower risk of complications (by avoiding the intra-abdominal organs) and its ease of subsequently being able to be converted into a video-assisted retroperitoneal necrosectomy (VARD) procedure if needed. The retroperitoneal route also avoids intraperitoneal contamination with infection from the infected necrosis cavity.
- Patient is sedated under monitored anesthesia in conjunction with local anesthesia. If needed, general endotracheal intubation anesthesia may be utilized.
- Patient is positioned based on the route of access to the cavity, and this may be supine for transperitoneal approach or right lateral decubitus position for the left retroperitoneal approach. A limited ultrasound or CT imaging may be performed to ensure the route chosen is still appropriate after patient positioning since the anatomy may be altered by positional shifts of intra-abdominal organs.
- Choice of catheter size: A minimum catheter size of at least 12 French is recommended based on the PANTER trial. Catheter can be upsized up to a 24 French catheter if needed.

- Under imaging guidance, the cavity is accessed by a large bore needle puncture and a guidewire passed into it.
- Using the Seldinger technique, over the guidewire subcutaneous dilation is performed to create a wide tract from the skin puncture site to the cavity. Serial dilation is performed until the diameter of the chosen catheter is reached.
- The chosen catheter is then passed over the guidewire, through the dilated tract and into the infected necrosis cavity and correct positioning in the cavity is confirmed by drainage of the infected pus and imaging confirmation.
- An attempt should always be made to drain most of the infected fluid during the procedure by aspiration.
- Drainage catheter is then secured in place with 2–0 Nylon or Prolene suture.
- Post-procedure, the catheter should be flushed regularly 3–4 times daily to avoid clogging.
- Drainage catheter upsizing and/or placement of additional drains may be necessary for adequate drainage of infected necrosis.
- Drain evaluation via contrast injection (drain sinogram) or CECT are used as needed to optimize the location and function of the drain.

Percutaneous Catheter Drainage Pitfalls
- Formation of pancreatico-cutaneous or pancreatico-entero-cutaneous fistula in approximately 20% of cases. Pancreatico-cutaneous fistula forms when there is main ductal communication with the infected necrosis cavity. As a result of this internal "pancreatico-cavity" fistula, there is drainage of pancreatic ductal fluid into the cavity. Percutaneous catheter placement converts this internal fistula into a pancreatico-cutaneous fistula. This also applies to cases of internal fistula between the alimentary tract and the necrosis cavity. These pancreatico-cutaneous or pancreatico-entero-cutaneous fistulae can usually be managed nonoperatively with prolonged drainage.
- Catheter dislodgement.
- Bowel perforation.
- Vascular injury with acute bleeding.
- Pneumothorax.
- Introduction of infection into the pleural cavity if the catheter traverses the lower pleural cavity. This may lead to infected pleural effusion/abscess.

Video-Assisted Retroperitoneal Drainage (VARD) Procedure

As mentioned above, catheter drainage is usually successful in 35–50% of cases of infected pancreatic necrosis and no additional necrosectomy is needed. If percutaneous catheter drainage is not successful in resolving sepsis or if symptoms arising from infected necrosis persist, a VARD procedure will be the next option in the step-up approach to management.

Pre-procedure and Preparation Pearls for VARD Procedure
- VARD procedure should always be preceded by percutaneous catheter drainage, per the PANTER trial protocol. In preparation for VARD procedure, these patients should be evaluated to ensure the percutaneous catheter drainage has failed, despite catheter optimization, prior to proceeding with VARD procedure.
- Most VARD procedures will be done after preceding left retroperitoneal catheter drainage. However, some patients may have bilateral retroperitoneal catheters if they have bilateral retroperitoneal extensions of the infected necrosis cavity. In these cases of bilateral catheters, a pre-VARD procedure evaluation should be done to determine if the patient can tolerate bilateral VARD procedures under the same general anesthetic or if the VARD procedure should be staged by doing a unilateral VARD first, followed by a later subsequent contralateral VARD procedure once the patient has recovered.
- A thorough review of updated imaging should be done to ensure the necrosis cavity has developed a mature wall around it to facilitate a safe necrosectomy.
- Standard VARD procedure is done using an open incision around the drainage catheter entry site into the cavity and then a laparoscope is passed through this into the cavity for visualization and graspers are used to perform necrosectomy.
- Below we will also describe our technique of pneumo-retroperitoneum-assisted VARD procedure (PRA-VARD).

Standard VARD Procedure Steps
- The VARD procedure is done under general anesthesia.
- For unilateral VARD procedure, usually the left side, the patient is positioned in a right lateral decubitus position.
- A flank incision is made on either side of the drain exit site.
- The drain is used as a guide to extend the incision deeper all the way into the necrosis cavity, with entry into the cavity confirmed by immediate release of purulent, often foul-smelling fluid. The fluid portion of the cavity contents is suctioned out.
- Any visible loose infected necrosis tissue is sequentially removed using grasping forceps until cleared.
- A 0° videoscope is then introduced into the necrosis cavity and used to guide further necrosectomy under direct visualization.
- Laparoscopic grasping instruments are used alongside the scope, to sequentially remove any loose and loosely adherent necrosis tissues from the cavity.
- Any firmly adherent tissue should be left in place to avoid debridement of viable tissue and avoid significant bleeding.
- Once debridement of loose necrosis tissue is completed, a cavity lavage with saline is performed and existing percutaneous drainage catheters are removed.
- At least two large bore (usually 19 French) surgical drains are placed into the cavity. Postoperative lavage may be performed through these drains.
- Drains are secured and the muscle layers and fasciae are approximated to close the necrosectomy incision.

- Given the contaminated field and incision site, the skin of the incision is left open for wet-to-dry dressing change.
- If bilateral VARD procedure is to be performed at the same time, the patient is repositioned with the left lateral decubitus position and a similar procedure is performed on the contralateral side. However, if the patient cannot tolerate bilateral VARD, the contralateral side is deferred for later.

Pneumo-Retroperitoneum-Assisted VARD (PRA-VARD) Procedure Steps (Figs. 4.6 and 4.7c).

- Procedure is done under general anesthesia. Initial steps are similar to standard VARD procedure.
- For unilateral VARD procedure, usually the left side, the patient is positioned in a right lateral decubitus position. The modifications of the VARD procedure into PRA-VARD procedure include the following steps:
- A flank incision measuring at least 6–7.5 cm is made on either side of the drain exit site (Fig. 4.7c, part A).
- The drain is used as a guide to extend the incision deeper all the way into the necrosis cavity, with entry into the cavity confirmed by immediate release of purulent, often foul-smelling fluid. The fluid portion of the cavity contents is suctioned out. The percutaneous drain is removed.
- A single incision laparoscopic device with wound protection device and cap to allow for multiport placement is then used to establish pneumo-retroperitoneum. The green ring of the small- or medium-sized wound retractor is inserted through the incision and deployed into the necrosis cavity. The white ring is then rolled inwards until the wound is fully retracted (Fig. 4.7c, part B).
- The wound protection device is then placed over the white ring and locked in place.
- One 12 mm, and two 5 mm balloon laparoscopic trocars are placed through the cap and insufflation is connected to establish pneumo-retroperitoneum.
- A 30° laparoscopic is then used to visualize the interior of the cavity and guide the necrosectomy.
- Laparoscopic grasping instruments are used to sequentially remove any loose and loosely adherent necrosis tissues from the cavity (Fig. 4.7c, part C).
- Any firmly adherent tissue should be left in place to avoid debridement of viable tissue and avoid significant bleeding.
- Once debridement of loose necrosis tissue is completed, a cavity lavage with saline is performed with laparoscopic suction irrigation.
- The cap, trocars, and wound protector are removed and large bore surgical drains are placed into the cavity.
- Drains are secured and the muscle layers and fasciae are approximated to close the necrosectomy incision.
- Given the contaminated field and incision site, the skin of the incision is left open for wet-to-dry dressing change.

- If bilateral PRA-VARD procedure is to be performed at the same time, the patient is repositioned with the left lateral decubitus position and a similar procedure is performed on the contralateral side. However, if a patient cannot tolerate bilateral PRA-VARD procedure, the other size is deferred for later.

Advantages of PRA-VARD procedure over the standard VARD procedure include:

- Closed space pneumo-retroperitoneum insufflation allows for a wider space-creation in the necrosis cavity, providing excellent visualization to ensure a more thorough, non-blind and potentially safer necrosectomy compared to standard VARD where such insufflation cannot be achieved (Fig. 4.6b).
- The GelPort® system allows placement of three trocars in a triangulating fashion to allow for an easier procedure with less instrument collision.

Pitfalls of VARD and PRA-VARD Procedures
- Pancreatico-cutaneous fistula
- Bowel perforation with enterocutaneous fistula
- Vascular injury to surrounding mesenteric vessels with acute intraop- or postoperative major bleeding
- Wound dehiscence and complications

Sinus Tract Necrosectomy

This was originally described by Carter et al. [32]. It is a form of minimally invasive necrosectomy that is akin to the standard VARD procedure but differs from the latter in the way the necrosis cavity is accessed.

Pre-procedure preparation is similar to VARD procedure as described above.

Sinus Tract Necrosectomy Procedure Steps
- Image-guided percutaneous catheter placement to the infected necrosis always precedes sinus tract necrosectomy.
- The drainage catheter tract is then serially dilated with increasing size of catheters until a 30 French catheter size is reached (10 mm diameter tract).
- A nephroscope is then used through this tract to enter the infected necrosis cavity and provide visualization for necrosectomy.
- Grasping laparoscopic instruments are then used to remove loose and loosely adherent necrotic tissues.
- Large bore surgical drain (s) is placed into the cavity for post-procedure lavage.
- Compared to standard VARD or PRA-VARD procedures, a limited extent of necrosectomy is achieved by a single sinus tract necrosectomy and usually multiple (3–6) sinus tract necrosectomy procedures are needed.
- If complete or adequate necrosectomy cannot be achieved, sinus tract necrosectomy can be converted to a standard VARD or PRA-VARD procedure.

Pitfalls of Sinus Tract Necrosectomy
- Pancreatico-cutaneous fistula
- Bowel perforation with enterocutaneous fistula
- Vascular injury to surrounding mesenteric vessels with acute intraop- or postoperative major bleeding
- Wound complications

Minimally Invasive (Laparoscopic and Robotic) Trans-Abdominal Necrosectomy

As discussed above, the retroperitoneal approach is the preferred approach to necrosectomy whenever feasible. However, in some cases, the location of the infected necrotizing pancreatitis cavity makes a retroperitoneal approach impractical and not feasible.

A trans-abdominal approach is the best option for infected necrosis cavities that are predominantly located in or extending to the anterior peritoneal cavity, with associated lateral and posterior displacement of the alimentary tract and other intra-abdominal organs (Figs. 4.4c and 4.8a–c). Given the origin of the necrosis in the lesser sac, the stomach is usually displaced anteriorly and cephalad while the transverse colon and transverse duodenum may be displaced caudad. In these cases, the retroperitoneal organs (kidneys, spleen, adrenals, etc.) remain in their usual location or may be laterally displaced.

As a result, a trans-abdominal approach provides the easiest access to the cavity. Transperitoneal necrosectomy can be accomplished by open, laparoscopic or robotic approach, depending on the available resources and surgeon's expertise and skills.

Our approach is a minimally invasive approach, with robotic trans-abdominal necrosectomy.

Pre-procedure Preparation Pearls for Minimally Invasive (Robotic/ Laparoscopic) Trans-Abdominal Necrosectomy Procedure
- Assess the patient's condition and the ability to tolerate general anesthesia and operative necrosectomy.
- A thorough review of updated imaging should be done to ensure the necrosis cavity has developed a mature wall around it to facilitate a safe necrosectomy.
- The relationship between the necrosis cavity and the stomach, transverse colon, duodenum, and small bowel should be reviewed to guide the approach to necrosectomy.

Robotic Necrosectomy Procedure Steps
- Since most of these infected necrosis collections are in the midline abdomen, the patient is positioned supine.

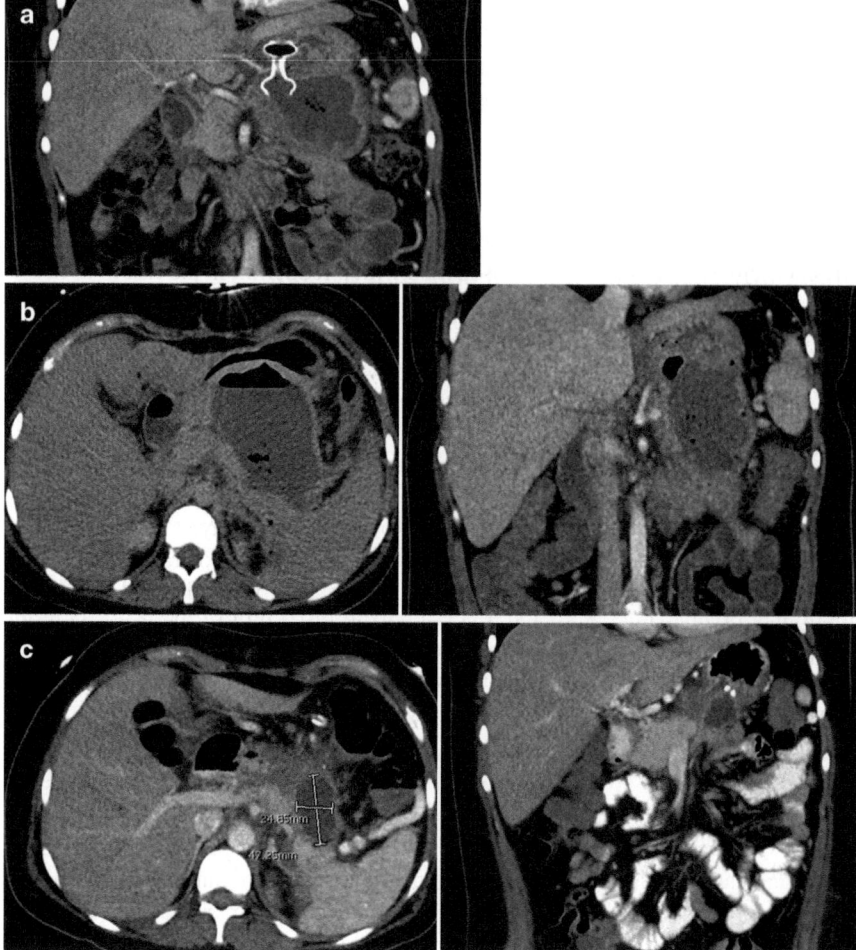

Fig. 4.8 The endoscopic cystogastrostomy stent is shown on CT done 2 weeks following EUS-guided cystogastrostomy procedure, showing incomplete drainage the cavity due to residual solid necrosis tissue (**a**). The stent was removed without endoscopic necrosectomy, and patient was discharged. The patient returned 3 weeks later with infected necrosis with sepsis, nausea, and emesis, with CT showing necrosis with air pockets (**b**). Patient underwent trans-abdominal robotic necrosectomy with cystogastrostomy. Postoperative day 7 CT showed near-complete resolution of the cavity (**c**)

- Trocar placement is variable depending on the location of the cavity and patient habitus; generally, a mid or lower abdominal placement is feasible, with four robotic trocars and a 12 mm assistant trocar placed in a transverse line across the abdomen. Placement should be such that access to the furthest extent of the cavity (usually the lesser sac region) can be reached.

- For large lesser sac collections displacing the stomach anteriorly, access to the cavity can be reached through the lesser sac or through a trans-gastric route.
- We often use a lesser sac approach through the gastrocolic ligament. The gastrocolic ligament is divided with an energy device. This is usually thickened and foreshortened due to peripancreatitis.
- Intraoperative ultrasound is performed to localize the infected necrosis cavity and guide the choice of the best site for a subsequent "cavitotomy."
- The cavitotomy should be created next to the posterior wall of the greater curvature of the stomach. Once the ideal site for a cavitotomy is chosen, the posterior wall of the stomach is exposed adjacent to the site chosen for cavitotomy.
- A cavitotomy is made with electrocautery hook/scissors or ultrasonic energy device and the infected pus is suctioned out of the necrosis cavity by the bedside assistant.
- A gastrotomy is made adjacent to the cavitotomy and an endoscopic stapler is used to create a large (preferably 60 mm) cystogastrostomy.
- Robotic graspers are used to remove loosely adherent necrosis tissue from the cavity, which is collected and contained on a sponge.
- Once necrosectomy is completed, the cavity is irrigated and the robotic camera may be used to visualize the interior of the cavity to confirm complete necrosectomy, drainage of pus, and hemostasis.
- The common cysto-gastric opening is then closed with a 3–0 barbed absorbable suture to complete the cystogastrostomy.
- If the necrosis cavity is not adjacent to the gastric wall to allow for cystogastrostomy, a cystojejunostomy can be performed if it is adjacent to the jejunum, similar to Fig. 4.3.
- If the necrosis cavity is not adjacent to the alimentary tract to allow for a cystogastrostomy or cystoenteric anastomosis, the debrided and drained cavity can be plugged with vascularized omentum and a surgical drain placed in it.
- The laparoscopic approach follows the same steps as the robotic approach detailed above. The difference lies in the trocar placement which should be chosen to allow for adequate triangulation and access.
- A minimally invasive trans-gastric approach to necrosectomy may also be used where the stomach is displaced anteriorly and therefore covers the anterior surface of the cavity. In this case, after ultrasound is performed to confirm posterior location of the cavity, an anterior gastrotomy is made with an ultrasonic energy device.
- Ultrasound is then used over the posterior gastric wall to ensure absence of significant vasculature posterior to the posterior gastric wall and apposition of the posterior gastric wall and the cavity wall.
- The necrosis cavity is accessed through a posterior gastrotomy and a stapled cystogastrostomy is created.
- Necrosectomy is then completed as the cavity is managed as detailed above.
- The anterior gastrostomy is then closed with a stapler or suture closure.

Minimally Invasive Necrosectomy Procedure Pitfalls
- Gastrocutaneous fistula
- Pancreatico-cutaneous fistula
- Gastroduodenal or splenic artery injury/pseudoaneurysm with subsequent gastrointestinal or intra-abdominal bleeding
- Colon or small bowel injury and fistula
- Wound complications including infection and dehiscence

Open Necrosectomy

Open necrosectomy had been the only procedure for infected necrosis for several decades. However, due to the high morbidity (up to 95%) and high mortality rates (10–40%) [20], as well as the dramatic evolution of percutaneous, endoscopic, and minimally invasive drainage techniques, it is reserved for cases that are not amenable to, or who do not respond to these other interventions. These contemporary approaches are associated with better outcomes and are now considered first for management of necrosectomy if feasible and resources allow, prior to considering open necrosectomy.

Open Necrosectomy Procedure Details
- A supine position is usually adequate for a trans-abdominal necrosectomy.
- Most necrosis cavities can be accessed through an upper midline incision. Rarely, a bilateral subcostal incision is needed.
- Access to the necrosis cavity can be gained through the lesser sac or through a trans-gastric approach, depending on the relationship of the stomach to the necrosis cavity.
- If the stomach overlies the anterior surface of the infected necrosis cavity, a trans-gastric approach is used through an anterior gastrostomy followed by ultrasound-guided posterior gastrotomy and cavitotomy, necrosectomy, and drainage of the cavity, and with stapled cystogastrostomy. The anterior gastrotomy is then closed.
- If the necrosis cavity is adjacent to the jejunum, a cystojejunostomy is performed instead after necrosectomy.
- If the cavity is not adjacent to the stomach or small bowel, it is plugged with vascularized omentum and drains placed.
- If the cavity is adjacent to the mesocolon, debridement and drainage occur through the mesocolon. Attention should be made to the blood supply to avoid inducing ischemia to segments of the colon. Colectomy may be necessary at the time of surgery in difficult cases.

Open Necrosectomy Pitfalls
- Gastrocutaneous or pancreatico-cutaneous fistula
- Duodenal perforation, leak
- Gastroduodenal artery injury/pseudoaneurysm with bleeding

Management of Pseudocyst

Pseudocysts are the chronic (>4 weeks old) forms of peripancreatic fluid collections that arise from acute pancreatitis without associated pancreatic or peripancreatic necrosis. Majority of these peripancreatic fluid collections resolve without any intervention. However, a few persist and transform into pseudocysts by developing a mature thick wall made of granulation, non-epithelialized tissue. Traditional management was based on chronicity and size with pseudocysts >4–6 cm and older than 6 weeks often being intervened on. However, intervention is reserved for symptomatic pseudocysts.

It is of critical importance to accurately differentiate a pseudocyst from a walled-off pancreatic necrosis (WOPN) since the management of each is vastly different (see above). Pseudocysts can present with either compressive symptoms that lead to pain, nausea, emesis, early satiety, bowel obstruction, or erosive symptoms including bleeding from vascular erosion or pseudoaneurysm, erosion into the biliary tree, and the alimentary tract with internal fistula.

The understanding of the pathophysiology of acute pancreatic and peripancreatic fluid collection that subsequently leads to pseudocyst formation is key to decision-making about their management. Acute peripancreatic fluid collections without associated necrosis arise from pancreatic main or side branch ductal disruption with pancreatic fluid leakage. A pseudocyst that develops from these collections may still retain communication with the pancreatic ductal system. As a result, a percutaneous drainage will result in a persistent pancreatico-cutaneous fistula.

Internal drainage into the alimentary tract is the preferred option, with endoscopic internal drainage being the first-line option.

Surgical Management of Pseudocyst by Surgical Cystogastrostomy

This is a second-line option to endoscopic approach and is only indicated for symptomatic often large pseudocysts. The choice between open and minimally invasive approach depends on a number of factors including the location of the pseudocyst (retroperitoneal vs. peritoneal), relationship with the alimentary tract, associated extent of inflammation and visceral adherence, and feasibility of establishment of pneumoperitoneum/pneumo-retroperitoneum (Fig. 4.9a).

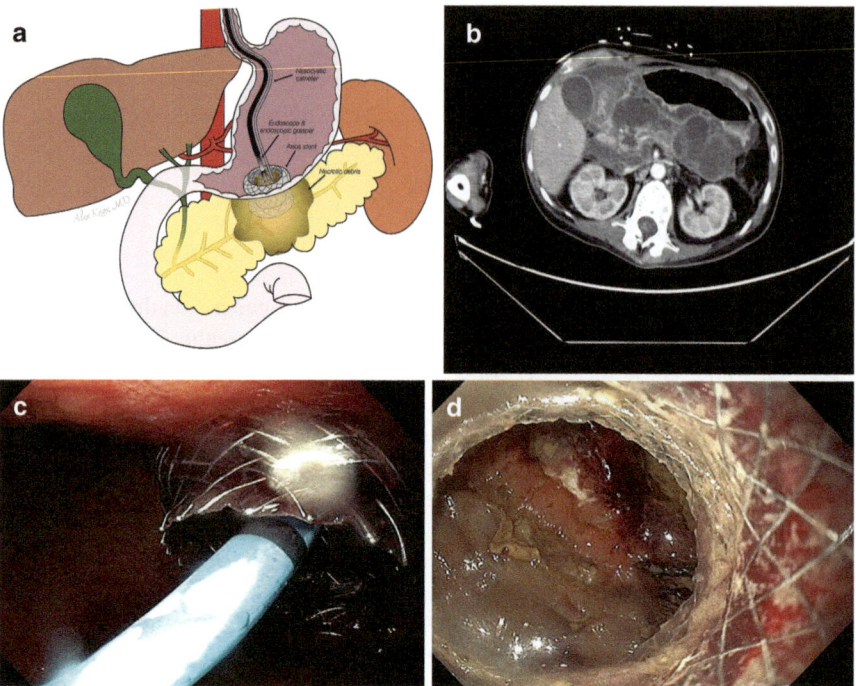

Fig. 4.9 (**a**) Parts *A–D*: CT abdomen showing a large WOPN with EUS of the same lesion showing anechoic cystic lesion with large amount of heterogeneous echogenic material within consistent with WOPN (*A* and *C*). LAMS and DPPS in situ of the WOPN, note hemorrhagic WON fluid exiting through LAMS (*C*). WOPN cavity 1 week after LAMS with necrotic debris (*D*). (**b**) Endoscopic cystogastrostomy. An axios stent is placed connecting the stomach with the necrotic peri-pancreatic cavity through which an endoscopic grasper can be used to remove necrotic debris

Open Trans-Gastric Cystogastrostomy

Pre-op Preparation Pearls
- A thorough review of the patient's preoperative imaging is critical to inform the operative intervention, including the anatomy around the pseudocyst.
- Nasogastric decompression should be done preoperatively if gastric outlet obstruction from the pseudocyst is present and is causing gastric dilation. This is both for patient safety to avoid aspiration during induction of general anesthesia, as well as facilitate easier performance of the trans-gastric cystogastrostomy.

Procedure Details

- Open internal drainage to the stomach is the best option for patients with large symptomatic pseudocyst with extrinsic compression of the stomach and associated frozen abdomen, all of which preclude endoscopic or minimally invasive approaches.
- In these cases, a thorough preoperative evaluation and review of imaging is performed to determine the best interventional approach. Supine position is usually best. A limited upper midline incision usually provides great access to the body of the stomach and the lesser sac and the most common location of pseudocyst in the mid pancreas. Intraoperative ultrasound is recommended to locate the best site of close apposition between the posterior gastric wall with the pseudocyst wall and confirm mature thick pseudocyst wall to anastomose to the stomach.
- Ultrasound evaluation is also used to ensure absence of vasculature traversing the site if intended cystogastrostomy.
- Once these conditions are met, an anterior gastrotomy is made preferably with an ultrasonic energy device. Once intragastric, pseudocyst bulge may be identified underneath the posterior gastric wall.
- Intraoperative ultrasound may again be performed to guide location of the posterior gastrostomy and pseudocyst puncture. Posterior gastrotomy and pseudocyst puncture is then performed, and the pseudocyst fluid is drained completely. A pseudocyst should have minimal to no debris.
- Examination of the cyst cavity is performed. The cystogastrostomy anastomosis can then be created using a stapler or running suture depending on surgeon's preference.
- The anterior gastrostomy is then closed by stapling or two-layer suture closure.
- If needed, cholecystectomy is performed if the patient had biliary pancreatitis. A drain may be placed if deemed necessary; however, this is usually not needed.

Postoperative Care and Follow-up

No upper gastrointestinal contrast study is necessary after operative cystogastrostomy. The patient can usually resume a liquid diet the day after surgery and be discharged on soft diet. If surgical drain is placed, this can be removed prior to discharge if drain fluid amylase if low. Endoscopic cystogastrostomy patients will usually need to repeat endoscopy in 2–4 weeks for stent removal (Figs. 4.9b and 4.10a–j). Patients should follow-up at 2–6 weeks postoperatively.

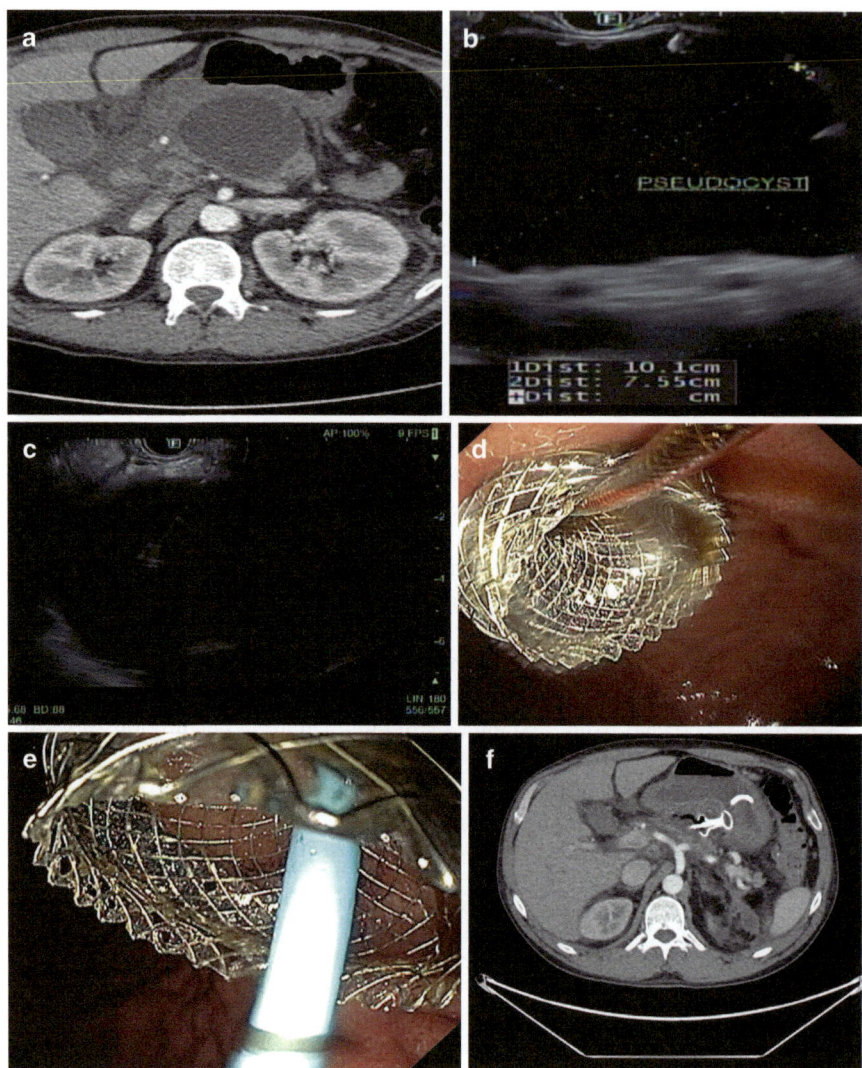

Fig. 4.10 CT abdomen and endoscopic ultrasound showing a large pseudocyst (**a** and **b**). EUS-guided LAMS placement in progress (**c**). LAMS deployed, notice serous fluid drainage through the LAMS (**d**) and LAMS+DPPS within pseudocyst (**e**). CT of the abdomen following LAMS + DPPS showing resolution of pseudocyst (**f**). CT abdomen following LAMS+DPPS showing resolution of pseudocyst (**g**). The LAMS is subsequently removed but the DPPS left in situ (**h**). CT abdomen and EUS 2 months after removal of the LAMS, showing no pseudocyst recurrence noted (**i** and **j**)

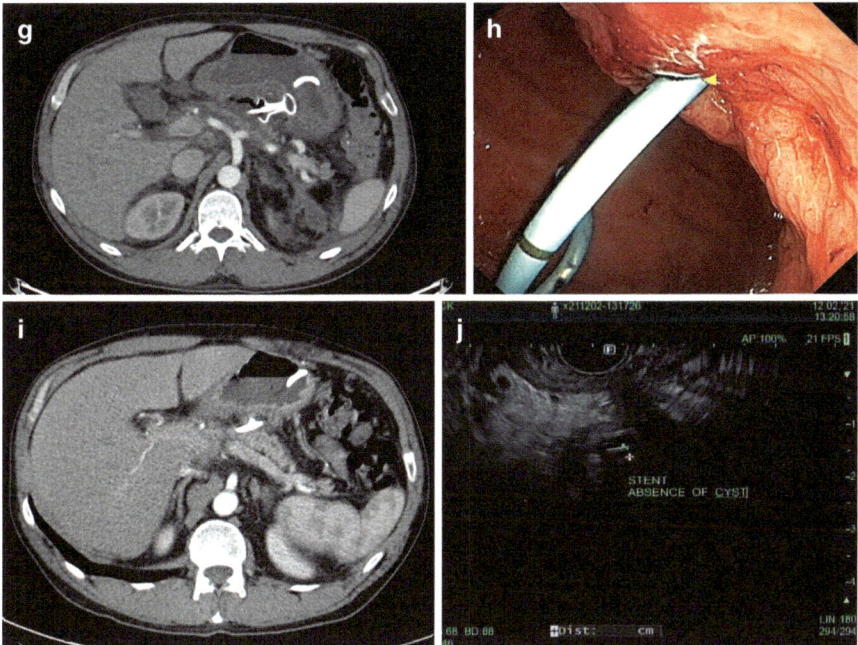

Fig. 4.10 (continued)

Disconnected Distal Pancreatic Duct Syndrome

Introduction

Disconnected distal pancreatic duct syndrome (DDPDS) or disconnected left pancreatic remnant refers to a sequelae of necrotizing pancreatitis whereby pancreatic neck/body necrosis leads to neck/body parenchymal and ductal disruption, and loss of the continuity of the pancreatic ductal system between the tail, body, neck, and head of the pancreas (Fig. 4.11). This results in an isolated viable upstream pancreatic distal body/tail parenchyma and ductal system that is not in continuity with the pancreatic head ductal system, and is therefore not connected to the alimentary tract [33, 34].

DDPDS usually occurs from necrotizing pancreatitis but can also occur from traumatic injury to pancreas, malignancy, postoperative complications, and chronic pancreatitis [34]. DDPDS occurs in 30–50% of cases of necrotizing pancreatitis. Maatman et al. in their retrospective review of 647 patients with necrotizing pancreatitis reported a DDPDS prevalence of 36% [33].

Disconnected pancreatic duct syndrome remains the most common cause of recurrent PFCs. The size of the disconnected viable pancreatic tail remnant varies depending on the extent of pancreatic neck/body necrosis and disruption. The most common site of necrosis and pancreatic ductal disruption is the pancreatic neck and

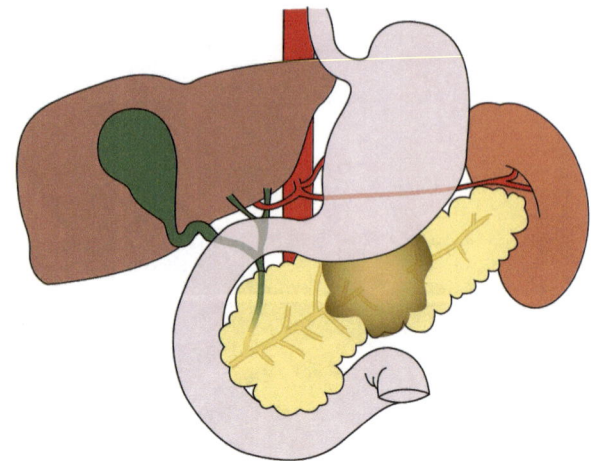

Fig. 4.11 Disconnected distal pancreatic duct syndrome. Central pancreatic necrosis with a large fluid collection containing necrotic debris leading to a discontinuous pancreatic duct between the body and tail of the pancreas

proximal body. This is due to the fact that this is a vascular watershed area that falls between the transverse pancreatic arteries from the splenic artery and the anterior and posterior pancreaticoduodenal arteries from the gastroduodenal and superior mesenteric arteries.

The diagnosis of DDPDS may be difficult to determine in the first week after onset of necrotizing pancreatitis since necrosis may still be patchy and not complete. After the first week, contrast-enhanced CT imaging will confirm the diagnosis by identifying the necrosis and showing a central pancreatic fluid collection of >2 cm that replaced the neck and body parenchyma and will be enlarging over time.

Management of DDPDS

Management depends on a number of factors including size of the disconnected viable distal pancreatic remnant, size of the intervening necrosis cavity between the pancreatic head and the viable distal pancreatic remnant, pancreatic head, and distal remnant pancreatic main ductal communication with the necrosis cavity, among others.

Management options include nonoperative intervention, cystogastrostomy/cysto jejunostomy, pancreaticojejunostomy, or distal pancreatic remnant resection [34].

(a) *Nonoperative Management*

Some cases of DDPDS will spontaneously resolve over time. This is likely in cases where the communication of the main pancreatic duct is maintained between the distal pancreatic remnant into the necrosis cavity, which also still maintains communication to the pancreatic duct in the head. This internal drainage may lead to spontaneous resolution over time. In these situations, the necrosis resolves over time and the continuity of the duct is restored via a fistula tract connecting the distal pancreatic duct to the pancreatic head duct into the alimentary tract.

(b) *Cystogastrostomy/cystojejunostomy*

Operative internal drainage should be considered for symptomatic DDPDS. Due to the common location in the mid pancreas in the retrogastric lesser sac, a cystogastrostomy following necrosectomy is a great option for managing mid pancreatic necrosis that is still communicating with the main duct of the distal pancreatic remnant duct. Cystojejunostomy may be done if the cavity is adjacent to the proximal jejunum and not in close apposition to the posterior gastric wall. Cystogastrostomy or cystojejunostomy allows for internal drainage into the alimentary tract. Procedure steps are the same as described above.

(c) *Distal Pancreaticojejunostomy*

Pancreaticojejunostomy is reasonable for patients with a sizable distal pancreatic duct remnant >5–6 cm who continue to have symptoms or develop recurrent distal remnant pancreatitis. Adequate time should be allowed between the acute necrotizing pancreatitis episode and the pancreaticojejunostomy, in order to allow the associated inflammation and scarring to resolve. This may be 6 months to a year. If the pancreatic remnant can be accessed and exposed, a jejunal Roux is used to create a distal pancreaticojejunostomy for internal drainage. Distal pancreaticojejunostomy should especially be considered for younger patients with substantial distal remnant pancreatic parenchyma volume and length to preserve and prevent future development of diabetes mellitus.

(d) *Distal Remnant Pancreatectomy*

Distal pancreatic remnant resection is an ideal option in patients with recurrent symptoms of distal remnant pancreatitis who have a small <5 cm viable pancreatic remnant. Due to the small size, internal drainage via pancreatico-enteric anastomosis is a great option. Due to preceding inflammation from necrotizing pancreatitis and the subsequent scarring, the surrounding tissue planes will be obliterated, and the remnant pancreas will likely be firmly adherent to the splenic vessels and splenic hilum. While an attempt may be made to preserve the spleen, splenic preservation is often extremely difficult due to dense post-inflammatory peripancreatic and splenic hilar scarring, and the scirrhous obliteration of normal planes that often leads to en bloc splenectomy. Due to this possibility of splenectomy, these patients should receive post-splenectomy vaccinations preoperatively.

References

1. Banks PA, Bollen TL, Dervenis C, et al. Classification of acute pancreatitis—2012: revision of the Atlanta classification and definitions by international consensus. Gut. 2013;62:102–11. https://doi.org/10.1136/gutjnl-2012-302779.
2. Kwong WT-Y, Ondrejková A, Vege SS. Predictors and outcomes of moderately severe acute pancreatitis—evidence to reclassify. Pancreatology. 2016;16:940–5. https://doi.org/10.1016/j.pan.2016.08.001.

3. Singh VK, Bollen TL, Wu BU, et al. An assessment of the severity of interstitial pancreatitis. Clin Gastroenterol Hepatol. 2011;9:1098–103. https://doi.org/10.1016/j.cgh.2011.08.026.
4. Sarr MG, Banks PA, Bollen TL, et al. The new revised classification of acute pancreatitis 2012. Surg Clin North Am. 2013;93:549–62. https://doi.org/10.1016/j.suc.2013.02.012.
5. Zaheer A, Singh VK, Qureshi RO, et al. The revised Atlanta classification for acute pancreatitis: updates in imaging terminology and guidelines. Abdom Imaging. 2013;38:125–36. https://doi.org/10.1007/s00261-012-9908-0.
6. Datir A, Niknejad M. Acute pancreatitis. Radiopaedia. 2008; https://doi.org/10.53347/rID-849.
7. Thoeni RF. The revised Atlanta classification of acute pancreatitis: its importance for the radiologist and its effect on treatment. Radiology. 2012;262:751–64. https://doi.org/10.1148/radiol.11110947.
8. Balthazar EJ, Freeny PC, vanSonnenberg E. Imaging and intervention in acute pancreatitis. Radiology. 1994;193:297–306. https://doi.org/10.1148/radiology.193.2.7972730.
9. Johnson MD, Walsh RM, Henderson JM, et al. Surgical versus nonsurgical management of pancreatic pseudocysts. J Clin Gastroenterol. 2009;43:586–90. https://doi.org/10.1097/MCG.0b013e31817440be.
10. Harris HW, Barcia A, Schell MT, et al. Necrotizing pancreatitis: a surgical approach independent of documented infection. HPB. 2004;6:161–8. https://doi.org/10.1080/13651820410033634.
11. Vege SS, Fletcher JG, Talukdar R, et al. Peripancreatic collections in acute pancreatitis: correlation between computerized tomography and operative findings. World J Gastroenterol. 2010;16:4291–6. https://doi.org/10.3748/wjg.v16.i34.4291.
12. Ashley SW, Perez A, Pierce EA, et al. Necrotizing pancreatitis: contemporary analysis of 99 consecutive cases. Ann Surg. 2001;234:572–80. https://doi.org/10.1097/00000658-200110000-00016.
13. Mofidi R, Duff MD, Wigmore SJ, et al. Association between early systemic inflammatory response, severity of multiorgan dysfunction and death in acute pancreatitis. Br J Surg. 2006;93:738–44. https://doi.org/10.1002/bjs.5290.
14. Leppäniemi A, Tolonen M, Tarasconi A, et al. 2019 WSES guidelines for the management of severe acute pancreatitis. World J Emerg Surg. 2019;14:27. https://doi.org/10.1186/s13017-019-0247-0.
15. Working Group IAP/APA Acute Pancreatitis Guidelines. IAP/APA evidence-based guidelines for the management of acute pancreatitis. Pancreatology. 2013;13:e1–15. https://doi.org/10.1016/j.pan.2013.07.063.
16. Garg PK, Singh VP. Organ failure due to systemic injury in acute pancreatitis. Gastroenterology. 2019;156:2008–23. https://doi.org/10.1053/j.gastro.2018.12.041.
17. Machicado JD, Gougol A, Tan X, et al. Mortality in acute pancreatitis with persistent organ failure is determined by the number, type, and sequence of organ systems affected. United Eur Gastroenterol J. 2021;9:139–49. https://doi.org/10.1002/ueg2.12057.
18. Baron TH, DiMaio CJ, Wang AY, et al. American gastroenterological association clinical practice update: management of pancreatic necrosis. Gastroenterology. 2020;158:67–75.e1. https://doi.org/10.1053/j.gastro.2019.07.064.
19. Rashid MU, Hussain I, Jehanzeb S, et al. Pancreatic necrosis: complications and changing trend of treatment. World. J Gastrointest Surg. 2019;11:198–217. https://doi.org/10.4240/wjgs.v11.i4.198.
20. van Santvoort HC, Besselink MG, Bakker OJ, et al. A step-up approach or open necrosectomy for necrotizing pancreatitis. N Engl J Med. 2010;362:1491–502. https://doi.org/10.1056/NEJMoa0908821.
21. Boxhoorn L, van Dijk SM, van Grinsven J, et al. Immediate versus postponed intervention for infected necrotizing pancreatitis. N Engl J Med. 2021;385:1372–81. https://doi.org/10.1056/NEJMoa2100826.
22. Bakker OJ, van Santvoort HC, van Brunschot S, et al. Endoscopic transgastric vs. surgical necrosectomy for infected necrotizing pancreatitis: a randomized trial. JAMA. 2012;307:1053–61. https://doi.org/10.1001/jama.2012.276.

23. van Brunschot S, van Grinsven J, van Santvoort HC, et al. Endoscopic or surgical step-up approach for infected necrotising pancreatitis: a multicentre randomised trial. Lancet. 2018;391:51–8. https://doi.org/10.1016/S0140-6736(17)32404-2.
24. van Grinsven J, van Dijk SM, Dijkgraaf MG, et al. Postponed or immediate drainage of infected necrotizing pancreatitis (POINTER trial): study protocol for a randomized controlled trial. Trials. 2019;20:239. https://doi.org/10.1186/s13063-019-3315-6.
25. Onnekink AM, Boxhoorn L, Timmerhuis HC, et al. Endoscopic versus surgical step-up approach for infected necrotizing pancreatitis (ExTENSION): long-term follow-up of a randomized trial. Gastroenterology. 2022;S0016—5085(22):00504–2. https://doi.org/10.1053/j.gastro.2022.05.015.
26. Arvanitakis M, Dumonceau J-M, Albert J, et al. Endoscopic management of acute necrotizing pancreatitis: European Society of Gastrointestinal Endoscopy (ESGE) evidence-based multidisciplinary guidelines. Endoscopy. 2018;50:524–46. https://doi.org/10.1055/a-0588-5365.
27. Rodriguez JR, Razo AO, Targarona J, et al. Debridement and closed packing for sterile or infected necrotizing pancreatitis: insights into indications and outcomes in 167 patients. Ann Surg. 2008;247:294–9. https://doi.org/10.1097/SLA.0b013e31815b6976.
28. Khreiss M, Zenati M, Clifford A, et al. Cyst gastrostomy and necrosectomy for the management of sterile walled-off pancreatic necrosis: a comparison of minimally invasive surgical and endoscopic outcomes at a high-volume pancreatic center. J Gastrointest Surg. 2015;19:1441–8. https://doi.org/10.1007/s11605-015-2864-6.
29. Munene G, Dixon E, Sutherland F. Open transgastric debridement and internal drainage of symptomatic non-infected walled-off pancreatic necrosis. HPB. 2011;13:234–9. https://doi.org/10.1111/j.1477-2574.2010.00276.x.
30. Trikudanathan G, Vege SS. Current concepts of the role of abdominal compartment syndrome in acute pancreatitis—an opportunity or merely an epiphenomenon. Pancreatology. 2014;14:238–43. https://doi.org/10.1016/j.pan.2014.06.002.
31. van Brunschot S, Schut AJ, Bouwense SA, et al. Abdominal compartment syndrome in acute pancreatitis: a systematic review. Pancreas. 2014;43:665–74. https://doi.org/10.1097/MPA.0000000000000108.
32. Carter CR, McKay CJ, Imrie CW. Percutaneous necrosectomy and sinus tract endoscopy in the management of infected pancreatic necrosis: an initial experience. Ann Surg. 2000;232:175–80. https://doi.org/10.1097/00000658-200008000-00004.
33. Maatman TK, Mahajan S, Roch AM, et al. Disconnected pancreatic duct syndrome predicts failure of percutaneous therapy in necrotizing pancreatitis. Pancreatology. 2020;20:362–8. https://doi.org/10.1016/j.pan.2020.01.014.
34. van Dijk SM, Timmerhuis HC, Verdonk RC, et al. Treatment of disrupted and disconnected pancreatic duct in necrotizing pancreatitis: a systematic review and meta-analysis. Pancreatology. 2019;19:905–15. https://doi.org/10.1016/j.pan.2019.08.006.

Chapter 5
Acute Pancreatitis: Complications

Jackson A. Baril, Rachel C. Kim, and Eugene P. Ceppa

Introduction

Acute pancreatitis (AP) is a systemic and local pathology that can affect nearly every organ system. Therefore, complications of AP occur both near the pancreas, its adjacent vessels and viscera as well as distant organs. These complications contribute significantly to the overall mortality associated with pancreatitis and warrant early recognition, careful monitoring, and prompt treatment. Many complications are mitigated by treatment of the underlying AP. However, some require specific complication-targeted interventions including medical therapy, therapeutic endoscopy, image-guided percutaneous interventions, and/or surgery via a multidisciplinary approach.

Visceral Artery Pseudoaneurysm and Hemorrhage

Arterial complications in AP are uncommon yet carry a profound risk of mortality up to 19–34% [1, 2]. The incidence of pseudoaneurysm or hemorrhagic complications of AP is between 1.3 and 10% [3–5]. The exact onset of arterial complications varies dramatically with a mean time of detection ranging from 64 days to 2.3 years after initial episode of pancreatitis [3, 5]. This correlates with other published data

J. A. Baril · R. C. Kim
Department of Surgery, Indiana University School of Medicine, Indianapolis, IN, USA
e-mail: jbaril@iu.edu; rckim@iu.edu

E. P. Ceppa (✉)
Department of Surgery, Indiana University School of Medicine,
Indianapolis, IN, USA
e-mail: eceppa@iu.edu

© The Author(s), under exclusive license to Springer Nature
Switzerland AG 2025
E. P. Ceppa et al. (eds.), *The SAGES Manual of Evolving Techniques in Pancreatic Surgery*, https://doi.org/10.1007/978-3-031-78409-5_5

showing arterial complications of AP most often occur in the setting of acute on chronic pancreatitis (92%) and less commonly during the index episode of pancreatitis (8%) [6].

The pathophysiology of pseudoaneurysm and hemorrhage from AP is thought to be from the compartmentalization of pancreatic fluid within the disrupted pancreatic capsule in the retroperitoneum. The proteolytic enzyme release in proximity of the visceral arteries combined with the systemic inflammatory environment of AP effectively serves as the perfect storm for arterial disruption. Disruptions in walled off necrosis or pseudocysts may also result in arterial bleeding [4]. Pseudoaneurysms are most common in the splenic artery (35–50%), followed by the gastroduodenal (20–30%) and pancreaticoduodenal (20–25%) arteries [4, 7]. Less common are the mesenteric, colic, and hepatic arteries, yet all are recognized sources [4, 8].

The most common presenting symptom of arterial pseudoaneurysm in AP is abdominal pain (62%) followed by gastrointestinal hemorrhage (26–29%) consistent with "hemosuccus pancreaticus." [6, 9] Abdominal or back pain and hypovolemia are presenting symptoms of AP, which make vascular complications of AP difficult to diagnose on history and physical alone. A high index of suspicion should be had with any patient presenting with acute on chronic pancreatitis and evidence of hypovolemia, anemia, or sudden onset pain. In patients with drains previously placed for the management of pancreatic fluid collections, a heraldic bleed via the drain in many cases is the initial sign of a pseudoaneurysm. In one series of 28 patients, bloody drain output was a common presenting symptom (32%) followed by asymptomatic patients whose pseudoaneurysm was incidentally found on CT scan (21%) [5].

Computed tomography (CT) is the initial diagnostic method of choice for detecting visceral artery pseudoaneurysm or acute hemorrhage given its availability, cost, and speed [10]. Compared with conventional angiography, cross-sectional CT angiography (CTA) detected bleeding in the setting of pancreatitis with a sensitivity and specificity of 94.7% and 90%, respectively [11] (Fig. 5.1). The practitioner's experience, knowledge of the patient, and index of suspicion should not be discounted when a CTA does not show an overt pseudoaneurysm; a visceral arteriogram should be performed if the patient's clinical picture matches that of hemorrhagic shock with an unremarkable CTA.

Treatment for visceral artery pseudoaneurysm or hemorrhage in the hemodynamically stable patient with AP is angiography with embolization. There is a breadth of literature supporting angiographic intervention with high rate of success to stop hemorrhage. Initial interventional radiology (IR) embolization is successful in 93–100% of published cases [5–7, 13]. However, rebleeding can occur in 3.5–12.5% of patients after successful embolization [1, 5–7, 14]. These data suggest that embolization is particularly successful with low associated morbidity. An alternative IR approach is percutaneous stenting of the celiac or common hepatic artery to preserve hepatic arterial blood supply while achieving proximal control of hemorrhage.

Percutaneous thrombin injection is an important adjunct treatment for pseudoaneurysm. There are case reports of thrombin injection to successfully embolize

Fig. 5.1 CTA showing a pancreatic pseudocyst eroding the splenic artery [12]

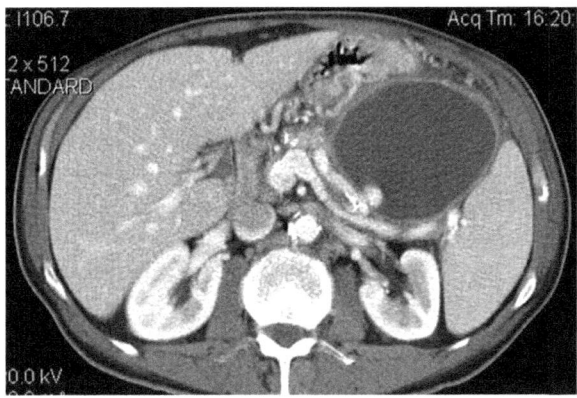

pseudoaneurysms. However, this subset likely has a selection bias for successful cases. Of the 23 patients published with percutaneous thrombin injection, four patients had repeat bleeding as the thrombin is thought to be precise and without collateral effects, yet is an absorbable, biodegradable embolization agent. Of those four, two underwent repeat thrombin injection and one underwent coil angioembolization [4].

Surgical intervention for arterial pseudoaneurysm or hemorrhage is rare due to poor outcomes when operating on patients in the setting of a massive systemic inflammatory condition. Surgery is indicated in the unstable patient after failed angioembolization. The most common surgery reported for refractory hemorrhage is distal pancreatectomy with or without splenectomy [15]. Prior to the advancement of IR techniques, surgery was more common for management of arterial complications with one-third to one-half of patients with bleeding pseudoaneurysm undergoing surgery. Appropriately, the rate of surgical intervention has fallen to 11% in more recent studies with improved overall survival [1, 5, 15].

Venous Thrombosis

Venous thrombosis is a more common complication of acute pancreatitis when compared with arterial bleeding. Among a meta-analysis of over 10,000 patients with acute and chronic pancreatitis, splanchnic venous thrombosis was found in 16.6% of patients with AP and 11.6% of patients with CP [16]. Another meta-analysis found rates of splenic vein thrombosis of 22.6% and 12.4% in AP and CP [17]. Venous thrombosis in AP is related to both local and systemic inflammation generating a prothrombotic state, and venous flow disruptions as a result of external compression during AP [18]. Often there is a clear association between the vessel with venous thrombosis and areas of necrosis and collections resulting from AP [19]. Thrombosis is most common in the splenic vein (11.2%), followed by the portal vein (6%) and mesenteric veins (2.7%) [16].

Portal venous thrombosis (PVT) is more easily diagnosed via transabdominal ultrasonography (US) (Fig. 5.2). Sensitivity and specificity for PVT is between 60 and 100% via US. Endoscopic ultrasound (EUS) has comparable sensitivity and specificity, 81 and 93%, but is more invasive and does not visualize the intrahepatic portal venous system with as much detail [20]. For venous thromboses outside the portal venous system, CT or magnetic resonance angiography are the diagnostic modalities of choice with sensitivities reaching 95%, improved from 71% in the early 2000s [8, 20] (Fig. 5.3).

Portal venous thrombosis is treated with either systemic anticoagulation or portal venous stenting. Image-guided portal vein stenting is currently used to treat malignant stenosis [21, 22]. Stenting is sometimes performed before or after surgery for pancreatic adenocarcinoma in cases of portal vein stenosis [23–25]. There is less published data on the use of portal vein stenting for PV thrombosis or compression

Fig. 5.2 US imaging showing thrombosed left portal vein (black arrow) [20]

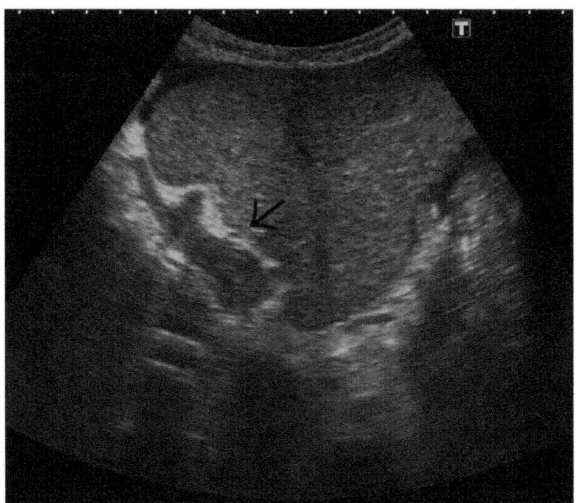

Fig. 5.3 Coronal oblique venous phase CT of a patient with AP with thrombosed splenic vein (white arrows) and a segmental branch of right portal vein (single white arrow) with hepatic artery buffer response in the form of differential hyperenhancement of the affected liver segment (black arrows) [20]

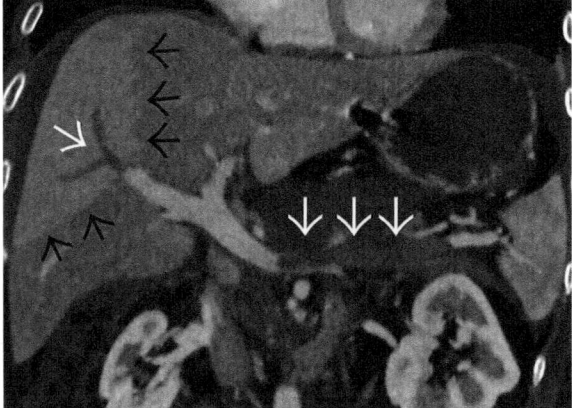

in AP; many cases focus on retroperitoneal decompression via percutaneous drains to alleviate pressure on the portal venous circulation.

Splenic vein thrombosis can usually be safely watched and treated with systemic anticoagulation. Complications of splenic vein thrombosis can include sinistral portal hypertension and esophageal varices. Gastroesophageal varices occur in up to 20% of patients with splenic vein thrombosis; however, bleeding from these is rare (12.3%) when compared to varices from those with hepatic cirrhosis [17]. In patients who have sinistral portal hypertension or asymptomatic gastric or esophageal varices secondary to splenic vein thrombosis as a result of acute on chronic pancreatitis, splenectomy is not routinely performed [8]. However, in such patients who are symptomatic or undergoing a planned pancreatic surgery, splenectomy can be performed during the same operation and does not lead to increased morbidity or mortality [26, 27]. Similarly, mesenteric vein thrombosis is usually treated with systemic anticoagulation. Surgery is reserved for cases of mesenteric ischemia with overt peritonitis which require emergent laparotomy and bowel resection [28].

Intra-Abdominal Hypertension

Intra-abdominal hypertension (IAH) is a unique complication of pancreatitis which can range in severity from asymptomatic to life-threatening. IAH, defined as sustained intra-abdominal pressures greater than 12 mm hg, may occur in severe AP. The incidence of IAH in severe AP ranges from 50% to 80% [29–33]. A combination of retroperitoneal inflammation, aggressive fluid resuscitation, visceral edema, ileus, and peripancreatic fluid collections result in IAH in AP [34].

Management of IAH includes correcting a positive fluid balance as able, evacuate intra-luminal gastrointestinal contents, evacuate extraluminal abdominal fluid, and improving abdominal wall compliance. Each management pillar has a range of interventions from nasogastric decompression and goal directed fluid management, to drainage of intra-abdominal collections and dialysis to achieve negative fluid balance [35]. Early recognition is key in preventing progression to abdominal compartment syndrome (ACS) and reducing morbidity and mortality.

ACS is defined as sustained IAH >20 mmHg with new organ dysfunction as a result [36]. Acute kidney injury (AKI) is the most common organ dysfunction seen in ACS and can rapidly progress to anuria requiring renal replacement therapy [35, 37]. Pulmonary complications include the inability to ventilate due to elevated IAH resulting in prohibitively high airway pressures. Conversely, increased PEEP is unlikely to contribute more than 1–2 mmHg to the intra-abdominal pressure [38]. Other signs of organ dysfunction include hemodynamic instability and metabolic derangements which can occur in severe AP without ACS. Organ dysfunction in severe AP is difficult to attribute to AP or ACS. Nonetheless, IAH and ACS should be measured early and treated aggressively with medical management and, when needed, surgical intervention.

Surgical decompression is necessary in patients with continued ACS despite maximal non-surgical management to decrease intra-abdominal pressures. Mortality can reach 50% in patients with AP and ACS [39]. Among patients with severe AP, the incidence of ACS is not well documented. However, among patients admitted to the intensive care unit with severe AP, incidence of ACS has been reported between 27 and 38% of patients [32, 39]. In a single-center study of 2345 episodes of AP, 226 required ICU admission of which 26 (11.5%) required surgical decompression for ACS [40]. Early laparotomy was associated with improved outcomes compared to patients with laparotomy >72 h after admission.

Thoracic Complications

Acute pancreatitis can have effects on the respiratory system ranging from asymptomatic pleural effusions to acute respiratory distress syndrome (ARDS). The presence of pleural effusion is a poor prognostic indicator in acute pancreatitis and is a criterion on the Bedside Index for Severity in Acute Pancreatitis (BISAP) score [41]. Pleural effusion is present in 4–17% of patients with AP with the majority being sympathetic in nature and requires thoracentesis only when symptomatic [42]. Rarely, in approximately 0.6% of AP, a pancreaticopleural fistula forms. These are most common in alcohol-induced pancreatitis and in pancreatic duct disruption. Treatment of duct disruption with endoscopic stenting can resolve the fistula, yet there are no clear treatment guidelines due to the paucity of the event [43]. Like with pleural effusion, addressing the pancreatitis is the primary treatment to mitigate additional pulmonary injury.

As a more severe sequela, ARDS occurs in severe AP as a result of inflammatory cytokines, endothelial and epithelial damage to pneumocytes and pulmonary vasculature, as well as interstitial neutrophil infiltration [44]. Defined as PaO_2/FiO_2 ratio of <200, ARDS has a high mortality between 30 and 60% and is the cause of early death in most elderly patients who die of severe AP [44]. Pancreatitis was the cause of 3.4% of ARDS cases from over 900,000 ARDS cases analyzed in the US between 2006 and 2014 [45] but has also been reported in 12.8% of ARDS admissions to ICUs in Beijing [46]. Like pleural effusions, treatment of ARDS should focus on supportive care and addressing the underlying pancreatitis. Effective measures include lung protective ventilation with lower tidal volumes, judicious use of fluids, reducing ventilator dyssynchrony, and prone positioning [47, 48]. High PEEP strategies (25–35 cm H_2O) to increase lung recruitment increases mortality in ARDS patients [49]. The use of steroids has not proven effective in reducing mortality in ARDS. [50]

Pancreatic pseudocyst can present in the mediastinum through the esophageal or aortic hiatus. Most frequently, this is due to pancreatic duct disruption (PDD) and presents with dysphagia or chest pain [43]. They are diagnosed by CT scan but can also be seen on upper EUS. Stenting of the pancreatic duct can often resolve the pseudocyst. However, drainage via EUS with transesophageal or transgastric methods are sometimes needed if duct stenting is not successful as mediastinal pseudocyst rarely spontaneously resolve.

Gastrointestinal Complications

Gastric outlet obstruction (GOO) is an uncommon complication of AP with an incidence of approximately 5%. In early pancreatitis, within four weeks of disease onset, GOO is most often caused by compression from pancreatic necrosis or pseudocyst and less commonly from edema of the stomach and/or duodenum [51]. Treatment previously was upfront surgery with gastrojejunostomy, but now minimally invasive techniques with gastric decompression, jejunal feeding, and drainage of fluid collections are successful in most cases [52, 53].

Colonic complications are rare and include fistula, necrosis, and stricture [54]. Bowel perforation secondary to necrosis warrants a colectomy with wide drainage and possible stoma creation. The colonic mesentery is at grave risk during any urgent acute pancreatitis-associated surgery. Colonic stricture often presents as a late complication following the episode of pancreatitis due to acute or chronic ischemia to segments of the colon. Among patients with colonic stricture, surgical resection may be performed successfully with a primary anastomosis in an elective setting after resolution of the acute pancreatitis episode [55–57].

References

1. Bergert H, Hinterseher I, Kersting S, Leonhardt J, Bloomenthal A, Saeger HD. Management and outcome of hemorrhage due to arterial pseudoaneurysms in pancreatitis. Surgery. 2005;137(3):323–8.
2. Flati G, Andrén-Sandberg A, La Pinta M, Porowska B, Carboni M. Potentially fatal bleeding in acute pancreatitis: pathophysiology, prevention, and treatment. Pancreas. 2003;26(1):8–14.
3. Balthazar EJ, Fisher LA. Hemorrhagic complications of pancreatitis: radiologic evaluation with emphasis on CT imaging. Pancreatology. 2001;1(4):306–13.
4. Evans RP, Mourad MM, Pall G, Fisher SG, Bramhall SR. Pancreatitis: preventing catastrophic haemorrhage. World J Gastroenterol. 2017;23(30):5460–8.
5. Maatman TK, Heimberger MA, Lewellen KA, Roch AM, Colgate CL, House MG, et al. Visceral artery pseudoaneurysm in necrotizing pancreatitis: incidence and outcomes. Can J Surg. 2020;63(3):E272–e7.
6. Zyromski NJ, Vieira C, Stecker M, Nakeeb A, Pitt HA, Lillemoe KD, et al. Improved outcomes in postoperative and pancreatitis-related visceral pseudoaneurysms. J Gastrointest Surg. 2007;11(1):50–5.
7. Kim J, Shin JH, Yoon HK, Ko GY, Gwon DI, Kim EY, et al. Endovascular intervention for management of pancreatitis-related bleeding: a retrospective analysis of thirty-seven patients at a single institution. Diagn Interv Radiol. 2015;21(2):140–7.
8. Mallick I, Winslet M. Vascular complications of pancreatitis. J Pancreas. 2004;5:328–37.

9. Tessier DJ, Stone WM, Fowl RJ, Abbas MA, Andrews JC, Bower TC, et al. Clinical features and management of splenic artery pseudoaneurysm: case series and cumulative review of literature. J Vasc Surg. 2003;38(5):969–74.
10. Kirby JM, Vora P, Midia M, Rawlinson J. Vascular complications of pancreatitis: imaging and intervention. Cardiovasc Intervent Radiol. 2008;31(5):957–70.
11. Hyare H, Desigan S, Nicholl H, Guiney MJ, Brookes JA, Lees WR. Multi-section CT angiography compared with digital subtraction angiography in diagnosing major arterial hemorrhage in inflammatory pancreatic disease. Eur J Radiol. 2006;59(2):295–300.
12. Donatini G, Iacconi P, De Bartolomeis C, Iacconi C, Caldarelli C, Caramella D, et al. Massive upper gastrointestinal bleeding from a pancreatic pseudocyst rupture: a case report. Cases J. 2009;2(1):6793.
13. Zabicki B, Limphaibool N, Holstad MJV, Juszkat R. Endovascular management of pancreatitis-related pseudoaneurysms: a review of techniques. PLoS One. 2018;13(1):e0191998.
14. Kalva SP, Yeddula K, Wicky S, Fernandez del Castillo C, Warshaw AL. Angiographic intervention in patients with a suspected visceral artery pseudoaneurysm complicating pancreatitis and pancreatic surgery. Arch Surg. 2011;146(6):647–52.
15. Udd M, Leppäniemi AK, Bidel S, Keto P, Roth WD, Haapiainen RK. Treatment of bleeding pseudoaneurysms in patients with chronic pancreatitis. World J Surg. 2007;31(3):504–10.
16. Xu W, Qi X, Chen J, Su C, Guo X. Prevalence of splanchnic vein thrombosis in pancreatitis: a systematic review and meta-analysis of observational studies. Gastroenterol Res Pract. 2015;2015:245460.
17. Butler JR, Eckert GJ, Zyromski NJ, Leonardi MJ, Lillemoe KD, Howard TJ. Natural history of pancreatitis-induced splenic vein thrombosis: a systematic review and meta-analysis of its incidence and rate of gastrointestinal bleeding. HPB (Oxford). 2011;13(12):839–45.
18. Valla DC, Condat B. Portal vein thrombosis in adults: pathophysiology, pathogenesis and management. J Hepatol. 2000;32(5):865–71.
19. Gonzelez HJ, Sahay SJ, Samadi B, Davidson BR, Rahman SH. Splanchnic vein thrombosis in severe acute pancreatitis: a 2-year, single-institution experience. HPB (Oxford). 2011;13(12):860–4.
20. Rajesh S, Mukund A, Arora A. Imaging diagnosis of splanchnic venous thrombosis. Gastroenterol Res Pract. 2015;2015:101029.
21. Park JH, Yeo JH, Kim YS, Ahn HK, Sym S, Shin D, et al. Portal vein stent for symptomatic malignant portal vein stenosis: a single-center experience. Curr Probl Cancer. 2020;44(2):100476.
22. Sakurai K, Amano R, Yamamoto A, Nishida N, Matsutani S, Hirata K, et al. Portal vein stenting to treat portal vein stenosis in a patient with malignant tumor and gastrointestinal bleeding. Int Surg. 2014;99(1):91–5.
23. You Y, Heo JS, Han IW, Shin SH, Shin SW, Park KB, et al. Long term clinical outcomes of portal vein stenting for symptomatic portal vein stenosis after pancreaticoduodenectomy. Medicine. 2021;100(39):e27264.
24. Shirata C, Nishioka Y, Sato J, Watadani T, Arita J, Akamatsu N, et al. Therapeutic effect of portal vein stenting for portal vein stenosis after upper-abdominal surgery. HPB (Oxford). 2021;23(2):238–44.
25. Scemama U, Birnbaum DJ, Ouaissi M, Turrini O, Moutardier V, Soussan J. Portal vein stent placement in five patients with chronic portal vein thrombosis prior to pancreatic surgery. J Vasc Interv Radiol. 2016;27(6):889–94.
26. Sakorafas GH, Sarr MG, Farley DR, Farnell MB. The significance of sinistral portal hypertension complicating chronic pancreatitis. Am J Surg. 2000;179(2):129–33.
27. Agarwal AK, Raj Kumar K, Agarwal S, Singh S. Significance of splenic vein thrombosis in chronic pancreatitis. Am J Surg. 2008;196(2):149–54.
28. Bala M, Kashuk J, Moore EE, Kluger Y, Biffl W, Gomes CA, et al. Acute mesenteric ischemia: guidelines of the world society of emergency surgery. World J Emerg Surg. 2017;12(1):38.
29. De Waele JJ, Hoste E, Blot SI, Decruyenaere J, Colardyn F. Intra-abdominal hypertension in patients with severe acute pancreatitis. Crit Care. 2005;9(4):R452.

30. Mifkovic A, Skultety J, Sykora P, Prochotsky A, Okolicany R. Intra-abdominal hypertension and acute pancreatitis. Bratisl Lek Listy. 2013;114(3):166–71.
31. Al-Bahrani AZ, Abid GH, Holt A, McCloy RF, Benson J, Eddleston J, et al. Clinical relevance of intra-abdominal hypertension in patients with severe acute pancreatitis. Pancreas. 2008;36(1):39–43.
32. Chen H, Li F, Sun JB, Jia JG. Abdominal compartment syndrome in patients with severe acute pancreatitis in early stage. World J Gastroenterol. 2008;14(22):3541–8.
33. Kurdia KC, Irrinki S, Chala AV, Bhalla A, Kochhar R, Yadav TD. Early intra-abdominal hypertension: a reliable bedside prognostic marker for severe acute pancreatitis. JGH Open. 2020;4(6):1091–5.
34. Radenkovic DV, Johnson CD, Milic N, Gregoric P, Ivancevic N, Bezmarevic M, et al. Interventional treatment of abdominal compartment syndrome during severe acute pancreatitis: current status and historical perspective. Gastroenterol Res Pract. 2016;2016:5251806.
35. De Laet IE, Malbrain MLNG, De Waele JJ. A Clinician's guide to Management of Intra-abdominal Hypertension and Abdominal Compartment Syndrome in critically ill patients. Crit Care. 2020;24(1):97.
36. Cheatham ML, Malbrain ML, Kirkpatrick A, Sugrue M, Parr M, De Waele J, et al. Results from the international conference of experts on intra-abdominal hypertension and abdominal compartment syndrome. II. Recommendations. Intensive Care Med. 2007;33(6):951–62.
37. Dalfino L, Tullo L, Donadio I, Malcangi V, Brienza N. Intra-abdominal hypertension and acute renal failure in critically ill patients. Intensive Care Med. 2008;34(4):707–13.
38. De Keulenaer BL, De Waele JJ, Powell B, Malbrain ML. What is normal intra-abdominal pressure and how is it affected by positioning, body mass and positive end-expiratory pressure? Intensive Care Med. 2009;35(6):969–76.
39. van Brunschot S, Schut AJ, Bouwense SA, Besselink MG, Bakker OJ, van Goor H, et al. Abdominal compartment syndrome in acute pancreatitis: a systematic review. Pancreas. 2014;43(5):665–74.
40. Mentula P, Hienonen P, Kemppainen E, Puolakkainen P, Leppäniemi A. Surgical decompression for abdominal compartment syndrome in severe acute pancreatitis. Arch Surg. 2010;145(8):764–9.
41. Gao W, Yang HX, Ma CE. The value of BISAP score for predicting mortality and severity in acute pancreatitis: a systematic review and meta-analysis. PLoS One. 2015;10(6):e0130412.
42. Browne GW, Pitchumoni CS. Pathophysiology of pulmonary complications of acute pancreatitis. World J Gastroenterol. 2006;12(44):7087–96.
43. Kumar P, Gupta P, Rana S. Thoracic complications of pancreatitis. JGH Open. 2019;3(1):71–9.
44. Zhou MT, Chen CS, Chen BC, Zhang QY, Andersson R. Acute lung injury and ARDS in acute pancreatitis: mechanisms and potential intervention. World J Gastroenterol. 2010;16(17):2094–9.
45. Eworuke E, Major JM, Gilbert McClain LI. National incidence rates for acute respiratory distress syndrome (ARDS) and ARDS cause-specific factors in the United States (2006–2014). J Crit Care. 2018;47:192–7.
46. Ge QG, Zhu X, Yao GQ, Wang C, Yin CH, Lü JQ, et al. Epidemiological investigation on acute respiratory distress syndrome occurring in intensive care units in Beijing from 1998 to 2003. Zhongguo Wei Zhong Bing Ji Jiu Yi Xue. 2007;19(4):201–4.
47. Howell MD, Davis AM. Management of ARDS in adults. JAMA. 2018;319(7):711–2.
48. Brower RG, Matthay MA, Morris A, Schoenfeld D, Thompson BT, Wheeler A. Ventilation with lower tidal volumes as compared with traditional tidal volumes for acute lung injury and the acute respiratory distress syndrome. N Engl J Med. 2000;342(18):1301–8.
49. Cavalcanti AB, Suzumura ÉA, Laranjeira LN, Paisani DM, Damiani LP, Guimarães HP, et al. Effect of lung recruitment and titrated positive end-expiratory pressure (PEEP) vs low PEEP on mortality in patients with acute respiratory distress syndrome: a randomized clinical trial. JAMA. 2017;318(14):1335–45.

50. National Heart, Lung, and Blood Institute Acute Respiratory Distress Syndrome (ARDS) Clinical Trials Network. Efficacy and safety of corticosteroids for persistent acute respiratory distress syndrome. N Engl J Med. 2006;354(16):1671–84.
51. Qu C, Yu X, Duan Z, Zhou J, Mao W, Wei M, et al. Clinical characteristics and management of gastric outlet obstruction in acute pancreatitis. Pancreatology. 2021;21(1):64–8.
52. Aranha GV, Prinz RA, Greenlee HB, Freeark RJ. Gastric outlet and duodenal obstruction from inflammatory pancreatic disease. Arch Surg. 1984;119(7):833–5.
53. Sugimoto M, Sonntag DP, Flint GS, Boyce CJ, Kirkham JC, Harris TJ, et al. Biliary stenosis and gastric outlet obstruction: late complications after acute pancreatitis with pancreatic duct disruption. Pancreas. 2018;47(6):772–7.
54. Mohamed SR, Siriwardena AK. Understanding the colonic complications of pancreatitis. Pancreatology. 2008;8(2):153–8.
55. Abcarian H, Eftaiha M, Kraft AR, Nyhus LM. Colonic complications of acute pancreatitis. Arch Surg. 1979;114(9):995–1001.
56. Mandal AK, Kafle P, Puri P, Chaulagai B, Hassan M, Bhattarai B, et al. Acute pancreatitis causing descending colonic stricture: a rare sequelae. J Invest Med High Impact Case Rep. 2019;7:2324709619834594.
57. Maisonnette F, Abita T, Pichon N, Lachachi F, Cessot F, Valleix D, et al. Development of colonic stenosis following severe acute pancreatitis. HPB (Oxford). 2003;5(3):183–5.

Part III
Chronic Pancreatitis

Chapter 6
SAGES Manual: Chronic Pancreatitis–Classification and Medical Management

Emily Hensler and Subhashini Ayloo

Classification of Chronic Pancreatitis

Chronic pancreatitis remains a significant challenge for medical practitioners because of its heterogeneity in clinical course and progression among patients [1]. Unlike acute pancreatitis, which has well-established systems for classification and severity scoring (e.g., the Atlanta classification [2], the Glasgow criteria [3], Ranson's criteria [4], and the APACHE II score [5]), no widely accepted and utilized system exists for the classification of chronic pancreatitis. Several classification systems have been proposed, but no single system has become standard in the management of this disease process. In addition, the majority of proposed classification systems lack rigorous prospective multi-institutional validation [1]. Many of the proposed classification systems are also less applicable in clinical practice owing to their focus on radiologic morphology or to the complexity of the classification system itself. Here, we review the Marseille, Cambridge, Rosemont, TIGAR-O, M-ANNHEIM, ABC, Manchester, Heidelberg, and Chronic Pancreatitis Prognosis Score (COPPS) classification systems and discuss the strengths and limitations of these systems.

E. Hensler · S. Ayloo (✉)
Department of Surgery, Warren Alpert Medical School of Brown University, Providence, RI, USA
e-mail: ehensler@lifespan.org

© The Author(s), under exclusive license to Springer Nature Switzerland AG 2025
E. P. Ceppa et al. (eds.), *The SAGES Manual of Evolving Techniques in Pancreatic Surgery*, https://doi.org/10.1007/978-3-031-78409-5_6

Marseille Classification

The initial Marseille conference on pancreatitis classification occurred in 1963, and the group classified pancreatitis into four categories: acute, acute relapsing, chronic relapsing, and chronic [6]. This classification was then revised at the Second International Symposium on the Classification of Pancreatitis in 1984 to eliminate the relapsing acute and chronic relapsing subcategories because of the difficulty of accurately differentiating between the two. This consensus group also differentiated acute pancreatitis from chronic pancreatitis based on clinical and morphological criteria, with the caveat that clinical presentation and morphological changes may not correlate in these patients.

The authors of the 1984 Marseille classification stated that acute pancreatitis presents clinically as acute attacks of abdominal pain associated with elevations in serum pancreatic enzymes, occurring either as an isolated episode or as recurrent attacks over time [6]. These attacks can lead to end organ damage and death, but patients typically recover without lasting morbidity or progression to chronic pancreatitis. The authors also describe a spectrum of disease, from mild acute pancreatitis, characterized by interstitial edema and some fat necrosis but typically without necrosis of the parenchyma, to severe acute pancreatitis, characterized by more extensive fat necrosis within the pancreas and surrounding tissues, necrosis of the pancreatic parenchyma, and even hemorrhage.

Chronic pancreatitis, in comparison, is often defined by persistent pain with or without evidence of endocrine or exocrine dysfunction (diabetes or steatorrhea, respectively). The morphologic changes in patients with chronic pancreatitis include complications such as pseudocyst formation, ductal dilation, and permanent scarring, which can lead to loss of functional pancreatic parenchyma. The authors break down classification of chronic pancreatitis based on these morphological changes (Table 6.1) with an additional category for obstructive chronic pancreatitis, which they describe as being caused by occlusion of the major duct by scarring or tumors, but rarely stones. Occlusion of the major duct leads to parenchymal atrophy throughout the pancreas as well as fibrosis—these changes often improve with resolution of

Table 6.1 Summary of the Marseille classification [6]

	Acute pancreatitis	Chronic pancreatitis
Description	Acute episode of pain + elevated enzymes, ± temporary pancreatic dysfunction, temporary morphologic changes	Recurrent pain with morphologic changes, ± pancreatic dysfunction
Morphologic changes	1. Mild: fat necrosis and edema, no parenchymal necrosis 2. Severe: fat necrosis, parenchymal necrosis, hemorrhage	1. Focal parenchymal necrosis 2. Segmental/diffuse parenchymal fibrosis 3. ± Pancreatic calculi 4. Obstructive: occluded duct leading to ductal dilation, parenchymal atrophy, diffuse fibrosis

the obstruction. Overall, this early classification system relies heavily on morphological changes to the pancreas, which the authors admit do not always correlate to a patient's clinical presentation and disease course. This limits the applicability and utility of the Marseille classification in routine clinical practice.

Cambridge Classification

The Cambridge working group met in 1983 and developed the Cambridge classification system for pancreatitis [7]. This system has since formed the basis for many revised or modified systems [1]. The authors focused on five aspects of disease in their development of this classification system: etiology, pancreatic exocrine function, imaging findings, histology, and surgery [7]. They concluded that acute and chronic pancreatitis are defined by the reversibility of pancreatic changes—acute pancreatitis may result in a temporary alteration in function, whereas chronic pancreatitis is defined by irreversible changes. Although etiology, exocrine function, and histology were deemed to be important in defining chronic pancreatitis, specific guidelines were not included for their use in this classification.

The Cambridge group specifically graded chronic pancreatitis based on imaging findings using endoscopic retrograde cholangiopancreatography (ERCP), ultrasound (US), or computed tomography (CT). They divided the findings into five groups: (1) normal; (2) equivocal; (3) mild; (4) moderate; and (5) marked. For ERCP, the grading system focused primarily on the location and number of abnormal duct branches, with marked chronic pancreatitis also including other changes such as pancreatic duct stones, obstruction, and gland enlargement. Similar to the Marseille classification, the authors acknowledge that the clinical course does not always mirror morphological changes, especially early in a patient's clinical course.

Rosemont Classification

The Rosemont classification is an imaging-based classification system published in 2009 [8]. It was developed by a consensus group of 32 endoscopic ultrasound (EUS) practitioners from North America and Japan. The group anonymously voted on statements focused on definitions and the predictive value of features seen on EUS and whether each feature should be considered a major or minor feature. Major features were further subdivided into A and B categories based on their predictive value. The threshold for consensus was deemed to be two-thirds of the participants.

The features were classed as parenchymal or ductal. The parenchymal features in this classification system include at least three areas of hyperechogenicity >2 mm with shadowing (major A), three or more >5-mm lobules in the body or tail of the pancreas (major B if contiguous, minor if not), three or more hyperechoic areas

>3 mm without shadowing (minor), >2-mm cysts (minor), and three or more hyper-echoic lines at least 3-mm long running in two or more directions in the same plane (also called strands; minor). The ductal features include calculi in any part of the main pancreatic duct (deemed to be the most predictive feature; major A), irregular-ity of the main duct in the body or tail (minor), at least three dilated side branches >1 mm that connect to the main duct in the body or tail (minor), dilation (>3.5 mm in the body, >1.5 mm in the tail) of the main pancreatic duct (minor), and hyper-echogenicity of the main duct wall across at least 50% of the portion of the duct in the body and tail (minor). These features were then combined to create a diagnostic classification system with four categories: consistent with, suggestive of, or indeter-minate for chronic pancreatitis, and normal (Table 6.2).

TIGAR-O Classification

Unlike earlier published classification systems, the TIGAR-O system focuses on the etiology of chronic pancreatitis [9]. The authors of this system assert that other clas-sification methods focus on the end result of the pancreatic damage seen in patients with chronic pancreatitis, whereas a focus on etiology allows for more precision to predict disease progression and to manage these patients. The potential etiologies are divided into the following categories: toxic-metabolic, idiopathic, genetic, auto-immune, recurrent severe acute pancreatitis, and obstructive. Patients with multiple risk factors are categorized based on the risk factor associated with the highest risk of developing chronic pancreatitis. The toxic-metabolic category includes

Table 6.2 Summary of imaging findings in chronic pancreatitis in accordance with the Cambridge classification [7]

Grade	ERCP findings	US/CT findings
1. Normal	No abnormalities	No abnormalities
2. Equivocal	<3 abnormal branch ducts	Dilated main pancreatic duct, enlarged gland, cavities, ductal irregularities, acute pancreatitis, hyperechoic duct, irregular head/body of gland, or heterogeneous pancreatic parenchyma
3. Mild	>3 abnormal branch ducts	At least two of the above criteria
4. Moderate	Main pancreatic duct and branch duct abnormalities	At least two of the above criteria
5. Marked	Main pancreatic duct and branch duct abnormalities AND >1 cm cavity, enlarged gland-filling defects/stones, obstruction or stricture, or neighboring organ involvement	At least two of the above criteria

ERCP endoscopic retrograde cholangiopancreatography, *US* ultrasound, *CT* computed tomography pancreatitis due to alcohol consumption, smoking, hypercalcemia, hyperlipidemia, medications, toxins, and chronic kidney disease. The idiopathic category includes minimal change pancreatitis and tropical pancreatitis. The genetic category includes mutations in *PRSS1* (autosomal dominant), *CFTR* (autosomal recessive), and *SPINK1* (autosomal recessive). The autoimmune category includes conditions that can be associated with chronic pancreatitis, such as inflammatory bowel disease, primary biliary cirrhosis, primary sclerosing cholangitis, and Sjögren syndrome. Recurrent severe acute pancreatitis occurs when patients experience an incomplete recovery from attacks of acute pancreatitis. These recurrent attacks can be due to a number of causes, including alcohol and hyperlipidemia. The obstructive category includes obstructive features associated with chronic pancreatitis, such as tumors, sphincter of Oddi dysfunction, fibrosis causing duct obstruction, trauma, or ana-tomical abnormalities such as pancreatic divisum.

Although different etiologies may indeed necessitate different management strategies or present unique treatment options, this classification system addresses only one aspect of the disease and does not consider symptom severity or pancreatic dysfunction.

M-ANNHEIM Classification

The M-ANNHEIM classification, published in 2007, sought to create a unified clas-sification system that combined risk factors, severity, and clinical course [10]. Specifically, this system classifies pancreatitis by risk factors, clinical staging, diag-nostic criteria, imaging criteria, and severity scoring. Although comprehensive, this system is limited by the large amount of data needed to accurately classify patients and its overall complexity [1].

The risk factors are grouped as follows: alcohol use, nicotine use, nutritional, hereditary, efferent duct factors, immunologic, and miscellaneous/metabolic [10]. Alcohol use is stratified by intake per day, with moderate intake defined as <20 g ethanol, increased intake as 20–80 g ethanol, and excessive intake as >80 g ethanol. Smoking history is quantified in pack-years. Nutritional factors include a history of hyperlipidemia or a diet high in fat or protein. Genetic factors include mutations in *PRSS1*, *SPINK1*, and *CFTR*, as well as patients with an apparent autosomal domi-nant inheritance pattern without an identified gene mutation. This hereditary cate-gory also includes idiopathic and tropical pancreatitis. Efferent duct factors include features that lead to obstruction, such as tumors, scarring, sphincter of Oddi dys-function, pancreas divisum, and congenital abnormalities. The immunologic cate-gory includes autoimmune diseases that can lead to chronic pancreatitis, including inflammatory bowel disease, Sjögren syndrome, primary sclerosing cholangitis, and primary biliary cirrhosis. Miscellaneous/metabolic factors include hypercalcemia, chronic kidney disease, toxins, and medications.

The authors describe a clinical-stage classification that ranges from stage 0 to IV, with each stage being further subdivided. Stage 0 is subclinical and includes patients without chronic symptoms. This can include patients who never develop symptoms (stage 0a), those who have a single acute episode (stage 0b), and those who have an acute episode with complications (stage 0c). Stage I includes patients without evidence of exocrine or endocrine insufficiency and is subdivided into patients with recurrent acute episodes (stage Ia), those with pain between acute attacks (stage Ib), and those who meet stage Ia or Ib and also have complications (stage Ic). Stage II patients have evidence of partial exocrine or endocrine insufficiency (but not both). Stage IIa patients do not have associated pain, stage IIb patients do have associated pain, and stage IIc patients meet stage IIa or IIb criteria with complications. Stage III patients have both endocrine and exocrine insufficiency, with stage IIIa including patients with pain and stage IIIb including patients with complications. Stage IV represents pancreatic burnout. These patients do not have pain but have both endocrine and exocrine dysfunction with or without complications.

For diagnostic criteria, the authors classified patients as having definite, probable, or borderline chronic pancreatitis based on imaging, functional, and histological characteristics. Definite chronic pancreatitis is defined as a typical symptom history plus at least one of the following: calcifications, Cambridge 4 or 5 duct abnormalities, steatorrhea that improves with pancreatic enzyme replacement, or histologic changes consistent with chronic pancreatitis. Patients with probable chronic pancreatitis have one or more of the following features: Cambridge 3 duct abnormalities, recurrent pancreatic pseudocysts, abnormal exocrine function, or abnormal endocrine function. Patients with borderline chronic pancreatitis have a typical symptom history without any of the previously described criteria. Pancreatitis due to alcohol use is also included as a separate subcategory based on the daily intake amount.

The imaging criteria were determined using CT, magnetic resonance imaging, magnetic resonance cholangiopancreatography, or EUS. CT, magnetic resonance imaging (MRI), and magnetic resonance cholangiopancreatography (MRCP) criteria were based on the Cambridge classification, while EUS criteria included the size of the pancreas, the presence of cysts, hypoechoic or hyperechoic areas, lobulations, hyperechogenicity of the wall of the main duct, main duct dilation or irregularity, dilated side branch ducts, or calcifications. The authors classified CT, MRI, or MRCP imaging as normal (no abnormalities), equivocal (one abnormality), mild (at least two abnormalities with a normal main duct), moderate (at least two abnormalities, including minor changes to the main duct), or marked (two or more abnormalities, with one of the "marked" criteria from the Cambridge classification). They proposed that EUS examinations with one to four abnormal findings should be classified as equivocal/mild, whereas those with at least five abnormal findings should be classified as moderate/marked.

The severity index assigns a numeric score in each of the following categories: subjective pain, use of pain medications, need for surgery, exocrine insufficiency, endocrine insufficiency, staging based on imaging, and presence of complications. Each category is scaled from 0 to 4, with complications and surgical interventions able to be counted multiple times if they occurred multiple times in the patient's clinical course. This generates a total score, with 0–5 points correlating to minor severity or M-ANNHEIM A, 6–10 points as increased severity or M-ANNHIEM B, 11–15 points as advanced severity or M-ANNHEIM C, 16–20 points as marked severity or M-ANNHEIM D, and >20 points as exacerbated severity or M-ANNHEIM E.

All these criteria taken together make up the M-ANNHEIM classification system. The authors stated that their goal was to create a comprehensive, simple-to-use system to classify patients with chronic pancreatitis to more easily compare patients' clinical courses and treatments. They also theorized that this system could be used to identify trends in disease progression from different etiologies. However, given the number of parameters included, this system is somewhat cumbersome for routine use.

ABC Classification

The ABC classification system was developed as a simple, noninvasive way to stratify patients with pancreatitis by disease severity, with the goal to group patients by clinical stage to determine treatment needs [11]. Patients are placed in group A if they have no pain, group B if they have pain but no complications, and group C if they have pain and complications. Complications include pseudocysts, obstruction of the biliary system or duodenum, portal hypertension, pancreatic ascites, and cancer. Each of the groups is further subdivided based on functional impairment (no impairment, endocrine only, exocrine only, or both endocrine and exocrine). Of note, this system does not include any imaging characteristics and, instead, focuses on the symptoms of pain and pancreatic insufficiency. The authors state that this is because imaging findings can be nonspecific and do not necessarily correlate with disease severity. This focus on symptomatology rather than imaging may make this a more clinically relevant classification system though it is also limited by its narrow focus.

Manchester Classification

The Manchester classification was developed as a clinical system and divides patients with pancreatitis into three stages based on symptoms and disease complications [12]. The authors retrospectively identified 41 patients with radiographic evidence of chronic pancreatitis (by MRCP, CT, or ERCP) and classified them into mild, moderate, or end-stage disease. Patients were categorized as mild if they had pain but did not require frequent pain medication. These patients also had preserved pancreatic functions (both endocrine and exocrine) and did not have any complications. Patients with moderate disease had pain that required at least weekly pain medication, and some level of pancreatic dysfunction, but no complications. Patients with end-stage disease had diabetes or steatorrhea, as well as evidence of a complication related to chronic pancreatitis, such as portal hypertension, duodenal stenosis, or stricture in the biliary tree.

Based on this classification method, 44% of the patients studied had mild disease, 46% had moderate disease, and 10% had end-stage disease. The authors then reviewed 10 years of clinical records for these patients and reclassified them to determine the amount of disease progression during this time period. After 10 years, no patients were considered to have mild disease. The rates of diabetes and steatorrhea also increased dramatically over the study period. At the initial time point, 5% of patients had steatorrhea, and this number rose to 27% at the 10-year time point. Initially, 5% of patients had diabetes, and this number rose to 61% by the end of the 10-year study period.

One of the strengths of this system is that it captures the progression of clinical disease that patients experience. It also considers that pain may not be present in end-stage disease without excluding patients who continue to experience pain. It is somewhat limited by its design, having been developed retrospectively and based on referrals to a tertiary care center. Its applicability may also be limited, as the majority of patients (78%) had disease resulting from alcohol use.

Heidelberg Classification

The Heidelberg classification sought to provide a simple method of categorizing patients with pancreatitis that would offer insight into treatment and prognosis, similar to the Child–Pugh classification in liver disease [13]. The Heidelberg system combines clinical and radiographic criteria for diagnosis and stratifies patients by disease severity (Table 6.3). Stage A is considered early chronic pancreatitis. These patients may have pain or recurrent acute episodes, but they do not exhibit disease complications. Patients in stage A also have overall preservation of their pancreatic function although they have mild dysfunction without overt symptoms. For example, these patients may have abnormal glucose tolerance without diabetes or mildly impaired exocrine function without steatorrhea.

Stage B is the intermediate stage. Patients in this group again have overall preservation of pancreatic function (no diabetes or steatorrhea) but have experienced complications of chronic pancreatitis. These complications include biliary or duodenal obstruction, vascular occlusion, clinically significant pseudocysts, pancreatic fistula or ascites, or a complication that impacts a neighboring organ (such as the spleen or colon). Stage C is considered an end-stage disease and is further subdivided into three categories: C1, patients with endocrine dysfunction (i.e., diabetes); C2, patients with exocrine dysfunction (i.e., steatorrhea); and C3, patients with both endocrine and exocrine dysfunction with or without complications.

The authors applied their classification system to 191 patients and then restaged the patients every 6 months for 3 years. They found that, at each time point, approximately 4% of patients had developed new disease complications, which suggested a steady rate of disease progression. However, all patients had received operative

Table 6.3 Summary of the Rosemont classification [8]

	Features
Consistent with chronic pancreatitis	– 1 Major A and ≥3 minor – 1 Major A and Major B – 2 Major A
Suggestive of chronic pancreatitis	– 1 Major A and <3 minor – Major B and ≥3 minor – At least 5 minor
Indeterminate for chronic pancreatitis	– 0 Major and 3–4 minor – Major B – Major B and <3 minor
Normal	– 0 Major and 0–2 minor

Major A criteria: at least three areas of hyperechogenicity >2 mm with shadowing; calculi in any part of the main pancreatic duct
Major B criteria: three or more contiguous >5-mm lobules in the body or tail of the pancreas
Minor criteria: three or more noncontiguous >5-mm lobules in the body or tail of the pancreas; three or more hyperechoic areas >3 mm without shadowing; >2-mm cysts; three or more hyperechoic lines at least 3-mm long running in two or more directions in the same plane; irregularity of the main duct in the body or tail; at least three dilated side branches >1 mm that connect to the main duct in the body or tail; dilation (>3.5 mm in the body, >1.5 mm in the tail) of the main pancreatic duct; hyperechogenicity of the main duct wall across at least 50% of the portion of the duct in the body and tail

Table 6.4 Summary of the Heidelberg classification [13]

Stage	Description
A	– Early chronic pancreatitis – Pain, recurrent acute pancreatitis episodes without complications – Preserved pancreatic function
B	– Intermediate – Preserved pancreatic function – Complications present (e.g., biliary or duodenal obstruction, vascular occlusion, clinically significant pseudocysts, pancreatic fistula or ascites, or a complication impacting a neighboring organ)
C	– End-stage – C1: endocrine dysfunction – C2: exocrine dysfunction – C3: both endocrine and exocrine dysfunction ± complications

intervention for their disease, so this trend of progression may not be indicative of the general population of patients with chronic pancreatitis (Table 6.4).

Chronic Pancreatitis Prognosis Score Classification

The COPPS was developed to evaluate the risk of hospital admission for patients with chronic pancreatitis and was modeled after the Child–Pugh score in liver disease [14]. This system uses multiple subjective and objective variables to generate a score that is correlated to a disease stage. The authors examined clinical, laboratory, and imaging variables and identified correlations with hospital readmissions over a 12-month period. These initial variables included levels of hemoglobin A1c, total and conjugated bilirubin, stool elastase, alanine aminotransferase (ALT), gamma-glutamyl transferase (GGT), international normalized ratio (INR), albumin, C-reactive protein (CRP), platelets, urea, mean corpuscular volume (MCV), and triglycerides, and the Cambridge score, pain rating, and body mass index (BMI).

Of these, only BMI and levels of hemoglobin A1c, CRP, and platelets correlated to hospital readmission. The authors included the pain rating in the scoring system because of its impact on patient quality of life, despite the lack of correlation to hospital readmission. Patients could receive 1–3 points for each variable, which depended on the reference ranges set by the authors based on an initial cohort of 91 patients, for a maximum of 15 points on this scale. Patients were considered to be COPPS A if they had 5–6 points, COPPS B with 7–9 points, and COPPS C with 10–15 points. In this initial cohort, the COPPS stage correlated with hospital readmissions (both in general and for pancreas-specific reasons), number of days spent in the hospital, and number of endoscopic treatments performed.

The authors then validated this scoring system in a second cohort of 129 patients, with similar results. This system is distinct from the other classification systems previously discussed in that it was developed using prospective recruitment of patients. However, the COPPS is limited in scope, as it only includes hospitalized patients and so may not be widely applicable.

Medical Management of Chronic Pancreatitis

Chronic pancreatitis is a complicated disease that can be very difficult to treat, given the number of etiologies, presenting symptoms, and lack of correlation between imaging and clinical course. The lack of a widely accepted classification system also contributes to the complexity of patient management. Overall, medical management is the first step to treat chronic pancreatitis and primarily focuses on reduction of the frequency of acute episodes, reduction of patient symptoms, and management of the effects of pancreatic dysfunction. A summary of treatment modalities is given in Fig. 6.1.

Reducing Frequency of Acute Pancreatitis

Acute episodes of pancreatitis can lead to chronic pancreatitis or worsen symptoms in those with chronic pancreatitis. Therefore, reduction in the frequency of these attacks is an important component of the medical management of pancreatitis [15]. Risk factor modification is the main method to reduce the frequency of acute attacks. Alcohol use is the primary modifiable risk factor for chronic pancreatitis, as it is one

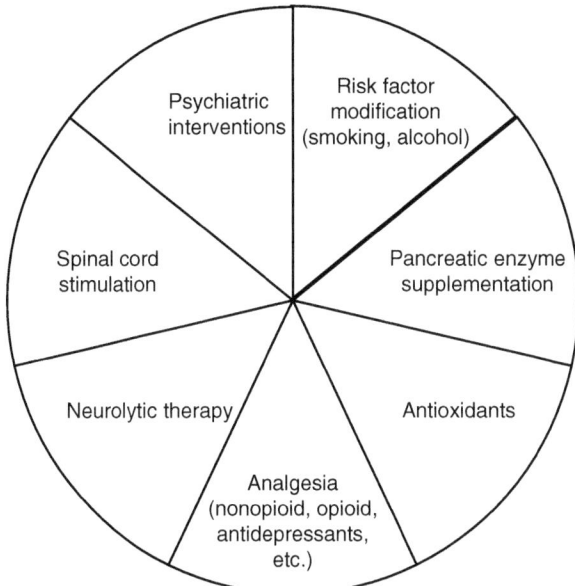

Fig. 6.1 Options for medical management of chronic pancreatitis, addressing pain, endocrine dysfunction, exocrine dysfunction, and nutritional deficiencies

of the most common etiologies for chronic pancreatitis and also leads to recurrent episodes of acute pancreatitis [16]. Therefore, cessation of alcohol use is recommended in patients with chronic pancreatitis or those at risk for its development caused by known genetic factors [15]. Similarly, smoking cessation is also recommended for these patients. While it was previously believed that the apparent link between smoking and chronic pancreatitis was due to the confounding effect of alcohol use, smoking has now been shown to be an independent risk factor for the development of chronic pancreatitis as well as for episodes of acute pancreatitis [17, 18].

Pain

Pain remains one of the most difficult symptoms to manage, especially in complicated disease processes like chronic pancreatitis, despite the availability of a wide range of pain management options [15]. Pain significantly impacts on patients' quality of life, which can be improved by reducing the frequency and intensity of attacks. Pain in patients with chronic pancreatitis can be caused by pancreatic inflammation, complications of the disease, or even neurogenic causes. Thus, medical management may need to be tailored to the individual patient and requires a multimodal approach.

The first step in the treatment of pain due to chronic pancreatitis is pain assessment. Several pain severity assessment tools have been validated in patients with chronic pancreatitis. The Brief Pain Inventory is one such tool and has been used in patients with chronic pain from a wide range of causes, including chronic pancreatitis [19]. Although the Brief Pain Inventory does include an assessment of pain severity, it also assesses how pain affects a patient's mood, sleep, ability to work, and relationships. This tool has been found to correlate well with the overall quality of life in patients with chronic pancreatitis. The McGill Pain Questionnaire is another tool that focuses on more than disease severity [20]. It uses descriptors of a patient's pain and asks the patient to choose from a list of words that apply to their pain and then to further describe their pain as mild, moderate, or severe [21]. Most of the pain descriptors are conventional words describing physical sensations, such as sharp, stabbing, and cramping, but others address other aspects of pain, including emotional responses, such as exhaustion, fear, cruelty, and sickening.

Quantitative sensory testing has also been used in patients with chronic pancreatitis to determine treatment effects [15]. Quantitative sensory testing involves the presentation of standardized noxious stimuli to patients and the evaluation of their responses. In patients with chronic pancreatitis, this method has allowed the comparison of treatment options and their effects on pain. For example, visceral pain is better managed by oxycodone than by morphine [22], and pregabalin can reduce patient hypersensitivity caused by central sensitization [23].

As described above, risk factor modification can be used as one facet of pain management in patients with chronic pancreatitis [15]. Alcohol abstinence is associated with a reduction in frequency of acute pancreatitis episodes. Smoking also correlates with an increase in acute episodes, but no studies have specifically examined a link between smoking cessation and a reduction in pain in patients with chronic pancreatitis.

Supplementation with pancreatic enzymes may also reduce pain. In healthy individuals, nutrient ingestion leads to secretion of cholecystokinin-releasing factor, which stimulates the release of cholecystokinin, which triggers normal pancreatic secretions. Some patients with chronic pancreatitis have an obstructed pancreatic duct; thus, ongoing pancreatic secretion stimulated by nutrient ingestion is hypothesized to increase pressure in the duct, which causes pain. However, supplemental pancreatic enzymes degrade cholecystokinin-releasing factor, preventing downstream pancreatic secretion. Several studies have shown a reduction in pain in patients treated with tablets of supplemental pancreatic enzymes, whereas several studies have shown no benefit [24]. However, the studies that showed no benefit used capsules that may not have dissolved in the duodenum because of an acid-protective coating [15].

Antioxidant therapy has also been shown to reduce pain in patients with chronic pancreatitis [25]. Specifically, combination therapy with β-carotene, vitamins C and E, selenium, and methionine leads to pain relief, whereas treatment with a single antioxidant has no significant benefit [15]. Combination antioxidant therapy with pregabalin has also been shown to reduce pain in patients who suffer from recurrent pain despite endoscopic or surgical intervention [26].

More traditional pain management options also exist. The World Health Organization provides a framework for escalation of pain management that was initially developed for the management of chronic pain in cancer patients [27]. The first level uses nonopioid medications, including acetaminophen, ibuprofen, and pregabalin. Antidepressants, which have been successfully used in patients with pain from neuropathic causes, are also included in this level. The second level uses weak opiates, such as tramadol or codeine, with or without the non-opiate medications from the first level. The third level includes stronger opiate medications, such as morphine, oxycodone, and methadone. Other medications such as octreotide, ketamine, benzodiazepines, clonidine, cannabinoids, and antipsychotics are also used as adjuvants at any level to assist in pain management.

Neurolytic therapy, such as a celiac plexus block, can also be used to control a patient's pain if other treatment options fail, but this is only a short-acting option with a risk of side effects [15]. Spinal cord stimulators have also been studied in patients with chronic pancreatitis, and most patients experiencing relief from pain using this method [28]. However, this option is invasive and carries the risk of complications from placement in the spinal cord region [15]. Transcranial magnetic stimulation has been studied as a treatment for depression in patients with chronic pancreatitis and may also have some effect on pain levels [29]. Psychiatric interventions, such as cognitive behavioral therapy and hypnosis, have also been successfully used in the management of chronic pain, but there is minimal data for their use in patients with chronic pancreatitis [15].

Endocrine Dysfunction

Endocrine dysfunction from chronic pancreatitis results in type 3c diabetes, also known as pancreatogenic diabetes [30]. Patients with type 3c diabetes also have impaired glucagon and pancreatic polypeptide secretion. This leads to low insulin sensitivity in the liver, which then increases glucose production. Patients with type 3c diabetes from chronic pancreatitis tend to have more brittle diabetes than patients with type 2 diabetes. The incidence of diabetes increases with the duration of chronic pancreatitis, and diabetes is also more common in patients who have undergone pancreatectomy. Management of endocrine dysfunction in patients with chronic pancreatitis requires close attention to nutrition and blood glucose levels. Patients must be especially careful to avoid hypo- and hyperglycemic episodes.

Exocrine Dysfunction

Exocrine dysfunction from chronic pancreatitis is a result of the loss of the acinar cells that normally produce pancreatic enzymes [30]. Steatorrhea is the hallmark of pancreatic exocrine dysfunction and puts these patients at a high risk of fat-soluble vitamin deficiencies and malnutrition. Steatorrhea occurs due to lipase deficiency, which leads to poor fat breakdown and malabsorption, therefore increasing fat excretion in stool. Symptoms include fatty diarrhea, cramping, bloating, and flatulence. It is important to note that subclinical exocrine dysfunction can also occur. Exocrine dysfunction can be diagnosed in several ways. Lipase secretion following hormone administration can be assessed by intubation of the duodenum, but this is an invasive option. More commonly, levels of fecal fat or fecal elastase-1 are measured.

The mainstay of treatment of exocrine dysfunction in patients with chronic pancreatitis is the replacement of pancreatic enzymes. Administration of these enzymes to patients results in improved fat breakdown and reduced malabsorption, leading to improved nutrition. As previously discussed, enzyme replacement may have the added benefit of pain reduction in this population. As the pancreas produces less bicarbonate under conditions of chronic pancreatitis, patients may also require acid-suppression treatment in order to reduce denaturation of pancreatic enzymes. In addition, enzyme replacement should be uptitrated as needed, as many patients may be inadvertently undertreated.

It was previously believed that patients must have a loss of at least 90% of their pancreatic function to exhibit signs of exocrine dysfunction [31], but the study that this is based on compared only patients with severe symptoms of exocrine dysfunction with healthy controls. Therefore, this study may have missed important information from patients with milder symptoms or even subclinical dysfunction [30]. There may be a delay in the management of exocrine dysfunction in patients with mild or subclinical exocrine dysfunction who may benefit from enzyme replacement.

Nutritional Deficiencies

Patients with chronic pancreatitis frequently suffer from nutritional deficiencies [30]. This can result from recurrent pain, ongoing alcoholism, and other gastrointestinal symptoms resulting from complications of the disease itself or medications used to manage it. Patients may have reduced muscle mass [30] and can be underweight, with the authors of the COPPS system noting an inverse relationship between BMI and severity of chronic pancreatitis [14]. Patients with chronic pancreatitis also suffer from osteopenia and osteoporosis as a result of low dietary vitamin D and calcium and chronic inflammation.

Chronic pancreatitis can also lead to poor absorption of fat-soluble vitamins, including vitamins A, D, E, and K, resulting in vitamin deficiencies. The quantification of vitamin deficiency incidence varies widely and has primarily focused on laboratory-identified deficiencies rather than clinically significant deficiencies. Clinical manifestations of various vitamin deficiencies in patients with chronic pancreatitis have been published as case reports [32–34], but the true incidence of significant vitamin deficiencies in patients with chronic pancreatitis is unknown [30].

Conclusion

Overall, chronic pancreatitis remains a challenge to classify and manage. While several classification systems have been proposed, they focus on a wide range of factors with varying degrees of clinical relevance, including imaging findings, clinical symptoms, laboratory tests, etiology, etc. These classification systems are also limited in that the majority have not been prospectively validated or tested in a multi-institutional setting. In addition, many of these classification systems only group patients with common findings, without providing guidance on treatment or prognosis. These limitations have likely contributed to the lack of a widely accepted and utilized classification system for this disease process. Medical management of chronic pancreatitis often requires a multi-pronged approach, targeting pain, endocrine dysfunction, exocrine dysfunction, and nutrition. Patients may present with varying degrees of these symptoms, necessitating individualized treatment plans.

References

1. Rahman A, O'Connor DB, Gather F, Koscic S, Gilgan J, Mockler D, et al. Clinical classification and severity scoring systems in chronic pancreatitis: a systematic review. Dig Surg. 2020;37(3):181–91.
2. Banks PA, Bollen TL, Dervenis C, Gooszen HG, Johnson CD, Sarr MG, et al. Classification of acute pancreatitis—2012: revision of the Atlanta classification and definitions by international consensus. Gut. 2013;62(1):102–11.
3. Blamey SL, Imrie CW, O'Neill J, Gilmour WH, Carter DC. Prognostic factors in acute pancreatitis. Gut. 1984;25(12):1340–6.
4. Ranson JH, Pasternack BS. Statistical methods for quantifying the severity of clinical acute pancreatitis. J Surg Res. 1977;22(2):79–91.
5. Larvin M, McMahon MJ. APACHE-II score for assessment and monitoring of acute pancreatitis. Lancet. 1989;2(8656):201–5.
6. Sarles H. Revised classification of pancreatitis—Marseille 1984. Dig Dis Sci. 1985;30(6):573–4.
7. Sarner M, Cotton PB. Classification of pancreatitis. Gut. 1984;25(7):756–9.
8. Catalano MF, Sahai A, Levy M, Romagnuolo J, Wiersema M, Brugge W, et al. EUS-based criteria for the diagnosis of chronic pancreatitis: the Rosemont classification. Gastrointest Endosc. 2009;69(7):1251–61.
9. Etemad B, Whitcomb DC. Chronic pancreatitis: diagnosis, classification, and new genetic developments. Gastroenterology. 2001;120(3):682–707.
10. Schneider A, Löhr JM, Singer MV. The M-ANNHEIM classification of chronic pancreatitis: introduction of a unifying classification system based on a review of previous classifications of the disease. J Gastroenterol. 2007;42(2):101–19.
11. Bank S, Singh P, Pooran N. Proposal for a new grading system for chronic pancreatitis: the ABC system. J Clin Gastroenterol. 2002;35(1):3–4.
12. Bagul A, Siriwardena AK. Evaluation of the Manchester classification system for chronic pancreatitis. Jop. 2006;7(4):390–6.
13. Büchler MW, Martignoni ME, Friess H, Malfertheiner P. A proposal for a new clinical classification of chronic pancreatitis. BMC Gastroenterol. 2009;9:93.

14. Beyer G, Mahajan UM, Budde C, Bulla TJ, Kohlmann T, Kuhlmann L, et al. Development and validation of a chronic pancreatitis prognosis score in 2 independent cohorts. Gastroenterology. 2017;153(6):1544–54.e2.
15. Drewes AM, Bouwense SAW, Campbell CM, Ceyhan GO, Delhaye M, Demir IE, et al. Guidelines for the understanding and management of pain in chronic pancreatitis. Pancreatology. 2017;17(5):720–31.
16. Samokhvalov AV, Rehm J, Roerecke M. Alcohol consumption as a risk factor for acute and chronic pancreatitis: a systematic review and a series of meta-analyses. EBioMedicine. 2015;2(12):1996–2002.
17. Maisonneuve P, Lowenfels AB, Müllhaupt B, Cavallini G, Lankisch PG, Andersen JR, et al. Cigarette smoking accelerates progression of alcoholic chronic pancreatitis. Gut. 2005;54(4):510–4.
18. Yuhara H, Ogawa M, Kawaguchi Y, Igarashi M, Mine T. Smoking and risk for acute pancreatitis: a systematic review and meta-analysis. Pancreas. 2014;43(8):1201–7.
19. Olesen SS, Juel J, Nielsen AK, Frøkjær JB, Wilder-Smith OH, Drewes AM. Pain severity reduces life quality in chronic pancreatitis: Implications for design of future outcome trials. Pancreatology. 2014;14(6):497–502.
20. Seicean A, Grigorescu M, Tanţău M, Dumitraşcu DL, Pop D, Mocan T. Pain in chronic pancreatitis: assessment and relief through treatment. Rom J Gastroenterol. 2004;13(1):9–15.
21. Melzack R. The McGill Pain Questionnaire: major properties and scoring methods. Pain. 1975;1(3):277–99.
22. Staahl C, Dimcevski G, Andersen SD, Thorsgaard N, Christrup LL, Arendt-Nielsen L, et al. Differential effect of opioids in patients with chronic pancreatitis: an experimental pain study. Scand J Gastroenterol. 2007;42(3):383–90.
23. Bouwense SA, Olesen SS, Drewes AM, Poley JW, van Goor H, Wilder-Smith OH. Effects of pregabalin on central sensitization in patients with chronic pancreatitis in a randomized, controlled trial. PLoS One. 2012;7(8):e42096.
24. Warshaw AL, Banks PA, Fernández-Del CC. AGA technical review: treatment of pain in chronic pancreatitis. Gastroenterology. 1998;115(3):765–76.
25. Ahmed Ali U, Jens S, Busch OR, Keus F, van Goor H, Gooszen HG, et al. Antioxidants for pain in chronic pancreatitis. Cochrane Database Syst Rev. 2014;(8):Cd008945.
26. Talukdar R, Lakhtakia S, Nageshwar Reddy D, Rao GV, Pradeep R, Banerjee R, et al. Ameliorating effect of antioxidants and pregabalin combination in pain recurrence after ductal clearance in chronic pancreatitis: results of a randomized, double blind, placebo-controlled trial. J Gastroenterol Hepatol. 2016;31(9):1654–62.
27. Jadad AR, Browman GP. The WHO analgesic ladder for cancer pain management. Stepping up the quality of its evaluation. JAMA. 1995;274(23):1870–3.
28. Kapural L, Cywinski JB, Sparks DA. Spinal cord stimulation for visceral pain from chronic pancreatitis. Neuromodulation. 2011;14(5):423–6; discussion 6–7
29. Fregni F, Potvin K, Dasilva D, Wang X, Lenkinski RE, Freedman SD, et al. Clinical effects and brain metabolic correlates in non-invasive cortical neuromodulation for visceral pain. Eur J Pain. 2011;15(1):53–60.
30. Duggan SN. Negotiating the complexities of exocrine and endocrine dysfunction in chronic pancreatitis. Proc Nutr Soc. 2017;76(4):484–94.
31. DiMagno EP, Go VL, Summerskill WH. Relations between pancreatic enzyme outputs and malabsorption in severe pancreatic insufficiency. N Engl J Med. 1973;288(16):813–5.
32. Yokota T, Tsuchiya K, Furukawa T, Tsukagoshi H, Miyakawa H, Hasumura Y. Vitamin E deficiency in acquired fat malabsorption. J Neurol. 1990;237(2):103–6.
33. Reynaert H, Debeuckelaere S, De Waele B, Meysman M, Goossens A, Devis G. The brown bowel syndrome and gastrointestinal adenocarcinoma. Two complications of vitamin E deficiency in celiac sprue and chronic pancreatitis? J Clin Gastroenterol. 1993;16(1):48–51.
34. Kurtulmus N, Yarman S, Tanakol R, Alagol F. Severe osteomalacia in a patient with idiopathic chronic pancreatitis. Scott Med J. 2005;50(4):172–3.

Chapter 7
Chronic Pancreatitis: Drainage Procedures (Open Vs. MIS)

Dhiresh Rohan Jeyarajah and Houssam G. Osman

Background

In the West, chronic pancreatitis (CP) is mostly seen in patients with alcohol abuse as well as smoking. However, CP can develop in patients for other reasons including genetic predisposition (hereditary pancreatitis), tropical pancreatitis, and pancreas divisum. It is important to note that biliary pancreatitis does not lead to CP in the absence of disconnected pancreatic duct which can result in recurrent pancreatitis attacks. The common end pathway is calcification of the gland itself, or stone formation within the pancreatic ducts, that do not allow for adequate drainage of the exocrine function of the gland. This results in inflammation, initially, and then a cycle of scarring and fibrosis that can result in large duct or small duct obstruction. There is associated irritation of the nerves in the retroperitoneum that results in a dull, boring, and unrelenting pain that typically radiates to the back. This is truly miserable for the patient and abstinence from alcohol or tobacco may improve some of the inflammatory changes but will not completely reverse it. This nerve pain can be managed in many ways, mostly using a combination of NSAID, narcotic, and nerve stabilizing agents such as gabapentin. Intervention with celiac ganglia blockade can be achieved with endoscopic ultrasound guidance or percutaneously. Psychiatric medications may be needed to manage the anxiety and depression that comes with chronic pain. Psychological tools, such as cognitive behavioral therapy (CBP) or biofeedback, can be very helpful in providing coping strategies for the patient with CP. It is imperative that the pancreatic surgeon have a working

D. R. Jeyarajah (✉)
Department of Surgery, Methodist Health System, Dallas, TX, USA

Department of Surgery, TCU Burnett School of Medicine, Fort Worth, USA
e-mail: drj@tscsurgical.com

H. G. Osman
Department of Surgery, Methodist Health System, Dallas, TX, USA

E. P. Ceppa et al. (eds.), *The SAGES Manual of Evolving Techniques in Pancreatic Surgery*, https://doi.org/10.1007/978-3-031-78409-5_7

knowledge of non-surgical management of chronic pain. One of the most common issues with these CP patients is the lack of insight into management of their pain syndrome. Unexperienced physicians will often withhold analgesics for patients that have been on high doses of narcotics at home; weaning a patient from their pain medications is not appropriate in the immediate postoperative period or during an admission for an acute episode of pancreatitis.

Exocrine pancreatic insufficiency (EPI) is a common and unrecognized issue with patients with CP. The usual manifestation of greasy stools can be easily identified by the caring physician. However, many caregivers miss that increased gas, bloating, and looser stools that float may indeed be a manifestation of EPI. Aggressive treatment of the EPI symptoms is essential in the CP patient. The authors will commonly find that the bathroom that the EPI patient uses cannot be used by any family member for days after the patient has used it! Such is the manifestation of fat malabsorption that makes stool smell so odious. The authors ask the patient to increase their pancreatic enzymes until they reach constipation, and then back off slightly. Constipation will occur when there is minimal fat content in the stool and is an easy sign that the patient has reached a state of fat absorption. Conversely, eating a high fat meal will require an increase in pancreatic enzyme supplementation. Many of these patients need to gain weight and avoiding all fat will make this tough. Of course, in the patient who has high triglycerides driving the CP process, the patient must be on a triglyceride lowering agent and obey a low-fat diet. Many of these patients will be diabetic also, and triglycerides will rise with blood sugar, making blood sugar control a critical element to their CP management.

Associated with EPI is vitamin malabsorption and, much like the post bariatric surgery patient, the CP patient must be watched carefully for vitamin deficiencies. The authors routinely place these patients on bariatric multivitamin replacement and check bariatric labs on an ongoing basis.

Endocrine insufficiency must also be watched carefully. The pancreatic surgeon must have a working knowledge of the current state of diabetic management, especially a grasp of the several types of insulin on the market. The CP patient may have delayed gastric emptying (DGE) based on pancreatic inflammation and diabetes mellitus (DM); one must use a fast-acting insulin in this case and evaluate glycemia 30 min after the meal to ensure that the patient does not become hypoglycemic. Questioning the patient regarding their "lows" will indicate how much glucagon "window" is available from the native pancreas. This will give the surgeon an idea of whether a total pancreatectomy will cause any disturbance to the existing glycemic control. The presence of significant swings in blood sugar with low readings frequently will tell the surgeon that the pancreas is effectively burnt out with lack of both insulin and glucagon production. In this case, the authors are more likely to consider total pancreatectomy. Understanding the severity of the patient's DM will help guide the pancreatic surgeon in selecting from the surgical options for therapy. The holistic approach to the patient with CP is critical. The authors attempt to identify a single idea that captures what success looks like for each patient. This cannot be a surgical measure of success, but rather a quality-of-life measure. For example, the patient enjoys playing with their grandchildren and wishes that to be their main aspect to return to after surgery. Returning to this activity would be the true endpoint of success, not a surgical outcome per se.

Indications for Surgery in the CP Patient

As has been the case for decades, the indication for surgery in the CP patient remains to treat pain or complications (e.g., bile duct obstruction, gastric outlet obstruction). Drainage procedures will allow preservation of pancreatic parenchyma with its exocrine and endocrine function compared to surgical resection, but there is no good data to support the suggestion that drainage procedures will allow for reversal of EPI or endocrine already lost. As such, it is important that the pancreatic surgeon counsel the patient and caregivers carefully with regard to the specific indication for surgery. The authors are careful to be very specific in the expectations for resolution of pain. In addition to the type of surgery performed, the pathophysiology of pain in a specific patient and abstinence from alcohol and tobacco play a major role in pain score improvement following surgery and duration of that improvement. The pain relief will take months and the patient must be prepared for this slow weaning off pain medications. This is a process that will be frustrating for all involved and clear expectations must be laid out at the start of the surgery planning. The authors will increase the dosing of gabapentin to 300 mg TID to maximize non-narcotic effects and nerve stabilizing effects. They will also add an SSRI, where appropriate, and try to encourage the patient and family to seek counseling for non-pharmacologic measures that can be very helpful. Working with a pain management physician is very helpful. However, this has become a real challenge as many anesthesia-pain management doctors have closed their practices in the private world. The surgeon who deals with these patients must have a working knowledge of pain management. Typically, the author will maximize non-narcotic medications. They will then add a shorter acting narcotic and eventually ramp up to a long-acting agent (usually fentanyl patch that lasts for 3 days with a constant level of drug), an intermediate acting agent, such as oxycontin ER, which lasts for 12 h, and a shorter acting agent that will be used for breakthrough pain, such as hydrocodone. The plan for weaning will be to gradually decrease the longest acting agent first and gradually work down to the short-acting agent. The aim is to gradually close the patients "pain gates" that have been wide open for a while with their chronic pain. The patients are counseled about the importance of quitting alcohol prior to surgical intervention. Smoking cessation is paramount to successful outcome and is considered a requirement by the authors prior to surgical intervention in CP patients.

A rare indication for surgery, but one that deserves some discussion, is the prevention of cancer. This can be an area of discussion for the hereditary pancreatitis and the tropical pancreatitis patient. The authors are reticent to take a non-diabetic patient and perform a total pancreatectomy. However, it is usual that the patients in these group have brittle DM by the time that they ask for this discussion. The authors have limited personal experience with total pancreatectomy in each of these groups. When this has been performed, the patients follow the recovery of any total pancreatectomy patient.

Procedures and Technical Details

Operative Approach for Pancreatic Ductal Drainage

The patient that is well suited for a drainage procedure is one that has chronic pain and a large, dilated main pancreatic duct (PD), but absence of inflammatory pseudotumor in the pancreatic head, that is often the dominant morphologic abnormality in CP. Pancreatic head inflammatory masses may be accompanied by biliary or duodenal obstruction, which also represent contraindications to a decompressive surgical approach. In fact, drainage procedures are less invasive compared to resection and aim at simply decompressing a dilated PD but fail to tackle situations where biliary or duodenal obstruction represents the "pacemaker," propagating pain development in the disease. The general thought in the choice of a drainage procedure is the presence of a PD greater than 7 mm in size. However, the duct can always be found even if smaller using several techniques that will be outlined below. A patient with such a favorable duct is shown in Fig. 7.1.

The most commonly performed decompressive procedures described in the literature include the Puestow procedure [1] and the Partington and Rochelle modification [2]. Both procedures include the transverse opening of the PD from tail to body followed by a lateral pancreaticojejunostomy. The original Puestow procedure also included pancreatic tail resection and splenectomy.

The Frey procedure (named for Charles Frey and first described by Frey and Smith) [3] is often referred to as a combined resection and drainage surgery but is substantially a variant of the Puestow procedure and can be considered a drainage procedure carried out more proximally to further decompress the PD. The primary purpose of the local resection in the Frey procedure is not to remove the inflamed tissue from the pancreatic head, but rather to "core out" the pancreatic parenchyma, which can improve the exposure of the proximal duct and facilitate the lateral

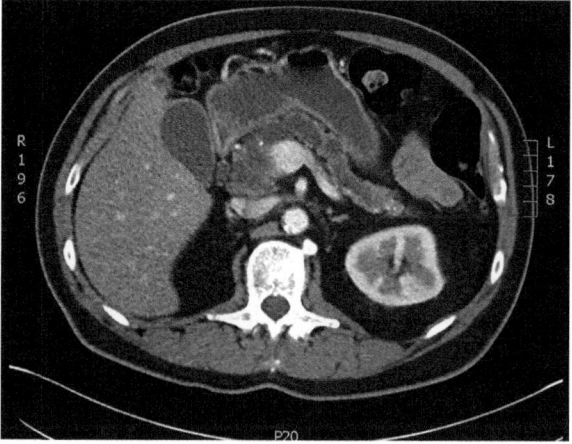

Fig. 7.1 Chronic pancreatitis patient with dilated pancreatic duct

pancreaticojejunostomy by preventing the dense pancreatic head tissue from naturally closing the longitudinal incision made in this part of the duct.

Preparation of the Patient

The patient is usually prepared through the ERAS pathway. This includes aggressive prehabilitation with physical therapy and nutritional interventions, especially in malnourished patients. The patient is started on gabapentin which is increased to at least 900 mg/day. They are then given a high carbohydrate drink 2 h prior to surgery unless they are diabetic or have DGE. In these latter cases, the patient is kept NPO for at least 8 h.

On the morning of the surgery, the patient's abdomen is clipped in the preoperative area, and they receive Alvimopan and Acetaminophen. They are taken to the surgical suite where appropriate antibiotics are given for a case that will involve entering the gastrointestinal tract.

The patient is generally positioned supine on the operating table with the right arm tucked. This allows for the self-retaining retractor to be positioned high enough on the bed that it will be out of the way of the operating surgeon standing on the patient's right side. In addition, when there are other learners in the room, they can comfortably stand above the surgeon on the right side without straddling an outstretched arm.

The surgeon must ensure that all anesthesia lines are not in the way of the railing on the side of the bed; this will result in cutting of critical lines when placing the retractor.

Operative Technique—Open Approach.

A midline incision is made in most circumstances. If the patient is very obese, a left-leaning bilateral subcostal incision may be necessary. In this case, the left arm is tucked so that the retractor can be placed on the left side of the patient and achieve greatest leftward retraction. The authors favor the former incision as closure is more straightforward; this exposure can be used in the future for other surgeries, and midline hernia repairs are more straightforward than a subcostal hernia. Important elements to placing the retractors are:

1. Place the post of the retractor far enough towards the patient's head, but do not place the post on the headpiece. This will tilt the headpiece upward when the blades are placed.
2. Angle the retractor bars downward so that the surgeons do not have to operate over the bars.
3. Achieve the greatest traction with the blades on the side that needs the greatest—left sided for left-sided surgery. Do not over-retract in the other direction as this will not allow for greatest exposure towards the side that you are focusing on.
4. If a subcostal incision is chosen, the inferior flap can be sewn with a number 2 nylon stitch to allow for inferior and constant retraction.

The steps of the drainage procedure are as follows:

1. Enter the lesser sac between the stomach and the colon.
2. Follow the right gastroepiploic vein to its origin from the superior mesenteric vein (SMV). This will allow you to find the SMV and know where the area of danger lies.
3. The authors leave the short gastric vessels alone and place a fenestrated retractor cephalad to hold the stomach upward and allow access to the lesser sac.
4. The ultrasound is then used to identify the pancreatic duct (PD). Use of the narrowest profile probe can be very helpful as the space is limited and long-axis view of the duct is really of critical importance.
5. Using a 21–25 gauge needle and using ultrasound in the long axis to follow the complete track of the needle, the duct is entered. A word of caution is to not get so excited when one sees pancreatic fluid in the syringe avoid the surgeon aspirating aggressively and collapsing the duct. One should stop aspirating when clear pancreatic fluid is seen in the syringe. Electrocautery is then used to cut down onto the needle to find the duct. A needle tip electrocautery may minimize charring and allow for better visualization and precise cut.
6. A right-angle clamp is then inserted longitudinally into the duct and cautery is used to spatulate the duct longitudinally towards the patient's left first. Care must be taken to stay in the center of the pancreatic parenchyma, as wandering cranially may cause injury to the splenic artery, which runs very close.
7. The ductotomy is carried towards the right of the patient. The gastroduodenal artery (GDA) will be encountered and the authors place two figure-of-eight suture cranially and caudad to control this vessel with permanent suture. The authors feel that the lack of efficacy of this procedure is related to lack of decompression of the pancreas head. The inexperienced surgeon will stop when they encounter bleeding at the GDA and will not adequately drain the head of the pancreas when indicated.
8. Adequate pancreatic ductotomy in the head of pancreas is paramount for a successful drainage procedure. The bile duct typically travels posterior to the pancreatic ductotomy plane, and the surgeon must not perform inadequate pancreatic head drainage in fear of enteric the bile duct.
9. When performing Frey procedure, the head of pancreas is then cored at this point. This addition can allow for greater decompression of the head of the gland, thought to be the pacemaker for pain in this disease. The authors favor resection and drainage options (see below) rather than the Frey procedure.
10. The roux limb is created and the anastomosis to the PD which has been opened for at least 10 cm is performed. The authors use a double-armed 4–0 polypropylene suture and start from the left side of the patient. The inferior aspect of the anastomosis is created first allowing for an easier cephalad aspect that is well visualized. It is sometimes necessary to use a 3–0 polypropylene on a CT-1 needle if there is very firm pancreatic parenchyma.
11. A drain is left and placed inferior to the anastomosis.

Minimally Invasive Approach to Pancreatic Drainage Procedures

The authors firmly believe that MIS adoption of any surgery must not limit the main principles of the surgery itself. Therefore, the key steps to the drainage procedure are as outlined above. Specific modifications to allow for easy MIS adaptation are mentioned below. The authors generally use robotic-assisted laparoscopy for operations that require significant suturing. The key areas of robotic adaptation are outlined below:

1. The patient is positioned supine with both arms tucked. There are securing straps on the thighs and chest, as well as a footboard. Positioning is checked to allow for 30 degrees of reverse Trendelenburg without the patient moving.
2. Prior to positioning, laparoscopy is used to identify and run the bowel distal to the Ligament of Treitz (LOT). The identified proximal loop of bowel (about 40 cm distal to LOT, but much dependent on body habitus and the thickness of the mesentery) is tacked in the left upper quadrant of the patient in preparation for the roux limb. Clear knowledge of proximal and distal is essential to allow for appropriate construction of the roux limb.
3. The patient is positioned as above, and the robot docked form the patient's left side.
4. The steps outlined above are performed and the loop of jejunum is anastomosed to the PD. One tip is that any larger needle (CT-1 for example) must be passed through a larger port such as a 10/12 mm port.
5. The Roux limb is constructed by running the bowel distally and constructing the jejunojejunostomy in the left upper quadrant using a stapler from the 12 mm port on the patient's right mid-clavicular line. This will allow for a greater distance from port to stapler device, allowing for use of the robotic stapler and the ability to manipulate intracorporeally. The enterotomy is then closed using a 3–0 self-locking suture.
6. The Roux limb is completed by dividing the bowel to the patient's left of the pancreaticojejunostomy. This makes the configuration a Roux from a loop.

Postoperative management of the patient will be discussed with resection below.

Resection for Patients with Chronic Pancreatitis

Indications for Resection

The authors believe that resection is the best option for the treatment of CP when possible. They believe that the pacemaker for pain in CP is the head of the gland, and therefore any reasonable way to achieve resection of this area is beneficial. The patient who is especially suited for a resection option is one that has dilation of both the bile duct and the PD. This patient will inevitably require a biliary drainage procedure and a pancreatic drainage procedure (double bypass) and so resection of the head will allow for successful dual drainage and resection of the pacemaker for pain.

While resection is optimal, it may not be possible due to anatomic reasons. This would mainly be related to occlusion of venous structures, namely the SMV/portal vein junction. Splenic vein occlusion can result in extrahepatic portal hypertension including huge gastric and peri-pancreatic varices that can make the procedure unsafe. In these cases, the HPB surgeon should back off to a dual drainage option.

The authors have popularized the "Whip-Stow" procedure where a pancreato-duodenectomy and a drainage procedure are achieved in the same surgery [4]. This will be the focus of this section.

The patient best suited for the "Whip-Stow" procedure needs surgery for chronic pain, dilated bile duct, dilated PD, and a firm gland texture (Fig. 7.2). The PD diameter does not matter in the case of a firm gland (usually present in CP). This is because the PD can always be found at the time of transection of the neck of the pancreas during resective surgery. The details will be outlined below.

Steps of the "Whip-Stow" procedure (see Fig. 7.3):

1- The surgeon should set up and proceed as for a Whipple procedure.
2- Once the resection is complete, the surgeon can place a Pean clamp into the cut edge of the pancreas. The PD is then opened along its length taking care to not veer off the gland and accidentally lacerate the splenic artery. This can be easy to do as the gland gets thinner towards the tail.
3- The aim is to provide as long a ductotomy as possible—ideally at least 10 cm.
4- Reconstruction of the pancreatoduodenectomy is performed as usual. The authors bring the transected jejunum in line with the resected duodenum during standard reconstruction for a pancreatoduodenectomy (i.e., jejunal limb lies under the SMA). However, when performing the pancreaticojejunostomy for the "Whip-Stow," the authors find that bringing the transected jejunum through the transverse mesocolon mesentery can allow for a more natural lay of the reconstruction loop.

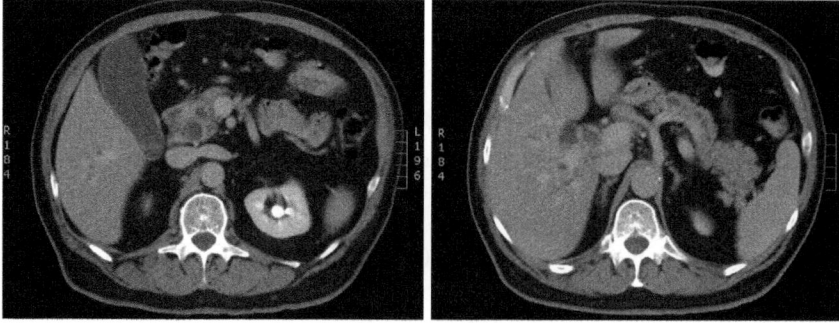

Fig. 7.2 Chronic pancreatitis patient with diseased head of pancreas and dilated duct

Fig. 7.3 Schematic representation of the Whip-Stow procedure

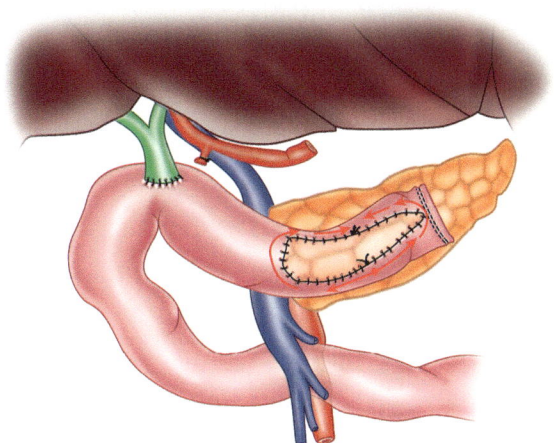

5- The authors use a single layer of 4–0 polypropylene on an SH needle for this anastomosis (as outlined above). Using a 3–0 on a CT-1 needle can be useful if the gland is very firm.

6- A close-suction drain is laid posterior to the pancreatic anastomosis.

Postoperative Care

The authors follow the general guidelines for post PD patients with an aggressive enhanced recovery after surgery (ERAS) pathway. This includes avoidance of naso-gastric tubes, aggressive removal of urinary catheters, advancement of diet based on patient desire, and aggressive weaning of opioids. Physical therapy and occupational therapy services are used to have patients mobilized within 4 h of surgery. Shower and self-care are encouraged immediately, but certainly at day 1 and thereafter. The authors do not use the intensive care unit, where the focus is not on mobilizing the patient and normalizing their activity. This is a very important aspect to recovery.

References

1. Puestow CB, Gillesby WJ. Retrograde surgical drainage of pancreas for chronic relapsing pancreatitis. AMA Arch Surg. 1958;76(6):898–907. https://doi.org/10.1001/archsurg.1958.01280240056009.
2. Partington PF, Rochelle RE. Modified Puestow procedure for retrograde drainage of the pancreatic duct. Ann Surg. 1960;152(6):1037–43. https://doi.org/10.1097/00000658-196012000-00015. PMID: 13733040; PMCID: PMC1613865

3. Frey CF, Smith GJ. Description and rationale of a new operation for chronic pancreatitis. Pancreas. 1987;2:701–7.
4. Jeyarajah DR, Khithani A, Curtis D, Galanopoulos CA. The 'Whip-Stow' procedure: an innovative modification to the whipple procedure in the management of premalignant and malignant pancreatic head disease. Am Surg. 2010;76(1):70–2. PMID: 20135943

Chapter 8
Chronic Pancreatitis: Resection

Jonathan C. DeLong and Brendan C. Visser

Background

Chronic pancreatitis is a slowly progressive, but unrelenting chronic condition in which patients without access to specialized gastrointestinal or surgical services become debilitated and often self-treat with escalating doses of opioid analgesics. The most common cause of chronic pancreatitis in the developed world is alcohol consumption and tobacco use. Other causes include gallstones, drugs (valproate, thiazides, estrogens), hypercalcemia conditions, obstruction of the main pancreatic duct due to scarring, post-ERCP pancreatitis, recurrent pancreatitis, or malignancy. Genetic predispositions to chronic pancreatitis include PRSS1, SPINK1, or CFTR genetic mutations. There is growing data that these patients may benefit from early referral for total pancreatectomy with islet cell autotransplantation (TPIAT) which is discussed in detail in Chap. 11.

The hallmark of this unyielding disease is severe abdominal pain which may be associated with exocrine insufficiency (bloating, excessive flatulence, steatorrhea, or a documented reduction in fecal elastase), endocrine insufficiency (diabetes mellitus), failure to thrive, and an increased risk for pancreatic malignancy. Histologically, the glandular structure of the pancreatic parenchyma is destroyed and replaced with interstitial fibrosis and necrosis due to the chronic and recurrent bouts of inflammation. However, the diagnosis is most frequently made from patient history and radiographic findings alone. The histological features are heterogeneous

J. C. DeLong (✉)
Division of Surgical Oncology, University of Tennessee Medical Center Knoxville, Knoxville, TN, USA
e-mail: jcdelong@utmck.edu

B. C. Visser
Division of Hepatobiliary and Pancreas Surgery, Stanford University, Stanford, CA, USA
e-mail: bvisser@stanford.edu

E. P. Ceppa et al. (eds.), *The SAGES Manual of Evolving Techniques in Pancreatic Surgery*, https://doi.org/10.1007/978-3-031-78409-5_8

and may include gland atrophy, pseudocyst formation, calcifications, necrosis, or ductal abnormalities. It is critical to consider malignancy in cases of pancreatitis, as a mass-lesion that is obstructing the pancreatic duct may in fact be the inciting factor for the disease.

Various theories exist to explain pathogenesis of the severe pain that is experienced in patients with chronic pancreatitis. One such theory is that chronic calcifications and fibrosis cause hypertension of the pancreatic duct. As such, some surgical interventions are aimed at decompressing the system. Surgical interventions are categorized as resection procedures, drainage procedures, or combined drainage and resection procedures. In this chapter, we will discuss the resection procedures (Whipple/pancreatoduodenectomy and distal pancreatectomy). An operation is often offered after failure of medical treatment or non-surgical interventions (opioid analgesics, neural blockade, exocrine replacement therapy). Non-surgical interventional strategies may include percutaneous drainage procedures or endoscopic interventions (cyst gastrostomy, luminal apposing metal stents with or without endoscopic necrosectomy, sphincterotomy with or without pancreatic duct stenting, and balloon dilation). Nutritional optimization is imperative when managing chronic pancreatitis and can be accomplished with enteral feeding with percutaneous gastrostomy, combined percutaneous gastrostomy-jejunostomy, or nasoenteric jejunal feeding tubes. Thoughtful attention to pancreatic enzyme replacement is necessary to absorb the nutrients from supplemental feeds. Many patients who ultimately undergo surgery for chronic pancreatitis have undergone one or more of these interventions.

There is no consensus among experts regarding the selection criteria for patients with chronic pancreatitis to undergo surgery, but pain relief and management of complications from chronic pancreatitis are the main indications. There are three potential goals of surgery. First, to reduce reliance on opioid analgesics to the point that patients can be weaned off narcotic pain medication entirely. Second, intervening early may reduce or halt ongoing parenchymal destruction and thus preserve the remaining pancreatic function. And finally, in some cases, resection is offered to rule out malignancy as a possible etiology for recurrent bouts of pancreatitis (where imaging characteristics are suggestive of an underlying mass). Understanding the location of disease through careful inspection of high-quality axial imaging is essential to offering the appropriate surgical intervention. In carefully selected patients, surgical intervention can offer pain reduction 80–90% of the time.

Indications for Resection

Head-Dominant Disease

In most patients with chronic pancreatitis, the source of inflammation and thus the main site of disease is located in the pancreatic head. This phenomenon has been termed the "pacemaker" effect that the pancreatic head plays in the disease (see

Fig. 8.1 "Pacemaker" type, head-dominant disease

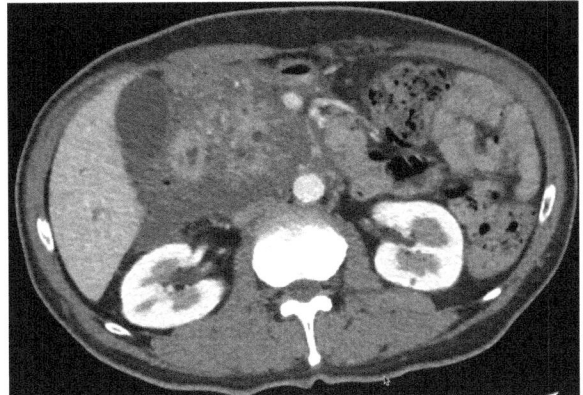

Fig. 8.2 "Normal" parenchyma in body and tail of the same patient

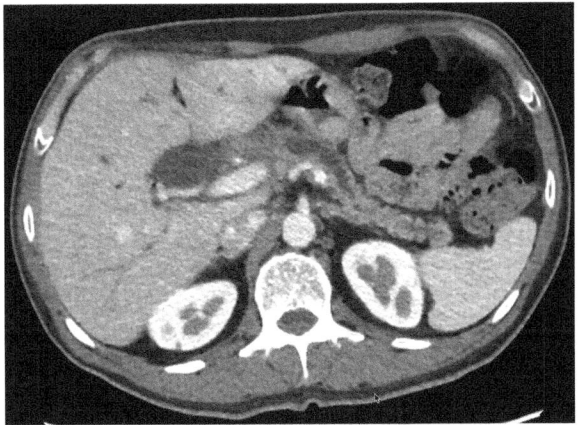

Figs. 8.1 and 8.2). Inflammatory enlargement of the pancreatic head can cause local complications including stricture of the pancreatic duct, common bile duct, and/or the duodenum.

There is growing evidence that early intervention may preserve pancreatic function by eliminating the cycle of inflammatory parenchymal destruction. Surgical intervention is superior to endoscopic decompression; yet, many patients undergo endoscopic balloon dilation, sphincterotomy, or pancreatic duct stenting prior to surgery. A Cochrane review of surgical resection for chronic pancreatitis for disease that is isolated to the pancreatic head found no difference in perioperative morbidity or mortality between pancreatoduodenectomy (Whipple) and duodenum-preserving pancreatic head resection (DPPHR) [1]. The latter is discussed in detail in Chap. 10. It should be noted that while pancreatoduodenectomy was at one time a mainstay in the treatment of chronic pancreatitis, both drainage/combined procedures and total pancreatectomy with islet cell autotransplantation (TPIAT) are performed with increasing frequency in contemporary pancreatic surgery [2].

The most common type of chronic pancreatitis is calcifying type which is characterized radiographically by calcifications and pancreatic ductal stones. There may be associated phlegmonous changes from repeated episodes of pancreatitis and the disease is often most severe in the head. Pancreatic head-dominant disease can be treated with a pancreatoduodenectomy.

Tail-Dominant Disease

Distal pancreatectomy for chronic pancreatitis is performed less frequently than pancreatoduodenectomy (Whipple). There are some specific indications where this is the procedure of choice. In the post-acute setting, some patients develop pancreatic necrosis of the body or neck of the gland such that the distal body and tail are in discontinuity. This is called disconnected left pancreatic duct remnant (DLPR) and is the most common indication for distal pancreatectomy for chronic pancreatitis (see Figs. 8.3, 8.4, and 8.5) [3]. DP may be warranted for patients with ongoing symptoms attributed to disease isolated to the tail or recurrent bouts of acute on chronic pancreatitis from isolated tail disease. Of note, patients with an asymptomatic isolated tail glandular change from chronic pancreatitis do not mandate intervention. The tail can atrophy over time making surgical intervention unnecessary. Another scenario that occasionally arises is necrosis of the tail that leads to recurrent, symptomatic pseudocyst formation arising from the tail of the gland. First-line treatment for these patients is internal endoscopic drainage. For the pseudocysts that recur after endoscopic transgastric cystgastrostomy, distal pancreatectomy can offer definitive management (see Fig. 8.6).

Other patients may develop a midbody stricture of the pancreatic duct or mass effect by a pseudotumor (non-neoplastic solid lesion of the pancreas following pancreatitis). The key point is that distal pancreatectomy is appropriate for patients

Fig. 8.3 Tail-dominant disease with abscess and phlegmon

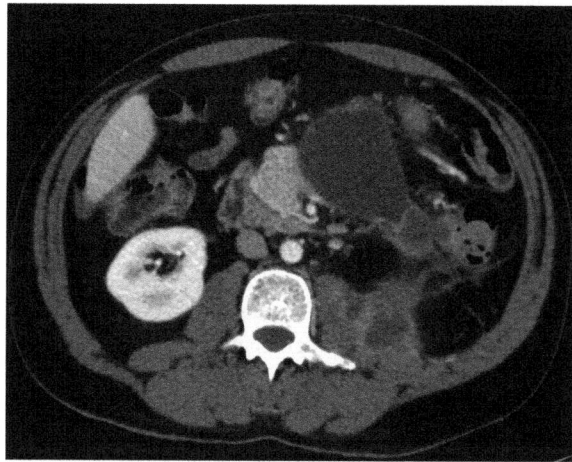

Fig. 8.4 Tail-dominant disease with abscess extending down psoas muscle

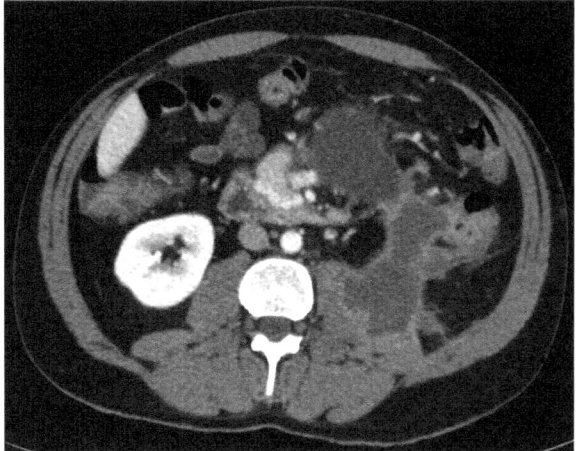

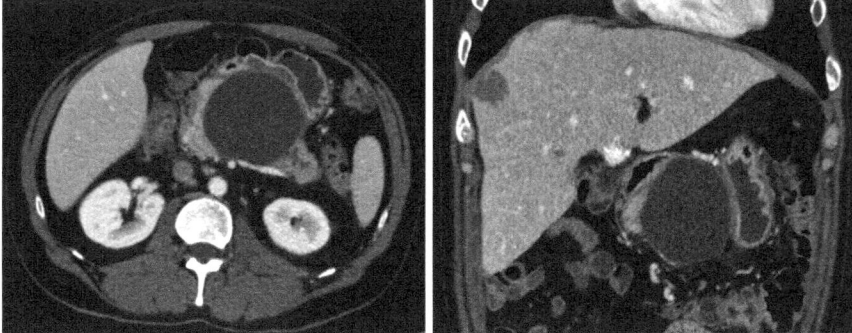

Fig. 8.5 Disconnected duct with pseudocyst abutting posterior wall of stomach

whose disease is confined exclusively to the tail of the gland, thus preserving normal pancreatic parenchyma at the pancreatic head. In patients with disease throughout the gland, an erroneously offered distal pancreatectomy will only partially solve their problem and lead to further sequelae of their disease.

Like patients with disease confined to the head of the pancreas, general indications for surgery include patients who have failed medical management, those with debilitating abdominal pain with or without dependence on opioid analgesics, and patients with failure to thrive. Most patients who undergo distal pancreatectomy for chronic pancreatitis will be offered an open operation. In one series of patients only 6.2% of distal pancreatectomies performed for chronic pancreatitis at a high-volume center were performed laparoscopically due to the degree of severe inflammation causing prohibitive risk for minimally invasive surgery. For this reason, electing to offer laparoscopic or robotic surgery for chronic pancreatitis should be done only in highly selected and carefully considered cases. It is the exception and not the rule.

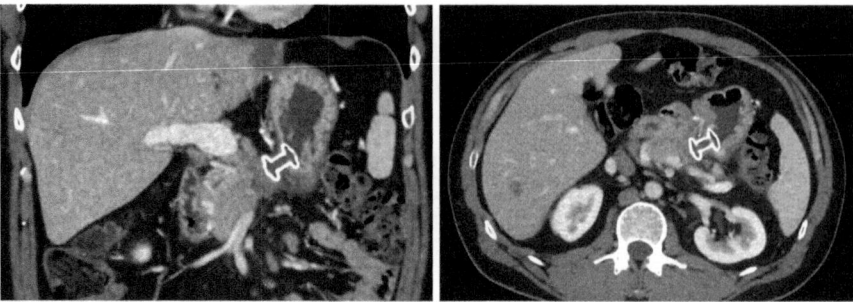

Fig. 8.6 Same patient as Fig. 8.5 after wall-opposing metal stent

Suspicion for Malignancy

As stated earlier, it may not be possible to differentiate radiographic sequelae of pancreatitis from a pancreatic mass. Mass effect from pancreatic cancer can be a cause of pancreatitis [4]. A thorough history including weight loss chronicity, new-onset diabetes mellitus, smoking, family history, or previous interventions should be taken. Upper endoscopy with endoscopic ultrasound (EUS) may be useful for a detailed examination of the pancreas parenchyma. Efforts to achieve a tissue diagnosis with fine needle aspiration are warranted given the higher complexity and perioperative morbidity of a PD in the setting of CP. There are some cases where malignancy cannot be ruled out and the diagnosis is made at the time of surgery due to the difficulty of determining pancreatic cancer histologically in the background of chronic pancreatitis.

Perioperative Management

Workup of a patient with chronic pancreatitis begins with a detailed history and physical exam. Approximately 20–30% of patients with acute pancreatitis will develop recurrent pancreatitis and another 10% of patients will ultimately progress to chronic pancreatitis. Questions including number of previous episodes, severity, previous hospitalizations, pain-free periods, and time since last episode will establish the timeline. Many patients who progress to chronic pancreatitis experience frequent or near-constant abdominal pain, so questions regarding the use of opioid analgesics including how much and for how long the patient has been taking opioids will be especially important for management in the postoperative period. Alcohol consumption is the most common inciting factor for chronic pancreatitis which is made worse by concurrent use of tobacco. A multidisciplinary approach to develop a realistic plan for alcohol cessation is important because postoperative outcomes in patients who continue to drink alcohol are poor.

A thorough patient history will also include questions regarding family history as an increasing number of genetic mutations have been found to predispose patients to chronic pancreatitis. This may be especially true in young patients or those with no known inciting factors (i.e., idiopathic). Genetic mutations such as PRSS1, SPINK-1, and CFTR among others are known to increase the risk of developing pancreatitis especially when combined with what would otherwise be considered modest alcohol consumption. Family history should also include questions regarding cancer in close relatives.

A common complication of chronic pancreatitis is failure to thrive, and poor nutrition in the preoperative period is associated with worse outcomes. Due to the location of the inflammation and associated changes, some patients may be unable to eat solid foods due to duodenal stricture or inflammatory-mediated dysmotility. Questions regarding quantity, composition, and frequency of meals, experience of postprandial emesis, or tolerance of a liquid-only diet may be suggestive of this problem. In patients with documented poor nutrition, enteral support in the form of tube feeding may be indicated. Small, flexible nasoenteric tubes with the weighted tip of the tube positioned in the proximal jejunum may provide temporary support in order to nutritionally optimize a malnourished patient prior to surgery. Percutaneous gastrostomy tubes with the addition of a jejunal feeding tube may also be appropriate for this indication. Enteric feeds are preferable to parenteral nutrition and every effort should be made to find an enteric solution. Of note, exocrine insufficiency is common in chronic pancreatitis patients and the resultant diarrhea may erroneously be attributed to tube feed intolerance.

Possible lab work for patients with chronic pancreatitis include prealbumin and transferrin to determine nutritional status, cancer antigen 19–9 (CA 19–9) and carcinoembryonic antigen (CEA) if malignancy is being considered, IgG4 for autoimmune causes of pancreatitis, and genetic testing for genetic mutations such as SPINK-1 and CFTR. A comprehensive metabolic panel (CMP) is useful to evaluate renal function, evidence of liver disease from alcohol consumption, and in cases of biliary stricture. A complete blood count (CBC) may reveal thrombocytopenia in patients with portal hypertension. A phosphatidylethanol test (PeTH) may be useful to confirm alcohol cessation. Routine serum amylase or lipase studies, which are acutely elevated during cases of acute pancreatitis, are not useful in patients with chronic pancreatitis.

High-quality axial imaging is essential for the management of this disease. Every effort should be made to obtain all of the abdominal imaging studies that a patient has received over the course of their disease. Reviewing these studies over time will provide valuable information regarding the overall course and pace of progression. New studies to obtain will include a contrast-enhanced triple phase computed tomography (CT) scan. A standard pancreas protocol CT scan includes late arterial, portal venous, and delayed phases. Special attention should be paid to the superior mesenteric vein/portal vein confluence for stenosis or thrombosis as well as other evidence of portal hypertension like splenomegaly or gastric varices.

Further information can be obtained from a secretin-enhanced magnetic resonance cholangiopancreatography (MRCP) which provides valuable information regarding ductal anatomy. Secretin stimulates the pancreas to secrete bicarbonate-rich fluid that improves the image resolution of T2-weighted images of the pancreatic duct resulting in an optimal non-invasive imaging of the pancreatic duct. In the modern era, MRCP provides anatomical imaging and endoscopic retrograde cholangiopancreatography (ERCP) is reserved for endoscopic interventions such as pancreatic duct stenting, balloon dilation, and sphincterotomy of the sphincter of Oddi [5].

Procedure Steps

Open Whipple

1. After making an upper midline incision and opening fascia, take the falciform off the anterior abdominal wall (this will be used later for flap coverage of the gastroduodenal artery stump).
2. Explore the abdomen for evidence of unrecognized malignant disease. Given chronic inflammation, there may be extensive adhesions requiring lysis.
3. Ultrasound is useful to identify key vascular landmarks. Doppler mode confirms patency and flow within vessels such as the splenic vein.
4. Open the gastrocolic ligament outside of the gastroepiploic arcade. Continue mobilization to the right taking down the hepatic flexure of the colon.
5. Perform a wide Kocher maneuver all the way to the aorta. Chronic inflammation replaces the typical thin, wispy plane with thick, fibrous tissue (Figs. 8.7 and 8.8).
6. Dissect down to the superior mesenteric vein (SMV). This is accomplished by lifting the stomach anteriorly and following the right gastroepiploic pedicle. The right gastroepiploic vein drains into the SMV just inferior to the inferior

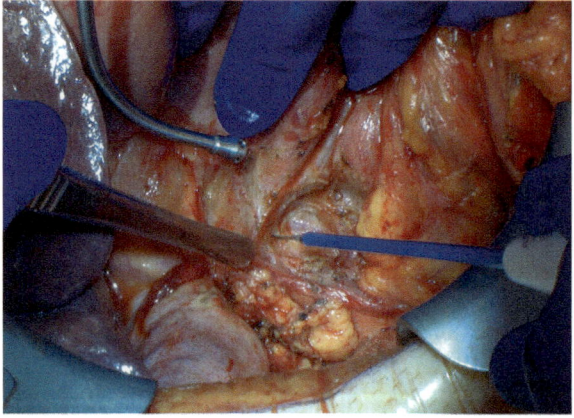

Fig. 8.7 Whipple Kocher maneuver with chronic inflammation

Fig. 8.8 Thickened
adventitia over IVC after
Kocherization (Pancreas
and Duodenum retracted
anteriorly)

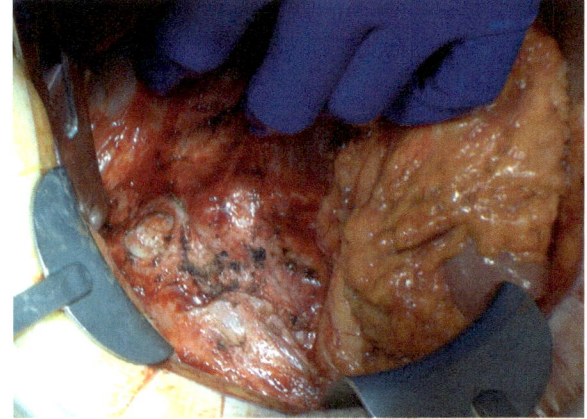

border of the pancreas. Follow this vein to expose the SMV. The right gastroepiploic vein is ligated and divided.

7. An attempt is then made to create a tunnel under the neck of the pancreas.
Depending on the degree of chronic inflammation, this may not be feasible, and
perseverance may lead to uncontrolled bleeding in a deep hole with poor access
and exposure. Attempts at a traditional tunnel between the pancreas neck and
SMV/PV may not be possible.

8. Then turn to the infracolic compartment where the proximal jejunum is divided
a short distance from the ligament of Treitz with a GIA stapler. The mesentery
is divided with a vessel sealer down to the root staying close to the bowel and
avoiding the first jejunal branch.

9. Then perform a top-down cholecystectomy.

10. Next, ligate the right gastric artery followed by the right gastroepiploic pedicle.
The duodenum is then divided with a linear stapler just distal to the pylorus.
Chronic inflammation may prevent mobilization of the duodenum in which
case a classic Whipple with distal stomach transection is performed.

11. The gastroduodenal artery is then divided. We use a vascular stapler load for
even, consistent compression along the diameter of the vessel.

12. The neck of the pancreas is then divided. If a tunnel was able to be created, then
this is done in the standard fashion. However, if severe inflammation precludes
this, then it may make sense to perform a progressive division of the neck in a
stepwise approach from above, slowly working down onto the portal vein. This
is done by making a little space, then dividing a little pancreas in an incremental
process.

13. A frozen section of the pancreatic margin is sent to pathology if there is any
concern for malignancy.

14. Next divide the bile duct. To prevent the spillage of bile, a bulldog can be placed
superiorly, and a silk tie is used to ligate the duct distally. A frozen section of
the bile duct is typically not done for this indication.

15. Next the uncinate is freed from the portal vein and superior mesenteric vein using a combination of blunt dissection, vessel sealer, and silk ties. If possible, vascular control should be obtained. A Kitner is a useful tool to peel the vein off the specimen. Prolene repair sutures should be loaded and ready because the avulsion of small venous branches can lead to significant hemorrhage. If bleeding does occur, lifting the specimen anteriorly against the PV/SMV can slow or stop the bleeding to assist with obtaining control.
16. The uncinate dissection is finished by taking the specimen off of the superior mesenteric artery (SMA). This is done using the vessel sealer and ties with frequent palpation of the SMA pulse to avoid iatrogenic injury.
17. After the dissection is complete, the reconstruction is performed in the standard fashion. We perform an end to side pancreaticojejunostomy using the Blumgart technique. For the inner layer, we use 6–0 PDS on a BV needle. We place a pancreatic stent through the anastomosis.
18. For the hepaticojejunostomy we use 5–0 PDS on an RB2 needle with interrupted sutures in the standard end-to-side fashion.
19. For the duodenojejunostomy, we hand sew using 3–0 PDS.
20. Two 15 Fr closed suction drains are positioned, one next to the hepaticojejunostomy and the other next to the pancreaticojejunostomy.

MIS Whipple

In our practice, we offer minimally invasive pancreatoduodenectomy (Whipple) procedures (for any indication) in carefully selected patients. In general, when a patient presents with a history of chronic pancreatitis, our standard practice is to offer an open operation. This is due to the increased difficulty of dissection from chronic inflammation, distortion of normal tissue planes, and risk of uncontrolled hemorrhage with limited access. Safety is paramount in these cases. It is our belief that not all cases should be attempted robotically, and the successful implementation of minimally invasive techniques in pancreatic surgery starts with good patient selection. We do offer minimally invasive pancreatic drainage procedures for chronic pancreatitis, as the risk profile is considerably less than that with a pancreatic head resection. These procedures will be discussed in detail elsewhere in the manual.

Open Distal Pancreatectomy

1. After the abdomen is prepped and draped, an upper midline incision is made from the xiphoid process down to the umbilicus. A self-retaining retractor is set up to maintain exposure.

2. The gastrocolic omentum is freed from the transverse colon, preserving the blood supply to the omentum so it can be used later as a flap. A vessel sealer is used to come around the splenic flexure. Short gastric arteries are similarly divided.
3. The stomach is then retracted anteriorly to gain access to the lesser sac. The subsequent steps are determined by the conditions and specific indications for distal pancreatectomy for chronic pancreatitis.
4. In the case of tail-dominant disease with an intact duct, the pancreas is mobilized to get around the gland in an area just proximal to the diseased segment.
5. The splenic artery followed by the splenic vein can be taken with a vascular staple load. The splenic vein is often fused to the back of the pancreas and cannot be safely mobilized off the gland. It can be taken together with the pancreas with a linear staple load.
6. The pancreas can typically be divided with a GIA black reinforced staple load. In some cases, the gland is too thick or firm to be divided in this manner. In that case, it can either be partially thinned with an energy device and then stapled or divided using a vessel sealer. An attempt should be made to find the duct and close with absorbable suture.
7. The tail of the pancreas is mobilized out of the retroperitoneum and removed along with the spleen. Considering the inflammatory adhesions between the pancreatic parenchyma and the splenic vessels, spleen preservation is usually not attempted. However, splenic vessel and spleen preservation should be considered as an option if technically feasible. Unlike for malignant tumors, where a right-to-left dissection is preferred, when the indication for distal pancreatectomy is chronic pancreatitis, a left-to-right dissection is equally appropriate. The safest and least distorted plane should be selected.
8. We often elect against drain placement, not because leaks are uncommon, but rather because a contained pseudocyst is often easier to manage than a prolonged pancreatic fistula.

MIS Distal Pancreatectomy

Unlike in a minimally invasive Whipple procedure, where chronic pancreatitis adds significant technical complexity and often prohibitive risk, a minimally invasive distal pancreatectomy in the setting of chronic pancreatitis is within the realm of possibility. It is reasonable to attempt a laparoscopic or robotic distal pancreatectomy for this indication while understanding that these operations will typically be harder than when the indication is for a tumor. It is our practice to offer splenic preservation whenever possible. However, with chronic pancreatitis, this is often not feasible, so a distal pancreatectomy and splenectomy is typically performed. In addition, unlike for tumor indications where a right-to-left or "antegrade" dissection is widely considered to be best practice, with chronic pancreatitis it is equally reasonable to use a left-to-right approach, as this may be a less hostile dissection plane.

1. The patient is positioned supine and carefully secured to the table which is positioned with a slight break to maximize the operative space. The abdomen and left flank are prepped and draped, and the robot is positioned for docking on the patient's left.
2. Port placement is determined by body habitus, the predominant site of disease, and surgical plan. In most cases, the camera port is placed slightly above and to the right of the umbilicus. The remaining robotic trocars are placed 7 cm apart in a linear position.
3. A 2 cm incision is made below the umbilicus and a small wound protector placed with a 12 mm assistant trocar through that which is ultimately used for specimen extraction. A 5 mm port is also placed for liver retraction initially, and later anterior stomach retraction to expose the lesser sac.
4. The robot is docked, and the camera is placed in arm 2 such that the surgeon has 1 left arm and 2 right arms.
5. The splenic flexure of the colon is carefully taken down with the vessel sealer. Inflammation from chronic pancreatitis can make this difficult and meticulous dissection is required to avoid colonic injury.
6. The stomach is lifted anteriorly and the gastrocolic omentum is opened close to the gastroepiploic arcade so excessive omentum doesn't hang down and obstruct the view. Short gastric vessels are taken with the vessel sealer.

   Note: in cases of splenic vein thrombosis, an effort should be made to preserve the short gastric vessels until the splenic artery has been divided, as these vessels provide the only outflow for the spleen. Alternatively, the spleen can be embolized preoperatively.

7. The triangular-shaped "snake" liver retractor is repositioned under the stomach with anterior retraction. An orogastric tube that was previously placed by anesthesia is positioned such that it is "bowing" along the greater curvature and terminates in the gastric antrum. This creates a lip for the retractor to sit under which prevents slipping of the stomach and maintains exposure.
8. Next the retroperitoneal plane behind the pancreas is developed starting from the bottom to the top of the gland, and extending laterally. If this proves challenging, and neoplasm is not suspected as the etiology of the chronic pancreatitis, a left-to-right approach can be considered.
9. The splenic artery is next identified at the superior border of the pancreas and divided with a vascular stapler.
10. The splenic vein will typically be fused to the back of the pancreas and isolation is not often possible. It can instead be taken together with the pancreas.
11. Next the pancreas is divided with a linear stapler with a reinforced black staple load. In order to use this staple load, the assistant trocar may need to be upsized to a 15 mm trocar. The stapler is closed and subsequently fired *very* slowly over the course of several minutes (at least 5).
12. The rest of the pancreas is subsequently freed from the retroperitoneum together with the spleen. The specimen is kept intact during the dissection and ultimately

placed in a strong specimen bag and removed. The extraction site may need to be extended depending on the size of the specimen.
13. The surgical site is inspected for hemostasis. The liver retractor is taken down and the trocars are removed.

Pitfalls and Pearls

While once considered to be the gold standard surgical resections for patients with chronic pancreatitis, pancreatoduodenectomy and distal pancreatectomy have less of a role in the management of chronic pancreatitis in the modern era of pancreas surgery. This is partly due to increased surgical options for pancreatitis, particularly the drainage procedures, but also due to the recognition of improved outcomes and growing enthusiasm for total pancreatectomy with islet cell autotransplantation (TPIAT) [6]. This is particularly true among patients with early to mid-stage disease, where there remains a sufficient number of islet cells for the procedure to be beneficial. However, these treatments are currently limited to specialized centers making access a significant limitation to this strategy.

Given the difficulty of the operation, chronicity of disease, and comorbidities in this patient population, complications after pancreatic resection for chronic pancreatitis are common. In fact, approximately one third of patients experience a significant complication (Clavian-Dindo Grade >/= to 3). Examples of the types of complications that are seen include clinically relevant postoperative pancreatic fistula (CR-POPF), surgical site infection, new onset diabetes, persistent opioid use, percutaneous drains, return to the operating room, readmission, and death. CR-POPF is higher in patients operated on for pancreatic necrosis, pseudocyst, or disconnected left pancreatic duct remnant than in patients who undergo distal pancreatectomy for neoplasm [7]. The development of new-onset diabetes in patients undergoing distal pancreatectomy for chronic pancreatitis is seen in 19–46% of patients.

Pearls

1. Surgical resection for chronic pancreatitis is harder than when the indication for surgery is a tumor. This is particularly true with a Whipple.
2. MIS techniques for chronic pancreatitis should be attempted with caution but may be appropriate for some patients undergoing distal pancreatectomy. If a patient with pancreatic head-dominant disease has mild inflammation to the degree that an MIS Whipple could be reasonably feasible, then TPIAT may be the superior surgical option.
3. Vascular pitfall for distal pancreatectomy is the celiac artery, for Whipple it is the superior mesenteric vein.

4. Unlike when the indication for surgery is tumor, a distal pancreatectomy can be performed left-to-right *or* right-to-left, depending on the most favorable conditions. Extending the resection deeper into the retroperitoneum (e.g., through Gerota's fascia) may also provide a less hostile plane.
5. In a left-to-right dissection when the spleen and pancreas are lifted anteriorly, you have better appreciation of the position of the celiac artery.
6. Splenic vein thrombosis is common. Do not divide short gastric vessels until the splenic artery has been taken. Alternatively, a splenectomy can be performed as a separate specimen. Dividing short gastric vessels prior to the splenic artery in the setting of splenic vein thrombosis leads to significant venous oozing in the operative field.
7. The splenic vein may not be able to be divided off the back of the pancreas to be taken separately so it can be taken together with the pancreas in the same staple load.
8. Sometimes the tissue of the pancreas may be too hard to divide even with the thickest staple load. The options in this scenario are to clamp, divide, and over-sew (if open) or to thin out the front of the gland and then staple (whether MIS or open).
9. The decision to drain for a distal pancreatectomy is based on surgeon prefer-ence and judgment, but in our practice we rarely leave a surgical drain (unless the GI lumen has been opened during the case) because it is our belief that in the setting of a leak a pseudocyst (no drain) is preferable to a pancreatic fistula (drain).
10. In a Whipple, creating the entire tunnel under the neck of the pancreas is often not feasible and persistence can result in bleeding with limited access. In the setting of profound chronic inflammation, it can make sense to divide the pan-creas in a stepwise approach whether from above or below, progressively exposing the vein.
11. When performing a Whipple for CP, if the head of the gland is *very* adherent to the SMV and PV (after division of the neck), consider obtaining proximal, dis-tal, and splenic vein control prior to persisting with blunt (ie Kittner) dissection.
12. In a pacemaker situation, if the tail of the gland is very atrophic, completion of the pancreaticojejunostomy is not necessary in all cases. An atrophic pancreatic remnant can be closed using a linear stapler (but leaves a small amount of endo-crine function).

References

1. Gurusamy KS, Lusuku C, Halkias C, Davidson BR. Duodenum-preserving pancreatic resec-tion versus pancreatoduodenectomy for chronic pancreatitis. Cochrane Database Syst Rev. 2016;2(2):CD011521. https://doi.org/10.1002/14651858.CD011521.pub2. PMID: 26837472; PMCID: PMC8278566
2. Diener MK, Hüttner FJ, Kieser M, Knebel P, et al., ChroPac Trial GroupPartial pancreato-duodenectomy versus duodenum-preserving pancreatic head resection in chronic pan-

creatitis: the multicentre, randomised, controlled, double-blind ChroPac trial. Lancet. 2017;390(10099):1027–37. https://doi.org/10.1016/S0140-6736(17)31960-8.
3. Siegel JB, Mukherjee R, Lancaster WP, Morgan KA. Distal pancreatectomy for pancreatitis in the Modern Era. J Surg Res. 2022;275:29–34. https://doi.org/10.1016/j.jss.2022.01.016. Epub 2022 Feb 23
4. Yadav D, Lowenfels AB. The epidemiology of pancreatitis and pancreatic cancer. Gastroenterology. 2013;144(6):1252–61. https://doi.org/10.1053/j.gastro.2013.01.068. PMID: 23622135; PMCID: PMC3662544
5. Rieder B, Krampulz D, Adolf J, Pfeiffer A. Endoscopic pancreatic sphincterotomy and stenting for preoperative prophylaxis of pancreatic fistula after distal pancreatectomy. Gastrointest Endosc. 2010;72(3):536–42. https://doi.org/10.1016/j.gie.2010.04.011. Epub 2010 Jul 3
6. Nathan JD, Yang Y, Eaton A, Witkowski P, et al. Surgical approach and short-term outcomes in adults and children undergoing total pancreatectomy with islet autotransplantation: a report from the prospective observational study of TPIAT. Pancreatology. 2022;22(1):1–8. https://doi.org/10.1016/j.pan.2021.09.011. Epub 2021 Sep 29. PMID: 34620552; PMCID: PMC8748311
7. Bassi C, Marchegiani G, Dervenis C, Sarr M, et al., International Study Group on Pancreatic Surgery (ISGPS)The 2016 update of the International Study Group (ISGPS) definition and grading of postoperative pancreatic fistula: 11 Years After. Surgery. 2017;161(3):584–91. https://doi.org/10.1016/j.surg.2016.11.014. Epub 2016 Dec 28.

Chapter 9
Combined Procedures (Open Vs. MIS)

Jörg Kleeff, Johannes Klose, and Ulrich Ronellenfitsch

Introduction

Given that the concept and pathogenesis of chronic pancreatitis had been poorly defined until the 1950s, surgical options were mostly limited to symptomatic measures [1]. Procedures to resolve cholestasis in the early twentieth century were all limited to extrapancreatic structures and included cholecystostomy, cholecystoenterostomy, and bilioenteric anastomosis. Although it was known that drainage and stone removal from the pancreatic duct led to pain relief, only in 1954 Zollinger and Duval introduce the first combined drainage and resection procedure, which included distal pancreatectomy with splenectomy and distal pancreatojejunostomy for internal drainage [2, 3]. However, such retrograde internal drainage usually provided little pain relief. Over time, the notion that the "pacemaker of pain" in chronic pancreatitis is most often located in the pancreatic head emerged [4]. While mere drainage operations came into clinical practice in the late 1950s and pancreatoduodenectomy was the established treatment for pancreatic head malignancies, in 1972 the first duodenum-preserving resection of the head of the pancreas was performed by Beger [5]. The aim of the procedure was to remove the pacemaker of pain, providing effective pancreatic drainage and removing cholestasis while at the same time preserving pancreatic tissue to the most possible extent. This concept has been further developed in technical and anatomical modifications to the procedure. Nowadays, combined resection and drainage procedures form an important cornerstone in the surgical treatment of chronic pancreatitis.

J. Kleeff (✉) · J. Klose · U. Ronellenfitsch
Department of Visceral, Vascular and Endocrine Surgery, University Hospital Halle (Saale),
Martin-Luther-University Halle-Wittenberg, Halle (Saale), Germany
e-mail: joerg.kleeff@uk-halle.de; johannes.klose@uk-halle.de;
ulrich.ronellenfitsch@uk-halle.de

E. P. Ceppa et al. (eds.), *The SAGES Manual of Evolving Techniques in Pancreatic Surgery*, https://doi.org/10.1007/978-3-031-78409-5_9

Indications for Combined Resection and Drainage Surgery for Chronic Pancreatitis and Choice of One Procedure Vs. the Other

Rationale for Surgery in Chronic Pancreatitis

The aim of surgery in patients with chronic pancreatitis is multi-faceted. Most importantly, relief from pain, which often severely disables patients in their daily activities, must be achieved. This can lead to a significant improvement in patients' quality of life. Secondly, preservation or restoration of gastrointestinal function, which comprises the integrity of the stomach and duodenum, the exocrine pancreas function as well as the biliary excretion into the intestinal tract, should be attained. Left-sided portal hypertension resulting from compression of the portal vein and the confluence of the superior mesenteric and the splenic vein should be resolved. Lastly, preservation of the pancreatic endocrine function is important. Keeping these goals in mind, the ideal surgical approach for chronic pancreatitis should both remove the "pacemaker of pain" [4], which is predominantly located in the pancreatic head and only rarely in the tail, and provide drainage of a pre-stenotic dilated pancreatic and/or biliary duct. Combined resection and drainage procedures are used to achieve these aims. In contrast to pancreatoduodenectomy, distal pancreatectomy, or total pancreatectomy, they limit the resection of pancreatic tissue to the diseased parts and maintain the maximal possible amount of healthy pancreatic tissue and the distal stomach and duodenum. At the same time, they provide effective drainage of the dilated pancreatic and/or biliary duct to the small intestine.

Procedures

Two combined resection-drainage operations are commonly used while one is rarely employed contemporarily. In addition, there are several modifications or combinations of these techniques.

The duodenum-preserving pancreatic head resection (DPPHR), also named *Beger* procedure after the German surgeon who first performed it in the 1970s and reported the first large case series in 1980 [5], includes a division of the pancreas at the level of the mesenteric-portal axis, which can release compression of the portal vein and thereby revert left-sided portal hypertension. The proximal pancreas is divided along the concave side of the descending part of the duodenum, preserving a layer of pancreatic tissue as well as the common bile duct and the papilla (Fig. 9.1). The intrapancreatic segment of the common bile duct is dissected along its anterior wall, which often leads to its decompression. The procedure results in removal of the pancreatic head and uncinate process while preserving a few millimeters wide remnant of the pancreatic head towards the duodenal wall. Subsequently, an

Fig. 9.1 Duodenum-preserving pancreatic head resection (DPPHR). Division of the proximal pancreas along the concave side of the descending part of the duodenum, preserving a layer of pancreatic tissue as well as the common bile duct and the papilla. (From [28])

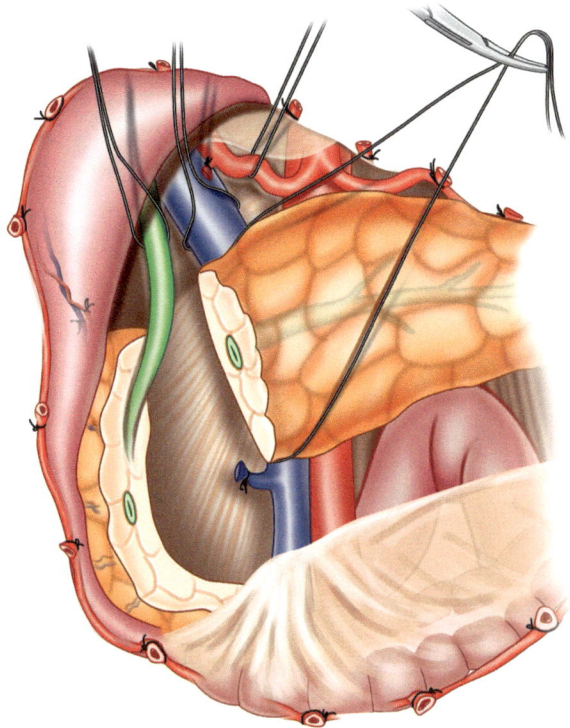

anastomosis of the divided pancreatic duct at the body, and optionally of the common bile duct to a small bowel loop, is performed as Roux-en-Y reconstruction.

The *Frey* procedure, named after the American surgeon who first described it in 1987 [6], can be regarded as a combination of DPPHR and the Partington-Rochelle operation. The extent of resection at the pancreatic head is smaller than in DPPHR since a posterior layer of pancreatic tissue is preserved. The pancreas is thus not transected at the level of the mesenteric-portal axis, which facilitates the operation especially in the presence of massive inflammatory adhesions. However, a possible left-sided portal hypertension cannot be resolved. It uses a long side-to-side pancreaticojejunostomy with Roux-en-Y reconstruction to drain the pancreatic duct (Fig. 9.2).

The *Duval* operation dates back to the 1950s, when it was first described independently by Duval and Zollinger [2, 3]. It involves drainage of the pancreatic duct towards its distal end by resecting the pancreatic tail and performing an anastomosis between the pancreatic remnant and a small intestinal loop. The procedure resects the "pacemaker of pain" only in the rare cases where it is located in the tail, and thus does not often lead to sustainable pain relief. This is the reason why it has been largely abandoned.

The *Hamburg modification* was described in 1998 by Izbicki et al. [7]. It represents a modification of the Frey procedure and involves a larger extent of pancreatic

Fig. 9.2 Frey procedure. Construction of a retrocolic long side-to-side pancreaticojejunostomy to drain the pancreatic duct. (From [28])

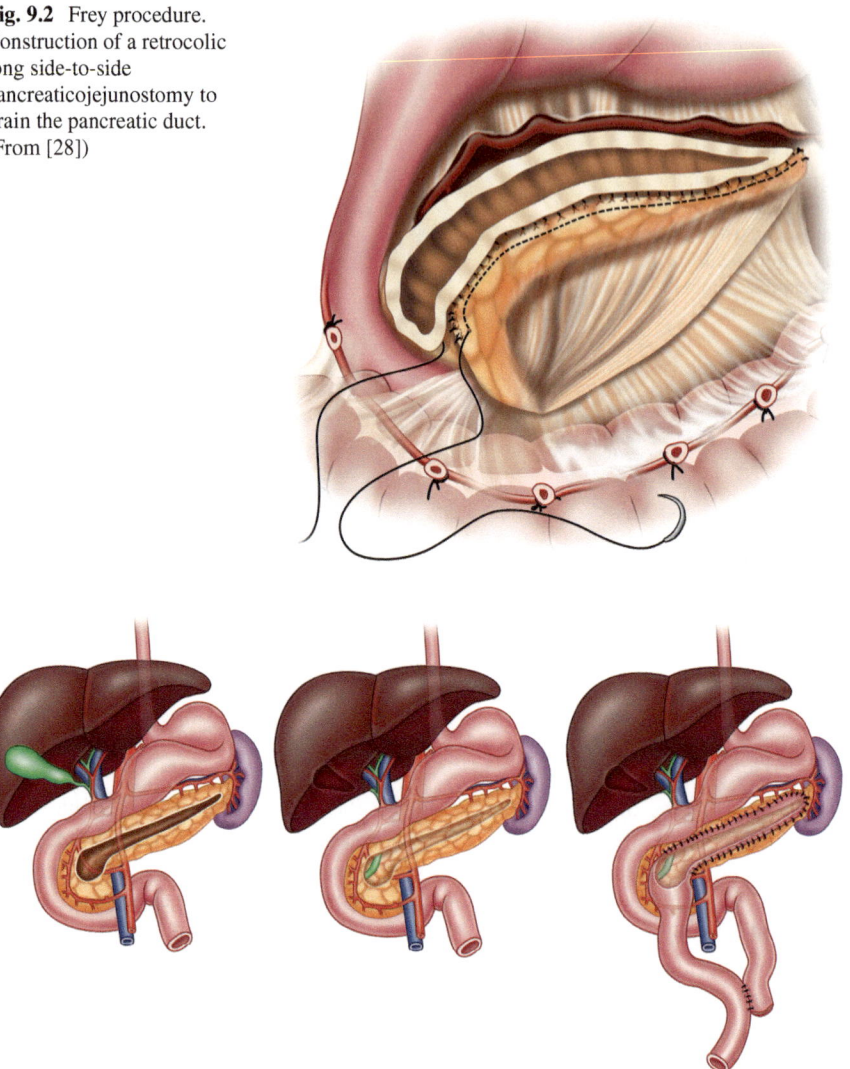

Fig. 9.3 Hamburg modification. A larger extent of pancreatic head including the uncinate process is resected, while division of the pancreas at the level of the mesenteric-portal axis is avoided. After pancreatic duct decompression, a long side-to-side pancreaticojejunostomy with Roux-en-Y reconstruction is performed. (From [29])

head resection reaching also into the uncinate process. It avoids division of the pancreas at the level of the mesenteric-portal axis in order to reduce the risk of vessel injury. The pancreatic duct is further decompressed by a V-shaped excision of the anterior pancreatic wall, and a long side-to-side pancreaticojejunostomy with Roux-en-Y reconstruction is performed (Fig. 9.3).

The *Berne modification* was described in 2001 by Gloor et al. and combines the Frey procedure with DPPHR [8]. It also avoids division of the pancreas at the level of the mesenteric-portal axis. Division is instead performed further towards the duodenum so that the anterior surface of the common bile duct is still completely dissected. Reconstruction is done similarly to DPPHR with pancreaticojejunostomy and a Roux limb (Fig. 9.4).

Indications

The indication for a combined resection and drainage procedure is the removal of an assumed "pacemaker of pain," usually located in the pancreatic head, with the expectation that a mere drainage operation cannot relieve the symptoms because compression of the pancreatic and bile duct would persist. Obstruction of the common bile duct or the pancreatic duct resulting in duct stones or pseudocysts, or of the portal vein resulting in left-sided portal hypertension can also constitute an indication for surgery, even in the absence of severe pain. Several meta-analyses showed that the long-term outcomes of surgery are superior to those of endoscopic treatment with regard to pain relief [9]. Given their lower invasiveness and risk of complications, endoscopic treatments are often the first treatment step. Usually, the indication for the operation is seen when repetitive endoscopic treatments fail to have a beneficial effect. The operation should not be delayed for too long, as pain can become chronic and refractory to therapy [10, 11]. Several studies showed that an operation early after first diagnosis leads to much stronger pain relief, and that a high number of endoscopic procedures as well as opioid use are associated with

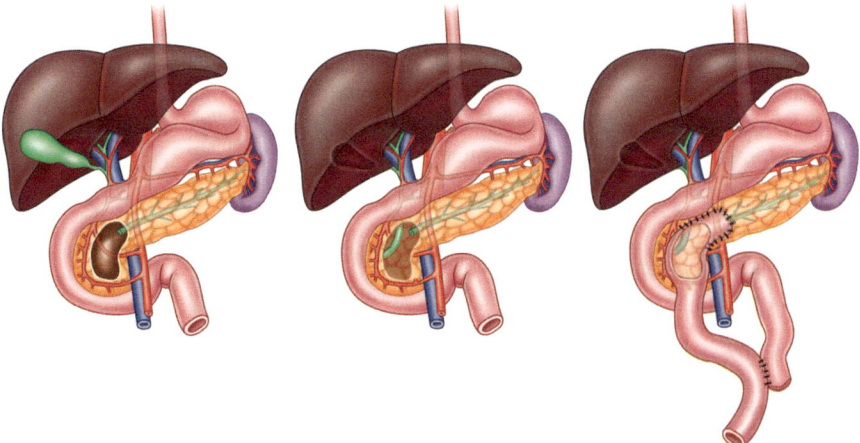

Fig. 9.4 Berne modification. In this combination of the Frey procedure with DPPHR, the pancreatic division is performed further towards the duodenum with the anterior surface of the common bile duct being completely dissected. (From [29])

worse pain relief [12, 13]. Endoscopic and isolated drainage procedures bear the risk that a malignant tumor is not detected and not removed. The risk of developing pancreatic cancer is markedly increased in patients with chronic pancreatitis. It reaches 4.6% at 5 years after and 14.0% at 25 years after first diagnosis of chronic pancreatitis. It is assumed that this risk can be reduced by 90% with a combined drainage and resection procedure [10, 11, 14]. However, lower estimates of cancer risk in chronic pancreatitis patients have lately been reported, and the risk reduction achieved by surgery has been disputed.

Contraindications

There are several relative and absolute contraindications towards combined resection and drainage procedures in chronic pancreatitis. A very limited physical status and severe comorbidities can represent contraindications against any larger abdominal surgery including combined resection and drainage procedures. Common comorbidities in patients with chronic pancreatitis are persistent alcohol abuse, often with liver cirrhosis, and addiction to opioids. Careful multidisciplinary assessment by the surgeon, the anesthesiologist, and other disciplines (e.g., gastroenterologists, cardiologists) is required to assess the operative risk. A pronounced lack of expected postoperative compliance, especially if exocrine or endocrine dysfunction is to be expected, is a relative contraindication to surgery. Finally, severe portal hypertension, often occurring due to complete occlusion of the superior mesenteric, splenic, or portal vein, with enlarged venous collaterals around the pancreas constitute a prohibitive risk of intraoperative hemorrhage or of destruction of portal venous drainage and subsequent hemorrhagic intestinal infarction. In such cases, complete pancreatic head resection is contraindicated, limiting the choice of feasible procedures. If malignancy is suspected based on imaging features or high Ca 19–9 serum levels without concomitant cholestasis, or even histologically confirmed, a combined resection and drainage procedure is not indicated. Rather, an oncological resection, usually pancreatoduodenectomy or total pancreatectomy, with systematic lymphadenectomy, must be performed.

Choice of Procedure

First, the choice between a mere resection procedure and a potentially parenchyma-sparing combined drainage and resection procedure should be made. A meta-analysis of randomized controlled trials published in 2016 showed no relevant differences between pancreatoduodenectomy and DPPHR in terms of morbidity and mortality, but a shorter hospital stay following DPPHR [15]. The available evidence was insufficient to allow for a comparison of postoperative pain relief. Results of the hitherto largest multicentric study, the ChroPac trial, were published in 2017

[16]. The trial showed no difference in its primary endpoint, quality of life 24 months after surgery, or in the secondary endpoints such as postoperative complications, length of hospital stay, and endocrine function, between the two procedures. Based on this evidence, no clear recommendation for either pancreatoduodenectomy on the one hand or parenchyma-sparing combined drainage and resection procedure on the other hand can be made [10, 11]. Although this recommendation is based only on expert consensus, DPPHR and modifications are to be favored over pancreato-duodenectomy in patients with severe portal hypertension and portal venous drainage via collaterals (Fig. 9.5) given the high risk of intraoperative bleeding and postoperative hemorrhagic intestinal infarction [10].

If a specific combined drainage and resection procedure is decided for, the choice which of the different procedures is most appropriate for a given patient is not easy and only partially supported by high-level evidence regarding selected clinical outcomes. The Duval procedure is only indicated in the rare cases in which the "pacemaker of pain" is suspected to be located in the pancreatic tail. A recently published network meta-analysis of the eleven hitherto conducted randomized controlled trials, which all showed at least one domain with a high risk of bias, aimed at comparing the different operations for chronic pancreatitis with the pacemaker supposedly located in the pancreatic head, i.e., pancreatoduodenectomy, DPPHR, the Berne modification, and the Frey procedure [17]. For none of the operations, a statistically significant advantage over another one was found for the outcomes pain relief, quality of life, pancreatic function, morbidity, and mortality. Probability ranking showed that for short-term pain relief, PPPD had the highest probability of being ranked first followed by the Berne, Frey, and DPPHR procedures, while for long-term pain relief the Berne modification was ranked first. For quality of life, the Frey operation had the highest probability of being ranked first. Both for exocrine and endocrine pancreatic function, the Berne and Frey procedures were ranked first. For postoperative morbidity and long-term mortality, the Berne modification had the highest probability of being ranked most beneficial followed by the Frey procedure, DPPHR,

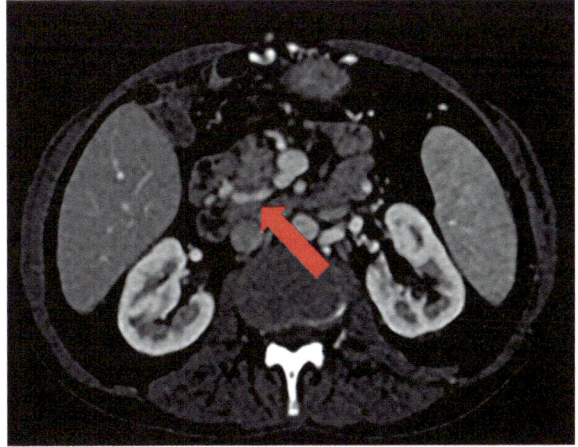

Fig. 9.5 Axial CT image of a patient with chronic pancreatitis, occlusion of the portal vein, and consecutive severe portal hypertension with portal venous drainage via retropancreatic collaterals (red arrow)

and PPPD. Another network meta-analysis including eight randomized controlled trials with 597 patients, all judged to have moderate to high risk of bias, ranked DPPHR best for pain relief and the Frey procedure best for quality of life and exocrine pancreatic function [18].

In summary, the available evidence cannot convincingly show that one single procedure is superior to the others with regard to the wide spectrum of clinical outcomes. Therefore, the indication for surgery and the choice of procedure requires an individualized approach, which is tailored to the morphological disease stage, comorbidities and overall physical status of the given patient. In particular, portal or superior mesenteric vein compression or occlusion and the presence of portal venous collaterals may constitute a contraindication against pancreatic head resection and thus against PPPD and DPPHR, leaving the choice between the Frey procedure and the Berne modification. In turn, as explained above, PPPD is mandatory if malignancy is suspected.

Pre-op and Preparation Pearls

Preoperative Workup

A thorough preoperative workup is key for a correct indication for surgery, for the best choice of the procedure, and for a good postoperative outcome. It should include the following items:

- Confirmed diagnosis of chronic pancreatitis, excluding non-pancreatic pain to the largest possible extent
- Treatment of the respective cause of pancreatitis

    - Alcohol cessation in alcoholic pancreatitis
    - Tobacco cessation since smoking is a known risk factor for chronic pancreatitis and accelerates disease progression
    - Cholecystectomy and removal of common bile duct stones in biliary pancreatitis
    - Immunosuppressive treatment in autoimmune pancreatitis
    - Cessation of causative drug in drug-induced pancreatitis

- Evaluation of pain (pain diary, visual analogue pain scale)
- Employment/work history
- Evaluation of quality of life with a validated instrument, for example, the EORTC QLQ-C30 and QLQ-PAN26 modules [19]
- Clinical evaluation:

    - Height and weight, body mass index
    - Jaundice
    - Ascites
    - Other clinical signs of liver failure

- Evaluation of exocrine (steatorrhea, fecal elastase measurements) and endocrine (glucose profile, HbA1c and C-peptide measurements, insulin dosage) pancreatic function
- Laboratory tests:
  - Complete blood count
  - Liver function tests (transaminases, albumin, cholinesterase)
  - Cholestasis indicators (direct and indirect bilirubin, alkaline phosphatase, gamma-glutamyl transferase)
  - Coagulation tests (INR, partial thrombin time)
  - Electrolytes
  - Kidney function tests
  - Ca 19–9
  - IgG4

- Triphasic CT with a specific focus on:
  - Pancreatic masses
  - Calcifications
  - Involvement of adjacent organs
  - Portal, superior mesenteric, and splenic vein patency
  - (Left-sided) portal hypertension with collaterals
  - Gallstones, common bile duct stones

- MRT/MRCP, endosonography to evaluate the biliary and pancreatic ducts (optional)
- Endosonography-guided biopsy if a mass/malignancy is suspected

Preparation for Surgery

Longer term and immediate preparation for the procedure should comprise:

- Ensuring sufficient postoperative compliance regarding the causative agent (alcohol abstinence, continuation of medical treatment)
- Smoking cessation
- Prehabilitation including improvement of nutritional status according to nutrition guidelines, if needed using enteral or parenteral supplementary nutrition, and physical activity
- Preparation of a sufficient number of blood group matched units of packed red blood cells
- Perioperative prophylactic antibiotic prophylaxis ("single shot") according to local standards

Key Steps

The procedures for chronic pancreatitis described above are usually performed as open surgery using a midline or transverse laparotomy. The evidence on minimally invasive approaches is limited to small case series from specialized centers and case reports [20–22]. These reports include very few patients who received an operation other than the Frey procedure. In cases with a more extensive procedure, the rate of conversion to open surgery was high [21]. Therefore, in light of the often-pronounced inflammatory adhesions and the relevant risk of hemorrhage in procedures involving pancreatic transection, minimally invasive surgery for combined resection, and drainage procedures for chronic pancreatitis cannot be generally recommended, but can be performed in experienced centers.

Open combined resection and drainage procedures for chronic pancreatitis require a setup equivalent to that of oncologic pancreatic resections. Patients require multiple large bore iv catheters, a central venous catheter when indicated and usually also an arterial line for continuous blood pressure management. A nasogastric tube is to be placed for the operation and may remain in situ postoperatively if needed. Placement of a Foley catheter allows for more accurate intra- and postoperative fluid management, but it should be removed shortly after the operation to facilitate early mobilization.

The most important surgical steps of the procedures can be summarized as follows.

Common Steps

- Timely antibiotic prophylaxis (see above)
- Supine position with the right or both arms at the sides
- Prepping and draping of the entire abdomen
- Midline or transverse laparotomy, depending on the configuration of the patient's abdomen/coastal arches and previous laparotomies
- Entering the lesser sac by dividing the gastrocolic ligament (caution must be exerted not to injure the gastroepiploic vascular arch)
- Mobilization of the caudal border of the pancreatic body and tail. The right gastroepiploic artery and vein usually need to be ligated and divided for exposure of the ventral plane of the pancreatic head and neck (caution: possible portal venous collaterals)
- Mobilization of the right colonic flexure and Kocher's maneuver, allowing for ventral and dorsal palpation of the pancreatic head (transduodenal biopsy of a suspicious mass for frozen section possible)
- Exposure of the portal and superior mesenteric vein at the caudal border of the pancreas and division of venous and arterial tributaries next to the pancreatic head and uncinate process
- Cholecystectomy (if not performed in a previous surgery)

Frey Procedure/Hamburg Modification

- Localization of the pancreatic duct by palpation or puncture with a small gauge needle and aspiration
- Incision of the ventral pancreas at the location of the duct, identification of duct orientation using an angulated clamp
- Opening of the duct to within 1.5 cm of the pancreatic tail and 1 cm of the ampulla, removal of all visible stones
- Verification of ampullary patency by placing a small probe through the ampulla into the duodenum (caution: due to invagination of the pancreatic head into the duodenum, the duct turns posterior-laterally from the ventral surface of the pancreas next to the duodenal margin until the ampulla is reached)
- Excision of the ventral portion of the pancreatic head up to the dorsal wall of the pancreatic duct; some tissue should be left along the duodenal curve and right of the superior mesenteric vein; frozen section of excised tissue is possible if malignancy cannot be ruled out
- **Hamburg modification:** V-shaped extension of excision into the uncinate process
- Identification and preservation of the intrapancreatic common bile duct, removal of periductal inflammations, thus relieving compression (in case of persisting stricture or duct injury, choledochojejunostomy can or must be performed)
- Roux-en-Y reconstruction with two-layered retrocolic pancreaticojejunostomy (outer layer: interrupted sutures, jejunal serosa and muscularis to pancreatic capsule; inner layer: continuous suture, full-thickness jejunum to the incised pancreatic surface) and end-to-side jejunojejunostomy 40 cm aborally from the pancreaticojejunostomy

DPPHR/Berne Modification

- Ligation of the gastroduodenal artery at its origin from the common hepatic artery
- Exposure of the common bile duct in the hepatoduodenal ligament up to the cranial pancreatic border
- Exposure of the confluence of the superior mesenteric vein and the splenic vein and of the portal vein dorsally to the pancreatic head (caution: adhesions of the pancreatic tissue to the veins, portal venous collaterals)
- Division of the pancreatic neck at the level of the mesenteric-portal axis
- **Berne modification:** no division of the pancreatic neck, avoiding complete dissection of the portal vein
- Subtotal excision of the pancreatic head by dividing small venous and arterial tributaries and dissecting the pancreatic tissue from the common bile duct towards the papilla and the uncinate process; frozen section of excised tissue is possible if malignancy cannot be ruled out

- Removal of inflammatory tissue around the common bile duct, thus relieving compression (in case of persisting stricture or duct injury, choledochojejunostomy can or must be performed); some pancreatic tissue must be left along the duodenal curve between the common bile duct and the duodenal wall
- Retrocolic Roux-en-Y pancreatojejunostomy: two-layered end-to-side anastomosis between the left pancreas and jejunum (outer layer: interrupted or continuous suture, jejunal serosa and muscularis to pancreatic capsule; inner layer: interrupted or continuous suture, jejunal mucosa to pancreatic duct)
- Latero-lateral pancreatojejunostomy between the same jejunal limb and the pancreatic head remnant (outer layer: interrupted or continuous suture, jejunal serosa and muscularis to pancreatic capsule; inner layer: interrupted or continuous suture, full-thickness jejunum to the incised pancreatic surface)
- End-to-side jejunojejunostomy 40 cm aborally from the pancreaticojejunostomy

Pitfalls/Tricks

- To facilitate dissection of the ventral side of the superior mesenteric and portal vein, a suture can be placed through the pancreatic tissue at the level of the neck in order to lift the pancreas ventrally.
- In case of pronounced hemorrhage during vessel dissection, compression of the pancreas can compress the portal and splenic vein and reduce blood flow, allowing for portal vein exposure and repair of its wall.
- To avoid injuring the common bile duct, a thin probe can be inserted through the orifice of the cystic duct (if no prior cholecystectomy had been performed) or through a small incision into the duct.

Specific Postoperative Outcomes

The postoperative complications specific to combined resection and drainage procedures for chronic pancreatitis mostly overlap with complications after pancreatic surgery for other indications (see dedicated chapters in this manual).

Local Complications

- Postoperative pancreatic fistula (POPF), classifiable according to the ISGPS consensus [23]
- Delayed gastric emptying (DGE), classifiable according to the ISGPS consensus [24]

- Postpancreatectomy hemorrhage (PPH), classifiable according to the ISGPS consensus [25]
- Postpancreatectomy Acute Pancreatitis (PPAP), classifiable according to the ISGPS consensus [26]
- Bile leak, classifiable according to the ISGPS consensus [27]
- Bile duct stricture with cholestasis
- Leak of the entero-enterostomy
- Chyle leak
- Surgical site infection

Systemic Complications

- Pneumonia
- Acute kidney failure
- Catheter infection/sepsis
- Endocrine pancreatic failure with newly onset or deteriorating diabetes mellitus
- Hypoglycemia in case of insulin overdosing and insufficient oral intake
- Exocrine pancreatic failure with bloating, abdominal pain, and malabsorption

Management of these complications is described in detail in other chapters of this manual.

References

1. Plagemann S, Welte M, Izbicki JR, Bachmann K. Surgical treatment for chronic pancreatitis: past, present, and future. Gastroenterol Res Pract. 2017;2017:8418372.
2. Duval MK Jr. Caudal pancreatico-jejunostomy for chronic relapsing pancreatitis. Ann Surg. 1954;140(6):775–85.
3. Zollinger RM, Keith LM Jr, Ellison EH. Pancreatitis. N Engl J Med. 1954;251(13):497–502.
4. Bockman DE, Buchler M, Malfertheiner P, Beger HG. Analysis of nerves in chronic pancreatitis. Gastroenterology. 1988;94(6):1459–69.
5. Beger HG, Witte C, Krautzberger W, Bittner R. Experiences with duodenum-sparing pancreas head resection in chronic pancreatitis. Chirurg. 1980;51(5):303–7.
6. Frey CF, Smith GJ. Description and rationale of a new operation for chronic pancreatitis. Pancreas. 1987;2(6):701–7.
7. Izbicki JR, Bloechle C, Broering DC, Kuechler T, Broelsch CE. Longitudinal V-shaped excision of the ventral pancreas for small duct disease in severe chronic pancreatitis: prospective evaluation of a new surgical procedure. Ann Surg. 1998;227(2):213–9.
8. Gloor B, Friess H, Uhl W, Büchler MW. A modified technique of the Beger and Frey procedure in patients with chronic pancreatitis. Dig Surg. 2001;18(1):21–5.
9. Boregowda U, Echavarria J, Umapathy C, Rosenkranz L, Sayana H, Patel S, et al. Endoscopy versus early surgery for the management of chronic pancreatitis: a systematic review and meta-analysis. Surg Endosc. 2022;36:8753–63.
10. Beyer G, Hoffmeister A, Michl P, Gress TM, Huber W, Algül H, et al. S3-Leitlinie Pankreatitis—Leitlinie der Deutschen Gesellschaft für Gastroenterologie, Verdauungs- und

Stoffwechselkrankheiten (DGVS)[1]—September 2021—AWMF Registernummer 021-003. Z Gastroenterol. 2022;60(3):419–521.

11. Löhr JM, Dominguez-Munoz E, Rosendahl J, Besselink M, Mayerle J, Lerch MM, et al. United European gastroenterology evidence-based guidelines for the diagnosis and therapy of chronic pancreatitis (HaPanEU). United European Gastroenterol J. 2017;5(2):153–99.

12. Ahmed Ali U, Nieuwenhuijs VB, van Eijck CH, Gooszen HG, van Dam RM, Busch OR, et al. Clinical outcome in relation to timing of surgery in chronic pancreatitis: a nomogram to predict pain relief. Arch Surg. 2012;147(10):925–32.

13. Willner A, Bogner A, Müssle B, Teske C, Hempel S, Kahlert C, et al. Disease duration before surgical resection for chronic pancreatitis impacts long-term outcome. Medicine (Baltimore). 2020;99(44):e22896.

14. Ueda J, Tanaka M, Ohtsuka T, Tokunaga S, Shimosegawa T. Surgery for chronic pancreatitis decreases the risk for pancreatic cancer: a multicenter retrospective analysis. Surgery. 2013;153(3):357–64.

15. Gurusamy KS, Lusuku C, Halkias C, Davidson BR. Duodenum-preserving pancreatic resection versus pancreaticoduodenectomy for chronic pancreatitis. Cochrane Database Syst Rev. 2016;2(2):Cd011521.

16. Diener MK, Hüttner FJ, Kieser M, Knebel P, Dörr-Harim C, Distler M, et al. Partial pancreatoduodenectomy versus duodenum-preserving pancreatic head resection in chronic pancreatitis: the multicentre, randomised, controlled, double-blind ChroPac trial. Lancet. 2017;390(10099):1027–37.

17. Mou Y, Song Y, Chen HY, Wang X, Huang W, Liu XB, et al. Which surgeries are the best choice for chronic pancreatitis: a network meta-analysis of randomized controlled trials. Front Surg. 2021;8:798867.

18. Ratnayake CBB, Kamarajah SK, Loveday BPT, Nayar M, Oppong K, White S, et al. A network meta-analysis of surgery for chronic pancreatitis: impact on pain and quality of life. J Gastrointest Surg. 2020;24(12):2865–73.

19. Pezzilli R, Bini L, Fantini L, Baroni E, Campana D, Tomassetti P, et al. Quality of life in chronic pancreatitis. World J Gastroenterol. 2006;12(39):6249–51.

20. Kilburn DJ, Chiow AKH, Leung U, Siriwardhane M, Cavallucci DJ, Bryant R, et al. Early experience with laparoscopic Frey procedure for chronic pancreatitis: a case series and review of literature. J Gastrointest Surg. 2017;21(5):904–9.

21. Nag HH, Nekarakanti PK, Arvinda PS, Sharma A. Laparoscopic versus open surgical management of patients with chronic pancreatitis: A matched case-control study. J Minim Access Surg. 2022;18(2):191–6.

22. Nakajima T, Fukumoto T, Tsukamoto T, Kanazawa A, Kodai S, Mori Y. Laparoscopic Frey's procedure for chronic pancreatitis in a Japanese patient. Am J Case Rep. 2020;21:e924206.

23. Bassi C, Marchegiani G, Dervenis C, Sarr M, Abu Hilal M, Adham M, et al. The 2016 update of the international study group (ISGPS) definition and grading of postoperative pancreatic fistula: 11 years after. Surgery. 2017;161(3):584–91.

24. Wente MN, Bassi C, Dervenis C, Fingerhut A, Gouma DJ, Izbicki JR, et al. Delayed gastric emptying (DGE) after pancreatic surgery: a suggested definition by the international study group of pancreatic surgery (ISGPS). Surgery. 2007;142(5):761–8.

25. Wente MN, Veit JA, Bassi C, Dervenis C, Fingerhut A, Gouma DJ, et al. Postpancreatectomy hemorrhage (PPH): an international study group of pancreatic surgery (ISGPS) definition. Surgery. 2007;142(1):20–5.

26. Marchegiani G, Barreto SG, Bannone E, Sarr M, Vollmer CM, Connor S, et al. Postpancreatectomy acute pancreatitis (PPAP): definition and grading from the international study group for pancreatic surgery (ISGPS). Ann Surg. 2022;275(4):663–72.

27. Koch M, Garden OJ, Padbury R, Rahbari NN, Adam R, Capussotti L, et al. Bile leakage after hepatobiliary and pancreatic surgery: a definition and grading of severity by the international study group of liver surgery. Surgery. 2011;149(5):680–8.

28. Traverso LW, Frey CF, Mayer K, Beger HG, Rau B, Schlosser W. Chronic pancreatitis. In: Clavien P-A, Sarr MG, Fong Y, Georgiev P, editors. Atlas of upper gastrointestinal and hepato-pancreato-biliary surgery. Berlin, Heidelberg, Springer; 2007. p. 849–84.
29. D'Haese J, Hüser N, Maak M, Friess H. Chronische pankreatitis: Chirurgische Therapie. In: Lehnert H, Schellong SM, Mössner J, Sieber CC, Swoboda W, Neubauer A, et al., editors. SpringerReference Innere Medizin: herausgegeben von Hendrik Lehnert. Berlin, Heidelberg, Springer Berlin Heidelberg; 2015. p. 1–9.

Chapter 10
Total Pancreatectomy with Islet Cell Autotransplantation

Jenny Chang, Robert Simon, and R. Matthew Walsh

History/Introduction

The first documented interest in total pancreatectomy dates from the late 1800s with experiments on canines by Joseph von Mering and Oska Minkowski of Strasbourg that demonstrated the lethality of the surgery due to severe hyperglycemia, as insulin was not available until 1922 [1]. Fifty years later, the first successful human total pancreatectomy was performed for hyperinsulinism by Dr. James Priestly at the Mayo Clinic in 1944 [1, 2]. The revolutionary work of isolating and transplanting islet cells in rodent and canine models turned into human trials of isolated islet transplantation from cadaveric donors which paved the foundation for the first reported human total pancreatectomy with islet cell autotransplantation (TPIAT) performed in 1977 by Dr. David Sutherland at the University of Minnesota [3, 4]. Specialized centers that perform TPIAT have evolved further with surgical innovation and improved outcomes.

Supplementary Information The online version contains supplementary material available at https://doi.org/10.1007/978-3-031-78409-5_10.

J. Chang · R. Simon · R. M. Walsh (✉)
Department of General Surgery, Digestive Disease Institute, Cleveland Clinic, Cleveland, OH, USA
e-mail: Changj7@ccf.org; walshm@ccf.org

Indications

Adults

The primary indications for TPIAT are intractable abdominal pain of visceral origin due to chronic pancreatitis or recurrent acute pancreatitis leading to impaired quality of life. The decision for TPIAT vs. other surgical procedures is an individualized one, based on the patient's etiology, disease morphology, comorbidities including diabetes, symptom burden, rate of disease progression, and thorough evaluation by a multidisciplinary team [5]. Patients with a known hereditary cause of chronic or recurrent acute pancreatitis such as alteration in the CFTR, SPINK1, and PRSS1 genes should be given special consideration as their disease is unlikely to remit and affects the entire gland making other surgical options untenable, while subjecting these patients to a lifetime risk of pancreatic cancer. Historically, TPIAT was considered after all other medical, endoscopic, and surgical therapies have failed. Currently, an argument can be made for earlier intervention to prevent lower islet cell yield from the fibrosis of ongoing pancreatitis or prior partial pancreatectomies. Additionally, an improved pain response may occur with earlier intervention for chronic pancreatitis, which is particularly inferred from experience in pediatric patients. Central sensitization from recurrent inflammation may permanently damage nociceptive neurons. Additionally, in those patients treated with chronic opioid therapy, earlier intervention can help eliminate the possibility of opioid-induced hyperalgesia, a lower threshold for pain that may be a consequence of a prolonged duration of chronic pain, and can be extremely problematic in this era of opioid crisis [5, 6].

Pediatrics

The indications for TPIAT in chronic pancreatitis are the same in children as in adults. Children have distinct considerations, ranging from a high rate of idiopathic and hereditary etiologies, small body size, higher caloric needs for growth, and crucial psychosocial developmental periods. The largest series of pediatric TPIAT is from the University of Minnesota, with an average age of 13.8 year old [7].

In pediatric populations, the most common causes of chronic pancreatitis cannot be altered because they include idiopathic and hereditary etiologies. Additional etiologies of chronic pancreatitis in children include trauma, congenital anatomic variations including pancreatic divisum and annular pancreas. Of children with hereditary etiologies, the lifetime estimated cumulative risk of pancreatic cancer is up to 40–70% [8]. Therapeutic intervention, endoscopic or surgical, as described in previous chapters should be considered when an accurate diagnosis has been established and significant alterations in quality of life are noted, which often include disruptions in schooling. Early treatment to prevent opioid dependency is advisable to avert impairment of growth and development.

Patient Selection

Pancreatitis Etiology and Preoperative Workup

A multidisciplinary team assessment of prospective candidates is ideal, and at our center, this includes involvement of the primary treating physician, gastroenterologist, endocrinologist, surgeon, chronic pain anesthesiologist, and clinical psychologist specializing in chronic pain.

A careful history and understanding of the underlying etiology of CP is required. Although the primary indication for TPIAT is pain relief, it is imperative to recognize that the degree of symptoms does not always correlate with morphologic changes. Minimal change disease is a form of chronic pancreatitis where minimal objective morphologic changes are notable, yet patients may report debilitating pain affecting their quality of life.

Patients with chronic pancreatitis often undergo multiple radiographic studies prior to presentation, variably including CT, MRI/MRCP, ERCP, and/or upper EUS. These imaging modalities are crucial for evidence of neoplasm, demonstration of fibrosis (diffuse or localized), and anatomical considerations such as pancreatic ductal obstruction.

A key factor in selecting patients for TPIAT is assessing the extent of islet cell dysfunction to predict future islet yields. There are varying prevalence estimates of patients with diabetes from chronic pancreatitis, ranging from 25% to 80% [9]. Diabetic patients are still candidates for the operation, provided their beta cell mass is sufficient to produce c-peptide. Evaluation of beta cell mass includes measurement of endogenous insulin production with the following labs: hemoglobin A1c (HbA_{1c}), fasting serum glucose, fasting plasma c-peptide levels, C-peptide with arginine, fasting insulin levels, and glucose with mixed meal tolerance tests.

Pancreatic exocrine function is evaluated with fecal elastase for enzymatic replacement to mitigate perioperative malnutrition. As portal hypertension and hepatic disease are a relative contraindication for TPIAT, LFTs are required. In our institution, prior liver transplant is not a contraindication for TPIAT.

Patients who have failed prior surgical intervention(s) are still candidates for TPIAT, and studies have demonstrated that 10–20% of TPIAT patients have undergone prior pancreatic resection [10]. A prior Whipple procedure has not demonstrated a consequential decreased yield in islets, as most pancreatic islets are concentrated in the body and tail [11]. However, because the method of islet isolation involves disruption of the main pancreatic duct, a prior lateral pancreaticojejunostomy or distal pancreatectomy will decrease up to 50% of the islet cell yield [5, 11].

As one of the main indications for this procedure is pain, confirmation that the pancreas represents the largest factor in the etiology of pain cannot be understated. A retrograde epidural differential neuroaxial blockade is a diagnostic test that allows differentiation of the visceral or non-visceral (centralized or somatosensory) origin of chronic abdominal pain based on the patient's response to injection of normal saline then local anesthetic via an epidural [12, 13]. A celiac plexus block is not a requirement prior to TPIAT, but can also be a useful therapeutic and diagnostic adjunct to target the visceral afferent pain fibers to the pancreas. At our institution, each patient undergoes a thorough standardized evaluation of the patient's pain, mood, and function with a psychologist specializing in chronic pain. Psychosocial factors such as pain catastrophizing, depression and anxiety, post-traumatic stress disorder and unaddressed prior trauma, as well as ongoing litigation are predictors of a chronic pain syndrome which is unlikely to remit after surgery, and therefore must be addressed prior to continuing workup for TPIAT.

Contraindications

Contraindications to TPIAT include active alcohol abuse, which can be determined by measurement of phosphatidylethanol (PEth), a direct alcohol biomarker with nearly 100% sensitivity and detectability for up to 3 weeks after consumption of alcohol [14]. Other contraindications include illicit substance use excluding moderate uses of marijuana, poorly controlled psychiatric illness, litigation related to pain, or the lack of support system that could impair the patient's ability to adhere to the complicated medical management including diabetes, pancreatic enzyme therapy, and opioid pain medication taper. Additionally, current smoking is a contraindication, as it is associated with lower rates of insulin independence after TPIAT [15], presumably due to fibrosis exacerbated by active habitual smoking in chronic pancreatitis and increased perioperative complications.

Because some acinar and ductal tissue is transplanted with islets, pancreatic cancer or precancerous lesions including IPMN is an absolute contraindication.

C-peptide negative diabetes and type 1 diabetes are contraindications to TPIAT as these patients do not have adequate islet yield. However, these patients may be candidates for a total pancreatectomy without islet cell autotransplantation.

Portal vein thrombosis, portal hypertension, or significant liver diseases are contraindications due to the injection of islets into the portal system although research into other islet repository sites, such as the peritoneal cavity, is ongoing.

Procedural Aspects

Preoperative Care

Prophylactic perioperative antibiotics according to local protocol are administered.

Total Pancreatectomy

There are several surgical variations to the total pancreatectomy and biliary and gastrointestinal reconstruction.

Removal of the pancreas as a single specimen vs. two sections is dependent on institutional preference, degree of pancreatic inflammation and fibrosis, and prior decompression or resection procedures.

Splenic preservation is of interest, yet associated splenic vein thrombosis, densely adherent splenic vessels in advanced forms of chronic pancreatitis, and the critical need to avoid prolonged warm ischemia time, limits most attempts at splenic preservation. In our institution, about 70% undergo splenectomy [16], but in one of the largest multicenter TPIAT consortiums (Prospective Observational Study of TPIAT, POST), 95% of adult and 100% of children have undergone splenectomy [10].

Our institution does not preserve the pylorus. Our research has demonstrated that the pylorus preserving technique has a higher rate of long-term complications, up to 55% compared to 15% of the classic technique, particularly due to marginal ulceration [16]. It is also of importance to preserve the coronary vein, which will remain as the only venous drainage of the stomach, and its sacrifice could lead to venous congestion, gastric ischemia, or delayed gastric emptying.

It is imperative to limit warm ischemia time, with ligation of the vascular flow of the pancreas only after complete mobilization and preparation for removal. Precise hemostasis in anticipation for full heparinization at the time of islet cell infusion must also be performed. The gastroduodenal artery (GDA) is test-clamped to confirm preservation of flow to the hepatic proper artery and is only ligated immediately prior to final dissection of the uncinate process and specimen removal.

Various approaches to gastrointestinal and biliary reconstruction have been described. At our institution, the jejunum is brought behind the mesenteric vessels through the aortomesenteric window to lie in the position of the native duodenum and an end-to-side hepaticojejunostomy with interrupted 4–0 polydioxanone suture (PDS) is created. An antecolic end-to-side loop gastrojejunostomy is then created with an inner layer of running 3–0 PDS and outer layer of 3–0 silk.

After completion of the gastrointestinal reconstruction, the fascia and skin are closed, and the patient is taken to the post-anesthesia care unit (PACU) intubated on a continuous insulin infusion for a planned reopening of recent laparotomy and islet infusion once islet cell isolation and purification is completed.

Islet Cell Isolation, Purification

Our institution successfully performs islet cell isolation with remote processing at a location 2 h drive time away. Once the pancreas is removed, the surgeon flushes the organ via the splenic artery and GDA with the University of Wisconsin or histidine-tryptophan-ketoglutarate (HTK) solution, both of which are commonly used for solid organ perseveration, for cold preservation prior to transportation. We believe that lack of onsite or local islet-processing facility should not be a barrier to TPIAT and have comparable outcomes in terms of islet yield and postoperative insulin independence [17]. There is an 8–10 h total time lapse between complete removal of specimen and islet infusion at our institution. Other institutions have reported up to 48 h intervals between specimen removal and islet infusion.

The pancreas undergoes enzymatic with collagenase and proteinase and mechanical digestion via the Ricordi digestion isolation changer to yield islet isolates [18]. To initiate tissue digestion and dissolution, collagenase and proteinase are infused under pressure into the main pancreatic duct to distend the intact gland. After disruption, the pancreas is sectioned and placed in a Ricordi digestion isolation chamber for gentle mechanical dispersion until the islets are separated from acinar tissue as detected by microscopic analysis with dithizone staining. The extent of islet purification is imprecise as a balance must be achieved between purifying the islets away from surrounding tissue (to reduce the volume of the infusate and minimize thrombogenic particulate matter) while preserving the absolute number of islets with each successive purification cycle. Purification is achieved through continuous density gradient centrifugation. Final islet counts can be determined using an automated islet counter or standard manual counting methods, commonly reported as a standardized islet equivalent and islet equivalent per kilogram of body weight. One islet equivalent is equal to the volume of an islet with a diameter of 150 μm. Mean islet yield from large case series are listed in Table 10.2. Before transplant, islet preparations are suspended in a 50:50 solution of 20% human serum albumin and transplant media with antibiotics solution, such as ciprofloxacin. Although there is bacterial contamination from the attached duodenum, there is no clinical benefit to routinely culture this islet preparation. In our retrospective analysis, up to 65% of patients will have positive intraoperative cultures with no difference in infectious complication rate [19].

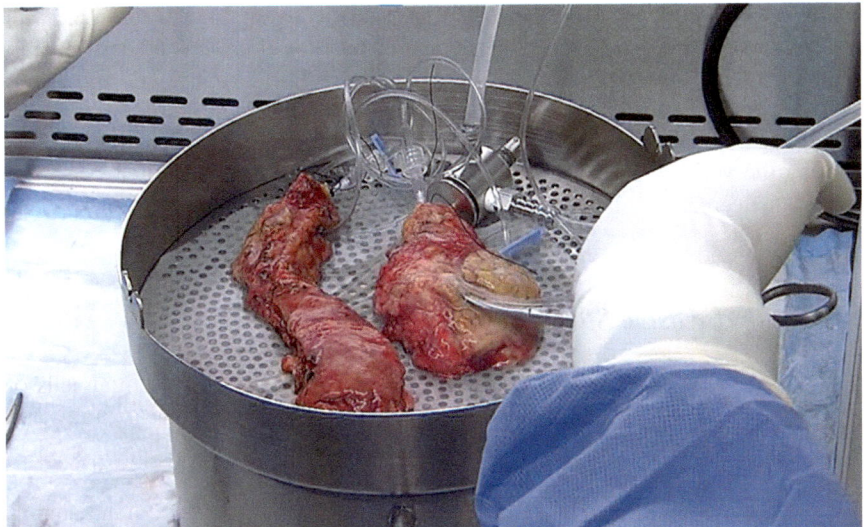

Islet Infusion

In our institution, a re-exploratory laparotomy is performed to confirm hemostasis and examine the biliary and gastrointestinal reconstruction. The portal system can be accessed through the catheterization of the splenic vein, mesenteric vein, umbilical vein in the falciform ligament, or transhepatic direct portal puncture. Our institution typically accesses the splenic vein remnant with a 10-gauge angiocatheter secured with a suture. If the splenic vein remnant is not appropriate, a mesenteric vein such as the inferior mesenteric vein is used. The superior mesenteric vein is a less preferred option as it requires oversewing of the site of venipuncture with 5–0 permanent monofilament suture. A transjugular intrahepatic portosystemic shunt (TIPS) performed by interventional radiology has also demonstrated to be a viable option while preserving portal vein pressure in our limited experience with liver transplant patients. Other institutions have also reported portal vein infusion via percutaneous transhepatic cannulation of the portal system, avoiding the need for a relaparotomy. The absolute volume of islets that can be delivered via intraportal infusion is dependent on the size of the liver and the degree of steatosis. Portal vein pressures are checked periodically with a manometer and if it reaches 25 cm H_2O, the infusion is stopped, and the remaining islets are placed in the peritoneal cavity. The major complications of portal access are portal hypertension and portal vein thrombosis. Weight-based systemic therapeutic heparinization with an initial bolus dosage of 60–70 units per kg is initiated immediately prior to islet infusion. Our research has demonstrated that there are no statistically significant differences in postoperative hemorrhage rates when compared by rates of lower (<60 units per kg) and higher (≥60 units per kg) rates of heparin dosing [19]. Prophylactic anticoagulation is continued postoperatively to help prevent portal vein thrombosis and platelet aggregation. Other current methods to reduce these complications include limiting the volume and rate of infusion and administering dextran for 48 h after surgery to decrease the inflammatory reaction in children [20].

Minimally Invasive Surgery (MIS)

The case complexity and need to minimize warm ischemia time has limited minimally invasive techniques for TPIAT. Publications on all the components of TPIAT (total pancreatectomy, gastrointestinal reconstruction, and AIT) are restricted to limited case series.

At Johns Hopkins University, about 60% of TPIAT operations are performed laparoscopically or laparoscopically assisted with an operative room equipped with an islet isolation laboratory for immediate processing [21]. They sequentially resect the pancreas into two stages—first the head and then the body and tail, which is extracted via the periumbilical 12 mm port. The hepaticojejunostomy is performed using a single layer of running 4–0 barbed sutures [22]. The gastrojejunal anastomosis is performed antecolic, retrogastric along the posterior wall of the stomach with a laparoscopic stapler in a side-to-side technique. Occasionally, a Braun jejunojejunostomy will be created to reduce bile reflux.

Once islet cells are ready for autotransplantation into the liver, a 15-gauge needle placed through a port site is guided into the portal vein. Once completed, the needle is removed, and direct pressure is applied to the site of the portal vein for hemostasis.

Most published literature regarding robot-assisted TPIAT are limited case reports [23]. There is one published series on robot-assisted TPIAT from the University of Arizona with six patients. Their technique is summarized below [24]. The University of Pittsburgh has published a successful case series on the robotic total pancreatectomy, including one case with TPIAT [25]. In the most recent ongoing POST consortium, 7% of adult TPIAT are performed robot-assisted, although their full data is yet to be published [10].

In the University of Arizona group, the pancreatic dissection is started from distal pancreas towards the head, dividing the splenic artery and vein distal to the pancreatic tail to aid the dissection of the body and the tail off the retroperitoneum, then dissection of the superior mesenteric vein, portal vein, and splenic vein confluence. A Kocher maneuver is then performed to mobilize and subsequently divide the duodenum and the pancreatic head, which is removed en-bloc via a Pfannenstiel incision. The hepaticojejunostomy is created over a 5 French stent with running 4–0

PDS sutures and the duodenojejunostomy is created with running 3–0 absorbable barbed sutures for the internal layer and running 3–0 nonabsorbable barbed sutures for the external layer. A stapled Braun jejunojejunostomy is created. A 14-gauge laparoscopic needle is inserted into the splenic vein (SV) stump. After completion of the infusion, the SV stump is double clipped.

There is institutional variation in the methods of islet infusion. Some centers may choose to use the inferior mesenteric vein or another colic vein branch; others have described performance of the islet infusion on the following day utilizing a transjugular approach into the hepatic veins or a percutaneous transhepatic portal vein infusion with the assistance of interventional radiology.

Postoperative Care

Patients are transferred to the intensive care unit (ICU) after surgery with a continuous insulin infusion, extubated the next morning, and subsequently transferred out of the ICU within 24 h on a standardized sliding scale algorithm with assistance from the endocrinology service. They are discharged on a basal bolus regimen to decrease the metabolic burden on the transplanted islets and allow for proper engraftment and revascularization.

All patients at our institution have a 10 French bridled nasojejunal feeding tube placed intraoperatively and are started on enteral feeds on postoperative day 1, which are continued until the patient demonstrates adequate oral intake.

Patients are also continued on deep vein thrombosis (DVT) prophylaxis while inpatient and discharged home on aspirin depending on the level of thrombocytosis from the splenectomy. Proton pump inhibitors are prescribed upon discharge for at least 3 months to prevent marginal ulceration and metoclopramide for 2 weeks to promote gastric motility. A taper to insulin independence is initiated in the outpatient setting with endocrinology.

The median postoperative length of stay is reported to be around 9–11 days for adults and 15 days for children [10, 16].

Lifelong pancreatic enzyme supplementation is required and annual nutritional monitoring for steatorrhea, body composition, and fat-soluble vitamins (A, D, and E), along with bone density is recommended.

Patients continue frequent follow-up with their endocrinologist for the first year after TPIAT, with eventual transition to annual testing for diabetes which includes fasting plasma glucose, hemoglobin A1C, and c-peptide levels. These variables combined with ongoing insulin requirements compromise of the BETA-2 Score which could be used to assess graft function [26].

Outcomes

Perioperative Data

Operative variables of mean operative time, estimated blood loss, and length of stay are listed in Table 10.1 comparing select studies on the open, laparoscopic, and robotic approach.

Perioperative Complications

TPIAT has one of the highest intrinsic complication rates of any elective operation. Immediate operative mortality has been reported to be 0–6% [11, 18]. Morbidity up to 50% has been described, with most commonly reported complications to be pneumonia, delayed gastric emptying, deep venous thrombosis, bleeding, and wound infection [16, 18, 19]. Thirty-day readmission rates range up to 25%, with the most common reason being surgical site infection and gastrointestinal issues (such as small bowel obstruction and delayed gastric emptying) [19]. Up to a 10% reoperative rate within 30 days of TPIAT has been reported, most commonly for bleeding [10]. Despite the risks of hemorrhage associated with this procedure, there is a complex coagulation and pro-inflammatory interface which increases thrombosis risk in these patients, due to the known smoldering inflammatory state that increases venous thromboembolism risk in chronic pancreatitis patients [29], major operation with risk of significant blood loss, and the instant blood-mediated inflammatory reaction with direct exposure of islets to plasma [20]. A complication specific to this procedure is portal vein thrombosis (PVT), which has been described in up to 10% in adults [10]. Some institutions such as the University of Minnesota routinely screen their patients for PVT with ultrasound within the first week of transplant [30], while ours does not.

Table 10.1 Perioperative data

	Open		Laparoscopic	Robotic
Study sample size	112	195	20	6
Mean operative time (min)	544	240	493	717
Mean estimated blood loss (mL)	548.8	589	627.5	630
Mean length of stay (days)	14	9	11	12.6
Citation (year)	Wilson (2014) [27]	Morgan (2018) [15]	Fan (2017) [28]	Galvani (2014) [24]

Endocrine Function

Most series report insulin independence in 20–40% of patients at 1–3 years with manageable insulin requirements for the remainder of patients [7, 11, 31, 32]. These results are summarized in Table 10.2. The number of islet equivalent per kilogram transplanted is the strongest predictor for insulin independence [31, 33, 34]. The incidence between obesity and insulin resistance is a known correlation, and it has been demonstrated that an absolute weight of 78 kg or a BMI greater than 28 may have an increased chance of requiring long-term insulin supplementation in TPIAT patients [31].

Unfortunately, the function of transplanted islet grafts will decline over time. This decrease in function is partially attributed to the proven immediate inflammatory response, termed instant blood-mediated inflammatory reaction, when islets are exposed to blood, along with islet hypoxia which leads to islet apoptosis [20, 35]. Research into alternative low inflammatory reaction transplant sites such as the omentum, muscle, and bone marrow as well as adjuvant agents such as tumor necrosis factor (TNF) blockers are ongoing [36].

Pain and Quality of Life

Multiple studies have demonstrated the reduction of pain in these patients. About 50% of patients are able to be independent from opioids 1 year after surgery, summarized in Table 10.3 below [7, 27, 33, 34]. Pain, per patient reported outcomes, persists or recurs in about 10–20% of patients after TPIAT [5, 37].

Overall, patients report improvements in their perceived physical and mental health, as measured by patient reported outcome surveys, with some institutions reporting up to 92% of patients reporting an overall improvement in health [15, 27, 34], and 60–70% improvement in depression and anxiety although improvement in

Table 10.2 Islet yield and glucose control following TPIAT

Center	University of Minnesota	University of Cincinnati	Medical University of South Carolina	University of Minnesota
Study sample size	215	112	195	75
Mean age (years)	35.7	37.3	40.3	13.8
Mean islet yield (IEG/kg)	3488	6027	3253	N/a
Insulin independence 1 year after TPIAT	27.0%	38%	29%	37%
Insulin independence 5 years after TPIAT	22.3%	27%	23%	N/a
Citation (year)	Bellin (2019) [34]	Wilson (2014) [27]	Morgan (2018) [15]	Chinnakotla (2014) [7]

Table 10.3 Pain control following TPIAT

Center	University of Minnesota	University of Cincinnati	Medical University of South Carolina
Study sample size	215	112	195
Preoperative mean oral morphine equivalents (MEQ/d)	N/a	118.9	208
Mean oral morphine equivalents 1 year after TPAIT (MEQ/d)	N/a	74.1	60
Narcotic independence 1 year after TPIAT	46%	55%	N/a
Narcotic independence 5 year after TPIAT	63%	73%	N/a
Citation (year)	Bellin (2019) [34]	Wilson (2014) [27]	Morgan (2018) [15]

quality of life is not always associated with decreased opioid use [37]. The need to start insulin also has not been associated with a lower quality of life [38]. However, to provide consistency in reporting this data varies, and to address these critical research gaps, a multicenter research consortium called POST was started on 2017 to prospectively collect data about pain, quality of life, glycemic control, and cost-effectiveness in patients undergoing TPIAT [10].

References

1. Schnelldorfer T, Adams DB, Warshaw AL, Lillemoe KD, Sarr MG. Forgotten pioneers of pancreatic surgery: beyond the favorite few. Ann Surg. 2008;247(1):191–202.
2. van Heerden JA. The first total pancreatectomy. Am J Surg. 1986;151(2):197–9.
3. Jahansouz C, Jahansouz C, Kumer SC, Brayman KL. Evolution of β-cell replacement therapy in diabetes mellitus: islet cell transplantation. J Transp Secur. 2011;2011:247959.
4. Najarian JS, Sutherland DE, Baumgartner D, Burke B, Rynasiewicz JJ, Matas AJ, et al. Total or near total pancreatectomy and islet autotransplantation for treatment of chronic pancreatitis. Ann Surg. 1980;192(4):526–42.
5. Bellin MD, Freeman ML, Gelrud A, Slivka A, Clavel A, Humar A, et al. Total pancreatectomy and islet autotransplantation in chronic pancreatitis: recommendations from PancreasFest. Pancreatology. 2014;14(1):27–35.
6. Pasricha PJ. Unraveling the mystery of pain in chronic pancreatitis. Nat Rev Gastroenterol Hepatol. 2012;9(3):140–51.
7. Chinnakotla S, Bellin MD, Schwarzenberg SJ, Radosevich DM, Cook M, Dunn TB, et al. Total pancreatectomy and islet autotransplantation in children for chronic pancreatitis: indication, surgical techniques, postoperative management, and long-term outcomes. Ann Surg. 2014;260(1):56–64.
8. Lowenfels AB, Maisonneuve P, DiMagno EP, Elitsur Y, Gates LK, Perrault J, et al. Hereditary pancreatitis and the risk of pancreatic cancer. International hereditary pancreatitis study group. J Natl Cancer Inst. 1997;89(6):442–6.

9. Hart PA, Bellin MD, Andersen DK, Bradley D, Cruz-Monserrate Z, Forsmark CE, et al. Type 3c (pancreatogenic) diabetes mellitus secondary to chronic pancreatitis and pancreatic cancer. Lancet Gastroenterol Hepatol. 2016;1(3):226–37.

10. Nathan JD, Yang Y, Eaton A, Witkowski P, Wijkstrom M, Walsh M, et al. Surgical approach and short-term outcomes in adults and children undergoing total pancreatectomy with islet autotransplantation: a report from the prospective observational study of TPIAT. Pancreatology. 2022;22(1):1–8.

11. Sutherland DER, Radosevich DM, Bellin MD, Hering BJ, Beilman GJ, Dunn TB, et al. Total pancreatectomy and islet autotransplantation for chronic pancreatitis. J Am Coll Surg. 2012;214(4):409–24.

12. Conwell DL, Vargo JJ, Zuccaro G, Dews TE, Mekhail N, Scheman J, et al. Role of differential neuroaxial blockade in the evaluation and management of pain in chronic pancreatitis. Am J Gastroenterol. 2001;96(2):431–6.

13. Bahuva R, Walsh RM, Kapural L, Stevens T. Morphologic abnormalities are poorly predictive of visceral pain in chronic pancreatitis. Pancreas. 2013;42(1):6–10.

14. Dasgupta A. Chapter 4—Alcohol biomarkers: an overview. In: Dasgupta A, editor. Alcohol and its biomarkers. San Diego, CA: Elsevier; 2015. p. 91–120. (Clinical Aspects and Laboratory Determination) https://www.sciencedirect.com/science/article/pii/B9780128003398000043.

15. Morgan KA, Lancaster WP, Owczarski SM, Wang H, Borckardt J, Adams DB. Patient selection for total pancreatectomy with islet autotransplantation in the surgical management of chronic pancreatitis. J Am Coll Surg. 2018;226(4):446–51.

16. Naples R, Walsh RM, Thomas JD, Perlmutter B, McMichael J, Augustin T, et al. Short- and long-term surgical outcomes of total pancreatectomy with islet autotransplantation: a comparative analysis of surgical technique and intraoperative heparin dosing to optimize outcomes. Pancreatology. 2021;21(1):291–8.

17. Johnston PC, Lin YK, Walsh RM, Bottino R, Stevens TK, Trucco M, et al. Factors associated with islet yield and insulin independence after total pancreatectomy and islet cell autotransplantation in patients with chronic pancreatitis utilizing off-site islet isolation: Cleveland Clinic experience. J Clin Endocrinol Metab. 2015;100(5):1765–70.

18. Rickert C, Lei J, Markmann J. Islet autotransplantation for chronic pancreatitis. In: Current surgical therapy. 12th ed. Elsevier Health Sciences. 2016.

19. Naples R, Perlmutter BC, Thomas JD, McMichael J, Bottino R, Solomina J, et al. Clinical significance of postoperative antibiotic treatment for positive islet cultures after total pancreatectomy with islet autotransplantation. Pancreas. 2021;50(7):1000–6.

20. Naziruddin B, Iwahashi S, Kanak MA, Takita M, Itoh T, Levy MF. Evidence for instant blood-mediated inflammatory reaction in clinical autologous islet transplantation. Am J Transplant. 2014;14(2):428–37.

21. Fackche N, Walsh CM, Singh VK, Makary MA. Total pancreatectomy with islet autotransplantation. In: Current surgical therapy. 13th ed. Elsevier Health Sciences; 2020.

22. Edil BH, Cooper MA, Makary MA. Laparoscopic pancreaticojejunostomy using a barbed suture: a novel technique. J Laparoendosc Adv Surg Tech. 2014;24(12):887–91.

23. Marquez S, Marquez TT, Ikramuddin S, Kandaswamy R, Antanavicius G, Freeman ML, et al. Laparoscopic and da Vinci robot-assisted total pancreaticoduodenectomy and intraportal islet autotransplantation: case report of a definitive minimally invasive treatment of chronic pancreatitis. Pancreas. 2010;39(7):1109–11.

24. Galvani CA, Rilo HR, Samamé J, Porubsky M, Rana A, Gruessner RWG. Fully robotic-assisted technique for total pancreatectomy with an autologous islet transplant in chronic pancreatitis patients: results of a first series. J Am Coll Surg. 2014;218(3):e73.

25. Zureikat AH, Nguyen T, Boone BA, Wijkstrom M, Hogg ME, Humar A, et al. Robotic total pancreatectomy with or without autologous islet cell transplantation: replication of an open technique through a minimal access approach. Surg Endosc. 2015;29(1):176–83.

26. Gołębiewska JE, et al. Assessment of simple indices based on a single fasting blood sample as a tool to estimate beta-cell function after total pancreatectomy with islet autotransplantation—a prospective study. Transpl Int. 2019;32(3):280–90. https://doi.org/10.1111/tri.13364.
27. Wilson GC, Sutton JM, Abbott DE, Smith MT, Lowy AM, Matthews JB, et al. Long-term outcomes after total pancreatectomy and islet cell autotransplantation: is it a durable operation? Ann Surg. 2014;260(4):659–67.
28. Fan CJ, Hirose K, Walsh CM, Quartuccio M, Desai NM, Singh VK, et al. Laparoscopic total pancreatectomy with islet autotransplantation and intraoperative islet separation as a treatment for patients with chronic pancreatitis. JAMA Surg. 2017;152(6):550–6.
29. Chung WS, Lin CL. Comorbid risks of deep vein thrombosis and pulmonary thromboembolism in patients with chronic pancreatitis: a nationwide cohort study. J Thromb Haemost. 2016;14(1):98–104.
30. Robbins AJ, Skube ME, Bellin MD, Dunn TB, Chapman SA, Berry KL, et al. Portal vein thrombosis after total pancreatectomy and islet autotransplant: prophylaxis and graft impact. Pancreas. 2019;48(10):1329–33.
31. Ahmad SA, Lowy AM, Wray CJ, D'Alessio D, Choe KA, James LE, et al. Factors associated with insulin and narcotic independence after islet autotransplantation in patients with severe chronic pancreatitis. J Am Coll Surg. 2005;201(5):680–7.
32. Webb MA, Illouz SC, Pollard CA, Gregory R, Mayberry JF, Tordoff SG, et al. Islet auto transplantation following total pancreatectomy: a long-term assessment of graft function. Pancreas. 2008;37(3):282–7.
33. Chinnakotla S, Radosevich DM, Dunn TB, Bellin MD, Freeman ML, Schwarzenberg SJ, et al. Long term outcomes of total pancreatectomy and islet auto transplantation for hereditary/genetic pancreatitis. J Am Coll Surg. 2014;218(4):530–43.
34. Bellin MD, Beilman GJ, Sutherland DE, Ali H, Petersen A, Mongin S, et al. How durable is total pancreatectomy and intraportal islet cell transplantation for treatment of chronic pancreatitis? J Am Coll Surg. 2019;228(4):329–39.
35. Barshes NR, Wyllie S, Goss JA. Inflammation-mediated dysfunction and apoptosis in pancreatic islet transplantation: implications for intrahepatic grafts. J Leukoc Biol. 2005;77(5):587–97.
36. Baldwin XL, Williams BM, Schrope B, Desai CS. What is new with total pancreatectomy and autologous islet cell transplantation? Review of current progress in the field. J Clin Med. 2021;10(10):2123.
37. Walsh RM, Saavedra JRA, Lentz G, Guerron AD, Scheman J, Stevens T, et al. Improved quality of life following total pancreatectomy and auto-islet transplantation for chronic pancreatitis. J Gastrointest Surg. 2012;16(8):1469–77.
38. Dorlon M, Owczarski S, Wang H, Adams D, Morgan K. Increase in postoperative insulin requirements does not lead to decreased quality of life after total pancreatectomy with islet cell autotransplantation for chronic pancreatitis. Am Surg. 2013;79(7):676–80.

Part IV
Preoperative Diagnosis and Surgical Indications

Chapter 11
Benign, Premalignant, and Malignant Duodenal Neoplasms

Matthew Hernandez, Paul Wong, and Laleh Melstrom

Introduction

Benign tumors of the duodenum represent 10–20% of all duodenal lesions and present asymptomatically in most patients [1]. However, depending on their anatomical location and etiology, these lesions may produce a variety of symptoms, including acute and chronic bleeding, abdominal pain, weight loss, nausea, and gastric outlet obstruction. Over the years, there has been an increased incidence of benign duodenal tumors that can be attributed to the recent improvements and greater use of gastrointestinal endoscopy.

Lesions of Epithelial Origin

Duodenal Adenomas

Duodenal adenomas are the most frequently seen polyp of the duodenum and derive their origins either sporadically or in conjunction with a hereditary genetic condition (e.g., familial adenomatous polyposis and MUTYH-associated polyposis). These adenomas have been reported in 0.3–4.6% of patients undergoing upper gastrointestinal endoscopy and are classified by their locations as ampullary or non-ampullary [2]. Duodenal adenomas are often asymptomatic and found incidentally on endoscopy. However, for ampullary adenomas, these lesions may be associated with obstruction of the biliary or pancreatic duct, leading to jaundice, cholangitis,

M. Hernandez (✉) · P. Wong · L. Melstrom
Department of Surgery, City of Hope National Medical Center, Duarte, CA, USA
e-mail: matthernandez@coh.org; lmelstrom@coh.org

© The Author(s), under exclusive license to Springer Nature
Switzerland AG 2025
E. P. Ceppa et al. (eds.), *The SAGES Manual of Evolving Techniques in Pancreatic Surgery*, https://doi.org/10.1007/978-3-031-78409-5_11

and pancreatitis. Other non-obstructive symptoms for duodenal adenomas may include bleeding, nausea, vomiting, weight loss, and abdominal pain.

Endoscopy remains the prominent diagnostic tool for duodenal adenomas, especially asymptomatic non-ampullary neoplasms. The diagnosis of duodenal adenomas is made based on the lesion's endoscopic appearance and histology. Duodenal adenomas are generally present as flat, small, white-colored lesions that appear slightly elevated when contrasted with the surrounding mucosa. Side-viewing endoscopy is required to obtain a complete evaluation of the lesion, and the features of benign lesions include regular borders, no ulceration, no spontaneous bleeding, and soft texture [3–5]. The histology of duodenal adenomas is classified based on the mucin phenotype, with intestinal type polyps representing 89% of cases and gastric type composing 11% [6, 7]. These phenotypes can be further stratified. Intestinal type polyps are subdivided into tubular and villous adenomas, and gastric type polyps are subclassified into pyloric gland and foveolar adenomas. Furthermore, similar to traditional serrated adenomas (TSA) in the colon, there have been reports of serrated adenomas possessing TSA-like features which possess an aggressive morphology that carries significant risk for malignancy [6, 8, 9].

Resection is often recommended for ampullary and non-ampullary duodenal adenomas given the malignant potential of these neoplasms. However, there are considerations for the method of resection that include size, location, morphology, and pathology of the adenoma. Endoscopic resection is preferred because less invasive, but surgical resection is considered if the adenoma is ≥2 cm, demonstrates severe dysplasia, suspicious carcinomatous infiltration, and recurrence after prior endoscopic resection [10, 11]. There has not been a consensus regarding the optimal endoscopic technique for resection, but the various methods include snare polypectomy, endoscopic mucosal resection, endoscopic submucosal dissection, and argon plasma coagulation ablation. While endoscopic resection provides a less invasive approach to remove the lesion, it comes with a risk of recurrence and complications, namely perforation and bleeding, due to the extensive arterial blood supply and thin walls of the duodenum [10]. Figure 11.1 demonstrates an ampullary adenoma before (a) and after (b) endoscopic resection. Following endoscopic resection,

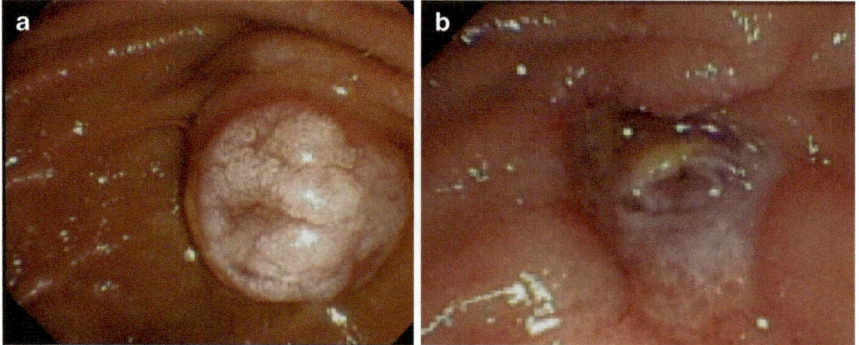

Fig. 11.1 Ampullary adenoma before (**a**) and after (**b**) endoscopic resection

surveillance endoscopy should be performed at 3–6 months which can be extended to 6–12 months if recurrence is not detected, after which patients should be followed with annual endoscopy for at least 2 years after initial endoscopic resection [10, 12–14].

If endoscopic resection is not feasible due to technical challenges of large and anatomically complex adenomas, surgical treatment of these lesions is the standard. Surgical approaches to resect these adenomas include pancreaticoduodenectomy, ampullectomy, and pancreas-preserving duodenectomy, transduodenal adenoma resections, and segmental duodenal resection but are associated with higher cost and greater risk for morbidity and mortality [15, 16]. Patients who receive surgical ampullectomy are recommended to undergo follow-up endoscopy due to the possibility of recurrence but those who undergo pancreaticoduodenectomy do not require further surveillance [5]. Lastly, noninvasive methods, such as non-steroidal anti-inflammatory drugs (NSAIDs) may be employed to treat duodenal adenomas, specifically in patients with familial adenomatous polyposis. In a randomized control trial consisting of 49 post-colectomy patients, there was significant reduction in duodenal polyposis seen after 6 months of treatment with celecoxib compared to a placebo [17].

In patients with familial adenomatous polyposis (FAP), extra caution should be given to ampullary and non-ampullary duodenal adenomas due to the increased risk of malignancy. Duodenal adenomas have been found in up to 90% of FAP patients, and these patients have demonstrated up to a 330-fold higher risk of developing duodenal cancer from these adenomas [16, 18]. In order to stratify risk for duodenal cancer in patients with FAP, the Spigelman Classification, which incorporates number and size of polyps, histology, and dysplasia, is utilized to identify frequency of endoscopic surveillance and need for prophylactic duodenectomy [19] (Table 11.1). Based on the Spigelman criteria, proposed surveillance strategies have advised patients with Stage 0 receive to repeat surveillance endoscopy every 4 years, those

Table 11.1 Spigelman Classification for duodenal adenomas in patients with Familial Adenomatous Polyposis (FAP)

Variables	1 point	2 points	3 points
Number of polyp	1–4	5–20	>20
Size of polyp (mm)	1–4	5–10	>10
Histology	Tubular	Tubulovillous	Villous
Dysplasia	Mild	Moderate	Severe

Spigelman score	Stage	Surveillance frequency
0	0	Every 4 years
1–4	I	Every 2–3 years
5–6	II	Every 2–3 years
7–8	III	Every 6–12 months, with surgical consideration
9–12	IV	Referral for surgery

with Stage I and II undergo endoscopy every 2–3 years, Stage III patients to receive endoscopy every 6–12 months with surgical consideration, and Stage IV patients to be referred for surgery [18, 20].

Duodenal Adenocarcinomas

The most common location for small bowel adenocarcinoma is the duodenum, which accounts for <1% of all gastrointestinal cancers [21]. The most common site within the duodenum is D2, followed by D3/4 [22]. Duodenal cancers in the first portion are quite rare [22, 23]. The clinical presentation is most often associated with pain, bleeding, and obstruction [23]. Patients may also present with weight loss and jaundice if there is ampullary obstruction.

Imaging is most often done in the form of contrast-enhanced computed tomography. Figure 11.2 demonstrates the infiltrative nature of duodenal adenocarcinomas that may lead to bleeding or obstruction. Endoscopy and endoscopic ultrasound further characterize these tumors and determine resectability. CDX2 on pathology which is a sensitive marker for colorectal cancer is more frequently expressed in duodenal adenocarcinomas [24]. Surgical management includes segmental resection and pancreaticoduodenectomy pending the location of the lesions. The importance of lymphadenectomy with a minimum pathologic evaluation of six lymph nodes is associated with improved survival [23, 25]. Adjuvant therapy most often involves systemic chemotherapy and the role of adjuvant radiotherapy has not been

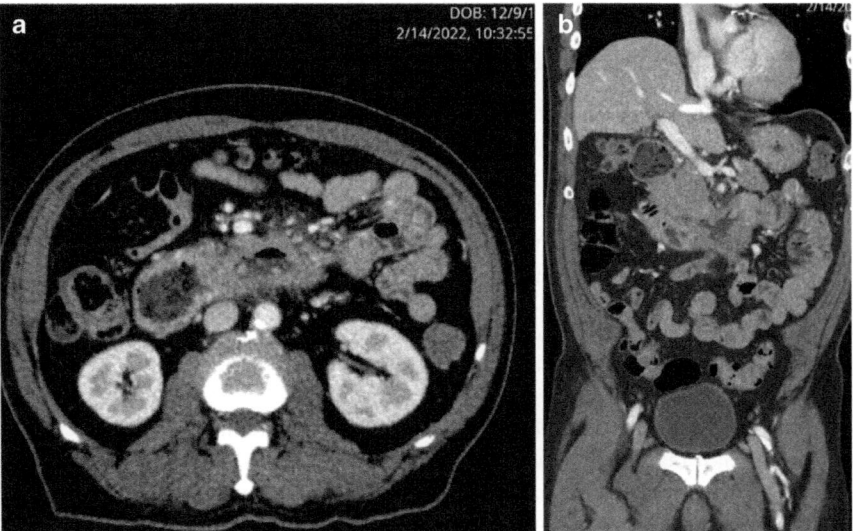

Fig. 11.2 Duodenal adenocarcinoma (**a**) axial and (**b**) coronal computed tomography view of invasive duodenal adenocarcinoma in the third portion of the duodenum

well defined [23]. In patients who are able to undergo resection, 10 year OS can be as high as 41% in some series [26].

Duodenal Neuroendocrine Tumors (D-NETs)

Duodenal neuroendocrine tumors (D-NETs) encompass 1–3% of NETs and specifically 11% of small intestinal NETs [27, 28], with most of these lesions being found in the first or second portions of the duodenum [29, 30]. These lesions can either form sporadically or are associated with familial multiple endocrine neoplasia, type 1 (MEN-1). Sporadic D-NETs are more likely to be solitary lesions, whereas multiple tumors usually raise suspicion of lesions arising in the context of MEN-1 [31].

Like other benign duodenal lesions, the majority of D-NETs are found incidentally on endoscopy. However, symptoms associated with D-NETs include abdominal pain, fatigue, and weight loss, but jaundice or pancreatitis can also be observed in ampullary or periampullary tumors [27]. In addition, excess hormonal expression can be indicative of functional tumors and is associated with clinical syndromes, such as Zollinger-Ellison Syndrome (ZES), carcinoid syndrome, and Cushing's disease [6, 30]. Specifically, ampullary and periampullary D-NETs often present at more advanced stages of disease and portend a worse survival than tumors found in other anatomical locations of the duodenum [30–32].

On endoscopic diagnosis, D-NETs possess a submucosal appearance as white or yellow-colored polyps with central dimpling or ulceration [28]. Endoscopic ultrasound (EUS) should also be conducted in order to confirm the size of the tumor and depth of invasion. Also, since lymph node involvement and liver metastases may be more frequently seen with the gastrinoma type of D-NETs, CT, and/or MRI can be conducted in order to assess the burden of disease [28, 32]. Based on histology subclassifications, 50–60% of D-NETs are gastrinomas, 15% are somatostatin-producing tumors, 19–27% nonfunctional serotonin-containing tumors, <3% are poorly differentiated neuroendocrine carcinomas, and <2% are gangliocytic paragangliomas [27]. Furthermore, histological grading of these lesions is essential for their diagnosis and management. The current standard for NET grading is from the World Health Organization (WHO), and it utilizes mitotic index and Ki-67 proliferation index to assess the relative risk of the tumor (Table 11.2).

Considerations for treatment are dependent on the size and location of the tumor, histological grade, and tumor type. While there is no consensus on the management of D-NETs, proposed algorithms have been based on the ENETS guidelines [27,

Table 11.2 World Health Organization (WHO) classification of neuroendocrine tumor grades

Grade	Mitotic rate (per 10 high power fields)	Ki-67 index
G1, Low	<2	<3%
G2, Intermediate	2–20	3–20%
G3, High	>20	>20%

32]. For non-ampullary or sub-centimeter Grade 1 lesions, endoscopic resection is recommended. Patients with periampullary D-NETs or lesions larger than 2 cm are recommended to receive surgical resection. In addition, D-NETs of any size with lymph node involvement should be considered for surgical resection. However, the management of lesions between 1 and 2 cm remains controversial, and the risks and benefits of endoscopic versus surgical resection should be weighed for these tumors. Fig. 11.3 demonstrates a 1.7 cm ampullary D-NET on MRI (a), endoscopy (b) and during robotic-assisted transduodenal resection.

For postoperative follow-up, the ENETS guidelines recommend abdominal ultrasound, EGD, or CT surveillance and plasma chromogranin A (CgA) levels at 6, 24, and 36 months for patients who underwent endoscopic resection [32]. For patients with surgically resected D-NETs, the recommended strategy includes CT scan, somatostatin receptor scintigraphy or 68Ga-DOTATATE PET/CT, and plasma CgA levels at 6- and 12-months following surgery, and then annually for a minimum of 3 years [32]. NCCN guidelines recommend surveillance of resected patients at 3–12 months, and then subsequent follow-ups every 6–12 months for 10 years.

Other Non-neoplastic Epithelial Lesions

Non-neoplastic lesions may also be present in the duodenum. The histological classifications of these lesions include Brunner's gland hyperplastic polyps, hamartomas, and cysts, along with ectopic gastric mucosa, pancreatic heterotopia, hyperplastic polyps, and inflammatory polyps [6]. Some lesions, such as hamartomatous polyps, are syndromic and have been shown to be associated with Peutz-Jeghers syndrome, Cronkhite-Canada syndrome, Cowden syndrome, and juvenile polyposis syndrome [6]. Endoscopic or surgical resection should be considered if these lesions become large, symptomatic, or demonstrate dysplastic characteristics.

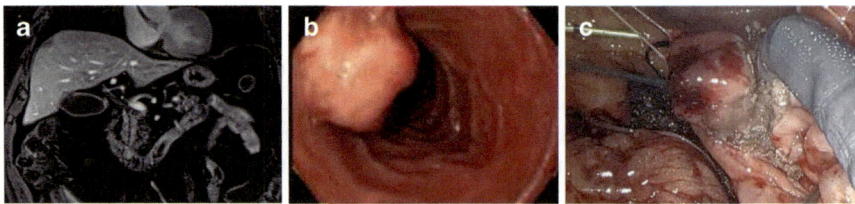

Fig. 11.3 Ampullary D-NET 1.7 cm ampullary D-NET on MRI (**a**), endoscopy (**b**) and during robotic-assisted transduodenal resection (**c**)

Lesions of Mesenchymal Origin

Duodenal Gastrointestinal Stromal Tumors (DGISTs)

Duodenal gastrointestinal stromal tumors (DGISTs) are rare neoplasms arising from interstitial cells of Cajal and are associated with high rates of malignancy [33]. While GISTs are the most common mesenchymal tumor found in the gastrointestinal tract, only 4–5% of these lesions are in the duodenum [34]. Most cases of DGISTs occur sporadically, but these tumors have also been linked to hereditary conditions, namely neurofibromatosis type 1 and Carney triad, in 5–10% of patients [35, 36]. These tumors may be found incidentally, especially if they are small in size, but common clinical presentations of DGISTs include gastrointestinal bleeding and nonspecific abdominal pain.

Preoperative diagnosis of DGISTs most commonly involves gastrointestinal endoscopy with forceps biopsy, especially for tumors possessing intramural growth or ulceration [37]. For extraluminal tumors, CT scans or MRI are most frequently utilized to diagnose the tumors. Endoscopic ultrasound (EUS) with fine-needle aspiration (FNA) was found to have significantly greater sensitivity and positive predictive value in the diagnosis of DGISTs than CT or MRIs [36]. Immunohistochemistry can also be utilized to discern the diagnostic difference between DGISTs and other mesenchymal lesions, as DGISTs are positive for c-Kit (CD117) and CD34, but negative for S-100 [34]. Notably, the histologic subtypes of DGISTs do not differ from GISTs found in other gastrointestinal locations, as these tumors usually present with spindle cell differentiation; the mitotic count of DGISTs has been shown to be lower than its gastric and small bowel counterparts [32].

In terms of treatment, traditional chemotherapy and radiation are not effective against DGISTs, and thus, surgical resection remains the treatment of choice. Current options for surgical resection of DGISTs include pancreaticoduodenectomy or limited resection (i.e., segment or wedge duodenectomy), but there remains controversy over the preferred method. Compared to limited resection, performing a pancreaticoduodenectomy allows for a wider resection margin that would mitigate the risk of positive margins and local recurrence [38, 39]. On the other hand, limited resection provides patients the opportunity to preserve pancreatic and gastrointestinal function, which would greatly reduce postoperative complications in the setting of non-dilated biliary and pancreatic ducts [40]. Because of the technical challenges and necessity for clear margins associated with DGISTs, endoscopic resections are generally not performed, but hybrid endo-laparoscopic surgical techniques may provide a less invasive approach to performing safe and effective resections for these tumors [41–43].

In addition to surgery, tyrosine kinase inhibitors (TKIs), such as imatinib mesylate, have shown great efficacy as neoadjuvant and adjuvant treatments to reduce morbidity and mortality associated with DGISTs. Specifically, the vascular tumors are transformed into cystic lesions and in some cases with reduction of size as well. Figure 11.4 demonstrates a large DGIST with a significant response to neoadjuvant

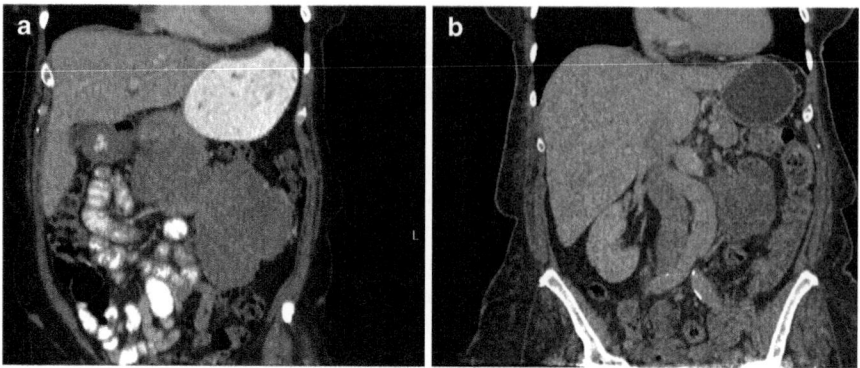

Fig. 11.4 Duodenal GIST as seen on CT on presentation (**a**) and after 6 months of neoadjuvant imatinib (**b**) with marked response and regression of tumor

imatinib. One of the major limitations of imatinib mesylate is tumor resistance; this is due to the development of additional c-KIT mutations in the tumor over time in the setting of continued Imatinib use for persistent disease [34].

The recommended follow-up strategies for patients following DGIST resection are dependent on patients' respective risk of recurrence and treatment conditions. For patients with less than intermediate risk of recurrence, annual abdominal CT scans are sufficient for surveillance [44]. In high-risk patients being treated with TKIs, follow-up imaging is suggested at 6-month intervals during treatment [44, 45]. Following the end of treatment, it is recommended for patients to receive imaging every 3–4 months during the first 2 years after adjuvant therapy, and then this interval is extended to every 6–12 months for up to 10 years. Patients who do not receive adjuvant therapy are recommended to obtain follow-up imaging every 3–4 months during the first few years following their surgery [45].

Leiomyoma

Leiomyomas of the duodenum are rare, benign neoplasms that arise from the smooth muscle. These tumors may present asymptomatically as incidental findings on radiological scans, but common manifestations of symptoms include gastrointestinal hemorrhage, abdominal pain, and obstruction [46]. Upper endoscopy plays a role in visualizing the lesion, and endoscopic biopsy can be utilized to obtain a histologic diagnosis. In addition, immunohistochemistry is essential in the diagnosis of these lesions, as leiomyomas are positive for smooth muscle actin and desmin but negative for S-100 protein [38]. The preferred treatment of choice for these tumors is surgery, with either local tumor excision, segmental duodenectomy, or pancreaticoduodenectomy. Less invasive techniques, such as endoscopic band ligation, may also play a role in providing a safe and effective resection for leiomyomas [47].

Lipoma

Lipomas of the duodenum are benign, slow-growing tumors that predominantly arise from the submucosa (90% of lesions) [48]. In addition, these lipomas are generally localized in the second portion of the duodenum and are often incidentally found on endoscopy or surgery [48, 49]. On endoscopy, these tumors are characterized as being round or ovoid-shaped soft masses, accompanied with regular or lobulated contours [50]. While most cases present asymptomatically, symptoms do occur depending on the lipoma's size and location, as lesions larger than 4 cm have been shown to lead to intussusception, bleeding, or obstruction [48]. Based on the size of the lipoma and associated symptoms, the recommended treatment is either endoscopic or surgical resection. Small, solitary lipomas have been shown to be effectively excised endoscopically through snare or endoloop-assisted polypectomy [49, 50]. Surgical resection is preferred for larger lesions due to technical challenges of endoscopy and potential risks of bleeding and perforation.

Neurogenic and Vascular Lesions

Neurogenic and vascular lesions of the duodenum are characterized as masses arising from the nerves or blood and lymph vessels, respectively. Neuromas constitute 3–6% of all small intestine tumors and may occur in patients with neurofibromatosis [51, 52]. These nerve tissue-derived lesions include neurofibromas, schwannomas, and gangliomas. On the other hand, vascular lesions predominantly feature hemangiomas and lymphangiomas. Neurogenic and vascular lesions are conventionally treated surgically with partial duodenectomy, but less invasive treatment strategies, such as endoscopic resection, may be employed to effectively treat these lesions [53].

Choledochal Cysts

Choledochal cysts represent a group of biliary cystic dilations of the extrahepatic duct, intrahepatic duct, or both [54]. These can cause considerable patient-related morbidity and mortality unless identified at an early stage and managed appropriately. Choledochal cysts are an uncommon congenital anomaly of the bile duct. The incidence of this is 1 in 100,000–150,000 live births worldwide [55]. However, the incidence has been reported to be as high as 1 in 13,500 individuals in the United States and nearly as high as 1 in 15,000 in Australia [55]. The incidence of a choledochal cyst is higher in the Asian population with an incidence of nearly 1 in 1000 individuals [55]. The majority of cases are reported to be from Japan.

Most choledochal cysts are diagnosed in childhood, yet nearly 25% can be detected during adulthood. Choledochal cysts are more common in females compared to males with the ratios being as high as 4:1 or 3:1 [56]. Choledochal cysts are classified according to location within the biliary tree and have been described previously by Todani et al. Patients who have a choledochal cyst often will report non-specific and vague symptoms such as abdominal pain [57]. Biliary cystic dilation complications due to local compression can include pancreatitis, cholangitis, secondary biliary cirrhosis, spontaneous rupture, and increase the risk of cholangiocarcinoma.

Choledochal cysts can be categorized into five types [54, 57]. Type I represents about 50 to 80% of all choledochal cysts, type II 2%, type III 1 to 4%, type IV 15–30%, type V 20%. Type I choledochal cyst can be classified into three additional phenotypes. Type Ia is a cystic dilation of the entire extrahepatic biliary tree that does not involve the intrahepatic ducts. Often the gallbladder and cystic duct will arise from a dilated common bile duct. Type Ib represents a focal segmental dilation of the extrahepatic biliary tree. Type Ic represents a fusiform dilation of the entire extrahepatic biliary tree that involves an intrahepatic duct. Type II choledochal cysts are a saccular diverticulum on the common bile duct. Type III choledochal cysts are also called choledochoceles, and these represent a cystic dilation of the intramural portion of the distal common bile duct that often will bulge into the duodenum. Type IV includes types IVa and IVb. Type IVa is the second most common choledochal cyst and it is represented by an intrahepatic and extrahepatic dilation of the biliary ducts. Type IVb represents multiple dilations of only the extrahepatic biliary tree. Type V choledochal cyst, also known as Caroli's disease, represents multiple dilations of the intrahepatic biliary ducts. This anatomic anomaly is often associated with congenital hepatic fibrosis which can present with cirrhosis and is termed Caroli's syndrome [58].

The etiology of choledochal cysts is an ongoing debate with both congenital and acquired proposed mechanisms. The most common is Babbitt's theory where choledochal cysts are thought to be due to an aberrant pancreaticobiliary ductal junction [59]. This manifests as the pancreatic duct joining the bile duct 1–2 cm proximal to the sphincter of Oddi. This length of a common channel can vary between 10 and 45 mm. A long common channel allows pancreatic juice to reflux into the biliary tree which increases intraluminal pressure and can in theory result in ductal dilation [60]. This is supported in that there is often a high amylase concentration within the bile samples of patients with choledochal cysts [60]. Further pancreatic enzyme reflux can lead to inflammation, epithelial breakdown, dysplasia, and subsequently malignancy. Despite this proposed mechanism, the long common channel is only observed in about 50–80% of patients with choledochal cysts. Another theory is due to obstruction of the distal common bile duct. Sphincter of Oddi dysfunction can predispose to the development of choledochal cysts.

Because most choledochal cysts present in childhood and about 25% will present in adulthood, it is important to recognize a set of classic symptoms. Often there is a triad which includes abdominal pain, palpable abdominal mass, and jaundice. This is seen altogether in about <20% of all cases. In children, 85% will have these two features of the triad whereas in adults only 25% will present with at least two features of the triad.

Due to chronic inflammation and subsequent bile stasis, stones and infections can develop. This can manifest in ascending cholangitis and obstructive jaundice. The symptoms of this include abdominal pain and fever. Chronic inflammation especially along the distal common bile duct can cause pancreatitis. Secondary biliary cirrhosis can be due to chronic biliary obstruction. There is an increased risk for malignancy in patients with choledochal cysts. The incidence of developing malignancy varies between 2% and 18% [61]. In a series of 38 adult patients this was reported to be as high as 21%. The incidence of malignancy increases with age [62]. Malignancy is often observed in the extrahepatic ducts and about 50–60% of patients, gallbladder in about 30–50% of patients, intrahepatic biliary ductal malignancies in about 2% of patients, and about <1% of patients with liver and pancreas malignancies [62].

Clinical investigation should be performed using imaging as well as liver function tests, serum amylase and lipase levels, INR and complete blood count to evaluate for obstructive jaundice or pancreatitis kidney function and altered coagulation profiles. Tumor biomarkers can be obtained including a CA 19–9 in patients who have suspicion for malignancy.

Diagnostic workup using imaging should be performed to assist with operative planning and complete excision of all choledochal cysts. Abdominal ultrasound is often a first step. Sensitivity of ultrasound is about 70–97% [63]. Ultrasounds can also be used for postoperative surveillance [64]. In addition to an ultrasound, contrasted MRI and MRCP can be used to delineate biliary anatomy [65]. HIDA scans can be used and have a sensitivity of 100% for type I choledochal cyst, meanwhile the sensitivity diminishes for the other types [66]. Computed tomography is highly accurate and can be used to help delineate arterial and vascular anatomy assisting in surgical planning [65]. CT scans can also be utilized to estimate cyst wall thickening which can be seen in malignancy. ERCP is extremely sensitive and diagnostic for choledochal cysts; the sensitivity decreases in patients who have developed considerable inflammation and scarring over time. ERCP is an invasive technique which can potentially cause cholangitis and pancreatitis [67]. MRCP is still considered the gold standard for diagnosis as the sensitivity is as high as 90 to 100% MRCP also avoids ionizing radiation and is noninvasive compared to ERCP [65]. MRCP can also be used with MRI imaging to evaluate surrounding vascular anatomy, presence of biliary sludge or stones and malignancies.

Management of choledochal cysts has changed considerably over time. Several decades ago, initial management consisted of a cyst enterostomy. However, this was associated with recurrence of symptoms and a high risk of malignancy within the remaining in situ cyst wall several decades later. There was an observed malignancy rate of nearly 30% in patients who had previously undergone a cyst enterostomy for the management of a choledochal cyst [62]. Complete excision of the biliary cyst was then recommended and reconstructed or diverted biliary tree was subsequently needed. Biliary diversion can be performed using a hepaticoduodenostomy or hepaticojejunostomy.

Complete excision of the cyst followed by Roux-en-Y hepaticojejunostomy is the standard of choice for the treatment of most choledochal cysts. This procedure can be performed via the open, laparoscopic, or robotic approach. Long-term surveillance and outcomes are dependent on complete cyst excision and appropriate surveillance.

Duodenal Lymphoma

Duodenal follicular lymphomas are often found incidentally [68]. Often upper endoscopic surveillance is performed for another reason and patients who have low stage follicular lymphomas often do not have overt clinical symptoms [68]. If the patient presents with symptoms it is often vague with abdominal pain. The mean age at diagnosis is 65 years [68]. There is no difference between male and female. Most commonly the second portion of the duodenum is involved.

At the time of endoscopy, a duodenal follicular lymphoma can be found as either a solitary or multiple nodular masses [69]. These can present as a polypoid lesion, and they are usually between 1 and 5 mm in size. As the masses grow, they can become ulcerated which can make endoscopic sampling easier. Multifocal disease is not uncommon with lesions located elsewhere in the jejunum or ileum [70]. On histologic evaluation, most follicular lymphomas of the duodenum are low grade [71]. On microscopy, these appear as well-circumscribed germinal centers with no visible macrophages and without mantle cell zones. Sheets of lymphoid cells that contain irregular nuclei are often present, and the lymphoma will involve the mucosa and submucosa [70]. The immunophenotype is similar to other low-grade follicular lymphomas and these will express CD20, CD10, BCL–6, BCL–2 and lack expression for CD5, CD23, CD43, BCL–1, and T-cell markers [72]. Often these lymphomas will have a low Ki-67 rate [72].

The classic genetic aberration often found is a translocation (14; 18)(q. 32; q. 21) for the genes of the immunoglobulin heavy chain and B-cell leukemia lymphoma [72]. Duodenal follicular lymphoma has a pathogenesis that is often related to repeat inflammation and antigen stimulation and shares some similarities with mucosa-associated lymphoid tissue (MALT) lymphomas [73]. Differential diagnosis includes MALT lymphoma, chronic lymphocytic leukemia, mantle cell lymphoma, and gastrointestinal involvement by systemic follicular lymphoma [74].

Duodenal follicular lymphomas often have a good prognosis with median survival exceeding 12 years [75]. The only treatment for this is chemotherapy. Patients who have limited stage follicular lymphomas within the duodenum can also be treated with radiation therapy [76, 77]. This is associated with a good overall outcome as relapse impacts subsequent outcomes. Even though treatment with radiotherapy to the duodenal lymphoma is quite successful most patients will not undergo treatment initially [78]. There is an option to watch and wait which has also been demonstrated to be effective as well. Other approaches for early stage disease consist of rituximab with chemotherapy, rituximab alone, combined modality therapies, or a variety of other systemic therapies [78].

Conclusion

Duodenal lesions span the spectrum of benign, premalignant, and malignant etiologies. Their presentation is often as obstruction, bleeding, or pain and their treatment is primarily endoscopic or surgical resection when appropriate.

References

1. Goh PMY, Lenzi JE. Benign tumors of the duodenum and stomach. In: Holzheimer RG, Mannick JA, editors. Surgical treatment: evidence-based and problem-oriented. Munich: Zuckschwerdt; 2001.
2. Basford PJ, Bhandari P. Endoscopic management of nonampullary duodenal polyps. Ther Adv Gastroenterol. 2012;5:127.
3. Baron TH. Ampullary adenoma. Curr Treat Options Gastroenterol. 2008;11:96–102.
4. Eswaran SL, Sanders M, Bernadino KP, et al. Success and complications of endoscopic removal of giant duodenal and ampullary polyps: a comparative series. Gastrointest Endosc. 2006;64:925–32.
5. Chini P, Draganov PV. Diagnosis and management of ampullary adenoma: the expanding role of endoscopy. World J Gastrointest Endosc. 2011;3:241.
6. Collins K, Ligato S. Duodenal epithelial polyps: a clinicopathologic review. Arch Pathol Lab Med. 2019;143:370–85.
7. Kővári B, Kim BH, Lauwers GY. The pathology of gastric and duodenal polyps: current concepts. Histopathology. 2021;78:106–24.
8. Rosty C, Campbell C, Clendenning M, Bettington M, Buchanan DD, Brown IS. Do serrated neoplasms of the small intestine represent a distinct entity? Pathological findings and molecular alterations in a series of 13 cases. Histopathology. 2015;66:333–42.
9. Rubio CA. Traditional serrated adenomas of the upper digestive tract. J Clin Pathol. 2016;69:1–5.
10. Lim CH, Cho YS. Nonampullary duodenal adenoma: current understanding of its diagnosis, pathogenesis, and clinical management. World J Gastroenterol. 2016;22:853.
11. Culver EL, McIntyre AS. Sporadic duodenal polyps: classification, investigation, and management. Endoscopy. 2011;43:144–55.
12. Abbass R, Rigaux J, Al-Kawas FH. Nonampullary duodenal polyps: characteristics and endoscopic management. Gastrointest Endosc. 2010;71:754–9.
13. Kakushima N, Tanaka M, Takizawa K, Ono H, Kanemoto H. Treatment for superficial nonampullary duodenal epithelial tumors. World J Gastroenterol. 2014;20:12501.
14. Apel D, Jakobs R, Spiethoff A, Riemann JF. Follow-up after endoscopic snare resection of duodenal adenomas. Endoscopy. 2005;37:444–8.
15. Ceppa EP, Burbridge RA, Rialon KL, et al. Endoscopic versus surgical ampullectomy: an algorithm to treat disease of the ampulla of Vater. Ann Surg. 2013;257:315–22.

16. Pavlovic-Markovic A, Dragasevic S, Krstic M, Stojkovic Lalosevic M, Milosavljevic T. Assessment of duodenal adenomas and strategies for curative therapy. Dig Dis. 2019;37:374–80.
17. Phillips RKS, Wallace MH, Lynch PM, et al. A randomised, double blind, placebo controlled study of celecoxib, a selective cyclooxygenase 2 inhibitor, on duodenal polyposis in familial adenomatous polyposis. Gut. 2002;50:857.
18. Brosens LAA, Keller JJ, Offerhaus GJA, Goggins M, Giardiello FM. Prevention and management of duodenal polyps in familial adenomatous polyposis. Gut. 2005;54:1034.
19. Spigelman AD, Talbot IC, Williams CB, Domizio P, Phillips RKS. Upper gastrointestinal cancer in patients with familial adenomatous polyposis. Lancet. 1989;334:783–5.
20. Groves CJ, Saunders BP, Spigelman AD, Phillips RKS. Duodenal cancer in patients with familial adenomatous polyposis (FAP): results of a 10 year prospective study. Gut. 2002;50:636.
21. Overman MJ, Hu C-Y, Kopetz S, Abbruzzese JL, Wolff RA, Chang GJ. A population-based comparison of adenocarcinoma of the large and small intestine: insights into a rare disease. Ann Surg Oncol. 2012;19:1439–45.
22. Ross RK, Hartnett NM, Bernstein L, Henderson BE. Epidemiology of adenocarcinomas of the small intestine: is bile a small bowel carcinogen? Br J Cancer. 1991;63:143–5.
23. Cloyd JM, George E, Visser BC. Duodenal adenocarcinoma: advances in diagnosis and surgical management. World J Gastrointest Surg. 2016;8:212.
24. Werling RW, Yaziji H, Bacchi CE, Gown AM. CDX2, a highly sensitive and specific marker of adenocarcinomas of intestinal origin: an immunohistochemical survey of 476 primary and metastatic carcinomas. Am J Surg Pathol. 2003;27:303–10.
25. Cloyd JM, Norton JA, Visser BC, Poultsides GA. Does the extent of resection impact survival for duodenal adenocarcinoma? Analysis of 1,611 cases. Ann Surg Oncol. 2015;22:573–80.
26. Poultsides GA, Huang LC, Cameron JL, et al. Duodenal adenocarcinoma: clinicopathologic analysis and implications for treatment. Ann Surg Oncol. 2012;19:1928–35.
27. Sato Y, Hashimoto S, Mizuno KI, Takeuchi M, Terai S. Management of gastric and duodenal neuroendocrine tumors. World J Gastroenterol. 2016;22:6817.
28. Yao JC, Hassan M, Phan A, et al. One hundred years after 'carcinoid': epidemiology of and prognostic factors for neuroendocrine tumors in 35,825 cases in the United States. J Clin Oncol. 2008;26:3063–72.
29. Hoffmann KM, Furukawa M, Jensen RT. Duodenal neuroendocrine tumors: classification, functional syndromes, diagnosis and medical treatment. Best Pract Res Clin Gastroenterol. 2005;19:675–97.
30. Randle RW, Ahmed S, Newman NA, Clark CJ. Clinical outcomes for neuroendocrine tumors of the duodenum and ampulla of Vater: a population-based study. J Gastrointest Surg. 2014;18:354–62.
31. Grin A, Streutker CJ. Neuroendocrine tumors of the luminal gastrointestinal tract. Arch Pathol Lab Med. 2015;139:750–6.
32. Delle Fave G, Kwekkeboom DJ, Van Cutsem E, et al. ENETS Consensus Guidelines for the management of patients with gastroduodenal neoplasms. Neuroendocrinology. 2012;95:74–87.
33. Hoeppner J, Kulemann B, Marjanovic G, Bronsert P, Hopt UT. Limited resection for duodenal gastrointestinal stromal tumors: surgical management and clinical outcome. World J Gastrointest Surg. 2013;5:16.
34. Miettinen M, Lasota J. Gastrointestinal stromal tumors: pathology and prognosis at different sites. Semin Diagn Pathol. 2006;23:70–83.
35. Andersson J, Sihto H, Meis-Kindblom JM, Joensuu H, Nupponen N, Kindblom L-G. NF1-associated gastrointestinal stromal tumors have unique clinical, phenotypic, and genotypic characteristics. Am J Surg Pathol. 2005;29:1170–6.
36. Cavallaro G, Polistena A, D'Ermo G, Pedullà G, De Toma G. Duodenal gastrointestinal stromal tumors: review on clinical and surgical aspects. Int J Surg. 2012;10:463–5.
37. Du H, Ning L, Li S, et al. Diagnosis and treatment of duodenal gastrointestinal stromal tumors. Clin Transl Gastroenterol. 2020;11:e00156.

38. Hou YY, Tan YS, Xu JF, et al. Schwannoma of the gastrointestinal tract: a clinicopathological, immunohistochemical and ultrastructural study of 33 cases. Histopathology. 2006;48:536–45.
39. Gervaz P, Huber O, Morel P. Surgical management of gastrointestinal stromal tumours. Br J Surg. 2009;96:567–78.
40. Chung JC, Kim HC, Hur SM. Limited resections for duodenal gastrointestinal stromal tumors and their oncologic outcomes. Surg Today. 2016;46:110–6.
41. Shen Z, Chen P, Du N, Khadaroo PA, Mao D, Gu L. Pancreaticoduodenectomy versus limited resection for duodenal gastrointestinal stromal tumors: a systematic review and meta-analysis. BMC Surg. 2019;19:1–9.
42. Lim KT. Current surgical management of duodenal gastrointestinal stromal tumors. World J Gastrointest Surg. 2021;13:1166.
43. Ojima T, Nakamura M, Hayata K, et al. Laparoscopic limited resection for duodenal gastrointestinal stromal tumors. J Gastrointest Surg. 2020;24:2404–8.
44. Joensuu H, Martin-Broto J, Nishida T, Reichardt P, Schöffski P, Maki RG. Follow-up strategies for patients with gastrointestinal stromal tumour treated with or without adjuvant imatinib after surgery. Eur J Cancer. 2015;51:1611–7.
45. Nishida T, Blay JY, Hirota S, Kitagawa Y, Kang YK. The standard diagnosis, treatment, and follow-up of gastrointestinal stromal tumors based on guidelines. Gastric Cancer. 2016;19:3.
46. Serraf A, Klein E, Schneebaum S, Davidson B, Herzig E, Ben-Ari G. Leiomyomas of the duodenum. J Surg Oncol. 1988;39:183–6.
47. Sun S, Jin Y, Chang G, Wang C, Li X, Wang Z. Endoscopic band ligation without electrosurgery: a new technique for excision of small upper-GI leiomyoma. Gastrointest Endosc. 2004;60(2):218–22. https://doi.org/10.1016/S0016-5107(04)01565-2.
48. Yaman I, Derici H, Paksoy S. Symptomatic duodenal lipoma with endoscopic snare polypectomy. Turk J Surg/Ulus Cerrahi Derg. 2014;30:103.
49. Aydin HN, Bertin P, Singh K, Arregui M. Safe techniques for endoscopic resection of gastrointestinal lipomas. Surg Laparosc Endosc Percutan Tech. 2011;21:218–22.
50. Pei MW, Hu MR, Chen WB, Qin C. Diagnosis and treatment of duodenal lipoma: a systematic review and a case report. J Clin Diagn Res. 2017;11:PE01.
51. Latos W, Kawczyk-Krupka A, Strzelczyk N, Sieroń A, Cieślar G. Benign and non-neoplastic tumours of the duodenum. Prz Gastroenterol. 2019;14:233.
52. Tishler JM, Han SY, Colcher H, Halpern NB. Neurogenic tumors of the duodenum in patients with neurofibromatosis. Radiology. 1983;149:51–3.
53. Nishiyama N, Mori H, Kobara H, et al. Bleeding duodenal hemangioma: morphological changes and endoscopic mucosal resection. World J Gastroenterol. 2012;18:2872.
54. Hewitt PM, Krige JEJ, Bornman PC, Terblanche J. Choledochal cysts in adults. Br J Surg. 1995;82:382–5.
55. Baison GN, Bonds MM, Helton WS, Kozarek RA. Choledochal cysts: similarities and differences between Asian and Western countries. World J Gastroenterol. 2019;25:3334–43.
56. Visser BC, Suh I, Way LW, Kang S-M. Congenital choledochal cysts in adults. Arch Surg. 2004;139:855–62.
57. Todani T, Watanabe Y, Narusue M, Tabuchi K, Okajima K. Congenital bile duct cysts: classification, operative procedures, and review of thirty-seven cases including cancer arising from choledochal cyst. Am J Surg. 2019;134:9–25.
58. Hussain SZ, Bloom DA, Tolia V. Caroli's disease diagnosed in a child by MRCP. Clin Imaging. 2000;24:289–91.
59. Babbitt DP. Congenital choledochal cysts: new etiological concept based on anomalous relationships of the common bile duct and pancreatic bulb. Ann Radiol. 1969;12:231–40.
60. Sugiyama M, Haradome H, Takahara T, et al. Biliopancreatic reflux via anomalous pancreaticobiliary junction. Surgery. 2004;135:457–9.
61. He X-D, Wang L, Liu W, et al. The risk of carcinogenesis in congenital choledochal cyst patients: an analysis of 214 cases. Ann Hepatol. 2014;13:819–26.

62. Madadi-Sanjani O, Wirth TC, Kuebler JF, Petersen C, Ure BM. Choledochal cyst and malignancy: a plea for lifelong follow-up. Eur J Pediatr Surg. 2019;29:143–9.
63. Shin HJ, Yoon H, Han SJ, et al. Key imaging features for differentiating cystic biliary atresia from choledochal cyst: prenatal ultrasonography and postnatal ultrasonography and MRI. Ultrasonography. 2021;40:301–11.
64. Hosokawa T, Hosokawa M, Shibuki S, et al. Role of ultrasound in follow-up after choledochal cyst surgery. J Med Ultrason. 2021;48:21–9.
65. Lewis VA, Adam SZ, Nikolaidis P, et al. Imaging of choledochal cysts. Abdom Imaging. 2015;40:1567–80.
66. Weissmann HS, Gold M, Goldstein RD, Sugarman LA, L. M. F. Choledochal cyst complicated by acute cholecystitis and bypass obstruction: diagnostic role of Tc-99m-HIDA cholescintigraphy. Clin Nucl Med. 1981;6:395–8.
67. Naga MI, Suleiman DN. Endoscopic management of choledochal cyst. Gastrointest Endosc. 2004;59:427–32.
68. Armitage JO, Weisenburger DD. New approach to classifying non-Hodgkin's lymphomas: clinical features of the major histologic subtypes. J Clin Oncol. 1998;16:2780–95.
69. Misdraji J, Harris NL, Hasserjian RP, Lauwers GY, Ferry JA. Primary follicular lymphoma of the gastrointestinal tract. Am J Surg Pathol. 2011;35:1255–63.
70. Takata K, Okada H, Ohmiya N, et al. Primary gastrointestinal follicular lymphoma involving the duodenal second portion is a distinct entity: a multicenter, retrospective analysis in Japan. Cancer Sci. 2011;102:1532–6.
71. Takata K, Sato Y, Nakamura N, et al. Duodenal follicular lymphoma lacks AID but expresses BACH2 and has memory B-cell characteristics. Mod Pathol. 2013;26:22–31.
72. Leich E, Salaverria I, Bea S, et al. Follicular lymphomas with and without translocation t(14;18) differ in gene expression profiles and genetic alterations. Blood. 2009;114:826–34.
73. Jegalian AG, Eberle FC, Pack SD, et al. Follicular lymphoma in situ: clinical implications and comparisons with partial involvement by follicular lymphoma. Blood. 2011;118:2976–84.
74. Sato Y, Ichimura K, Tanaka T, et al. Duodenal follicular lymphomas share common characteristics with mucosa-associated lymphoid tissue lymphomas. J Clin Pathol. 2008;61:377–81.
75. Kahl BS, Yang DT. Follicular lymphoma: evolving therapeutic strategies. Blood. 2016;127:2055–63.
76. Wilder RB, Jones D, Tucker SL, et al. Long-term results with radiotherapy for stage I-II follicular lymphomas. Int J Radiat Oncol Biol Phys. 2001;51:1219–27.
77. Guadagnolo BA, Li S, Neuberg D, et al. Long-term outcome and mortality trends in early-stage, Grade 1-2 follicular lymphoma treated with radiation therapy. Int J Radiat Oncol Biol Phys. 2006;64:928–34.
78. Jacobson CA, Freedman AS. Early stage follicular lymphoma, current management and controversies. Curr Opin Oncol. 2012;24:475–9.

Chapter 12
Endoscopic Duodenal Resection

Catherine Vozzo and Ashley Faulx

Introduction

Endoscopic duodenal resection of lesions and polyps is a complex topic. This is due to the variety of pathology encountered in the duodenum, their proximity to the ampulla, and the unique anatomical considerations within the duodenum including its robust blood supply, thin muscle layer, and scope positioning. In addition, the management of lesions will vary depending on the presence or absence of polyposis syndromes [1]. Careful consideration and thought must be given to each case prior to scheduling a patient for endoscopic resection.

Pre-procedural Considerations

Pre-procedural discussion will include thorough discussion of risks, benefits, and alternatives to the procedure. The patient's comorbidities, surgical history, and medications should be reviewed prior to the procedure. Anticoagulant and antiplatelet agents should be held according to society guidelines based on risk of bleeding [2]. The sedation plan should be discussed with the patient and anesthesiologist (if applicable).

C. Vozzo · A. Faulx (✉)
Division of Gastroenterology, University Hospitals of Cleveland, Case Western Reserve University School of Medicine, Cleveland, OH, USA
e-mail: catherine.vozzo@uhhospitals.org; Ashley.faulx@uhhospitals.org

© The Author(s), under exclusive license to Springer Nature
Switzerland AG 2025
E. P. Ceppa et al. (eds.), *The SAGES Manual of Evolving Techniques in Pancreatic Surgery*, https://doi.org/10.1007/978-3-031-78409-5_12

Indications

Careful endoscopic evaluation should take place prior to resection of any lesion. The lesions may appear mucosal or subepithelial. The lesion's proximity to the ampulla should be noted because endoscopic resection technique is vastly different if the lesion is considered ampullary or non-ampullary. Finally, the patient's medical history should be evaluated for genetic polyposis syndromes as the management of a sporadic duodenal polyp will differ from a patient with familial adenomatous polyposis or MUTYH-associated polyposis. As discussed in Chap. 11, some duodenal lesions may harbor malignant potential, whereas others are benign. Lesions should be considered for resection if they are pre-malignant or if they are symptomatic, such as bleeding or obstruction [1]. Lesions with malignant potential include gastrointestinal stromal tumors, carcinoids, solitary Peutz-Jeghers polyps, leiomyomas, and adenomas. Benign lesions include lipomas, gastric metaplasia, inflammatory polyps, and Brunner's glands or hamartomas (Fig. 12.1) [1, 3].

Table 12.1 outlines a suggested broad approach for various polyps encountered in the duodenum. However, the remainder of this chapter will primarily focus on resection of ampullary and non-ampullary adenomas.

Endoscopic Assessment of Non-ampullary Adenomas

Detection and characterization of duodenal polyps can be challenging because the duodenum is a fixed structure in the retroperitoneum. Distal attachment of a cap to the endoscope may improve stability, allow for better visualization of the papilla, and identify polyps in between folds [4]. It may be necessary to utilize a

Fig. 12.1 Previously bleeding duodenal polyp in second portion of the duodenum, marked with clip and tattoo, pathology ultimately positive for Brunner's gland hamartoma

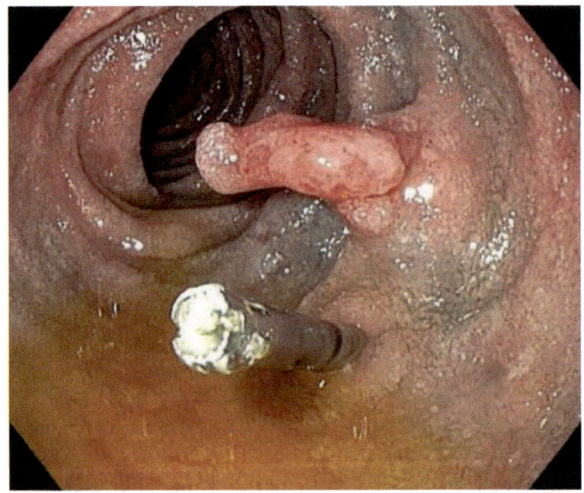

Table 12.1 Approach by polyp type

Polyp type	Resection approach
Non-ampullary adenomas	<6 mm in size: Cold snare polypectomy >6 mm in size: Endoscopic mucosal resection (EMR) technique
Ampullary adenomas	Endoscopic retrograde cholangiopancreatography and endoscopic ultrasound to assess extension with endoscopic papillectomy
Brunner's gland hamartoma	Cold snare polypectomy or EMR only if symptomatic
Gastric heterotopia	No intervention required. Consider *H pylori* testing
Inflammatory fibroid polyp	Cold snare polypectomy or EMR only if symptomatic
Lipoma	Cold snare polypectomy only if symptomatic
Carcinoid	If no evidence of invasion of the muscularis layer and 1 cm or less in size can be removed via EMR
Gastrointestinal stromal tumors	Endoscopic ultrasound-guided FNB for diagnostic purposes, but in most cases endoscopic resection is not considered (refer to GI surgeon)
Solitary Peutz-Jeghers polyp	Cold snare polypectomy

Table modified from Culver and Mcintyre [3]

Table 12.2 Paris classification (Major variants of type 0 neoplasia)

0-Ip	Protruded, pedunculated
0-Is	Protruded, sessile
0-IIa	Slightly elevated
0-IIb	Flat
0-IIc	Superficial, shallow, depression
0-III	Excavated (ulcer)

Table adapted from Ref. [6]

side-viewing endoscope to clearly outline the location of the polyp in relation to the papilla and should be photo documented prior to intervention [5]. The polyp's macroscopic appearance is typically milk white or reddish mucosa. Once the polyp is identified, tumor size should be estimated with an open biopsy forceps or snare. Inspection using high-definition white light endoscopy and definition should be provided according to the Paris classification (Table 12.2) [7]. Endoscopic example of a non-ampullary duodenal adenoma is seen in Fig. 12.2.

Histologic assessment varies depending on the region of the world in which you are practicing. When magnifying endoscopy with narrow-band imaging is available, biopsy of the lesion may not be necessary. This technique, not available in the United States, may distinguish neoplastic from non-neoplastic lesions in addition to low- and high-grade dysplasia [8, 9]. Features concerning for advanced histology include the size of the adenoma larger than 1 cm, the degree of involved mucosal circumference, and relation to the ampulla. Features concerning for submucosal invasion are Paris IIc, surface ulceration, and non-lifting after submucosal injection (Fig. 12.3). The role of EUS in small duodenal adenomas is minimal but may impact the management of polyps <2 cm, or in cases where metastases are noted [5].

Fig. 12.2 Fifteen millimeter sessile polyp in the second portion of the duodenum consistent with non-ampullary duodenal adenoma

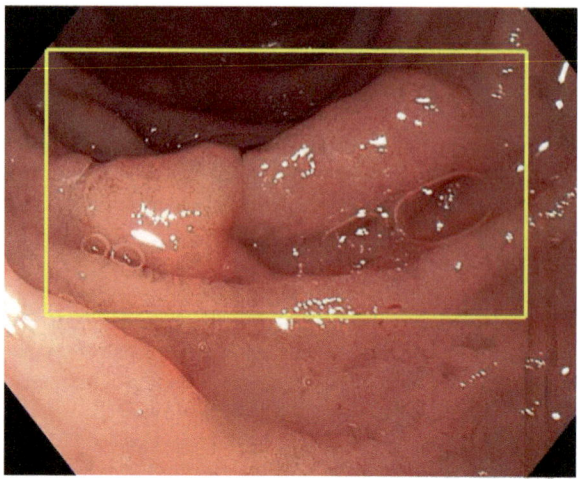

Fig. 12.3 Non-lifting after submucosal injection. In this setting, the adenoma was non-lifting secondary to scarring from prior resection. Photo courtesy of Brooke Glessing, MD

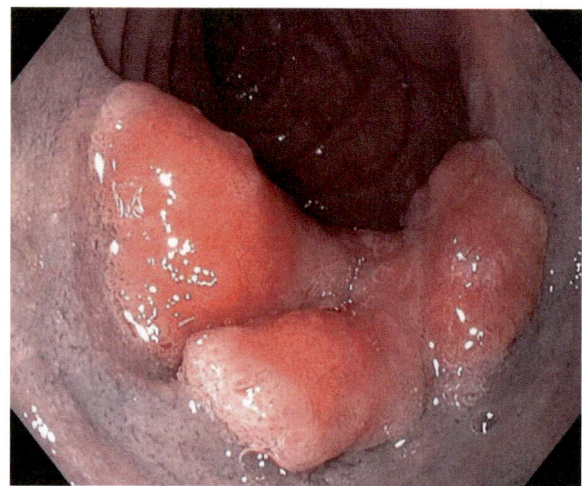

Any lesions with suspected invasive neoplasia are not suitable for endoscopic resection. Biopsy sampling should be limited to the surface of the polyp to avoid submucosal scarring and fibrosis that will make endoscopic resection difficult [10].

Endoscopic Assessment of Ampullary Adenomas

Ampullary adenomas are adenomas involving the major papilla and can be sporadic or related to a polyposis syndrome. Unlike non-ampullary polyps, ampullary lesions may cause symptoms due to their location including jaundice, abdominal pain, duodenal obstruction, pancreatitis, or bleeding [3]. It can be difficult to distinguish benign, pre-malignant, and malignant lesions around the ampulla. Features of concern include bleeding, firmness, and non-lifting after submucosal injection. Forceps biopsy and histological examination are mandatory in the diagnosis of ampullary tumors prior to considering resection approach [5, 11]. Diagnostic accuracy of biopsies is variable (ranging from 38% to 85%) and should be minimized by sampling tissue at least 10 days following sphincterotomy to minimize cytologic atypia that can occur and obtaining at least six biopsy samples [5]. While pancreatitis is possible following biopsy, overall this is regarded as low risk with a good safety profile [12].

Several factors should be noted prior to considering surgical or endoscopic resection of an ampullary lesion. This includes staging, assessment for intraductal extension of adenoma, and presence of pancreas divisum. Multiple modalities have been studied in literature and include transabdominal ultrasound, computed tomography (CT), magnetic resonance cholangiopancreatography (MRCP), endoscopic retrograde cholangiopancreatography (ERCP), endoscopic ultrasound (EUS), and intraductal US (IDUS). European Society of Gastrointestinal Endoscopy (ESGE) guidelines support the use of EUS and MRCP for staging given their marginally higher accuracy, reproducibility, and safety [11].

Sporadic ampullary tumors should be referred for surgical management if the lesion size is larger than 2–3 cm or intraductal extension exceeds 1–2 cm [5, 11]. Figure 12.4 is an ampullary adenoma with moderately differentiated adenocarcinoma in a background of adenomatous change with high-grade dysplasia.

Endoscopic Assessment in Polyposis Syndromes

Assessment of duodenal polyps (ampullary and non-ampullary) in adenomatous polyposis syndromes begins at age 25 years. The Spigelman classification for duodenal polyps helps predict cancer risk and outlines surveillance intervals (Table 12.3) [13]. Stage 0 patients will require repeat endoscopy in 4 years, stage I will require repeat endoscopy in 2–3 years, stage II will require repeat endoscopy in 1–3 years, and stage III will require repeat endoscopy in 6–12 months. Patients with stage IV should have surgical evaluation [14].

Fig. 12.4 Ampullary adenoma ultimately found to have invasive moderately differentiated adenocarcinoma. Photo courtesy of Brooke Glessing, MD

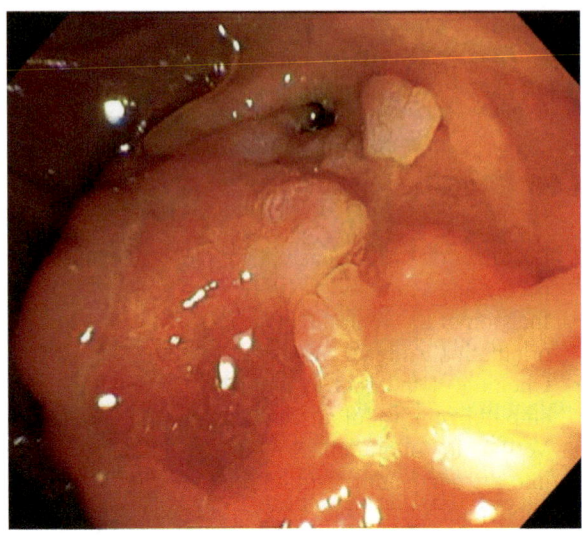

Table 12.3 Spigelman classification

Criteria	Points		
	1	2	3
Polyp number	1–4	5–20	>20
Polyp size (mm)	1–4	5–10	>10
Histology	Tubular	Tubulovillous	Villous
Dysplasia	Mild	Moderate	Severe

Stage 0 = 0 pts; stage I = 1–4 pts, stage II = 5–6 pts, Stage III = 7–8 pts, stage IV = 9–12 pts
Adapted from Spigelman et al. [13]

Resection Techniques

Sporadic Non-ampullary Adenomas: Cold Snare Polypectomy

Resection technique is similar to that of polypectomy in the right colon due to thinness of the duodenal wall. Cold snare polypectomy is recommended for small (<6 mm lesions). Hot snare polypectomy has been associated with delayed bleeding, perforation, and post polypectomy syndrome and therefore not preferred [15].

Technique: A snare trap is placed on a suction device prior to polypectomy. The lesion should be oriented at the 5-o'clock position. The snare is opened and positioned over the lesion. To obtain adequate tissue apposition, a combination of scope tip deflection and advancement of the snare is advised. One millimeter of normal tissue around the lesion helps to ensure lesion capture. The lesion is cut by closing the snare and returning the snare into the suction channel to facilitate easier retrieval of the polyp. The polypectomy site is examined carefully. A submucosal cord is often visible and need not be further resected. Bleeding is normal but should resolve spontaneously after some time. If bleeding continues, consider placement of a hemostatic clip [16].

Sporadic Non-ampullary Adenomas: EMR

Conventional EMR: Conventional EMR is used as first line for endoscopic resection of non-cancerous large non-ampullary duodenal adenomas (>6 mm).

Technique: This is usually completed with a forward-viewing endoscope fitted with a distal cap, yet a side-viewing duodenoscope may be required for lesions in the medial part of the descending duodenum. Dye or virtual chromoendoscopy may be used to outline the lesion prior to resection and is used to separate the muscularis propria from the lesion to reduce the chance of perforation. Marking the lesion with a snare tip cautery is recommended. Submucosal injection can be performed with dye saline solution or specific macromolecular solution. The volume injected is dependent on the size of the lesion, and repeat injection may be required if the cushion dissipates. Epinephrine can be added to the solution to prevent post-procedural bleeding (1:100,000 dilution). Snare size should be selected based on lesion size (usually 10 mm, 15 mm, or 25 mm) and should be enhanced with electrocautery. The polyps may require piecemeal resection (overlapping snare resections) if the lesion is larger than 2 cm [17].

Other emerging EMR techniques include cap-assisted EMR, cap-band-assisted EMR, and underwater EMR. Cap-assisted EMR and cap-band-assisted EMR can be used specifically for lesions that do not lift well or are difficult to capture with a snare [18]. In both of these techniques, the polyp is suctioned into cap and resected with a dedicated snare. Underwater EMR is an emerging technique that employs water immersion (rather than air or carbon dioxide). The lumen is less distended during polypectomy; therefore, there is no need for submucosal injection because the wall maintains its innate thickness [1]. Water acts to "float" the lesion and decrease the risk of capturing muscle in the snare.

Sporadic Non-ampullary Adenomas: ESD

The use of endoscopic submucosal dissection (ESD) in non-ampullary duodenal lesions is generally not supported in the guidelines because of the high risk of perforation [5, 15]. The higher risk of perforation in the duodenum is related to the thin muscularis propria layer. Retrospective studies comparing EMR vs ESD show a better en bloc resection rate with ESD but no difference in long-term outcomes and a higher rate of intra- and post-procedural perforation [19–21].

Technique: A high-definition therapeutic gastroscope with a single large (3.7 mm) instrument channel is the preferred endoscope for ESD. Prior to beginning the resection, the borders of the lesion should be marked with electrocautery. A long lasting lifting agent is then injected into the submucosal layer. The mucosa is incised, and the perimeter of the lesion is cut using a specialized electrosurgical knife. The submucosa is further injected and then dissected along this plane in a freehand manner [22].

Sporadic Non-ampullary Adenomas: Full-Thickness Resection Device

The feasibility of endoscopic full-thickness resection (EFTR) of duodenal lesions with a full-thickness resection device has been described in both the upper and lower GI tract [23, 24]. In a study of duodenal EFTR, the bleeding risk is similar to that of EMR without any observed perforations [25]. Randomized trials are required to directly compare EMR to EFTR in the duodenum. It should also be noted that ampullary adenomas cannot be resected via this approach as it would lead to obstruction of the bile and pancreatic ducts.

Ampullary Adenomas: Endoscopic Papillectomy

Commonly referred to in the literature as an ampullectomy, but more properly described as endoscopic papillectomy, refers to the removal of the major papilla via endoscopic means. The goal of endoscopic papillectomy is en bloc resection, allowing margins to be assessed.

Technique: A side-viewing duodenoscope is utilized to optimally visualize the papilla during endoscopic papillectomy. Lesions that spread beyond the ampulla may require submucosal injection; otherwise, injection should be avoided due to a ballooning effect that occurs around the adenoma given the natural tethering of the pancreatic and biliary orifices [26]. The general approach for resection is the fulcrum technique. The snare is opened partially inside the working channel. The tip of the snare is at the apex of the lesion/ampulla and is aligned slightly to the right of the lesion to avoid losing scope control. The snare is fully opened, and duodenoscope is pushed distally over the lesion. Once fully captured, the snare is closed completely. The snare should be moved back and forth to confirm that deeper layers have not been encircled prior to resection. The lesion should be cut with electrocautery, endocut mode with standards for polypectomy [27]. The specimen should be captured with snare quickly to ensure it does not migrate distally. Post polypectomy inspection should examine for bleeding, perforation, and en bloc resection. Pancreatic duct stent following endoscopic papillectomy is supported to help prevent post-procedural pancreatitis in addition to rectal indomethacin [11]. Some endoscopists prefer injection of contrast with methylene blue prior to ampullectomy to help locate pancreatic duct orifice after resection. Biliary cannulation is only

Fig. 12.5 Completed
ampullectomy. Cannulation
of biliary orifice completed
post-ampullectomy;
however, PD could not be
located. Photo courtesy of
Amitabh Chak, MD

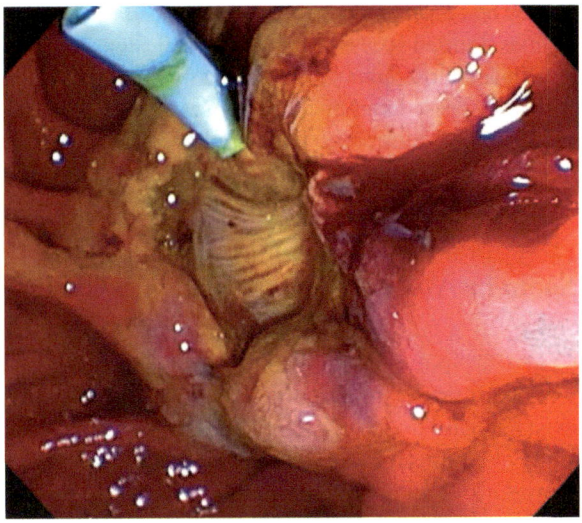

suggested if there is concern for perforation, bleeding, or suspected delay in biliary drainage [28]. Completed ampullectomy can be seen in Fig. 12.5.

There are some notable modifications to standard endoscopic papillectomy. Notably, balloon-catheter-assisted endoscopic snare papillectomy is a useful technique which is advantageous for flat lesions. A balloon catheter and snare are inserted into the bile duct via the accessory channel of a duodenoscope, and snare resection was performed while pulling the expanded balloon toward the lumen [29]. Underwater EMR of papilla has been described in the instance of a neuroendocrine tumor [30]. Finally, in some instances, the endoscopist may opt to cannulate the pancreatic duct and leave an insulated wire prior to papillectomy given how challenging it can be to locate and cannulate the PD after resection is complete [31].

Post-procedural Care, Adverse Events, and Recurrence Rates

The post-procedural level of care following upper GI endoscopy for a duodenal resection is largely dependent on the modality of resection. In the recovery area, the patient is monitored for sedation and procedural-related complications which may include bleeding, perforation, infection, or pancreatitis. The patient can usually be discharged on the same day of the procedure once vital signs are stable and the patient is alert. The patient should be counseled against driving, operating heavy machinery, or signing legal documents on the day of their procedure. The patient should be discharged home with a driver.

Post-procedural management after endoscopic papillectomy is more aggressive due to the high risk nature of the procedure and likelihood of adverse events. Patients should be considered for hospital admission if they have multiple medical comorbidities, limited access to care, or large lesion resection [5].

While endoscopy with polypectomy carries an exceptional safety profile, for the reason discussed earlier in this chapter, duodenal resections have higher rates of bleeding and perforation compared to other areas of the GI tract. Each resection modality has a different adverse event rate as discussed below.

Sporadic Non-ampullary Adenomas: Cold Snare Polypectomy

Cold snare polypectomy for small duodenal polyps (<6 mm) can be performed without difficulty and low rate of reported complications. Although very little data exist in regard to the procedural outcomes and recurrence rates, a single prospective study by Maruoka et al. examined outcomes for cold forceps or cold snare polypectomy for duodenal polyps <6 mm in size. There were no complications (delayed bleeding or perforation). The recurrence rate of adenomas at 3 months was also zero [32].

Sporadic Non-ampullary Adenomas: EMR

A number of retrospective and a single prospective study have examined the adverse event rate associated with non-ampullary duodenal polyp EMR. Immediate bleeding rates range from 0% to 43%, and immediate perforation rates range from 0% to 5.5%. The delayed complications of bleeding and perforation range from 0% to 17% and 0% to 4.4%, respectively. Recurrence rates after resection ranged from 0% to 37%. The rate of adverse events increased with increasing lesion size [17]. Intraprocedural bleeding should be managed immediately with cautery (snare tip or coagulating forceps). Clips may be used but can be challenging to place with a duodenoscope and may obscure the remainder of the resection field. Delayed bleeding can occur up to 7 days following the procedure and should be managed with emergent upper endoscopy [10]. Immediate perforations can usually be managed endoscopically. Delayed perforations can occur following the procedure and usually related to thermal damage to the muscular propria. These are difficult to manage and requires a multidisciplinary discussion with the goal to either observe versus close the defect surgically or endoscopically depending on anatomical location (peritoneal vs. retroperitoneal) and severity of patient's clinical condition. These are the most feared complications because they carry a 1% mortality rate [10].

Recurrence rates following EMR of non-ampullary adenomas vary widely in the literature from 0 to 37% [10, 33, 34]. A single prospective study by Probst et al. found a recurrence rate of 20% of duodenal adenomas ranging from 4 to 70 mm (mean 15 mm) with a complete resection rate of 94% on initial EMR after 48 months of follow-up [35].

Sporadic Non-ampullary Adenomas: ESD and EFTR

As discussed previously, ESD is generally avoided due to high complication rates. Notably, 9–36% risk of perforation and 2–15% rate of emergency surgery. Although ESD may provide a higher en bloc resection rate, safety should be considered over this finding and should only be utilized at expert centers in select cases.

EFTR has limited data yet has revealed a favorable adverse event rate. Prior studies reported a 16–20% minor-moderate bleeding rate, but no major bleeding events or perforations [24, 25]. With this newer device, data in the duodenum had been limited. Bauder et al. examined recurrence following EFTR at 12 months and found recurrence in 2/19 cases [25].

Endoscopic Papillectomy

Endoscopic papillectomy carries a similar adverse event profile to that of endoscopic retrograde cholangiopancreatography. A systematic review and meta-analysis by Spadaccini et al. included 29 studies with 1751 patients undergoing ampullectomy found an overall adverse event rate of 25% [36]. Adverse events may be early (pancreatitis, bleeding, and perforation) or delayed (papillary/biliary stenosis or duodenal luminal stenosis). Mortality is rare and reported to be 0.3% [27].

Adverse events may be effectively minimized and/or managed with prophylactic endoscopic hemostasis with either clip or cautery to high-risk bleeding areas. In addition, rectal indomethacin and pancreatic duct stent placement can be performed to reduce the risk of pancreatitis. Finally, immediate bleeding may occur, and the endoscopist should be prepared to employ standard techniques for hemostasis and include interventional radiology/angiography for hemorrhage refractory endoscopic means [11].

Recurrence rates in a 2020 systematic review with pooled analysis included 14 studies with at least 50 patients and found a pooled recurrence rate of 12% at 10–85 months [36]. Recurrence rates in patients with FAP may be higher, 58% or 14/24 patients in a single 10-year retrospective study [37].

Surveillance

Surveillance strategies following endoscopic resection of non-ampullary and ampullary tumors are lacking. A guidelines supported surveillance strategy is outlined in Table 12.4.

Table 12.4 Surveillance guidelines for duodenal adenomas

	ASGE [5]	ESGE [11, 15]
Ampullary adenoma	Initial: 1–6 months Every 3–12 months for 2 years OR Follow CRC surveillance guidelines	Initial: Within first 3 months Second: 6–12 months Yearly × 5 years
Non-ampullary adenoma	No interval provided Individualized based on adequacy of resection, dysplasia, underlying comorbid conditions	Initial: 3 months Second: 1 year Then individualized based on size/ dysplasia, villous component, and patient factors

Both societies support that a screening colonoscopy be offered to patients who have duodenal or ampullary adenomas

References

1. Gaspar JP, Stelow EB, Wang AY. Approach to the endoscopic resection of duodenal lesions. World J Gastroenterol. 2016;22(2):600.
2. Abraham NS, Barkun AN, Sauer BG, et al. American College of Gastroenterology-Canadian Association of Gastroenterology clinical practice guideline: management of anticoagulants and antiplatelets during acute gastrointestinal bleeding and the periendoscopic period. J Can Assoc Gastroenterol. 2022;5(2):100–1.
3. Culver EL, Mcintyre AS. Sporadic duodenal polyps: classification, investigation, and management. Endoscopy. 2011;43:144–55.
4. Kallenberg FGJ, Bastiaansen BAJ, Dekker E. Cap-assisted forward-viewing endoscopy to visualize the ampulla of Vater and the duodenum in patients with familial adenomatous polyposis. Endoscopy. 2017;49(2):181–5. https://doi.org/10.1055/s-0042-118311.
5. ASGE Standards of Practice Committee, Chathadi KV, Khashab MA, et al. The role of endoscopy in ampullary and duodenal adenomas. Gastrointest Endosc. 2015;82:773–81. https://doi.org/10.1016/j.gie.2015.06.027.
6. The Paris endoscopic classification of superficial neoplastic lesions: esophagus, stomach, and colon: November 30 to December 1, 2002. Gastrointest Endosc. 2003;58(6):S3–43.
7. Goda K, Kikuchi D, Yamamoto Y, et al. Endoscopic diagnosis of superficial non-ampullary duodenal epithelial tumors in Japan: multicenter case series. Dig Endosc. 2014;26:23–9.
8. Yoshimura N, Goda K, Tajiri H, Ikegami M, Nakayoshi T, Kaise M. Endoscopic features of nonampullary duodenal tumors with narrow-band imaging. Hepato-Gastroenterology. 2010;57(99–100):462–7.
9. Yamasaki Y, Takeuchi Y, Kanesaka T, et al. Differentiation between duodenal neoplasms and non-neoplasms using magnifying narrow-band imaging – do we still need biopsies for duodenal lesions? Dig Endosc. 2020;32(1):84–95. https://doi.org/10.1111/den.13485.
10. Amoyel M, Belle A, Dhooge M, et al. Endoscopic management of non-ampullary duodenal adenomas. Endosc Int Open. 2022;10(01):E96–108. https://doi.org/10.1055/a-1723-2847.
11. Geoffroy Vanbiervliet A, Strijker M, Arvanitakis M, et al. Endoscopic management of ampullary tumors: European Society of Gastrointestinal Endoscopy (ESGE) guideline. Endoscopy. 2021;53:429–48. https://doi.org/10.1055/a-1397-3198.
12. Mehta NA, Shah RS, Yoon J, et al. Risks, benefits, and effects on management for biopsy of the papilla in patients with familial adenomatous polyposis. Clin Gastroenterol Hepatol. 2021;19(4):760–7.
13. Spigelman AD, Talbot IC, Williams CB, Domizio P, Phillips RKS. Upper gastrointestinal cancer in patients with familial adenomatous polyposis. Lancet. 1989;334(8666):783–5.

14. Syngal S, Brand RE, Church JM, Giardiello FM, Hampel HL, Burt RW. ACG clinical guideline: genetic testing and management of hereditary gastrointestinal cancer syndromes. Am J Gastroenterol. 2015;110(2):223–62; quiz 263. https://doi.org/10.1038/ajg.2014.435.
15. Vanbiervliet G, Moss A, Arvanitakis M, et al. Endoscopic management of superficial nonampullary duodenal tumors: European Society of Gastrointestinal Endoscopy (ESGE) guideline. Endoscopy. 2021;53(5):522–34. https://doi.org/10.1055/a-1442-2395.
16. Tips and tricks: cold snare polypectomy for removal of colonic lesions. World Endoscopy Organization (WEO) [Internet]. [cited 2022 Aug 13]. Available from: https://www.worldendo.org/2021/12/15/tips-and-tricks-cold-snare-polypectomy-for-removal-of-colonic-lesions/
17. Tomizawa Y, Ginsberg GG. Clinical outcome of EMR of sporadic, nonampullary, duodenal adenomas: a 10-year retrospective. Gastrointest Endosc. 2018;87(5):1270–8. https://doi.org/10.1016/j.gie.2017.12.026.
18. Draganov PV. Pearls and pitfalls of endoscopic resection of duodenal adenomas. Gastroenterol Hepatol (N Y). 2020;16(3):149–51.
19. Pérez-Cuadrado-Robles E, Quénéhervé L, Margos W, et al. Comparative analysis of ESD versus EMR in a large European series of non-ampullary superficial duodenal tumors. Endosc Int Open. 2018;6(8):E1008.
20. Na HK, Kim DH, Ahn JY, et al. Clinical outcomes following endoscopic treatment for sporadic nonampullary duodenal adenoma. Dig Dis. 2020;38(5):364–72. https://doi.org/10.1159/000504249.
21. Esaki M, Haraguchi K, Akahoshi K, et al. Endoscopic mucosal resection vs endoscopic submucosal dissection for superficial non-ampullary duodenal tumors. World J Gastrointest Oncol. 2020;12(8):918–30. https://doi.org/10.4251/wjgo.v12.i8.918.
22. ASGE Technology Committee, Maple JT, Abu Dayyeh BK, et al. Endoscopic submucosal dissection. Gastrointest Endosc. 2015;81(6):1311–25. https://doi.org/10.1016/j.gie.2014.12.010.
23. Mão De-Ferro S, Castela J, Pereira D, Chaves P, Dias Pereira A. Endoscopic full-thickness resection of colorectal lesions with the new FTRD system: single-center experience. GE Port J Gastroenterol. 2019;26(4):235–41.
24. Hajifathalian K, Ichkhanian Y, Dawod Q, et al. Full-thickness resection device (FTRD) for treatment of upper gastrointestinal tract lesions: the first international experience. Endosc Int Open. 2020;8(10):E1291.
25. Bauder M, Schmidt A, Caca K. Endoscopic full-thickness resection of duodenal lesions—a retrospective analysis of 20 FTRD cases. United European Gastroenterol J. 2018;6(7):1015.
26. Menees SB, Schoenfeld P, Kim HM, Elta GH. A survey of ampullectomy practices. World J Gastroenterol. 2009;15(28):3486.
27. de Campos ST, Bruno MJ. Endoscopic papillectomy. Gastrointest Endosc Clin N Am. 2022;32(3):545–62.
28. Bourke M, Bassan M. Endoscopic ampullectomy: a practical guide. J Interv Gastroenterol. 2012;2(1):23–30. https://doi.org/10.4161/jig.20131.
29. Aiura K, Imaeda H, Kitajima M, Kumai K. Balloon-catheter-assisted endoscopic snare papillectomy for benign tumors of the major duodenal papilla. Gastrointest Endosc. 2003;57(6):743–7.
30. Keshava VE, Henien SR, Kumar AR. Endoscopic ampullectomy of a large neuroendocrine tumor using underwater EMR technique. VideoGIE. 2020;5(7):314–7. https://doi.org/10.1016/j.vgie.2020.03.004.
31. Pohl J. Ampullary adenoma - wire-guided ampullectomy. Video J Encycl GI Endosc. 2013;1(2):425–6. https://doi.org/10.1016/S2212-0971(13)70190-0.
32. Maruoka D, Matsumura T, Kasamatsu S, et al. Cold polypectomy for duodenal adenomas: a prospective clinical trial. Endoscopy. 2017;49(8):776–83. https://doi.org/10.1055/s-0043-107028.
33. Valli PV, Mertens JC, Sonnenberg A, Bauerfeind P. Nonampullary duodenal adenomas rarely recur after complete endoscopic resection: a Swiss experience including a literature review. Digestion. 2017;96(3):149–57. https://doi.org/10.1159/000479625.
34. Abbass R, Rigaux J, Al-Kawas FH. Nonampullary duodenal polyps: characteristics and endoscopic management. Gastrointest Endosc. 2010;71(4):754–9.

35. Probst A, Freund S, Neuhaus L, et al. Complication risk despite preventive endoscopic measures in patients undergoing endoscopic mucosal resection of large duodenal adenomas. Endoscopy. 2020;52(10):847–55. https://doi.org/10.1055/a-1144-2767.
36. Spadaccini M, Fugazza A, Frazzoni L, et al. Endoscopic papillectomy for neoplastic ampullary lesions: a systematic review with pooled analysis. United European Gastroenterol J. 2020;8(1):44–51. https://doi.org/10.1177/2050640619868367.
37. Tianle M, Jang EJ, Zukerberg LR, et al. Recurrences are common after endoscopic ampullectomy for adenoma in the FAP syndrome. Surg Endosc. 2014;28(8):2349.

Chapter 13
Surgical: Transduodenal Resection (Open vs Minimally Invasive)

Ann Polcari, Aram Rojas, and Melissa E. Hogg

Introduction

The duodenum is the most common location of small intestinal tumors [1]. Lesions in the duodenum pose a challenge for the surgeon, given the complex anatomic relation to the pancreas, liver, and biliary system (Fig. 13.1). Choosing a method for resection of a duodenal lesion is nuanced; it requires an understanding of the tumor's biology, location within the duodenum, size, and proximity to the ampulla of Vater. Distinguishing between benign and malignant lesions and the likelihood for lymph node involvement is key for decision-making, as malignant adenocarcinomas require a pancreatoduodenectomy (Whipple procedure) due to the high risk of lymph node metastasis. Benign lesions, pre-malignant lesions, small neoplastic lesions with low likelihood of lymph node metastasis, and low-grade tumors that do not metastasize to lymph nodes, on the other hand, are often amenable to less extensive and thus less invasive operations in experienced hands.

Of note, there are no evidence-based consensus guidelines regarding the role of transduodenal resections for masses of the duodenum. It is widely accepted that benign lesions of the duodenum, especially ampullary tumors, should be resected to avoid obstruction. However, the operations are technically challenging and thus require an experienced surgeon. Halsted was the first to describe the open

Supplementary Information The online version contains supplementary material available at https://doi.org/10.1007/978-3-031-78409-5_13.

A. Polcari
University of Chicago, Chicago, IL, USA

A. Rojas · M. E. Hogg (✉)
NorthShore University HealthSystem, Evanston, IL, USA
e-mail: MHogg@Northshore.org

© The Author(s), under exclusive license to Springer Nature Switzerland AG 2025
E. P. Ceppa et al. (eds.), *The SAGES Manual of Evolving Techniques in Pancreatic Surgery*, https://doi.org/10.1007/978-3-031-78409-5_13

Fig. 13.1 Pancreas
anatomy and relations

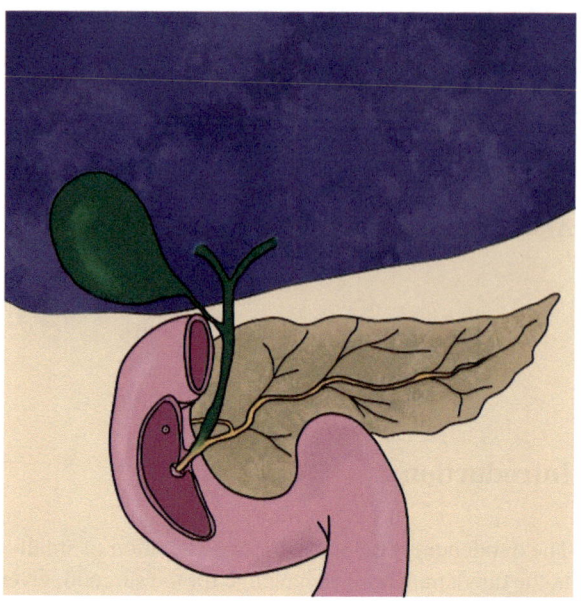

transduodenal ampullectomy (TDA) in 1899, but the procedure was largely abandoned as the pancreatoduodenectomy became the gold standard for resecting duodenal and ampullary cancers [2]. Transduodenal resections remained appealing for
benign lesions, given the morbidity associated with the Whipple procedure, but
existed as a primarily open operative technique. Though attempted laparoscopically
in 2003, the lack of articulating instruments and 2D visualization associated with
laparoscopic surgery limited the uptake of the minimally invasive technique [3].

More recently, the advancement of minimally invasive procedures for gastroenterologists and surgeons, alike, has changed the landscape for resection of duodenal
tumors. Advanced endoscopy is now an accepted tool for resecting small, superficial duodenal tumors. Robotic-assisted surgery has enabled increased opportunity
of minimally invasive approaches for transduodenal resection of ampullary and
duodenal masses. The first robotic-assisted transduodenal ampullectomy was successfully completed in 2015 and has since become a widely accepted approach to
resecting amenable benign duodenal lesions; flexibility of the instruments and
improved ergonomics for the surgeon make the robotic approach more enticing [3].

Of course, every surgeon should know when to choose the appropriate technique—whether endoscopic, open, minimally invasive, or a hybrid—in addition to
considering the full spectrum of procedures—from mucosal resections to the
Whipple procedure—based on tumor characteristics and individual patient factors.
In this chapter, we will focus on the management of duodenal tumors amenable to
transduodenal resection. We will discuss both the technique for transduodenal
wedge resections and surgical ampullectomy.

Duodenal Masses Amenable to Transduodenal Surgery

The lesions typically considered for transduodenal resection are non-adenocarcinomas. Incidence of these tumors has been growing, likely due to the increased use of endoscopy to assess upper gastrointestinal symptoms. On these exams, hyperplastic polyps are frequently found, but are usually small and amenable to endoscopic resection.

Benign Tumors

There are several mesenchymal-derived benign tumors found in the duodenal sub-mucosa, which can be excised via a transduodenal approach. Leiomyomas, derived from smooth muscle layers within the bowel wall, are often discovered during workup for anemia in middle-aged men—ulceration of the tumor's overlying mucous membrane can cause bleeding [1]. These tumors should be biopsied to rule out leiomyosarcoma, which is malignant and when small is amenable to transduodenal resection. Lipomas, which arise from the fatty submucosa of the small bowel wall, are also found in the duodenum. Lipomas are typically initially asymptomatic and are usually discovered after progressing to duodenal obstruction [1]. A well-defined mass of blood vessels found in the submucosa of the duodenum is the hemangioma. As one might assume, hemangiomas can cause significant bleeding, which ultimately leads to their diagnosis [1]. Lymphangiomas have been described, as well, though these tumors are rare. A host of neuron-derived tumors can also exist in the duodenum's wall and require resection, including neurofibromas (most common), schwannomas, and gangliomas.

Genetic Syndromes

Patients with familial adenomatous polyposis (FAP) syndrome and Peutz-Jeghers disease often develop polyps in the duodenum. Patients with FAP typically develop adenomas found in the more distal duodenum; these patients require regular surveillance as these polyps can lead to cancer [1]. The hamartomas developed in Peutz-Jeghers disease are usually benign and the duodenum is a rare location for these lesions [1]. Given small bowel lesions occur early in life in patients with these genetic conditions, young adults with duodenal polyps or tumors should be further evaluated specifically for these syndromes.

Pre-Malignant Tumors

The most common benign tumor found in the duodenum are adenomas, typically located in D2 and therefore amenable to transduodenal resection. Adenomas are derived from the epithelium. They are categorized as serrated, tubular, tubulovillous, and villous. These tumors can be sporadic, occur in inherited polyposis syndromes, or are derived from Brunner's glands. Adenomas have been proven to progress to cancer, so early excision is paramount. Large adenomas, especially, should be considered for removal via transduodenal resection, as endoscopic biopsy often misses portions of the polyp containing carcinoma in situ. Transduodenal resection is accepted for adenomas that display carcinoma in situ on biopsy.

Low-Grade Malignancies

Gastrointestinal stromal tumors (GISTs), which arise from the interstitial cells of Cajal and are distinguished by *c-kit* mutations, can also grow intramurally and obstruct the duodenal lumen or ulcerate through the mucosa and bleed; surgical resection is required for these tumors [4]. It is well accepted that GISTs can be removed via transduodenal surgical techniques, both wedge resection and ampullectomy (Supplementary Videos 13.1 and 13.2).

Another rare duodenal tumor requiring resection and potentially amenable to transduodenal resection is a neuroendocrine tumor (NET). These comprise <3% of all duodenal tumors but are increasingly found as abdominal imaging modalities improve. NETs can be aggressive tumors; however, small (<2 cm), well-differentiated Grade 1 periampullary NETs without evidence of lymph node metastasis can be resected via transduodenal resection.

Please refer to Chap. 11 for more in-depth discussion on benign, pre-malignant, and malignant duodenal neoplasms.

Indications for Transduodenal Resection

Alternatives

Adenocarcinomas of the duodenum are straightforward—tumors with biopsy or imaging-proven disease greater than Tis (carcinoma in situ) require a pancreatoduodenectomy. This is largely driven by the possibility of upstaging on final pathology, especially given the high risk of lymph node invasion. Please refer to Chaps. 19, 20, and 21 for in-depth review of open, laparoscopic, and robotic pancreatoduodenectomy.

Resection of other duodenal masses, on the other hand, is less cut-and-dry due to the variety of local excision techniques available. Duodenal masses of the descending portion of the duodenum (D2) are most often amenable to endoscopic and transduodenal approaches. Please refer to Chap. 12 for a more in-depth review of endoscopic duodenal resection. Non-cancerous and some cancerous lesions of the proximal duodenal segment (D1) and those that are infra-ampullary (in D3 and D4) typically require a more extensive resection such as the partial sleeve duodenectomy (PSD) [5]. This operation, like transduodenal approaches, can be completed open, laparoscopic, or robotically and is pancreas-sparing, but requires proximal small bowel reconstruction. Also, D1 and D3 lesions on the antimesenteric surface of the duodenum are amenable to a wedge resection. Please refer to Chap. 14 for more in-depth review of segmental duodenal resection (open vs MIS). For this chapter, we will focus on surgical options for D2 lesions.

Inclusion Criteria

Currently, the literature suggests that endoscopic mucosal resections (EMR), endoscopic submucosal dissections (ESD), or endoscopic papillectomy be reserved for benign lesions <2 cm in size; there should be no more than high-grade dysplasia on preoperative biopsy of the lesion, and it should not extend beyond the papilla into the common bile or pancreatic ducts [6, 7]. Some studies have reported mandatory transduodenal resection only after the tumor has reached 4 cm in size [6]. However, the primary goal of operative intervention is to achieve complete pathologic resection. Thus, if a lesion cannot be resected en bloc endoscopically, a transduodenal approach should be employed instead [2]. In fact, transduodenal resection is indicated for tumor recurrence or lack of clear margins after endoscopic resections. Lesions that reach the muscularis propria of the duodenal wall, encompass more than one-third of the duodenum circumference, or incorporate the common bile and/or pancreatic duct are reasons to perform a pancreatoduodenectomy. Of note, endoscopic resections can be considered as a palliative approach for patients who are poor surgical candidates.

Once a transduodenal operation is deemed appropriate, selection of the approach is largely contingent upon the proximity of the tumor to the ampulla [8]. A transduodenal wedge resection, in which the tumor is removed with a full-thickness portion of the duodenal wall, is possible if there is a clear margin between the lesion and the ampulla. This is most often done for D2 lesions on the antimesenteric wall of the duodenum located at least 2 cm from the ampulla. True periampullary lesions may require a transduodenal mucosal resection to avoid a full-thickness wedge that encroaches on the ampulla. A lesion that involves the common bile and/or pancreatic ducts within the ampulla necessitates a transduodenal ampullectomy.

An interesting new hybrid approach, called laparoscopic and endoscopic co-operative surgery (LECS), has been recently described by Hiki et al. and was tested in 12 patients by Ichikawa et al. [9, 10]. During this procedure, both ESD and laparoscopy are performed together. LECS is reserved for resection of non-ampullary tumors with the goal of reducing the common complications related to ESD. For example, the ESD resection bed is oversewn laparoscopically to avoid hemorrhage and leak after perforation. While we do not describe this technique in detail in this chapter, it appears to be a safe and feasible option for non-ampullary tumors.

Preoperative Planning

Surgical options for a patient with a duodenal tumor are largely dependent on findings during the preoperative workup, which typically consists of an upper endoscopy with biopsy, endoscopic ultrasound (EUS), computed tomography (CT) scan, and/or magnetic resonance imaging with cholangiopancreatography (MRI/MRCP). CT scan can be better to optimize understanding of vasculature and MRCP can be helpful to better depict the common bile duct (CBD and pancreatic duct. Both are not usually necessary and is surgeon preference.

Upper endoscopy is key in determining location of the tumor, particularly with respect to the ampulla and the physical characteristics of the tumor, such as size and shape (Fig. 13.2). Biopsy of the lesion during upper endoscopy is also essential in determining the required operative intervention. If the tumor is benign, such as an adenoma with features of dysplasia, or only contains carcinoma in situ, a

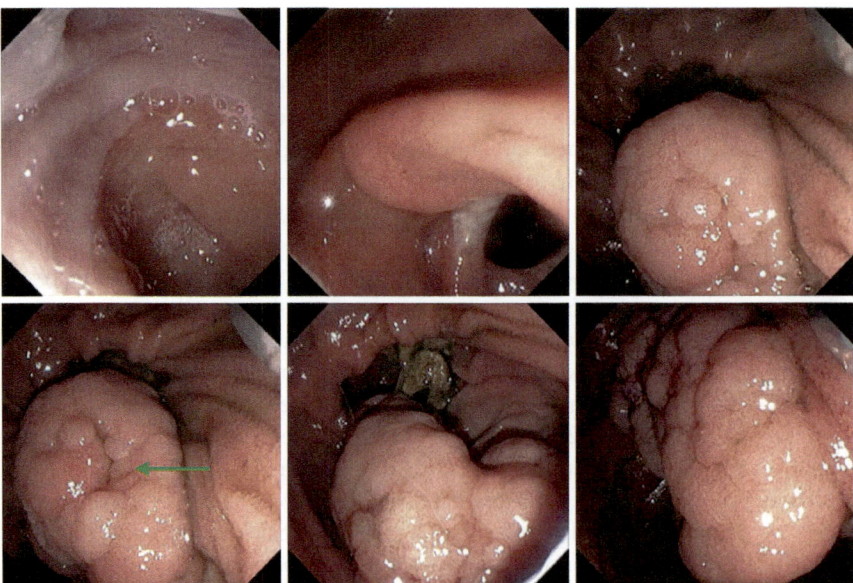

Fig. 13.2 GD Endoscopy showing duodenal mass (green arrow)

pancreatoduodenectomy may be avoided. It is often essential to get a second endoscopy as the first one may not completely delineate (1) mesenteric vs. antimesenteric location, (2) circumference of the wall involved, (3) proximity to the ampulla with pictures, and (4) complete size with measurements. If possible, requesting video footage of or being present during the preoperative endoscopy is recommended. Tattooing is not always helpful as this can disperse and enter the abdominal cavity widely.

Upper endoscopic ultrasound is important in identifying lymph node metastasis for cancerous lesions and is also extremely valuable in determining whether benign lesions can undergo endoscopic resection versus a transduodenal approach. EUS can evaluate the depth of invasion into the duodenal wall, as well as extension into the CBD or pancreatic duct for ampullary lesions (Fig. 13.3). Ultimately, it determines the approach by which a lesion is considered resectable.

CT (Fig. 13.4) and MRI/MRCP (Fig. 13.5) can further assist in decision-making by providing a map of the tumor and its association to the common bile and pancreatic ducts, in addition to revealing any local anatomic variations.

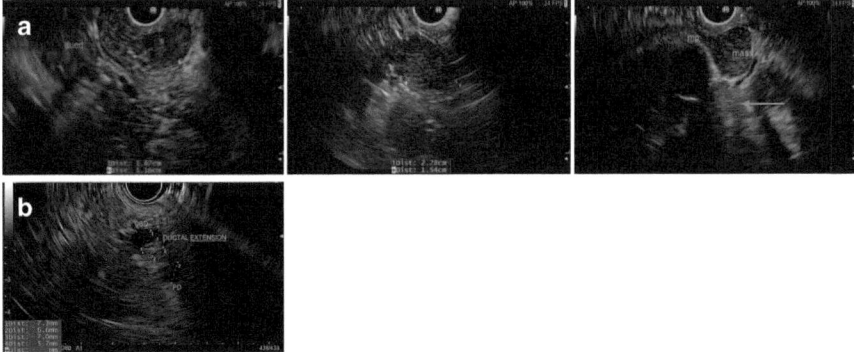

Fig. 13.3 (**a**) Endoscopic ultrasound showing duodenal mass (green arrow). (**b**) Eus in patient with tumor of the Ampulla

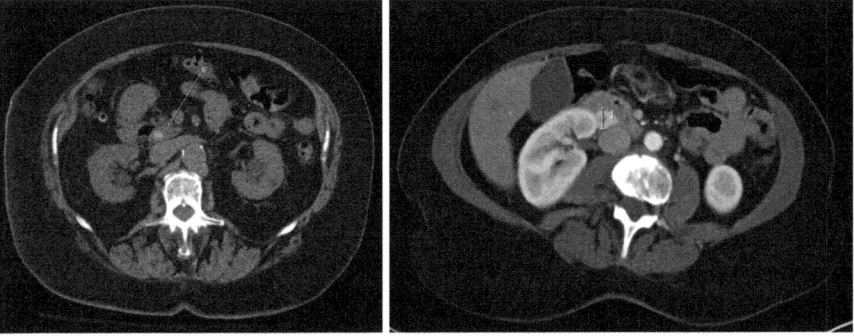

Fig. 13.4 CT scan showing duodenal mass (green arrow)

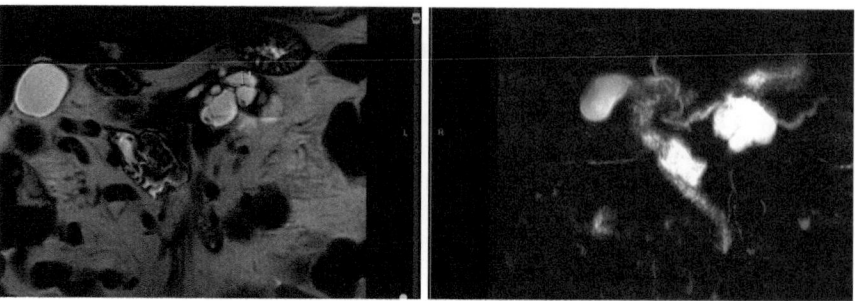

Fig. 13.5 Magnetic resonance imaging with cholangiopancreatography

Fig. 13.6 ERCP

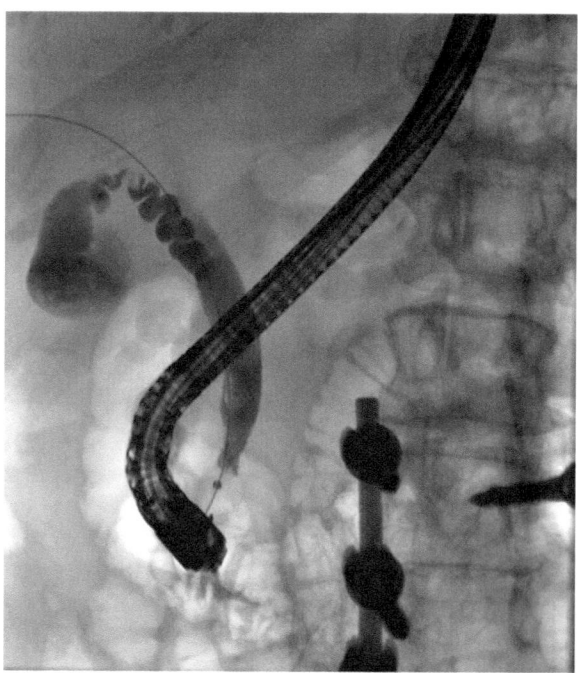

A few groups have reported using preoperative ERCP to place a stent in the CBD to assist in identification of the ampulla prior to duodenotomy during a minimally invasive transduodenal resection. The stent can help precisely target the duodenotomy using intra-operative ultrasound. This step is surgeon-dependent and not required preoperatively. However, it may be useful for ampullary tumors causing obstruction or in patients who are at high risk for cholangitis while awaiting surgery. When a patient presents with jaundice, a pause is necessary before considering an ampullectomy due to concern for malignancy. Careful attention should be paid to MRCP to look for stones, to EUS for identification of small masses, and to cholangiogram on ERCP to identify stricture (Fig. 13.6). It is possible to present with jaundice for benign etiologies, but one must perform due diligence.

Always consent the patient for a possible Whipple procedure. With careful workup and planning and in experienced hands this hopefully would not be necessary, but in the event that all the anatomy cannot be appropriately delineated or the reconstruction could compromise the lumen or the ducts, then a Whipple may be the safest option. In the setting of an adenoma, always discuss the possibility the tumor will be upstaged on final pathology and another operation may be necessary.

Surgical Techniques and Outcomes

Open Transduodenal Submucosal and Wedge Resection

1. The patient should be positioned supine on the operating table with both arms out at 90 degrees.
2. After intubation and initiation of general anesthesia, a nasogastric tube and urinary catheter should be placed in addition to pneumatic compression devices for DVT prophylaxis. Patient should be prepped according to hospital protocol.
3. Both a generous midline incision and right subcostal incision are acceptable. A midline incision is recommended for patients who may require adhesiolysis due to prior surgical history.
4. Palpate the liver and inspect the rest of the peritoneum to rule out evidence of metastatic disease.
5. After the surgeon's preferred self-retaining retractor is placed, mobilize the hepatic flexure of the colon.
6. Perform an extensive Kocher maneuver to expose the entirety of D2—lysing the duodenum's retroperitoneal attachments from the foramen of Winslow to the Ligament of Treitz and posteromedial to the root of the superior mesenteric artery (SMA). The posterior wall of the duodenum should be visible after completion of this maneuver.
7. Physically palpate the duodenal wall in a bimanual fashion to identify the target lesion and the ampulla. *TIP: For small tumors that may not be easily palpable, Hashimoto et al. describe a preoperative duodenoscopy with clip placement on the duodenal mucosa opposite the tumor to assist in determining the site of duodenotomy [11]. It is important to limit insufflation to avoid extensive dilation of the small bowel. Additionally, carbon dioxide insufflation may assist in limiting bowel distension.*
8. At this time, stay sutures may be placed through the duodenal wall lateral to the lesion and planned site of duodenotomy in order to maintain adequate exposure throughout the operation. *TIP: A laparotomy sponge can be placed behind the duodenum to facilitate positioning prior to making the duodenotomy.*
9. Using cautery, make a 2–4 cm longitudinal duodenotomy on the antimesenteric border of D2, opposite the lesion.

10. Prior to resection of mucosal or submucosal lesions, saline or epinephrine can be injected in the submucosal space to lift the lesion from the exterior layers of the duodenal wall.
11. A figure of eight suture can be placed through the lesion itself once visible to assist in retraction and visualization of the ducts [12]. *TIP: A 5 Fr pediatric feeding tube or small catheter can be placed into the CBD to ensure safe dissection of lesions near the ampulla* [11].
12. Wide local excision is performed using electrocautery, generally 5 mm to 1 cm margin in a clockwise manner circumferentially around the lesion. Tumors that are mucosal or submucosal in origin and periampullary or peri-pancreatic can be lifted off the duodenal wall via dissection in the subcutaneous space. Lesions with deeper origin and far from the ampulla (>2 cm) should undergo full-thickness wedge resection, removing the duodenal wall circumferentially around the lesion. *TIP: Abe* et al. *describe using indigocarmine dye solution to assist in visualizing tumor margins* [13]. *In this series, the solution is mixed with epinephrine and injected into the submucosa to help lift the tumor.*
13. Close the submucosal defect with interrupted, absorbable suture (e.g., 3-0 Vicryl™). Close the duodenotomy transversely in two layers—we use an inner absorbable suture and a permanent silk suture to Lembert the outer layer. *TIP: If the resection defect is too large to be closed primarily (e.g., 50% of the duodenal wall), one should consider proximal GI reconstruction* [13]. *Other alternatives such as a duodenal sleeve or pancreas preserving duodenectomy are options described in a later chapter.*

Minimally Invasive (Robotic-Assisted) Transduodenal Submucosal and Wedge Resection

1. The patient should be positioned supine on the operating table with both arms out at 90 degrees. The authors also choose to split the patient's legs (Fig. 13.7).
2. After intubation and initiation of general anesthesia, a nasogastric tube and urinary catheter should be placed in addition to pneumatic compression devices for DVT prophylaxis. The patient should be prepped according to hospital protocol.
3. After entry into the abdomen, set pneumoperitoneum to 10–15 mmHg.
4. Perform diagnostic laparoscopy of the liver and peritoneum to rule out metastatic lesions.
5. Robotic ports for the Xi (Intuitive Surgical, Sunnyvale California) should be placed as follows: 8 mm port in the left upper quadrant, 8 mm port above the umbilicus, 8 mm port in the left mid-clavicular line, and an 8 mm port in the left mid-axillary line.
6. At least one laparoscopic 12 mm assistant port is required for passing: ultrasound probe, sutures, and mini-lap pads. An additional 5 mm assistant trocar can be placed as well if needed for suction or retraction of the colon, which may be more critical in patients with central obesity.

Fig. 13.7 Patient positioned with split legs

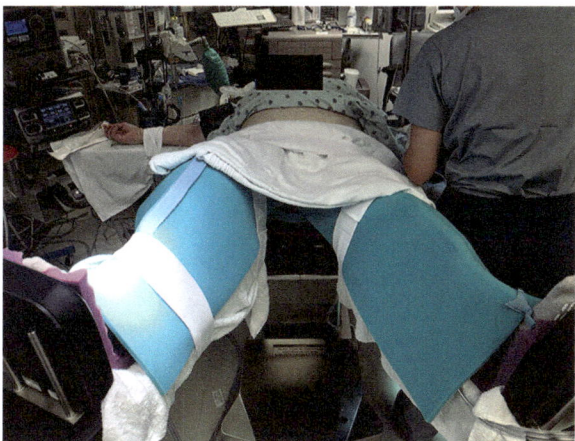

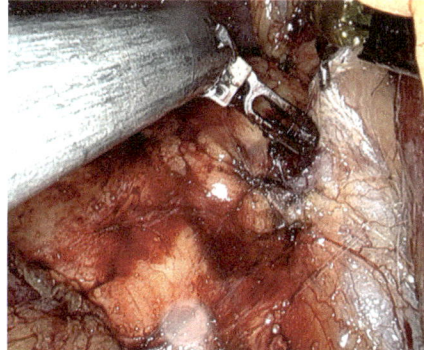 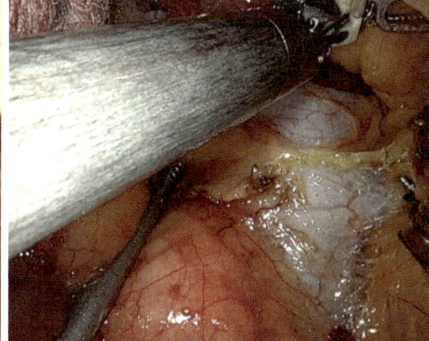

Fig. 13.8 Complete Kocher maneuver

7. Dock the robot. This can be done a variety of ways, but the authors prefer to dock from the patient's left, in the upper abdomen configuration of the Xi robot.
8. Mobilize the hepatic flexure of the colon.
9. Perform an extensive Kocher maneuver to expose the entirety of D2—lysing the duodenum's retroperitoneal attachments from the foramen of Winslow to the Ligament of Treitz and posteromedial to the root of the SMA (Fig. 13.8). The posterior wall of the duodenum should be visible after completion of this maneuver and duodenum should be mobilized away from hepatoduodenal ligament.
10. Since the lesion cannot be reliably palpated, the lesion is identified and its relationship to the ampulla assessed using intra-operative ultrasound. Given advancements in robotic-assisted technology, one can also use indocyanine green (ICG) to locate the CBD (Fig. 13.9) [14]. While the bile duct is patient dependent, it can sometimes be visualized through the intra-pancreatic portion of the bile duct.

Fig. 13.9 ICG

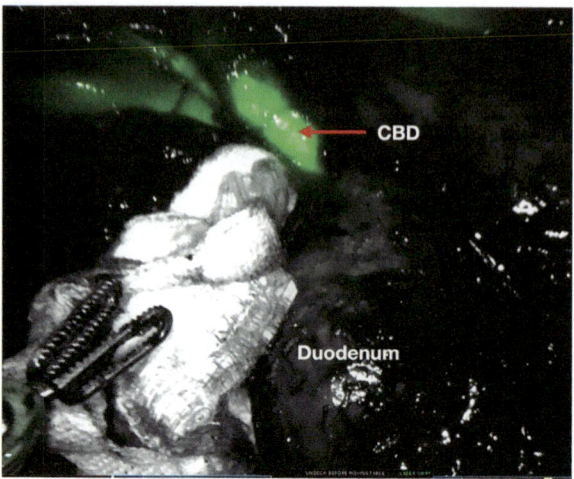

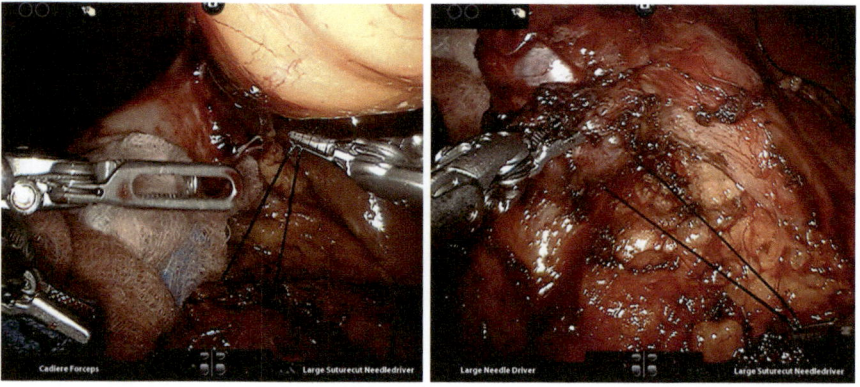

Fig. 13.10 Stay sutures

11. Stay sutures may be placed through the lateral walls of the duodenum near the lesion (Fig. 13.10). These can assist in closure and can be retracted by the third robot arm to give more exposure. Laparotomy sponges can also be used to bump up the duodenum, bringing the mass to the forefront.
12. Wide local excision is performed using electrocautery, generally a 5 mm to 1 cm margin in a clockwise manner circumferentially around the lesion starting at 3 o'clock (Fig. 13.11). Tumors that are mucosal or submucosal in origin and periampullary or peri-pancreatic can be lifted off the duodenal wall via dissection in the submucosal space. Lesions with deeper origin and enough distance from the ampulla should undergo full-thickness wedge resection, removing the duodenal wall circumferentially around the lesion (Fig. 13.12).
13. Place the specimen in bag for removal through the umbilical port.

**Fig.
13.11** Circumferential
demarcation around the
lesion

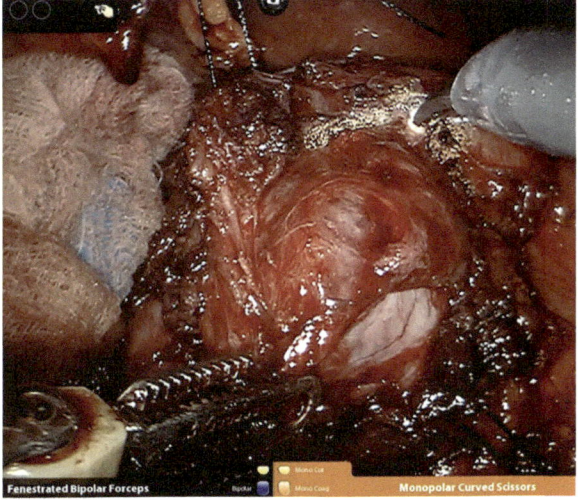

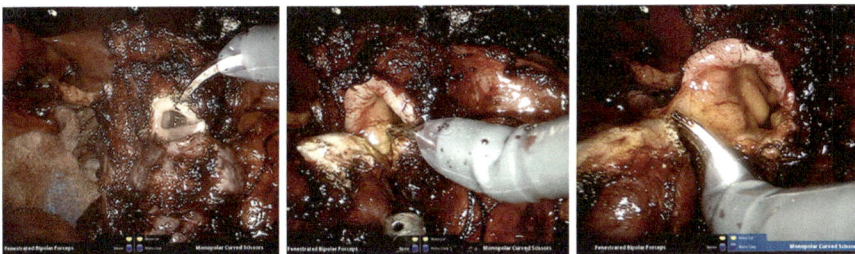

Fig. 13.12 Full-thickness resection removing the duodenal wall

14. Close any submucosal defects with interrupted, absorbable suture (e.g., 3-0 Vicryl™).
15. Close the duodenotomy in two layers—we use an inner absorbable barbed suture (Fig. 13.13) and a permanent silk suture to Lembert the outer layer (Fig. 13.14).

Open Transduodenal Ampullectomy

1. Patient should be positioned supine on the operating table with both arms out at 90 degrees.
2. After intubation and initiation of general anesthesia, a nasogastric tube and urinary catheter should be placed in addition to pneumatic compression devices for DVT prophylaxis. Patient should be prepped according to hospital protocol.
3. Both a midline incision and an extended right subcostal incision are acceptable. A midline incision is recommended for patients who may require adhesiolysis

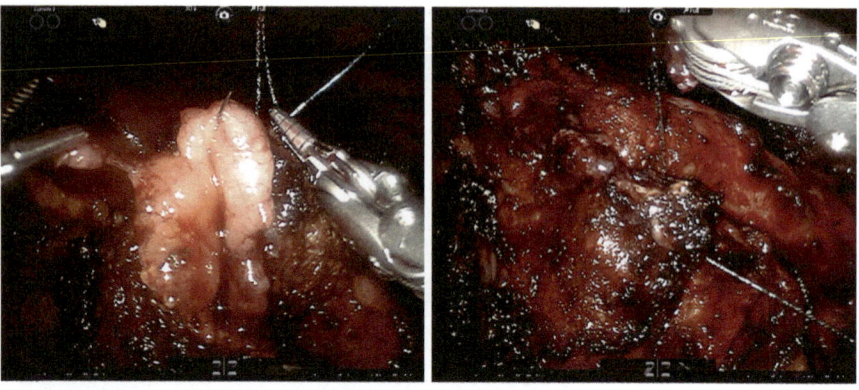

Fig. 13.13 Duodenum closure: first layer with barbed suture

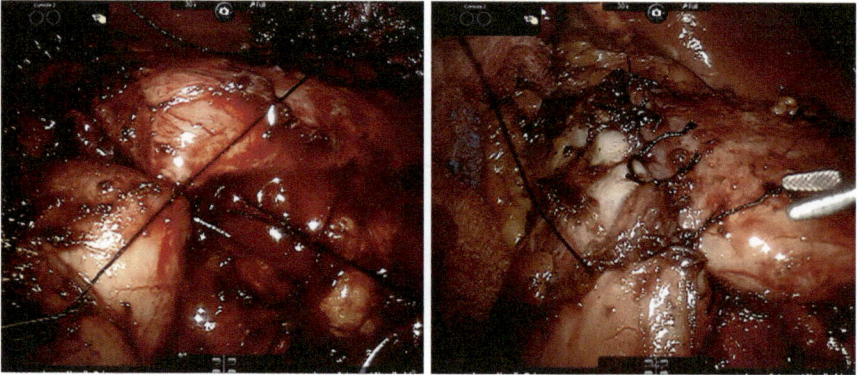

Fig. 13.14 Duodenum closure: second layer with silk

due to prior surgical history. Some authors will also make a reversed "L" incision [15].

4. Palpate the liver and inspect the rest of the peritoneum to rule out evidence of metastatic disease.
5. After the surgeon's preferred self-retaining retractor is placed, mobilize the hepatic flexure of the colon.
6. Perform an extensive Kocher maneuver to expose the entirety of D2—lysing the duodenum's retroperitoneal attachments from the foramen of Winslow to the Ligament of Treitz and posteromedial to the root of the SMA. The posterior wall of the duodenum should be visible after completion of this maneuver.
7. Physically palpate the duodenal wall in a bimanual fashion to identify the target lesion and the ampulla. *TIP: Several authors also describe creating a cystic ductotomy and passing a catheter into the duodenum to assist in identifying the ampulla, especially if the bile duct is small [15–17]. A cholecystectomy must then be performed.*

8. At this time, stay sutures may be placed through the duodenal wall lateral to the lesion and planned site of duodenotomy to maintain adequate exposure throughout the operation. *TIP: A laparotomy sponge can be placed behind the duodenum to facilitate positioning prior to making the duodenotomy.*

9. Using cautery, make a 2–4 cm longitudinal duodenotomy on the antimesenteric border of D2, opposite the ampulla.

10. Resect the ampulla. Use electrocautery to incise the mucosa 5 mm to 1 cm reaching the submucosal plane. Dissect in the submucosal plane starting at the 11 o'clock position and moving clockwise until reaching the CBD. Mark the duct with a suture on its superior edge. Continue dissecting clockwise until reaching the pancreatic duct, typically at the 4–6 o'clock position. Complete the dissection circumferentially until margins are grossly clear. *TIP: Jung et al. prefer to use the needle point electrocautery device on cutting (monopolar) mode to avoid distorting the margins for pathology* [18].

11. Reconstruct the ampulla; this is the most challenging step. Using 5-0 absorbable monofilament suture (i.e., 5-0 PDS), sew the ducts back to the duodenal wall using interrupted sutures. Start with the CBD and work toward the pancreatic duct. It is important to suture the septum between the two ducts together, as well. *NOTE: Some authors also describe reconstructing the ampulla in conjunction with dissection of the lesion (i.e., combining Steps 10 and 11 above, or "suturing as you go"). Papalampros et al. place serial sutures from the duodenal wall to the CBD and pancreatic duct as dissection of the mass progresses, leaving only re-approximation of the two ducts to be completed after the mass in completely removed* [12, 17].

12. Stent the bile duct. Sometimes this is done prior to resection, for reconstruction, or at the end. Occasionally, suturing the stent with lesion can allow manipulation of the lesion without touching it. For the end, 4–7 French stents that are designed to pass are used. Some surgeons suture these in place with absorbable suture.

13. Mathiel et al. note that there is typically an extra fold of duodenal tissue due to a larger duodenal defect than duct area; this defect can be closed with simple interrupted sutures [17].

14. Close the duodenotomy transversely in two layers—the authors use an inner absorbable suture and a permanent silk suture to Lembert the outer layer.

Minimally Invasive (Robotic-Assisted) Transduodenal Ampullectomy

1. Patient should be positioned supine on the operating table with both arms out. The authors also choose to split the patient's legs.

2. After intubation and initiation of general anesthesia, a nasogastric tube and urinary catheter should be placed in addition to pneumatic compression devices for DVT prophylaxis. Patient should be prepped according to hospital protocol.

3. After entry into the abdomen, typically via Veress needle at the umbilicus or at Palmer's point followed by an optical separator entry, set pneumoperitoneum to 10–15 mmHg.
4. Perform diagnostic laparoscopy of the liver and peritoneum to rule out metastatic lesions.
5. Robotic ports for the Xi (Intuitive Surgical, Sunnyvale California) should be placed as follows: 8 mm port in the left upper quadrant, 8 mm port above the umbilicus, 8 mm port in the left mid-clavicular line, and an 8 mm port in the left mid-axillary line (Fig. 13.15).
6. At least one laparoscopic 12 mm assistant port is required for passing: ultrasound probe, sutures, and mini-lap pads. An additional 5 mm assistant trocar can be placed as well if needed for suction or retraction of colon which may be more critical in patients with central obesity.
7. Dock the robot. This can be done a variety of ways, but the authors dock from the patient's left, in the upper abdomen configuration of the Xi robot (Fig. 13.16a, b).
8. Mobilize the hepatic flexure of the colon.
9. Perform an extensive Kocher maneuver to expose the entirety of D2—lysing the duodenum's retroperitoneal attachments from the foramen of Winslow to the Ligament of Treitz and posteromedial to the root of the SMA to mobilize the entire duodenum. The posterior wall of the duodenum and pancreas should be visible after completion of this maneuver.
10. Interrogate the duodenal wall for the target lesion and the ampulla. This may not be possible in minimally invasive fashion given lack of haptic feedback; adjuncts include ICG, ultrasound, and catheters via the cystic duct (Figs. 13.17 and 13.18; *see Tips and Tricks below*).
11. Stay sutures may be placed through the lateral walls of the duodenum near the pancreas at the level of the ampulla on either side of where the duodenotomy is planned to maintain exposure and later close the duodenum (Fig. 13.19).

Fig. 13.15 Robotic ports placement

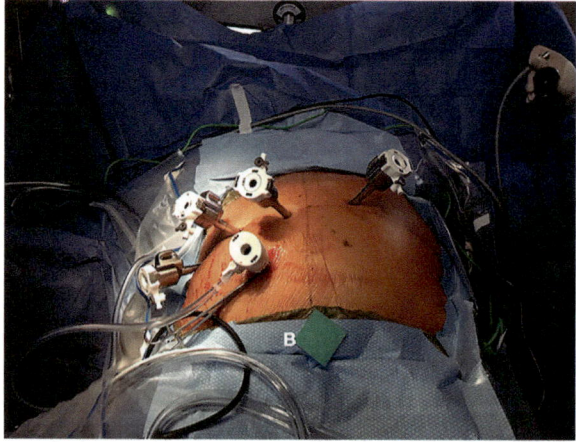

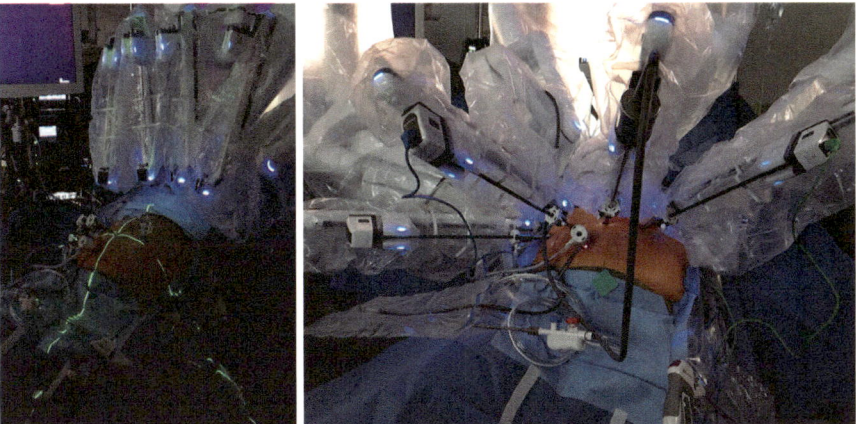

Fig. 13.16 Docking

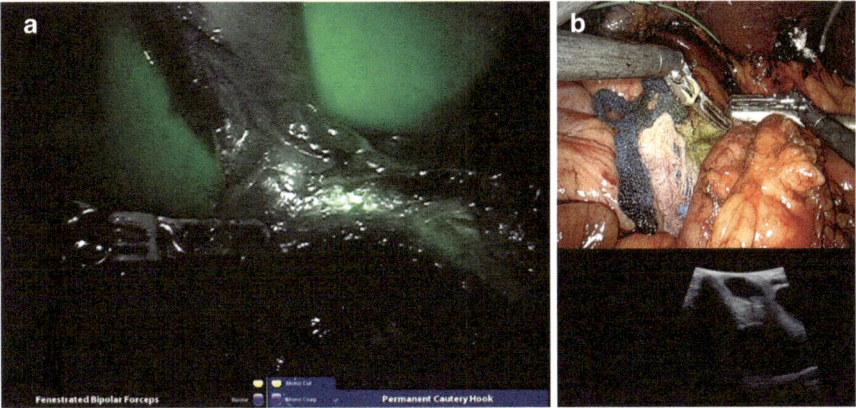

Fig. 13.17 (**a**) Fluorescence, (**b**) Ultrasound

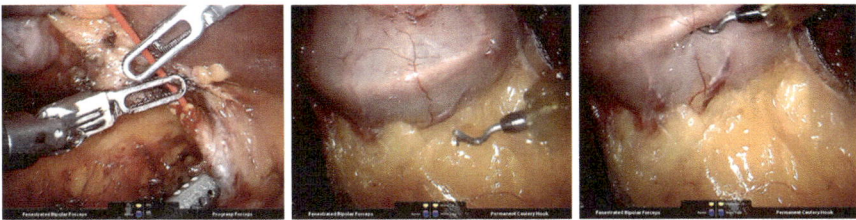

Fig. 13.18 Fogarty Catheter via the cystic duct

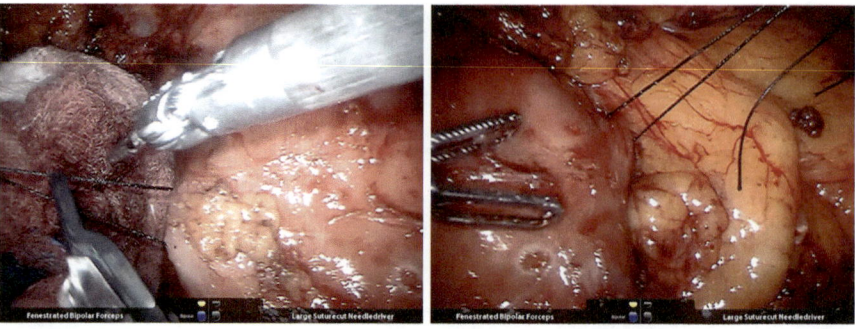

Fig. 13.19 Stays sutures placed on both sides of the duodenal wall

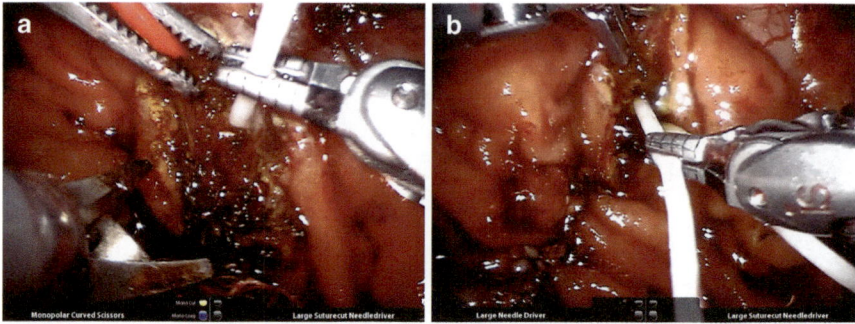

Fig. 13.20 (**a**) stent placed in the pancreatic duct. (**b**) Stent placed in the CBD

12. Using cautery, make a 2–4 cm longitudinal duodenotomy on the antimesenteric border of D2, opposite the ampulla. *TIP: A few mini-laparotomy sponges can be placed behind the duodenum to facilitate positioning prior to making the duodenotomy.*

13. Resect the ampulla. Use electrocautery to incise the mucosa 5 mm to 1 cm reaching the submucosal plane. Dissect in the submucosal plane starting at the 6 o'clock position and moving clockwise until reaching the CBD ~12 o'clock. Mark the duct with a suture on its superior edge. Continue dissecting clockwise until reaching the pancreatic duct, typically at the 4–6 o'clock position. Complete the dissection circumferentially until margins are grossly clear. *TIP: Using stents within the bile and pancreatic duct are helpful to the dissection and reconstruction* (Fig. 13.20). *Sometimes suturing the stent to the bile duct can create a handle to manipulate the ampulla without touching the adenoma. A four French stent is left unsutured in the PD to pass soon after the case. Its primary purpose helps avoid back-walling the duct during suturing.*

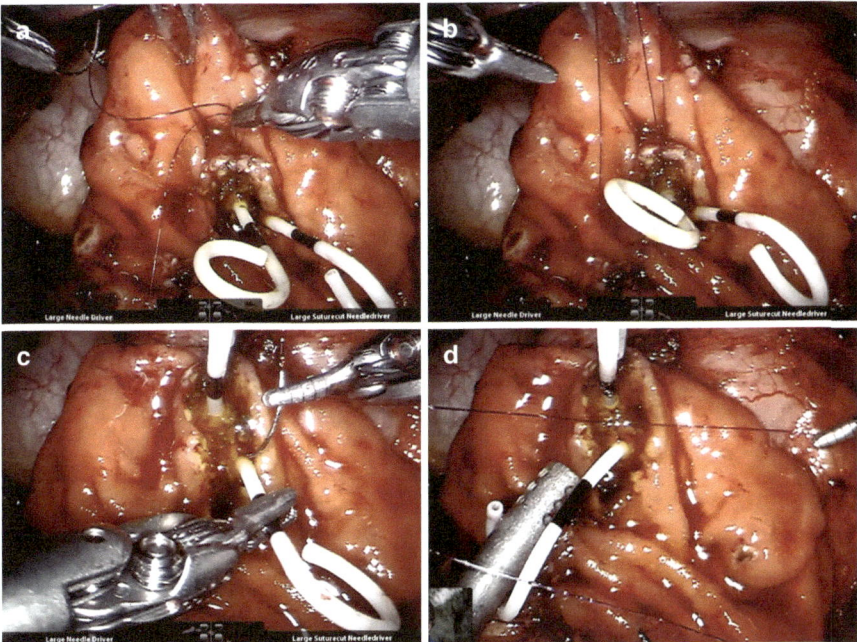

Fig. 13.21 Reconstruction of the ampulla: (**a**, **b**) First stitch 12 o'clock. (**c**, **d**) Second stich between bile duct and pancreatic duct

14. Place specimen in bag for removal through the 12 mm port.
15. Reconstruct the ampulla; this is the most challenging step. 5-0 absorbable monofilament (i.e., PDS) cut to 5 inches allows for use 2–3 times. The first stitch placed is 12 o'clock at the top of the bile duct (Fig. 13.21a, b). Then, the third robotic arm can retract this anteriorly. Place the second stitch inferior on the bile duct and superior on the pancreas duct for a septoplasty to unite the ducts (Fig. 13.21c, d). Next sew the ducts full thickness to the mucosa of the duodenal wall using interrupted sutures.
16. Stent the CBD and pancreatic duct—as describe previously if not already done.
17. Close the duodenotomy transversely in two layers—we use an inner absorbable barbed suture and a permanent silk suture to Lembert the outer layer (Fig. 13.22a–c).

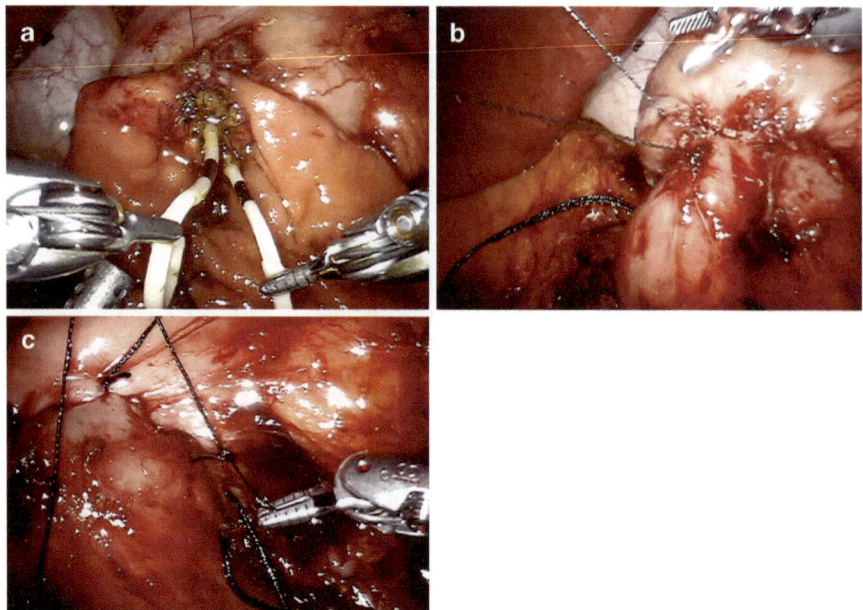

Fig. 13.22 (**a**) Stents in pave. (**b**) Duodenum closure first layer with V-lock suture. (**c**) Second layer with silk

Minimally Invasive Tips and Tricks

Finding the Ampulla Preoperative stenting can be helpful but is not necessary. A few adjuncts include:

1. Use of ICG to be given prior to the procedure. In the right patient, the bile duct will be visible within the pancreas all the way to its exit in the duodenum.
2. Use of ultrasound. Start in the porta hepatis to identify the portal triad "Mickey Mouse" head and follow the CBD (the upper left circle) into the pancreas and then out to the duodenum (Fig. 13.23).
3. Use of a wire or catheter through the cystic duct, down the CBD, and into the duodenum (Fig. 13.24). This makes palpation and identification easier.

Frozen Section This decision may be due to how close the gross margin appears on resection. If there is any concern for cancer, a Whipple may be the more appropriate operation. One can consider having pathology take a representative slice for inspection, but this may not be high yield. Some pathologists will allow you to place a STAT order on the permanent specimen so that if upgraded from adenoma to cancer on final pathology, then another operation can be done immediately. However, with proper patient selection, sending the bile duct margin to rule out adenoma or high-grade dysplasia will determine if you need to resect higher on the duct.

Fig. 13.23 Portal traid

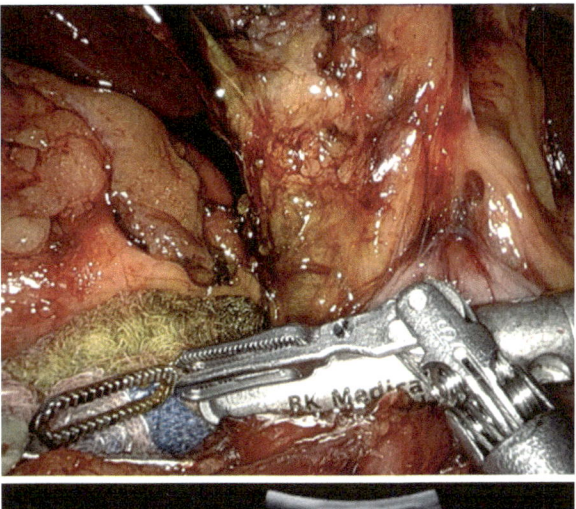

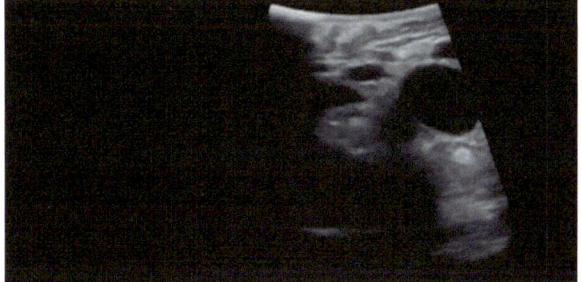

Fig. 13.24 Fogarty
catheter

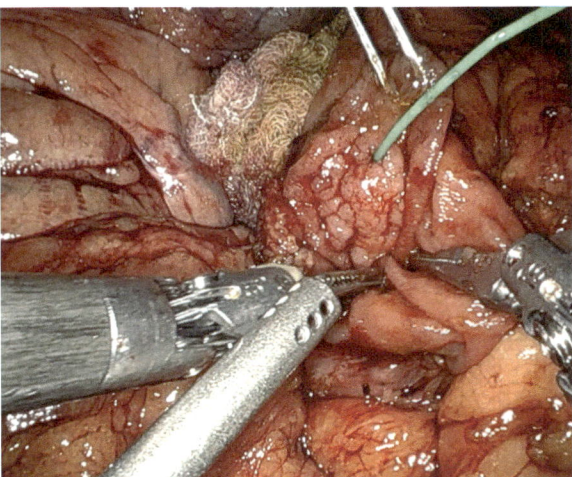

Fig. 13.25 4 fr. Hobbs
Medical stents

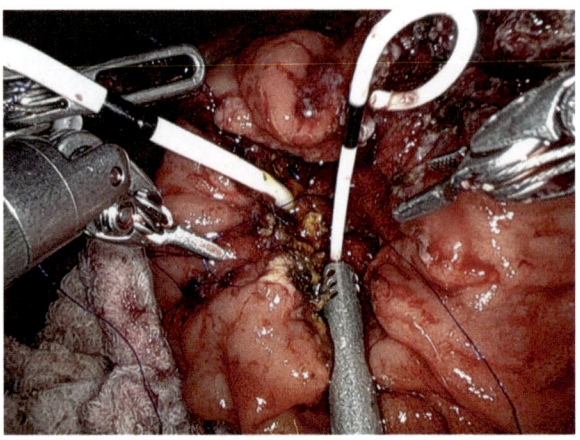

Stents The authors' preference for duct stents are 4-Fr Hobbs Medical stents (Stafford Springs, CT) (Fig. 13.25). These are helpful to avoid back-walling the duct and to note the trajectory of the duct. These can be stitched in place with a chromic or Vicryl™ suture (but do not need to be).

Leak Test The authors do not routinely perform a leak test with endoscopy after closure of the duodenotomy unless there is a concern about the integrity of the closure or concern over narrowing of the duodenum.

Drains Drains are not necessary but are the preference of the authors. A 19-Fr Blake drain is left, and a serum amylase is checked post-op day #1—if this is less than three times the serum amylase and the drain is not bilious, it is removed after the patient tolerates a diet. The diet is clear liquid for one meal followed by a low residue diet. If there is concern for duodenal narrowing, a full liquid or soft diet can also be used. It is possible to discharge patients on post-op day #1.

Falciform Flap Depending on the location of the duodenotomy and the size of the falciform ligament, this can be buttressed over the duodenotomy closure like a Graham Patch.

Follow-Up Typically, gastroenterology is asked to perform an upper endoscopy 6–12 months postoperatively to look at the surgical neo-papilla and to evaluate for possible recurrence (Fig. 13.26).

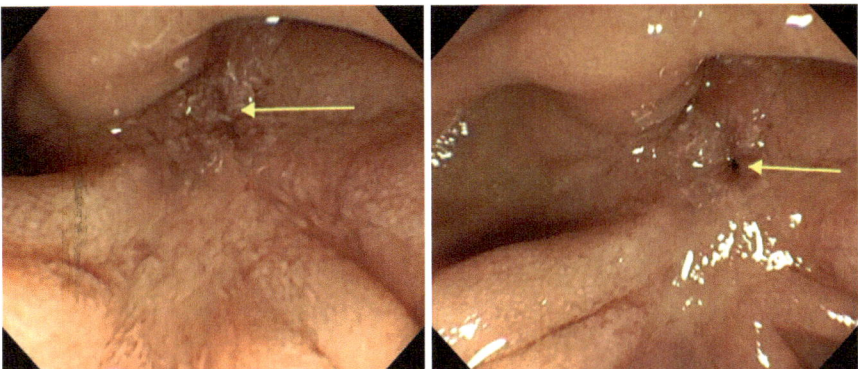

Fig. 13.26 Ampulla site post robotic amupullectomy

Outcomes

In general, patients have favorable outcomes after both transduodenal wedge resection and ampullectomy, regardless of open or minimally invasive technique. Given the rarity of these tumors and resections, data for each operation is sparse and inconsistent. There are several retrospective, single-center studies describing outcomes after open transduodenal resection. Most of these operations appear to take between 2 and 4 h and have minimal blood loss (50–100 mL). Length of stay, when reported, is typically well over 1 week and the 90-day mortality rate in recent literature approaches zero. Given the technical challenges associated with laparoscopic transduodenal resections, only case reports and small case series appear in the literature. Despite similar blood loss to the open procedure, operative times are an hour longer on average and length of stay is closer to 1 week. Nienty-day mortality is also zero for these cases. Since robotic surgery is the newest technique, it is also most often documented as case reports. Robotic-assisted cases appear to have shorter operative times and decreased length of stay compared to open and laparoscopic data though without an appreciable difference in overall mortality, morbidity, or recurrence. More studies are needed to parse out differences in the minimally invasive compared to open techniques, especially as robotic surgery becomes more prevalent.

The most common complications reported in recent literature are similar among all techniques and includes duodenal leak, duct stricture (especially after ampullectomy), intra-abdominal abscess, and rarely pancreatitis and cholangitis. Table 13.1 summarizes a brief literature review of outcomes for transduodenal wedge resection and ampullectomy.

Table 13.1 Literature review of outcomes for transduodenal ampullectomy and transduodenal wedge resections of benign tumors as identified via PubMed search for "transduodenal ampullectomy," "open transduodenal ampullectomy," "robotic transduodenal ampullectomy," "transduodenal wedge," "transduodenal wedge benign," "transduodenal submucosal resection"

Author, year	Study design	Cases included	Benign tumors or Tis on final path (%)	Tumor size (cm)	Resection type	Technique	Duration of operation (min)	Estimated blood loss (mL)	Length of stay (days)	Severe complications; Clavien-Dindo IIIa or greater	Recurrence (%) at mean follow-up time	90-day re-admission	90-day mortality
Logarajah et al., 2022 [16]	Retrospective single center	15	15 (100%)	2.8 (mean)	Ampullectomy	Open	122.9 (mean)	100 (median)	7 (mean)	None reported	2 (13.3%) at 21.3 months	N/A	–
	Retrospective single center	46	31 (55.7%)	1.74 (mean)	Ampullectomy	43 open, 1 laparoscopic, 2 robotic	218.5 (mean)	50 (median)	14.9 (mean)	4; duct strictures and wound dehiscence	–	6 (13%); cholangitis, stricture, SSI, SBO	0 (0%)
Jung et al., 2021 [18]	Retrospective single center	27	23 (85%)	–	Ampullectomy	Open	212.3 (mean)	–	14.3 (mean)	2; not reported	1 (3.7%) at 6 months	–	0 (0%)
	Retrospective single center	16	14 (87.5%)	2.3 (mean)	Ampullectomy	Open	238.5 (mean)	125 (mean)	12.5 (mean)	2; intra-abdominal abscess, duodenal leak	1 (6.3%) at 22 months	3 (18.8%)	1 (6.3%); palliative resection
	Retrospective single center	24	24 (100%)	2.7 (mean)	6 (25%) Ampullectomy, 6 (25%) wedge	Robotic	204 (mean)	50 (mean)	5 (median)	3 (12%); duodenal leak, hemorrhage	0 (0%) at 16.5 motnhs	2 (8%)	0 (0%)
	Retrospective single center	10	8 (80%)	1.7 (mean)	Ampullectomy	Open	–	–	–	0 (0%)	0 (0%) at 70 months	–	0 (0%)
Hong et al., 2018 [15]	Retrospective single center	26	22 (85%)	2.0 (mean)	Ampullectomy	22 open, 4 laparoscopic	250.9 (mean)	–	(mean)	1 (3.8%); hemorrhage	3 (11.5%) at 72 months	2 (7.7%); duodenal leak & stenosis	0 (0%)
	Case report	1	1 (100%)		Ampullectomy	Robotic	250	20	7	0 (0%)	0 (0%) at 1 year	0 (0%)	0 (0%)
	Retrospective single center	21	17 (81%)	1.5 (median)	Ampullectomy	Open	–	100 (median)	20 (median)	2 (9.5%); T-tube leak, CBD stricture	0 (0%) at 8 months		0 (0%)

Papalampros et al., 2017 [12]	Retrospective single center	14	11 (78.6%)	—	Ampullectomy	Open	145 (mean)	85 (mean)	11.6 (mean)	1 (7%); duodenal leak	0 (0%) at 26.5 months	—	0 (0%)
	Retrospective single center	11	6 (54.5%)	—	Ampullectomy	Open	—	—	—	0 (0%)	1 (9%) at 36 months	—	0 (0%)
	Retrospective single center	73	70 (96%)	—	Ampullectomy	Open	—	—	10 (median)	8 (11%); abscess, duodenal leak, necrotizing pancreatitis, cholangitis	1 (2.3%) at 54 months	—	0 (0%)
	Retrospective dual center	26	26 (100%)	2.9 (median)	Ampullectomy, wedge, sleeve, segmental duodenectomy	Robotic	240 (median)	50 (median)	6 (median)	4 (15%); abscess, duodenal leak, hemorrhage		5 (19.2%)	0 (0%)
Kim et al. 2011 [2]	Retrospective single center	21	20 (95%)	—	Ampullectomy	Open	—	—	9 (median)	5 (24%); dehiscence, duct stenosis	1 (5%) at 33 months	—	0 (0%)
	Case series	1	1 (100%)	2	Ampullectomy	Laparoscopic	200	50	8	0 (0%)	—	—	—
		1	1 (100%)	1	Ampullectomy	Laparoscopic	250	50	9	0 (0%)	—	—	—
	Case report	1	1 (100%)	—	Ampullectomy	Laparoscopic	240	50	6	0 (0%)	0 (0%) at 3 months	0 (0%)	0 (0%)
	Case series	1	1 (100%)	3	Ampullectomy	Open	166	70	10	0 (0%)	—	—	—
		1	1 (100%)	1.4	Ampullectomy	Laparoscopic	296	100	15	0 (0%)	—	—	—
		2	2 (100%)	1.75	Ampullectomy	Robotic	328.5	75	8.5	0 (0%)	—	—	—

(continued)

Table 13.1 (continued)

Author, year	Study design	Cases included	Benign tumors or Tis on final path (%)	Tumor size (cm)	Resection type	Technique	Duration of operation (min)	Estimated blood loss (mL)	Length of stay (days)	Severe complications; Clavien-Dindo IIIa or greater	Recurrence (%) at mean follow-up time	90-day re-admission	90-day mortality
Linn et al., 2021 [3]	Case report	1	1 (100%)	2.0	Ampullectomy	Robotic	305	50	27	1 (100%); DGE req. TPN, hepatic tuberculosis	0 (0%) at 6 months	1 (100%)	0 (0%)
	Case series	6	5 (83%)	1.9 (median)	Ampullectomy	Robotic	200 (median)	160 (median)	6 (median)	0 (0%)	0 (0%) at 20 months	1 (16.7%)	0 (0%)
	Case report	1	1 (100%)	3.5	Wedge	Laparoscopic	287	10		0 (0%)	0 (0%) at 12 months	0 (0%)	0 (0%)
	Case report	1	1 (100%)	1.8	Wedge	Open	–	–	–	–	0 (0%) at 67 months	–	0 (0%)
Hashimoto et al., 2016 [11]	Retrospective single center	4	2 (50%)	1.55 (median)	Wedge	Open	140.5 (mean)	26.5 (median)	–	0 (0%)	0 (0%) at 18 months	–	0 (0%)
	Case series	1	0 (0%)	1.4	Wedge	Laparoscopic	169	15	7	0 (0%)	–	–	–
		1	1 (100%)	1.3	Wedge	Laparoscopic	133	10	8	0 (0%)	–	–	–
		1	1 (100%)	1.5	Wedge	Laparoscopic	162	25	8	0 (0%)	–	–	–

Conclusions

Transduodenal resections serve as an intermediate option between endoscopic resection and pancreatoduodenectomy for patients with antimesenteric duodenal masses and ampullary lesions with good outcomes. Appropriate preoperative workup can identify a subset of a patients with duodenal and ampullary tumors amenable to transduodenal resection, thus sparing the more morbid Whipple procedure. Transduodenal wedge resection and ampullectomy can be successfully completed using minimally invasive (both laparoscopic and robotic-assisted) techniques, which may improve patient experience postoperatively. Transduodenal resections will continue to have a role in excision of benign, pre-malignant, and non-adenocarcinoma malignant masses of the duodenum.

References

1. Latos W, Kawczyk-Krupka A, Strzelczyk N, Sieroń A, Cieślar G. Benign and non-neoplastic tumours of the duodenum. Prz Gastroenterol. 2019;14(4):233–41. https://doi.org/10.5114/pg.2019.90250.
2. Kim J, Choi SH, Choi DW, Heo JS, Jang KT. Role of transduodenal ampullectomy for tumors of the ampulla of Vater. J Korean Surg Soc. 2011;81(4):250–6. https://doi.org/10.4174/jkss.2011.81.4.250.
3. Linn YL, Wang Z, Goh BKP. Robotic transduodenal ampullectomy: case report and review of the literature. Ann Hepatobiliary Pancreat Surg. 2021;25(1):150–4. https://doi.org/10.14701/ahbps.2021.25.1.150.
4. Popivanov G, Tabakov M, Mantese G, et al. Surgical treatment of gastrointestinal stromal tumors of the duodenum: a literature review. Transl Gastroenterol Hepatol. 2018;3:71. https://doi.org/10.21037/tgh.2018.09.04.
5. García-Molina FJ, Mateo-Vallejo F, Franco-Osorio JD, Esteban-Ramos JL, Rivero-Hernández I. Surgical approach for tumours of the third and fourth part of the duodenum. Distal pancreas-sparing duodenectomy. Int J Surg. 2015;18:143–8. https://doi.org/10.1016/j.ijsu.2015.04.051.
6. Scroggie DL, Mavroeidis VK. Surgical ampullectomy: a comprehensive review. World J Gastrointest Surg. 2021;13(11):1338–50. https://doi.org/10.4240/wjgs.v13.i11.1338.
7. Sekine M, Watanabe F, Ishii T, et al. Investigation of the indications for endoscopic papillectomy and transduodenal ampullectomy for ampullary tumors. J Clin Med. 2021;10(19):4463. https://doi.org/10.3390/jcm10194463.
8. Codjia T, Roussel E, Monge M, Gagnat G, Tuech JJ, Schwarz L. Pancreas-sparing surgery for benign duodenal lesions: four surgical techniques (with video). Ann Surg Oncol. 2021;28(6):3219–22. https://doi.org/10.1245/s10434-020-09238-3.
9. Hiki N, Yamamoto Y, Fukunaga T, et al. Laparoscopic and endoscopic cooperative surgery for gastrointestinal stromal tumor dissection. Surg Endosc. 2008;22(7):1729–35. https://doi.org/10.1007/s00464-007-9696-8.
10. Ichikawa D, Komatsu S, Dohi O, et al. Laparoscopic and endoscopic co-operative surgery for non-ampullary duodenal tumors. World J Gastroenterol. 2016;22(47):10424–31. https://doi.org/10.3748/wjg.v22.i47.10424.
11. Hashimoto D, Arima K, Chikamoto A, et al. Limited resection of the duodenum for nonampullary duodenal tumors, with review of the literature. Am Surg. 2016;82(11):1126–32.

12. Papalampros A, Moris D, Petrou A, et al. Non-Whipple operations in the management of benign, premalignant and early cancerous duodenal lesions. Anticancer Res. 2017;37(3):1443–52. https://doi.org/10.21873/anticanres.11468.
13. Abe N, Suzuki Y, Masaki T, Mori T, Sugiyama M. Surgical management of superficial non-ampullary duodenal tumors. Dig Endosc. 2014;26(Suppl 2):57–63. https://doi.org/10.1111/den.12272.
14. Paterakos P, Rojas AE, Choi SH. Robotic transduodenal ampullectomy: tips for safe reimplantation of biliary and pancreatic duct. J Gastrointest Surg. 2022;26(7):1550–1. https://doi.org/10.1007/s11605-022-05305-0.
15. Hong S, Song KB, Lee YJ, et al. Transduodenal ampullectomy for ampullary tumors—single center experience of consecutive 26 patients. Ann Surg Treat Res. 2018;95(1):22–8. https://doi.org/10.4174/astr.2018.95.1.22.
16. Logarajah S, Cho EE, Deleeuw P, Osman H, Jeyarajah DR. Transduodenal resection for duodenal adenomas may be an underutilized tool—a single institution experience. Heliyon. 2022;8(4):e09187. https://doi.org/10.1016/j.heliyon.2022.e09187.
17. Maithel SK, Fong Y. Technical aspects of performing transduodenal ampullectomy. J Gastrointest Surg. 2008;12(9):1582–5. https://doi.org/10.1007/s11605-008-0474-2.
18. Jung YK, Paik SS, Choi D, Lee KG. Transduodenal ampullectomy for ampullary tumor. Asian J Surg. 2021;44(5):723–9. https://doi.org/10.1016/j.asjsur.2020.12.021.

Chapter 14
Segmental Duodenectomy

Domenech Asbun, John Stauffer, and Horacio J. Asbun

Introduction

Although uncommon, a wide spectrum of neoplastic lesions arises in the duodenum, from benign lesions such as leiomyomas and hamartomas, to premalignant adenomas, to malignant adenocarcinoma or neuroendocrine tumors [1, 2]. The extent of disease dictates the appropriate treatment approach. Smaller benign lesions, adenomas, and intramucosal carcinomas are often amenable to endoscopic approaches, such as snare polypectomy or endoscopic mucosal resection [3]. Malignant lesions in the second portion of the duodenum involving the ampulla or pancreas require pancreatoduodenectomy (PD), while benign lesions of the ampulla may be treatable with an ampullectomy or pancreas-preserving total duodenectomy [4–6].

Duodenal lesions not involving the ampulla and not treatable endoscopically can often be resected with a segmental duodenectomy. This approach spares the patient the morbidity of a PD while having similar survival outcomes, even in the setting of malignancy [7–9]. This chapter will focus on technical aspects of a proximal segmental duodenectomy (PSD) and distal segmental duodenectomy (DSD). PSD is a resection of the first portion of the duodenum and possibly distal antrum/pylorus, for treatment of supra-ampullary lesions. DSD involves resection of the third and/or

Supplementary Information The online version contains supplementary material available at https://doi.org/10.1007/978-3-031-78409-5_14.

Asbun (✉) · H. J. Asbun
Division of Hepatobiliary and Pancreas Surgery, Miami Cancer Institute, Miami, FL, USA
e-mail: domenech.asbun@baptisthealth.net

J. Stauffer
Department of Surgery, Mayo Clinic Florida, Jacksonville, FL, USA

fourth portion of the duodenum, for infra-ampullary lesions. Both PSDs and DSDs preserve part of the duodenum and are inherently pancreas-preserving, meaning they do not involve pancreatic resection. Instead, the pancreatoduodenal complex is separated and a segment of duodenum resected in isolation. A similar approach has been described by the authors to perform total duodenectomy with reimplantation of the biliopancreatic duct complex [10]. However, this chapter will focus on PSD and DSD, in which the ampulla is not resected.

Anatomy

The duodenum is approximately 25–30 cm long and in direct continuity with the pylorus, marking the start of the small intestine. It continues from the pylorus later- ally and then inferiorly in a "C" shape along the lateral edge of the head of the pancreas, before turning medially. It is suspended upwards at the root of the mesen- tery by the suspensory muscle of the duodenum, or Ligament of Treitz, which marks the duodenojejunal flexure and thus the transition from duodenum to jejunum. This "ligament" is a band of fibrous and sometimes muscular fibers arising from the right crus of the diaphragm. After this point, the jejunum continues caudad through the base of the transverse mesocolon into the infracolic abdomen.

The first portion of the duodenum (D1) is approximately 2–4 cm long and is generally not adhered to the head of the pancreas. D1 receives blood supply from the supraduodenal and gastroduodenal arteries. The proximal portion of D1 can be enlarged and is often called the duodenal "bulb." As the second portion of the duo- denum (D2) begins its C-loop curve around the head of the pancreas, it transitions from intraperitoneal to retroperitoneal, and is attached to the pancreas. D2 is per- fused by perforating arteries from the head of the pancreas. It is roughly midway along D2 that the pancreatic and biliary ducts typically join at the ampulla of Vater to insert into the duodenum, via the major duodenal papilla. In some patients, the accessory pancreatic duct of Santorini empties into the minor papilla proximal and somewhat anterior to the major papilla.

The third portion (D3) continues to the left after the C-loop, passing anterior to the vena cava and aorta and with blood supply from the uncinate process. D3 simul- taneously passes posterior to the root of the bowel mesentery, which envelopes the superior mesenteric artery (SMA) and vein (SMV). The fourth portion (D4) contin- ues to the duodenojejunal flexure, often behind other sizable mesenteric blood ves- sels, receiving perfusion from branches off the superior mesenteric artery. There are folds of parietal peritoneum reflecting off D4 which form the paraduodenal fossa. D1, D2, D3, and D4 are also referred to as the superior, descending, transverse, and ascending portions of the duodenum, respectively, which summarizes their courses.

D2, D3, and D4 are retroperitoneal, and as such their mobilization requires inci- sion of overlying peritoneum. There are multiple layers of connective tissue that surround the duodenum and pancreatic head, which are remnants of embryologic structures. Most anteriorly is the parietal peritoneum, and as dissection proceeds

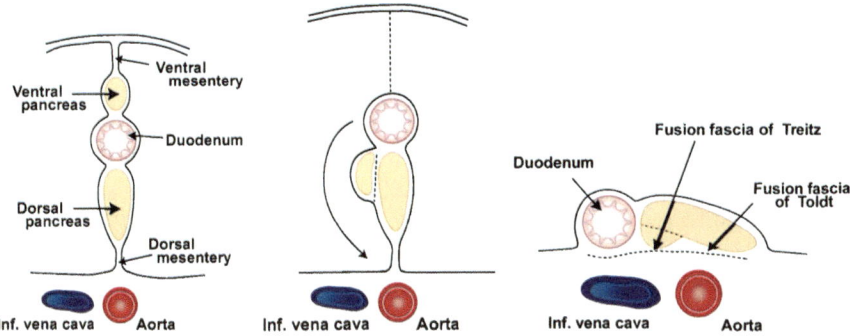

Fig. 14.1 Embryologic origins of periduodenal connective tissue. Far left image shows earliest structure origins, far right image shows fully developed anatomy [12]

deeper along the lateral edge of the duodenum, the so-called fusion fascia of Treitz is encountered [11–13]. The fusion fascia of Treitz is a fusion of multiple layers of connective tissue membrane that cover the ventral and dorsal mesenteric buds during embryologic development. These membranes also overlie the inferior vena cava and aorta (Fig. 14.1). During medial mobilization of D2 and D3 (Kocher maneuver), this fascia remains adherent to the pancreatoduodenal complex and not to the vena cava or aorta. The SMA pierces through this fascia after takeoff from the aorta (Fig. 14.2).

There is also a connective tissue plane between the head of the pancreas, D2/D3, and the bile duct (Fig. 14.3). This "groove" is the location of groove pancreatitis, an uncommon clinical entity characterized by pancreatitis that extends primarily into this potential space [15, 16]. This plane is critical to identify and follow during segmental duodenectomy.

Preoperative Preparation and Pearls

Many duodenal lesions are asymptomatic, especially those not involving the ampulla. Most common symptoms attributable to duodenal lesions include crampy abdominal pain and gastric outlet obstruction. Signs of biliary obstruction such as jaundice should raise concerns for an ampullary neoplasm. Some lesions may present as obvious or occult gastrointestinal bleeding, most characteristically gastrointestinal stromal tumors or adenocarcinomas with associated mucosal ulceration.

Cross-sectional abdominal imaging is important to evaluate for signs of locoregional or distant spread, with specific workup depending on the type of neoplasm diagnosed. It is important for computed tomography (CT) or magnetic resonance imaging (MRI) to have appropriate contrast phases and thin radiographic cuts at the level of the duodenum, which is usually a part of pancreatic imaging protocols. This is important to better assess the relationship of the lesion to the neighboring

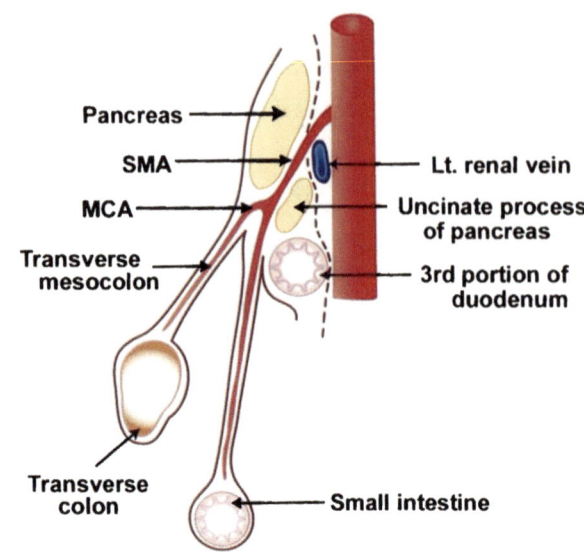

Fig. 14.2 Sagittal view of third portion of duodenum and its relation to mesenteric vessels and surrounding structures. Fusion fascia of Treitz represented by dotted red line [12]. *MCA* middle colic artery, *SMA* superior mesenteric artery

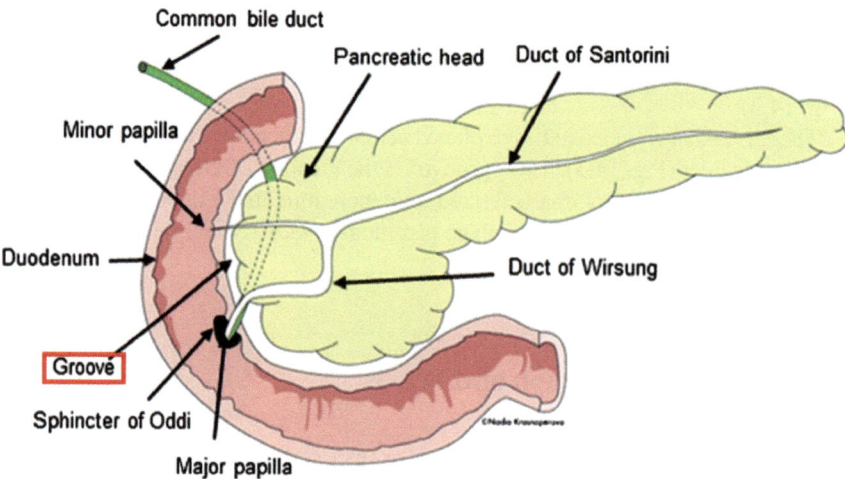

Fig. 14.3 Relations between different structures of the pancreatoduodenal complex. Pancreatoduodenal groove outlined in red on the left [14]

pancreatic parenchyma. MRIs should include diffusion-weighted phases. Oral contrast can be helpful, especially when evaluating the cause of an intestinal obstruction, but is not as important as properly timed intravenous contrast. Oral contrast can be given as part of a CT or MRI, or as a separate upper gastrointestinal X-ray series, although these series are of less utility once the diagnosis of a duodenal lesion is made.

Fig. 14.4 Endoscopic appearance of a duodenal mass. Major papilla labeled at top. With permission from HJ Asbun

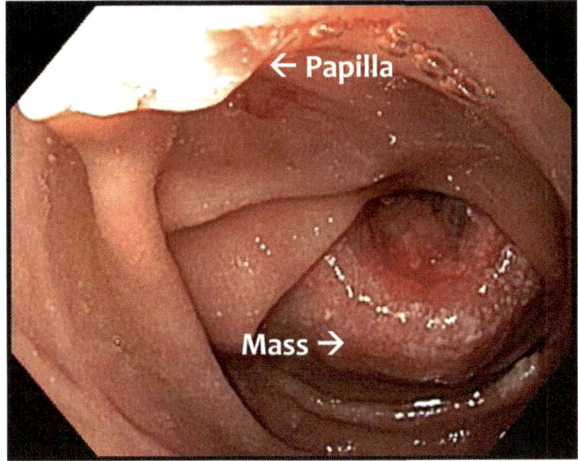

The majority of duodenal lesions should be worked up with an esophagogastroduodenoscopy (EGD) and biopsy by a skilled endoscopist (Fig. 14.4). Additionally, endoscopic ultrasound (EUS) can provide important information regarding the duodenal lesion's depth of invasion, the appearance of periduodenal lymphadenopathy, and the presence of other suspicious masses in the area (Fig. 14.5). Tissue diagnosis is most commonly made from tissue biopsy during EGD.

Endoscopic submucosal tattooing of the lesion is an important part of preoperative workup [17]. For this reason, it is important for the endoscopist and the surgeon to be in regular communication, ideally before endoscopy for a suspected duodenal malignancy. At time of EGD, a tattoo is placed proximal and distal to the lesion. These two tattoos, visible from inside the peritoneum during surgery, guide the lines of transection across the duodenum. It is thus important for the endoscopist to take care to accurately place the tattoos adjacent to where the lesion starts and ends, but not on the lesion or its edges. Ideally, only a small amount of dye is injected. Overinjection of dye can have excessive submucosal spread, making it harder to identify the specific location being tattooed.

As with other neoplasms, multidisciplinary discussion is imperative, preferably during multidisciplinary tumor board conferences. The management of duodenal neoplasms can be complex and may involve chemotherapy or other treatment modalities depending on the diagnosis [18, 19].

Fig. 14.5 Endoscopic ultrasound of the duodenum showing a mass (circled in white). With permission from HJ Asbun

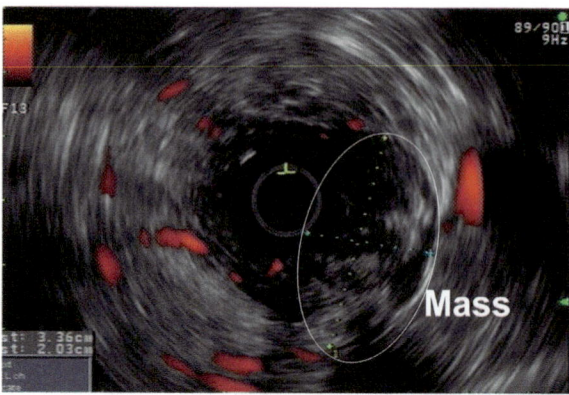

Fig. 14.6 Port placement for segmental duodenectomy. With permission from D Asbun

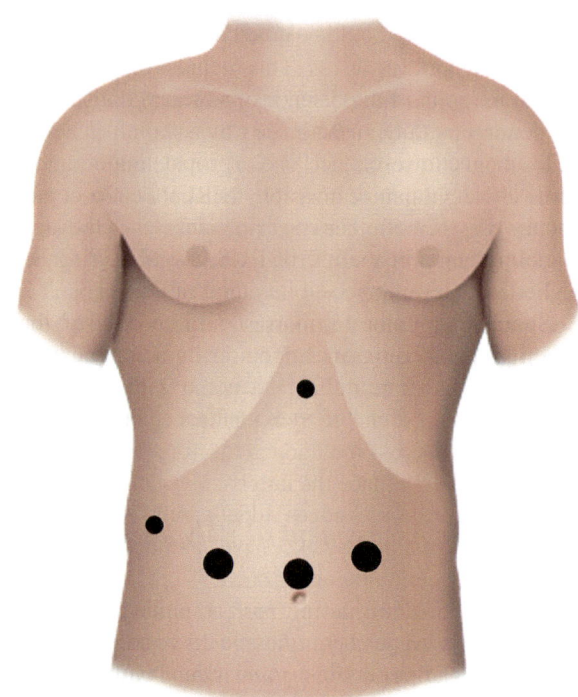

Laparoscopic Segmental Duodenectomy

Patient Positioning and Port Placement

The patient is positioned supine with legs split and arms tucked. Ports are placed as shown in Fig. 14.6, with a total of two 5 mm and three 12 mm ports. The subxiphoid 5 mm port is solely for the surgical assistant. The other ports are positioned to allow for triangulation towards the duodenum with adjustment of surgical instruments and camera depending on what portion of the duodenum is being dissected. Patient positioning and port placement is the same for both PSD and DSD.

Technique: Laparoscopic Proximal Segmental Duodenectomy (Figs 14.7 and 14.8)

Key Steps:

- Enter lesser sac, mobilize colon, expose duodenum (Video 14.1)
- Transect proximal duodenum with pyloric preservation (Video 14.2) (or gastric antrum if pylorus included in resection)
- Limited Kocher maneuver, mobilize proximal duodenum (Video 14.2)
- Dissect within pancreatoduodenal groove (Video 14.3)
- Confirm location of ampulla with IOC (Video 14.4)
- Transect duodenum distally (Video 14.4)
- Duodenojejunostomy (or gastrojejunostomy) (Video 14.5)
- Cholecystectomy

After insufflation and port placement, the gastrocolic ligament is incised and the lesser sac is entered. Dissection proceeds to the right, preserving the gastroepiploic arcade, until the greater omentum is separated from the distal stomach and pylorus. Any adhesions from the omentum to the hepatoduodenal ligament or gallbladder are taken down. The parietal peritoneum lateral to the duodenum is incised and the avascular plane between the transverse mesocolon and retroperitoneum is entered. Dissection along this plane mobilizes the transverse mesocolon inferiorly away

Fig. 14.7 Proximal segmental duodenectomy with pylorus preservation. Gray area represents segment resected. With permission from D Asbun

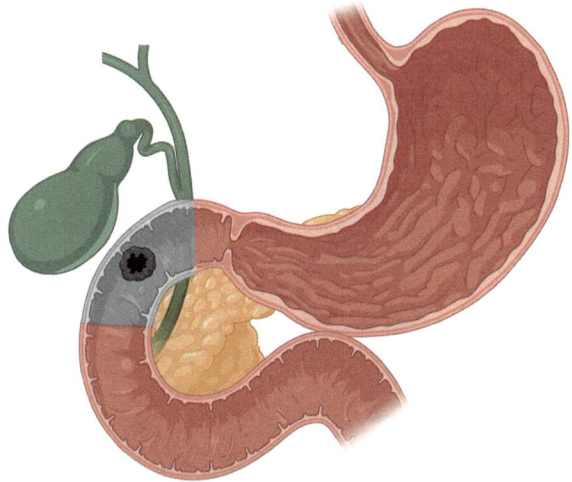

Fig. 14.8 Proximal
segmental duodenectomy
with resection of pylorus
and distal stomach. Gray
area represents segment
resected. With permission
from D Asbun

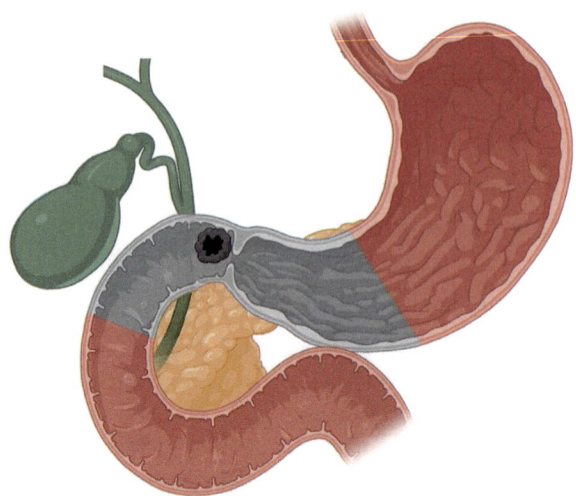

from the duodenum. It can be followed laterally to take down the hepatic flexure and upper ascending colon as needed for adequate exposure of the duodenum.

Adhesions to the posterior aspect of the stomach and pylorus are taken down with a surgical energy device. The gastroepiploic pedicle containing the gastroepiploic vein and artery is identified, isolated, and divided en bloc using a surgical stapler with a vascular load. Skeletonization of the vessels is not necessary. Alternatively, clips can be used. Dissection proceeds distally, mobilizing the proximal duodenum until arriving at the junction between duodenum and pancreas. Care is taken to avoid inadvertently incising the pancreatic capsule or serosa of the duodenum. The superior edge of the pylorus and duodenum are also mobilized by incising the pars flaccida of the gastrohepatic ligament near the pylorus. The course of the gastric arteries along the lesser curve is preserved although the right gastric artery may need to be sacrificed if it reaches the lesser curve too far distally.

The duodenum is divided approximately 2–3 cm distal to the pylorus as long as an adequate margin can be assured proximal to the tattoo (Fig. 14.7). Nasogastric tubes are withdrawn prior to duodenal transection, and perfusion to the proximally divided duodenum is assessed. If the duodenal lesion is too close to the pylorus to allow for transection 2–3 cm beyond the pylorus, the pylorus is sacrificed and the gastric antrum is transected (Fig. 14.8).

A Kocher maneuver is performed to medialize the proximal duodenum. This maneuver is carried out to the extent that allows adequate exposure of the duodenal segment to be resected, and a full Kocher maneuver is often not necessary. The duodenum is reflected medially and the peritoneum adjacent to the duodenum is incised. Dissection continues posteriorly along the avascular plane between the duodenum and the retroperitoneum, while progressive medial traction is applied. Once the segment of duodenum marked with the distal tattoo is free from the retroperitoneum, it is not necessary to further medialize the more distal duodenum.

Strong anterolateral traction is applied to the duodenum. This tension helps expose the plane between the pancreas and the duodenum, entering the pancreato-duodenal groove. Takedown of the anterior connective tissue layer leads the dissection along this connective tissue plane, exposing the fibrovascular attachments between the pancreas and duodenum (Fig. 14.9). Dissection proceeds carefully from proximal to distal, and the duodenum is gradually separated from the pancreatic head. The authors prefer ultrasonic shears during this dissection. Taking very small bites with the use of a hemostatic energy device is essential to control the perforating vessels that traverse this between the pancreas and the duodenum. Dissection is precise to avoid deviation beyond the plane and into the pancreas or duodenum.

The extent of dissection is determined by the location of the distal tattoo and the calculated location of the ampulla. It must proceed beyond the distal tattoo, but without crossing into the periampullary region. As dissection nears the periampullary region, there is often an increase in perforating vessels, signaling the vicinity of the common bile duct.

Once sufficient dissection is achieved, the hepatocystic triangle is dissected to expose the cystic duct, which is clipped and cannulated distally with a cholangiogram catheter. A bowel clamp is then placed across the duodenum at the planned distal transection margin. An IOC is performed with the clamp in place to confirm that the ampulla is not occluded by the bowel clamp. The clamp is replaced by a laparoscopic surgical stapler, assuring the wider stapler is not placed beyond the distal edge of the bowel clamp. The IOC can be repeated with the stapler in place if the surgeon has doubts about the patency of the ampulla (Fig. 14.10). The distal duodenum is stapled and transected.

The specimen is placed in an endoscopic retrieval bag, oriented so as to present one of the stapled edges first. It can usually be extracted by enlarging one of the 12 mm port sites an extra 2–4 cm. If the specimen is larger, it can be extracted through a Pfannenstiel incision. The peritoneum at the extraction site is reapproximated afterwards to allow for re-insufflation, with trocar usually replaced through it.

Fig. 14.9 View of pancreatoduodenal groove during dissection of a proximal duodenal lesion. *D* duodenum, *P* pancreas, *Red arrow* pancreatoduodenal groove. With permission from HJ Asbun

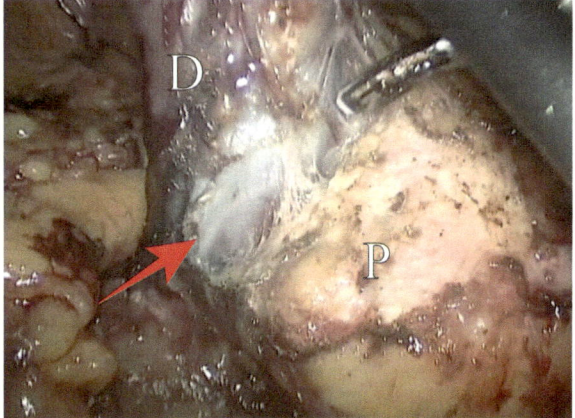

Fig. 14.10 Intraoperative cholangiogram with a surgical stapler clamped across planned duodenal transection line during a proximal segmental duodenectomy. Contrast flows freely through the patent ampulla into the duodenum. With permission from HJ Asbun

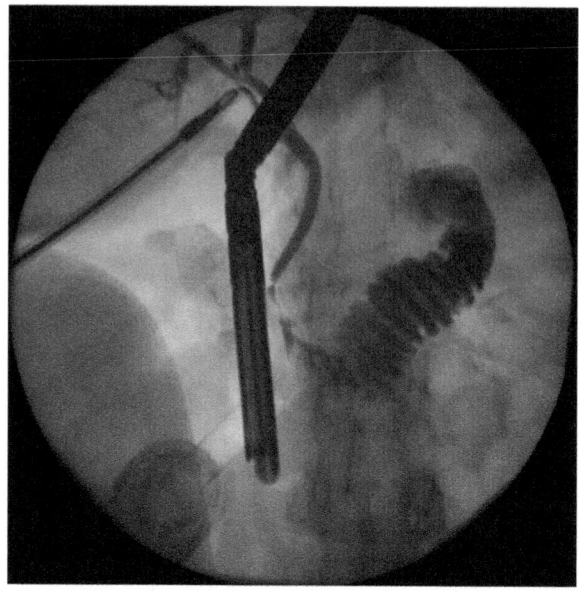

If the pylorus was preserved, a loop of jejunum approximately 30–40 cm distal to the ligament of Treitz is positioned antecolic, and an end-to-side duodenojejunostomy is performed. The pylorus is gently dilated prior to anastomosis. The authors perform a two-layer duodenojejunostomy using absorbable barbed suture for both layers. Small but full-thickness bites are important, including the staple line in the posterior suture line. If the pylorus was sacrificed, a stapled gastrojejunostomy is performed, either in a Roux-en-Y fashion, or Billroth II fashion. A Braun jejunojejunostomy may be added to the Billroth II to decrease the chance of excessive bile reflux into the stomach.

A cholecystectomy is completed following dissection in the hepatocystic triangle started with the IOC. The duodenojejunal (or gastrojejunal) anastomosis is inspected for proper perfusion and closure. Fluorescent angiography can aid in assuring proper perfusion to the anastomosis, and an air leak test can also be performed to further assure anastomotic integrity.

Technique: Laparoscopic Distal Segmental Duodenectomy (Fig. 14.11)

Key Steps:

– Enter lesser sac, mobilize colon, expose duodenum (Video 14.1)
– Wide Kocher maneuver, takedown ligament of Treitz (Video 14.6)
– Pull jejunum into right upper quadrant, transect jejunum (Video 14.7)

Fig. 14.11 Distal segmental duodenectomy. Gray area represents segment resected. With permission from D Asbun

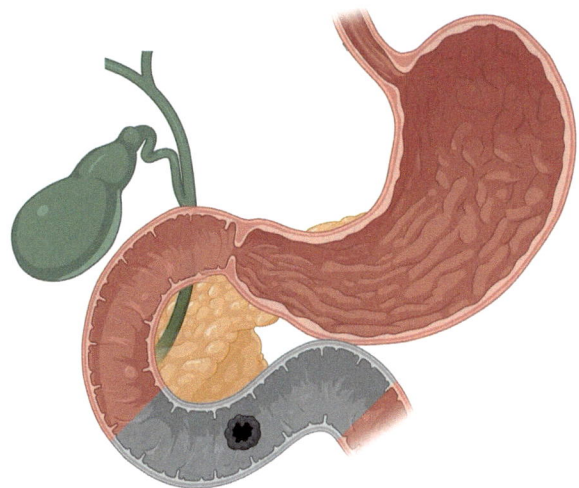

- Dissect within pancreatoduodenal groove (Video 14.8)
- Confirm location of ampulla with IOC (Video 14.9)
- Transect proximal duodenum (Video 14.9)
- Duodenojejunostomy (Video 14.10)
- Cholecystectomy

The lesser sac is entered and the colon mobilized using the same method as for PSD. However, for DSD a full Kocher maneuver is generally performed, with medialization of the duodenum such that the inferior vena cava and insertion of the left renal vein is exposed. Dissection continues distally along an avascular plane between the duodenum and the transverse mesocolon. In this plane, there are adhesions to the antimesenteric side of the duodenum, which is followed close to the duodenum. Deviation away from these antimesenteric adhesions risks injury to duodenal or colonic mesentery. Eventually the duodenojejunal flexure is reached and the ligament of Treitz is taken down from right to left. Both the proximal and distal tattoos should have been identified.

At this point, D4 should be free from its attachments and the duodenojejunal flexure taken down. The proximal jejunum is pulled up into the right upper quadrant. This jejunum is transected beyond the distal tattoo on the duodenum using a surgical stapler. The small bowel mesentery proximal to the staple line is cut with a surgical energy device adjacent to the proximal jejunum/distal duodenum. This continues until the duodenum is found to join with the pancreatic head.

The duodenum is pulled anterolaterally to expose the pancreatoduodenal groove, and the connective tissue plane is entered with ultrasonic shears (Fig. 14.12). Dissection along this plane is performed as described for PSD but from distal to proximal. It is continued proximally until just past the proximal tattoo, but without entering the periampullary area. Careful use of an energy device is important, as perforating vessels from the pancreas to the duodenum will be encountered and

Fig. 14.12 View of
pancreatoduodenal groove
during dissection of a
distal duodenal lesion. *D*
duodenum, *P* pancreas,
Red arrow
pancreatoduodenal groove.
With permission from D
Asbun

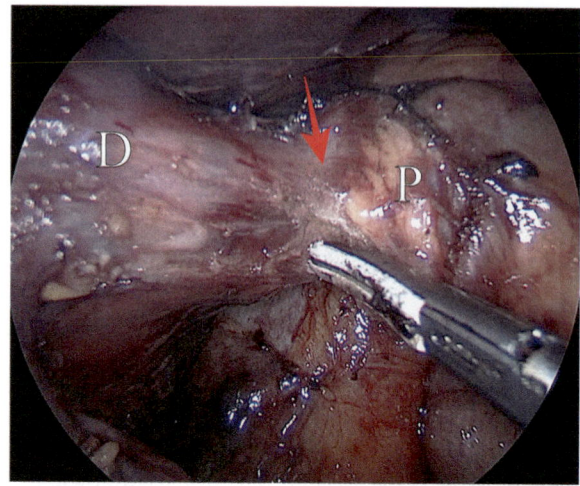

Fig. 14.13 Intraoperative
cholangiogram with a
laparoscopic bowel clamp
across planned duodenal
transection line during a
distal segmental
duodenectomy. Contrast
flows freely through the
patent ampulla into the
duodenum. With
permission from HJ Asbun

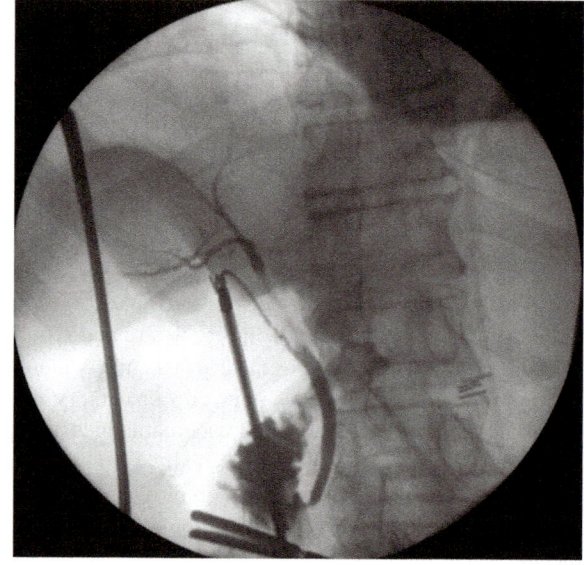

transected. Meticulous dissection ensures the surgeon remains in the pancreatoduodenal groove without deviating into the duodenum or pancreas.

A bowel clamp is placed across the planned transection line and—after identification, clipping, and cannulation of the cystic duct—an IOC is obtained (Fig. 14.13). Free flow of contrast into the duodenum assures the ampulla is not near the bowel clamp and will not be included in the staple line. Less frequently, an EGD can be performed and the ampulla visualized directly. The authors recommend this only for patients in whom IOC cannot be performed, as endoscopic visualization of the ampulla can be challenging, and endoscopy may potentially apply undue traction on the dissected duodenum. After confirming the ampulla is patent, the clamp is replaced with a stapler and the proximal duodenum transected as described for PSD. Specimen extraction likewise is as described above.

Reconstruction is usually performed as a stapled side-to-side duodenojejunostomy. The jejunum is brought up behind the mesenteric vessels to lay adjacent to the remaining duodenum. The antipancreatic side of the duodenum is anastomosed to the antimesenteric side of the jejunum in a side-to-side stapled duodenojejunostomy. Care is taken to avoid leaving a blind loop of stapled duodenum distal to the anastomosis. The common enterotomy is closed in two layers of absorbable suture, or with a transverse firing of a surgical stapler.

A cholecystectomy is completed following dissection in the hepatocystic triangle started with the IOC. The duodenojejunal anastomosis is inspected for proper perfusion and closure. Fluorescent angiography can aid in assuring proper perfusion to the anastomosis, and an air leak test can also be performed to further assure anastomotic integrity.

Robotic Segmental Duodenectomy

Patient Positioning and Port Placement

The patient is positioned supine with legs split and arms tucked. Robotic trocars and assistant ports are placed as shown in Fig. 14.14. Two robotic instrument trocars are in the right hemiabdomen, the camera periumbilical, and one robotic instrument trocar in the left. A 12 mm assistant port is placed roughly between the camera and the left-sided robotic trocar, to aid with passing of sutures, surgical sponges, and surgical staplers (if robotic surgical staplers are not used). Another 5 mm port is placed in the right infracostal region for a self-retaining liver retractor. This setup can be used for both PSD and DSD.

Technique

Abdominal entry/insufflation, inspection, and lysis of any adhesions is started laparoscopically. Once the robotic platform is docked, the technical steps for the robotic-assisted segmental duodenectomy mirror the steps in the laparoscopic PSD and DSD described above.

The primary robotic instruments are generally the robotic monopolar scissors or hook for the right hand, and fenestrated bipolar graspers for the left. Alternatively, robotic harmonic shears can be used in the right hand if available. The secondary left-sided instrument is an atraumatic grasper. During transection of the mesentery, a bipolar vessel-sealing instrument should be used in the right hand.

Fig. 14.14 Trocar placement for robotic segmental duodenectomy. *A* assistant's 12 mm trocar, *C* camera robotic trocar, *L* liver retractor 5 mm trocar, *R1–R3* robotic instrument trocars. With permission from D Asbun

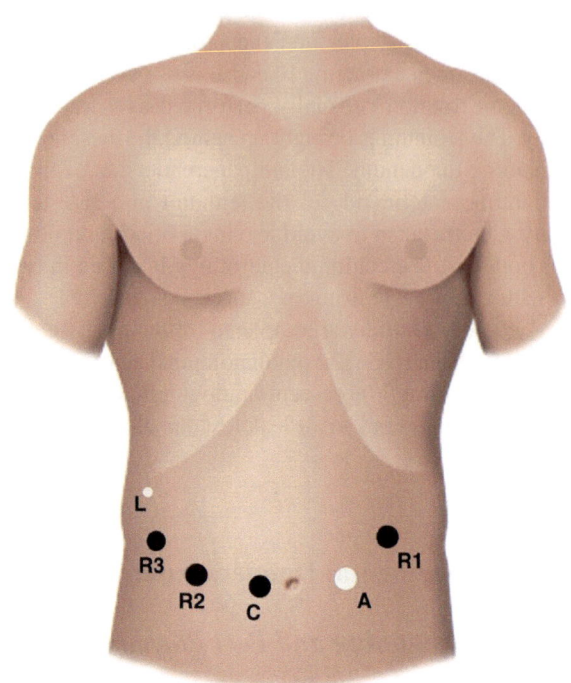

For transection of the duodenum and jejunum, a robotic stapler can be used in either the right or left hand of the surgeon although the left may provide a better angle for transection. Alternatively, the assistant can pass a laparoscopic stapler through the 12 mm assistant port.

Open Segmental Duodenectomy

Patient Positioning

The patient is positioned supine with arms out.

Technique

A midline laparotomy incision is made, with adequate length usually extending from just under the xiphoid to just above the umbilicus. A wound protector is placed around the wound. A self-retaining retractor, such as a Bookwalter retractor, is important for adequate exposure.

The subsequent technical steps follow those described in the laparoscopic PSD and DSD. Bimanual palpation and manipulation of the pancreatoduodenal complex and the bowel facilitates certain aspects of the operation, such as bowel mobilization and exposure. However, the open approach lacks the magnified view from various angles that is possible during a laparoscopic or robotic approach, and meticulous dissection along the correct planes is paramount.

Postoperative Management and Outcomes

Nasoenteric tubes and abdominal drains are not routinely used postoperatively although this is left at the discretion of the surgeon. In cases with difficult dissection in the pancreatoduodenal groove and concerns for pancreatic injury, a closed-suction drain can be left in place.

Usually sips of clear liquids are allowed after surgery, with advancement to liquid diet on postoperative day 1. The patient is not advanced to a soft diet until approximately 5 days after tolerating a liquid diet. Patients are placed on enhanced recovery pathways, which include measures such as minimizing opioid use and early ambulation. If there are concerns over the integrity of the anastomosis (due to difficult dissection, friable tissue, etc.), an upper gastrointestinal X-ray series with water-soluble contrast can be obtained in the early postoperative period before allowing unrestricted access to a clear liquid diet.

Early postoperative complications specific to PSD and DSD include delayed gastric emptying, pancreatitis, anastomotic bleeding, and anastomotic leak. Pancreatic fistulas have been reported but are rare, as dissection should not involve pancreatic parenchymal disruption. Longer term complications include anastomotic stricture, marginal ulceration, and cancer recurrence. Surveillance is dependent on the primary pathology.

Several studies have shown favorable outcomes after segmental duodenectomy for duodenal neoplasms, with PD providing no clear benefit over segmental duodenectomy [20–22]. Although most series are single-center, retrospective reviews, a population-level analysis of the Surveillance, Epidemiology, and End Results (SEER) database supported these findings [7]. It evaluated patients with duodenal adenocarcinoma who underwent resection between 1988 and 2010, comparing those with simple resection (duodenal only) with those who had a radical resection (duodenum and surrounding organs, meant to represent PD). A radical resection was not associated with an improved overall or disease specific survival, even after adjusting for confounding factors. These findings are supported by a more recent systematic review and meta-analysis [9].

Pearls and Pitfalls

- Alternative methods of identifying the duodenal lesion include intraoperative EGD or intraoperative ultrasound. In the author's experience, these may be more prone to error than preoperative endoscopy with tattooing.
- Port positioning, especially in laparoscopic procedures, may need to be adjusted based on body habitus. For example, patients with an obese abdomen may require the ports to be slightly more cephalad. Patients with a smaller abdomen or narrow costal margin may require some ports to be placed more laterally/ inferiorly to allow for adequate space between ports.
- Repositioning the bed as necessary is important to allow gravity to aid in retraction, especially in minimally invasive approaches. The bed is positioned in reverse Trendelenburg position with left side down during early dissection and medialization of the duodenum. The bed is more level during separation of the duodenum from the pancreas, duodenal transection, and reconstruction.
- If the transverse colon protrudes into the surgical field despite adequate mobilization, it can be gently retracted downward for better exposure. This is done with a blunt grasper or a snake-type liver retractor from the epigastrium/left upper quadrant, held by the assistant or by a static retractor secured to the bed.
- Division of the gastroepiploic pedicle in PSD can be challenging in patients with excessive intra-abdominal fat, peri-pyloric adhesions, or omental adhesions to the duodenum/pylorus. Careful takedown of these adhesions and exploiting known anatomic planes is helpful. A finger-type esophageal retractor can be helpful to gently encircle the pedicle from behind and create a window through which a Penrose drain can be placed. This window can be enlarged prior to passing a stapler.
- For transection of the duodenum and jejunum, a stapler with approximately 1.5 mm closed staple height is usually adequate.
- The proximal duodenum in PSD is usually adequately perfused through collateral blood flow coming from the stomach. If there are concerns for ischemia, indocyanine green or other methods of intraoperative assessment of perfusion can be employed.
- Difficulty in taking down the ligament of Treitz from right to left during DSD can be made easier by identifying and taking down the ligament of Treitz from inferior to the transverse mesocolon. Dissection will meet with the prior dissection performed superior to the mesentery.
- In patients who have had a prior cholecystectomy, it is necessary to identify the cystic duct stump to perform the IOC.
- If the duodenal lesion is in the more distal aspect of D4, it may be amenable to an inframesocolic approach. The colon is lifted cephalad, the ligament of Treitz identified and taken down, and the distal duodenum mobilized from caudal to cephalad. Care must be taken to avoid inadvertent injury to the mesenteric vessels, either by traction or dissection. Attempts are made to preserve the inferior mesenteric vein although it may be sacrificed if necessary.

Conclusion

A partial duodenectomy is a feasible procedure for a variety of duodenal lesions. It has good outcomes and spares patients the morbidity associated with more extensive resections. There are inherent technical challenges associated with the procedure. However, with a thorough understanding of anatomy, technical expertise, and good preoperative planning, surgeons can offer their patients the benefits of this operation.

References

1. Bilimoria KY, Bentrem DJ, Wayne JD, Ko CY, Bennett CL, Talamonti MS. Small bowel cancer in the United States: changes in epidemiology, treatment, and survival over the last 20 years. Ann Surg. 2009;249(1):63–71.
2. Hatzaras I, Palesty JA, Abir F, et al. Small-bowel tumors: epidemiologic and clinical characteristics of 1260 cases from the Connecticut tumor registry. Arch Surg. 2007;142(3):229–35.
3. Ochiai Y, Kato M, Kiguchi Y, et al. Current status and challenges of endoscopic treatments for duodenal tumors. Digestion. 2019;99(1):21–6.
4. Onkendi EO, Boostrom SY, Sarr MG, et al. 15-year experience with surgical treatment of duodenal carcinoma: a comparison of periampullary and extra-ampullary duodenal carcinomas. J Gastrointest Surg. 2012;16(4):682–91.
5. Schneider L, Contin P, Fritz S, Strobel O, Büchler MW, Hackert T. Surgical ampullectomy: an underestimated operation in the era of endoscopy. HPB (Oxford). 2016;18(1):65–71.
6. Vega EA, Salehi O, Nicolaescu DC, et al. Laparoscopic pancreatic head preserving total duodenectomy: the parenchymal sparing alternative to a whipple. Ann Surg Oncol. 2021;28(1):131–2.
7. Cloyd JM, Norton JA, Visser BC, Poultsides GA. Does the extent of resection impact survival for duodenal adenocarcinoma? Analysis of 1,611 cases. Ann Surg Oncol. 2015;22(2):573–80.
8. Bakaeen FG, Murr MM, Sarr MG, et al. What prognostic factors are important in duodenal adenocarcinoma? Arch Surg. 2000;135(6):635–41; discussion 641–2.
9. Meijer LL, Alberga AJ, de Bakker JK, et al. Outcomes and treatment options for duodenal adenocarcinoma: a systematic review and meta-analysis. Ann Surg Oncol. 2018;25(9):2681–92.
10. Stauffer JA, Adkisson CD, Riegert-Johnson DL, Goldberg RF, Bowers SP, Asbun HJ. Pancreas-sparing total duodenectomy for ampullary duodenal neoplasms. World J Surg. 2012;36(10):2461–72.
11. Skandalakis JE. Congenital anomalies and variations of the pancreas and pancreatic and extraphepatic bile ducts. The Pancreas. 1998;1:27–59.
12. Kimura W. Surgical anatomy of the pancreas for limited resection. J Hepato-Biliary-Pancreat Surg. 2000;7(5):473–9.
13. Yi SQ, Nagakawa Y, Ren K, et al. The mesopancreas and pancreatic head plexus: morphological, developmental, and clinical perspectives. Surg Radiol Anat. 2020;42(12):1501–8.
14. Mittal PK, Harri P, Nandwana S, et al. Paraduodenal pancreatitis: benign and malignant mimics at MRI. Abdom Radiol (NY). 2017;42(11):2652–74. https://doi.org/10.1007/s00261-017-1238-9.
15. Stolte M, Weiss W, Volkholz H, Rösch W. A special form of segmental pancreatitis: "groove pancreatitis". Hepato-Gastroenterology. 1982;29(5):198–208.
16. Tezuka K, Makino T, Hirai I, Kimura W. Groove pancreatitis. Dig Surg. 2010;27(2):149–52.
17. Rex DK. The appropriate use and techniques of tattooing in the colon. Gastroenterol Hepatol (N Y). 2018;14(5):314–7.

18. Puccini A, Battaglin F, Lenz HJ. Management of advanced small bowel cancer. Curr Treat Options in Oncol. 2018;19(12):69.
19. Ocasio Quinones GA, Khan Suheb MZ, Woolf A. Small bowel cancer. In: StatPearls [Internet]. Treasure Island (FL): StatPearls Publishing; 2022 [cited 2022 Oct 5]. Available from: http://www.ncbi.nlm.nih.gov/books/NBK560725/
20. Stauffer JA, Raimondo M, Woodward TA, Goldberg RF, Bowers SP, Asbun HJ. Laparoscopic partial sleeve duodenectomy (PSD) for nonampullary duodenal neoplasms: avoiding a whipple by separating the duodenum from the pancreatic head. Pancreas. 2013;42(3):461–6.
21. Bartel MJ, Puri R, Brahmbhatt B, et al. Endoscopic and surgical management of nonampullary duodenal neoplasms. Surg Endosc. 2018;32(6):2859–69.
22. Kaklamanos IG, Bathe OF, Franceschi D, Camarda C, Levi J, Livingstone AS. Extent of resection in the management of duodenal adenocarcinoma. Am J Surg. 2000;179(1):37–41.

Chapter 15
Cystic Neoplasms

G. Corvino, G. Perri, R. Salvia, and G. Marchegiani

Abbreviations

EUS   Endoscopic ultrasound
IPMN   Intraductal papillary mucinous neoplasm
MCN   Mucinous cystic neoplasm
SCN   Serous cystic neoplasm
SPT   Solid pseudopapillary tumor

Overview

Despite being defined as rare entities in the past, pancreatic cystic neoplasms (PCNs) are common, with a prevalence of up to 50% of the population and an incidence estimated to be 12%. The risk of developing a PCN increases with age [1]. Most patients are asymptomatic and diagnosed incidentally [2]. Due to the extensive use of cross-sectional imaging, while the early diagnosis is growing, the size of newly diagnosed PCNs is reducing. Therefore, the clinical approach toward PCNs is changing over time, with a relative decrease in surgical resections in favor of the

G. Corvino · R. Salvia
Department of General and Pancreatic Surgery, The Pancreas Institute Verona, University of Verona Hospital Trust, Verona, Italy

G. Marchegiani (✉) · G. Perri
Hepatopancreatobiliary and Liver Transplant Surgery, Department of Surgery, Oncology and Gastroenterology (DiSCOG), University of Padua, Padua, Italy
e-mail: giovanni.marchegiani@unipd.it

enrollment of patients in surveillance protocols, with some critical implications for sustainability and cost to healthcare systems.

According to World Health Organization (WHO) classification [3], PCNs can be sub-classified into benign, precursors, and malignant entities (Table 15.1).

Intraductal Papillary Mucinous Neoplasm (IPMN)

IPMNs are defined as preinvasive, intraepithelial, mucin-producing neoplasms that grow within the ducts of the pancreas, representing around 80% of PCNs [2, 4, 5]. Their typical appearance (at least in the early phases) is secondary to excessive mucin secretion that produces cystic dilatation of the pancreatic ducts [4]. The prevalence and the risk of malignant progression increase with age, while there are no differences by gender or location [6]. Most IPMNs are asymptomatic and in patients defined as "symptomatic," the symptoms are usually nonspecific (bloating, abdominal heaviness, postprandial fullness, and flatulence) and difficult to correlate directly with the disease, at the point of questioning the actual existence of such a correlation. A prospective study did not find any differences in the prevalence of pain in cases of presumed mucinous cystic neoplasm (MCN), serous cystic neoplasm (SCN), or IPMN, compared to the general population [7]. In a minority of patients, specific signs and symptoms directly related to the presence of IPMNs can be found (especially in the presence of a solid component), namely recurrent acute pancreatitis, obstructive jaundice, new-onset or worsening diabetes mellitus, and steatorrhea

Table 15.1 WHO classification, 2019 [3]

Histological classification of pancreatic cystic tumors
Benign and precursors
• Serous cystadenoma
• Serous cystadenocarcinoma
• Glandular intraepithelial neoplasia, low grade
• Glandular intraepithelial neoplasia, high grade
• Intraductal papillary mucinous neoplasm with low-grade dysplasia
• Intraductal papillary mucinous neoplasm with high-grade dysplasia
• Intraductal papillary mucinous neoplasm with an associated invasive carcinoma
• Intraductal tubulopapillary neoplasm (ITPN)
• Intraductal tubulopapillary neoplasm (ITPN) with associated invasive carcinoma
• Intraductal oncocytic papillary neoplasm (IOPN)
• Intraductal oncocytic papillary neoplasm (IOPN) with associated invasive carcinoma
• Mucinous cystic neoplasms with low-grade dysplasia
• Mucinous cystic neoplasms with high-grade dysplasia
• Mucinous cystic neoplasms with associated invasive carcinoma
Malignant
• Acinar cell carcinoma
• Solid pseudopapillary neoplasm
• Pancreatoblastoma

due to endocrine or exocrine insufficiency [7]. However, among these symptoms, only jaundice appears to be an independent predictor of high-grade dysplasia (HGD) or invasive cancer (IC) [8]. Acute pancreatitis symptoms are believed to be due to temporary partial or complete occlusion of the main pancreatic duct with viscid mucin. Persistent occlusion may result in pancreatic insufficiency, presenting with diabetes, steatorrhea, or both [4]. Obstructive jaundice could be present in case of an invasive solid component in the pancreatic head [7, 9].

Two different classifications of IPMNs are described: one is morphological, depending on the relationship with the ductal system, and another one is histological.

According to morphology, IPMNs can be classified as:

- Main duct IMPN (MD-IPMN): It is defined by the presence of segmented or diffuse dilation of the main pancreatic duct (MPD) ≥5 mm in diameter, without any other evident cause of obstruction
- Branch duct IPMN (BD-IPMN): dilatation of a secondary duct ≥5 mm without the involvement of MPD
- Mixed type IPMN (MT-IPMN): both main and branch ducts are involved

Different subtypes bear different risks of malignancy, the lowest being in case of BD-IPMN (6–46%) and the higher in case of MD- or MT-IPMN (60–92%) [10, 11]. However, it must be noticed that these data are extrapolated from surgical series and risk is therefore overestimated due to selection bias. The malignancy risk development during follow-up of BD-IPMN, in a recent systematic review, was indeed as low as 2.7%, with an overall malignancy rate of 3.5% [12].

According to histology [13–15], IPMNs can be further sub-classified depending on:

- The degree of atypia of the epithelial cells: low-grade dysplasia (LGD), HGD, and IC.
- The types of differentiation of epithelial cells are intestinal, gastric, pancreato-biliary, and oncocytic. Furthermore, IC arising from IPMNs is subtyped according to cytological characteristics: ductal/tubular (usually arising from gastric and pancreato-biliary type), colloid/muco-nodular (usually arising from intestinal type), and oncocytic (arising from oncocytic type) [16, 17].

The most frequent BD-IPMNs are of the gastric subtype with LGD and low risk of progression to develop IC, but when this occurs, it is usually of the tubular type, with a similar prognosis to that of pancreatic ductal adenocarcinoma (PDAC). MD-IPMNs, on the other hand, are generally of the intestinal subtype which presents a higher risk of progression to IC but when it occurs, it is often of the colloid type, with a relatively less dismal prognosis. Intraductal oncocytic papillary neoplasm (IOPN) has been recognized by the current WHO classification as rare lesions, distinct from IPMNs [3]. They are more frequent in males and usually involve the MPD. Although IOPNs are associated with invasive carcinoma in up to 30% of cases and high risk for recurrence, even many years after surgical resection, survival outcome is extremely favorable [18, 19]. A positive resection margin was the only independent factor for remnant pancreatic recurrence [20]. Long-term surveillance for IOPN is needed [21]. Different histologic types and distinct invasive components can coexist in the same IPMN; nonetheless, it is important to keep in mind that, if a concomitant PDAC (i.e., a lesion separated from the IPMN by an uninvolved segment of pancreatic parenchyma) is also present, this does not imply that it originates from the IPMN [22]. The rate of the development of concomitant PDAC was found to be 0.8%, ranging from 0% to 7% [23]. The traditional idea of the adenoma-to-carcinoma sequence is not the only accepted model of IPMNs progression [24]. Omori et al. [25] described three different pathways:

- The sequential type, where all driver mutations are shared by PDAC and co-occurring IPMNs
- The branch-off type, where some driver mutations are shared by PDAC and co-occurring IPMNs
- The de novo type, where PDAC has driver mutations not shared with co-occurring IPMNs

This underlines that IPMNs are not per se precursors of adenocarcinoma and that the pancreas of some patients with IPMNs may have an increased risk of developing PDAC ("field cancerization" hypothesis) [22]. The branch-off PDAC subtype had a better prognosis than patients with de novo or the sequential PDAC subtypes [25].

MCN

MCNs are considered either premalignant or already malignant entities. MCN is found almost exclusively in women in the fourth/fifth decade of life and more frequently in the body-tail location [26]. The characteristic location, the prevalence in the female sex, and the ovarian-like stroma invariably present at pathology examination support the hypothesis of a derivation of MCN from the ovarian primordium. MCNs are generally small, unifocal, round cysts and, by definition, without a connection to the pancreatic ductal system. From a clinical point of view, they can be totally asymptomatic. Once they become significantly large, undefined epigastric pain or sense of abdominal fullness is found to be due to compression of adjacent anatomical structures. It is not always possible to distinguish MCNs from other unilocular cystic lesions such as SCN or BD-IPMN, particularly once dealing with a small cyst. The misdiagnosis rate in a recent, large surgical series was as high as 19.2%, and surgery could have been avoided in 8.3% of patients. In older studies where almost all suspected MCNs were submitted to surgery, only 10–12% of resected MCNs harbored either HGD or invasive cancer, questioning the appropriateness of liberal policies in terms of surgical indications [27]. In very recent years, the follow-up of MCN of small size (<3 cm) has been advocated by several centers [28].

SCN

Serous cystadenomas are benign cystic tumors of the pancreas, usually discovered incidentally in 50–70-year-old females (sex ratio 2:1) without preferential location between pancreatic head or body/tail [26]. SCNs are usually sporadic, but they could also develop in the setting of a Von Hippel–Lindau syndrome (VHL syndrome), occurring in 60–80% of VHL patients [29].

Despite some "malignant entities" have been described in previous reports, SCNs are completely benign, as a recent clinicopathological review clarified how cases reported as "malignant" or "invasive" appear to no longer qualify for the recent WHO definition of "malignancy" [30].

As for MCNs, there is a lack of communication with the pancreatic ductal system. Unlike the mucin-producing counterparts, they have no potential to evolve into malignancy, so size becomes crucial in predicting the possible development of symptoms. Because of their growth, patients may present with nonspecific symptoms like abdominal pain, abdominal mass, gastric outlet obstruction, and rarely jaundice [7, 31, 32].

According to the morphology, five SCN subtypes [33] are described:

- Microcystic: thin wall multiple cysts measuring <2 cm separated by fibrous septa oriented toward the center of the lesion. A calcified central scar may be present (15% of cases). Sometimes if small and numerous cysts are present, they can mimic a honeycomb or a sponge.
- Macrocystic: (<10%): coalescing cysts ≥2 cm.
- Mixed (microcystic and macrocystic): a combination of the former patterns.
- Solid: absence of cystic spaces on histopathology, cells arranged in nests, sheets, and trabeculae separated by thick fibrous bands.
- Unilocular: single cyst without septations [33].

The macrocystic and unilocular variants are associated with the highest risk of misdiagnosis, particularly in young individuals and those located in the body tail. In general, in the absence of typical radiological characteristics (central scar and high-signal-intensity microcysts on T2-weighted images on magnetic resonance imaging, MRI), the execution of EUS-FNA is recommended, especially once FNA is performed to define the presence of serum or mucin in the cyst. If a SCN is suspected or confirmed, surgery is indicated only if severe abdominal symptoms related to the tumor (e.g., severe abdominal pain, obstructive jaundice, and gastric outlet obstruction) are present. In asymptomatic patients, cyst size alone is not considered an indication for resection, while during surveillance crossover to surgery may be considered in patients presenting with fast growth, as frequently fast growing SCN represents other misdiagnosed premalignant entities [31].

The European guidelines suggest surveillance discontinuation after 12 months from diagnosis but considering the risk of potential diagnostic mistakes, and the absence of specific guidelines on SCN, surveillance should probably continue with wider intervals (e.g., 24 months) and stopped only in patients unfit for surgery. If radiologically or clinically suspicious features develop during surveillance, follow-up intervals are shortened to 3–6 months [33].

SPT

Solid pseudopapillary tumor (SPT) is defined by the WHO classification [3] as "indolent tumors with low malignant potential," but their etiology remains unknown. They are rare entities, accounting for only 1–2% of all pancreatic tumors and 10–15% of cystic tumors of the pancreas [3]. They are more frequent in young women with a median age of 25–35, without a preferential pancreatic location. Due to its slow growth, SPT often remains asymptomatic. It generally has an expansive rather than infiltrative growth pattern, and when the nearby structures are involved, the most common presenting symptoms are abdominal pain, vomiting, abdominal discomfort, and a palpable mass. Other symptoms could be weight loss and only rarely jaundice. Typically, SPT presents as a mass >5 cm with both solid and cystic components but, in some cases, it can have a wide range of morphologies, from smaller completely solid tumors to larger mostly or completely cystic lesions [34, 35]. Approximately 10–15% of SPTs are metastatic at diagnosis, and the liver is the most common site, followed by lymph nodes and peritoneum. Ductal obstruction is rare and, when present, if associated with a solid mass, makes the differential diagnosis with adenocarcinoma challenging [36–38].

SPTs should always receive aggressive surgical treatment, as an excellent prognosis is achievable also in case of locally advanced, metastatic or recurrent disease, reaching a 5-year disease-free and disease-specific survival of around 98%. Disease recurrence after surgical resection is extremely uncommon, being reported between 3% and 9% and infiltrative growth pattern, invasion of the capsule, and pancreatic parenchyma invasion being the main predictors [34, 38, 39]. In selected cases, due to the young age, a parenchyma-sparing surgery may be considered [38].

Differential Diagnosis of PCNs

General Concepts

To date, the widespread use of diagnostic techniques such as computed tomography (CT) and MRI has greatly increased the prevalence of PCNs. In a study conducted in Germany, 49.1% of participants who underwent magnetic resonance cholangio-pancreatography (MRCP) had the incidental finding of at least one PCN [1]. Nevertheless, the accuracy of radiological imaging in identifying specific PCN subtypes remains low [40]. Therefore, at diagnosis, it is not always possible to discriminate between different types of PCNs or between benign and malignant ones. Salvia et al. reported a rate of incorrect diagnosis in 22% of cases, with rare PCNs such as cystic neuroendocrine tumor (NET) being the most misdiagnosed (46.7%). A high rate of misdiagnosis was also observed for BD-IPMN (28%) and SCN (26.1%). The higher diagnostic accuracy occurred in the case of SPT. Surprisingly, 5% of the cysts were found to be PDAC and 9% of the resected cysts were histologically non-neoplastic. Although resected MD-IPMN had a correct preoperative diagnosis in 94% of cases, 42.2% of misdiagnosed lesions received a preoperative diagnosis of MD- or MT-IPMN and were found to be non-neoplastic cysts on final histological examination [40]. BD-IPMNs have been associated with a high rate of misdiagnosis, with 20% of them having indeed a main pancreatic duct extension (MT-IPMN). A high rate of misdiagnosis has also been found for MCN. Hence, having a comprehensive diagnostic evaluation is critical and diagnostic accuracy should be implemented through the use of endoscopic ultrasound (EUS) +/− fine needle aspiration (FNA) with cystic fluid analysis and contrast-enhanced endoscopic ultrasound (CE-EUS), a real-time EUS evaluation after the peripheral intravenous administration of a US contrast agent, if possible [28]. Cytology might help only when malignant cells are identified. However, no definitive conclusions can be drawn if no malignant cells are directly observed [40].

The Role of Cross-Sectional Imaging (CT, MRI, MRCP)

Among different cross-sectional imaging techniques, MRI/MRCP and CT represent the imaging techniques of choice. CT showed sensitivity and specificity of about 70% and 90%, respectively, for detecting malignant PCNs but the accuracy for a specific diagnosis is still low, ranging from 39% to 44% [41]. Sainani et al. demonstrated an increased accuracy with higher resolution CT and a pancreas-specific protocol [42]. Waters and colleagues suggest that MRI/MRCP is superior in diagnosing and classifying PCNs and the type and extent of IPMN in particular. The real advantage of this technique is the differentiation from other lesions mimicking an IPMN, the evaluation of MPD involvement, and the identification of small branch-duct-type lesions. MRI/MRCP has an accuracy of 40–50% for specific diagnosis but a sensitivity and specificity of around 90% in assessing MPD communication. For this reason, it is considered the first-level technique of choice to study PCNs [41, 43].

The Role of EUS

EUS represents a second-level technique allowing for high-resolution imaging of the pancreas. EUS alone showed low accuracy in distinguishing mucinous from non-mucinous cysts with better performance (accuracy between 40% and 96%)

when histology is used [44, 45]. When it comes to diagnosing the specific subtype of PCN, Giannone et al. reported a misdiagnosis rate of 18.5%. This rate is reduced to 16% when EUS is performed. The accuracy in detecting the specific type of cyst differs between IPMN (96%), SPT (80%), MCN (71%), and SCN (58%). Among diagnostic accuracy, MPD dilatation, enhanced mural nodule, cyst dimension, and cytologic sampling are associated with a higher rate of correct diagnosis [46].

A considerable advantage of this method is the possibility to obtain an FNA for cytology and cystic fluid that can be used for amylase, lipase, carcinoembryonic antigen (CEA), glucose levels, and molecular analysis.

Current diagnostic evaluation of pancreatic lesions can be improved including CE-EUS [44] and contrast-enhanced harmonic EUS (CH-EUS), a real-time EUS evaluation after the peripheral intravenous administration of a US contrast agent performed under a dedicated contrast-harmonic mode, which represents the gold standard in identifying MNs and ensures the best performance for predicting malignancy. In detail, the CH-EUS performance for the characterization of MN has a sensitivity of 97% and a specificity of 90%. Moreover, a negative CH-EUS performed with dedicated contrast-harmonic could rule out malignant lesions with a very low risk of error (2–2.5%) [47]. Cytology can be diagnostic, but FNA is not always performed, and the sensitivity is limited by the scant cellularity. Furthermore, the sample may not represent the entire lesion and no definitive conclusions can be drawn if no malignant cells are observed directly [48–50]. Recently, a systematic review evaluated the diagnostic performance and safety of a novel imaging technique, needle-based confocal laser endomicroscopy (nCLE), that allows for real-time microscopic imaging of the cyst wall, showing a diagnostic accuracy of 99% with a low rate of adverse events [51]. The evaluation of cyst fluid should include CEA, amylase, glucose, and potentially novel biomarkers. Although traditional EUS sampling includes measurement of CEA, low pancreatic cyst fluid glucose is associated with high sensitivity and specificity with significantly improved diagnostic accuracy compared with CEA alone for the diagnosis of mucinous versus non-mucinous pancreatic cystic lesions. The lower level of glucose within the pancreatic cyst may reflect more metabolic activity in mucinous lesions, thus allowing for thresholds of <50 mg/dL to be considered a reasonable cut-off to identify mucinous lesions. Intracystic glucose measurements offer several potential advantages due to availability and very low cost. CEA (using the threshold of 192 mg/dL) is a marker that distinguishes mucinous from non-mucinous cysts, but is unable to distinguish IPMN from MCN and can't identify malignant cysts. Very low CEA levels (<5 ng/mL), instead, are more specific for SCN, pseudocyst, or cystic NET; the main limitation is CEA variations existing among different assays. Amylase is historically used to exclude a pseudocyst if <250 U/L. [52, 53]

Novel Biomarkers

With recent advancements in molecular technologies, investigators are now able to detect variations in DNA, RNA, protein, and small molecules from limited amounts of tissue. Such techniques have recently been introduced in cystic fluid analysis [54].

DNA-Based Biomarkers

KRAS mutations are present in almost every PDAC (90%), being one of the earliest mutations in pancreatic cancer tumorigenesis, and KRAS mutations combined with multiple allelic losses were found to be associated with high specificity in detecting advanced neoplasia within a mucinous PCN [55]. The combination of KRAS and GNAS mutations was detected with good sensitivity and specificity in IPMNs. While IPMNs are in general associated with KRAS, GNAS, and RNF43 mutations, MCNs do not present with GNAS mutations [56]. VHL mutations are typically associated with SCA and SPT which lack all of the above mentioned but show those of CTNNB1 [57].

TP53, PIK3CA, PTEN, CDKN2A, and SMAD4 are typically present in advanced neoplasia within a mucinous PCN [58–60].

Jones et al. showed that molecular studies using appropriate panels of genes could change the diagnosis in 12% of cases [61]. In the same way, Singhi et al. have identified a genetic panel which allowed the diagnosis of mucinous cysts with good sensitivity and specificity [62].

MiRNA

Upregulation and downregulation of miRNA could be the other potential biomarkers for early detection of malignancy. Ryu et al. reported that miR-21 could potentially differentiate mucinous from non-mucinous with good sensitivity and specificity. IPMNs could be associated with the upregulation of miR-155 and miR-21 with the upregulation of both showing a correlation with the degree of dysplasia [63]. Matthei et al. reported a miRNA panel that could differentiate IPMN with HGD from IPMN with LGD with a sensitivity and specificity of 89 and 100%, respectively [64].

Protein-Based Biomarkers

The presence of MUC5AC is associated with mucinous cysts and elevated concentrations of MUC2 and MUC4 to mucinous PCNs with advanced neoplasia [65]. Furthermore, Marker et al. found elevated serum MUC5AC concentrations in patients with mucinous PCNs with advanced neoplasia [66]. Many others protein such as plectin-1, SPINK1, and Das1 could be potential biomarkers [67–69].

Radiologic Features of Specific Subtypes of PCNs

IPMNs

IPMNs radiologically appear as a cystic dilation involving the ductal system. According to this, MD- or BD-IPMNs are defined. In MD-IPMNs, ductal dilation could be present along the entire length of the duct or segmental (Fig. 15.1). BD-IPMNs can present as unilocular or multilocular cystic lesions (cluster shape-like), that appear hyperintense on T2-weighted, separated by thin septa communicating with the MPD; MRCP has the highest accuracy to assess this communication [70]. In MT-IPMNs, both branch and the main ducts are involved (Fig. 15.2).

MCNs

MCNs are usually unilocular or oligo-locular (≤6 cysts), round, cystic lesions with viscous mucinous content that makes the lesion variably hypodense at CT, depending on mucin concentration, and slightly hyperintense on T2-weighted images at MRI. At CT, MCNs show irregular thick walls (>2 mm) and sometimes internal septa that enhance after contrast medium administration and, occasionally, peripheral calcifications "eggshell" (10–25% of cases) [71, 72].

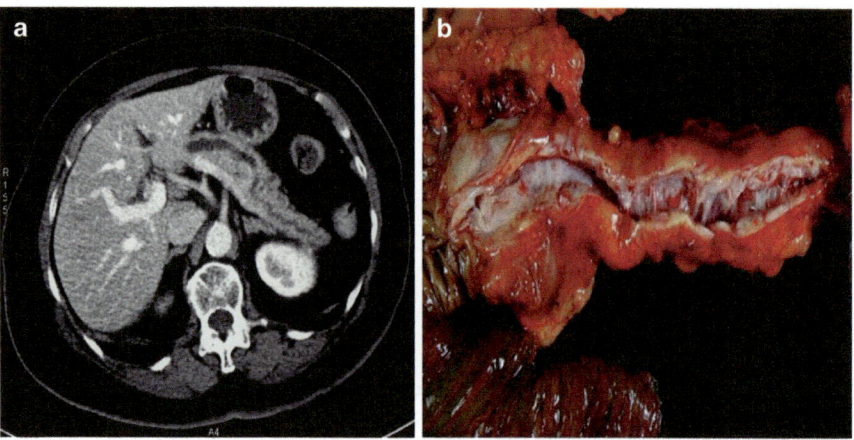

Fig. 15.1 (a) Contrast-enhanced CT of panductal MD-IPMN. (b) Gross Image of panductal MD-IPMN

Fig. 15.2 MRCP showing a MT-IPMN

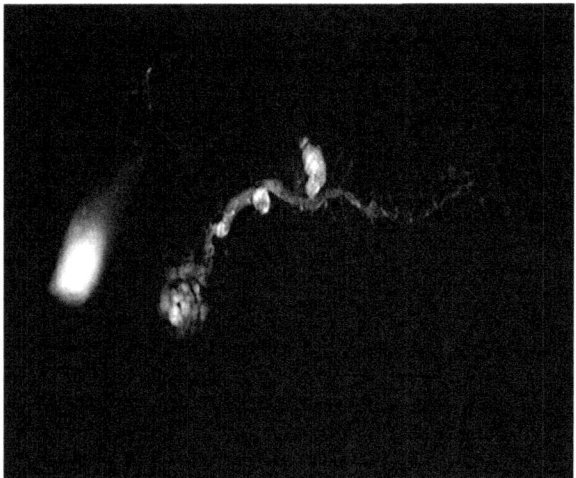

Fig. 15.3 T2-weighted MRI showing a typical SCN with central scar of the pancreatic head

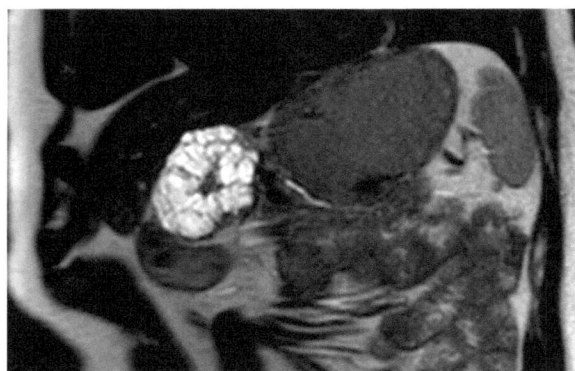

SCNs

Radiological criteria of presumed SCN are central scar and/or high-signal-intensity microcysts on T2-weighted images on MRI without communication with the MPD (Fig. 15.3). The majority of SCNs present as a microcystic variant; a well-demarcated lesion, with plurilocular shapes characterized by the presence of numerous sub-centimeter cysts separated by thin fibrous septa, which usually converge toward a central fibrous scar; this latter may present calcifications. These lesions can be multifocal in VHL patients. After the administration of medium contrast, it is possible to appreciate the vascularization of the septa [33, 73]. In atypical SCN variants (e.g., oligocystic, macrocystic, solid, and unilocular), highly suspicious for other PCNs or pancreatic solid neoplasms, EUS should be considered, and FNA of cyst fluid analysis should be performed at the operator's discretion. When FNA is performed, the results are considered consistent with SCN if cuboidal cells on the specimen and low CEA levels (<5 ng/mL) in the cystic fluid are present [29].

Fig. 15.4 Typical MRI
image of pancreatic
body-tail SPT

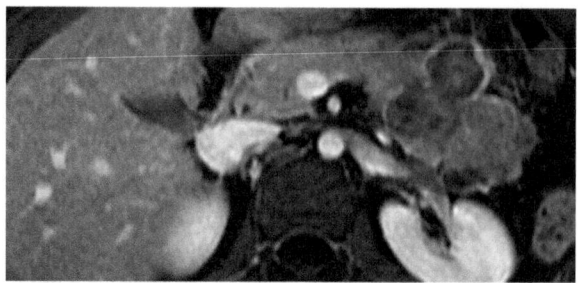

SPTs

SPTs present as large well-encapsulated masses with varying solid and cystic components, and sometimes completely solid or completely cystic masses can be encountered (Fig. 15.4). They could be misdiagnosed as neuroendocrine tumors (NET) but, differently from these, the enhancement of an SPT should be inferior to that of the pancreatic parenchyma. Calcifications and enhancing solid areas may be present at the periphery of the mass [36, 74]. In case of entirely or partially cystic lesions, MRI should be preferred and differential diagnosis with other PCNs should be considered (Table 15.2). Specific for the diagnosis could be the identification of blood products that appear as hyperintense areas on T1-weighted images and homogeneously or inhomogeneously hypointense areas on T2-weighted images [75]. Of note, the absence should not exclude the diagnosis [76].

At CE-EUS, SPT typically shows capsule rim enhancement, with non-enhancing areas inside the lesions [76–78].

The Management of PCNs

Regarding PCNs' decision-making, three guidelines are currently available, namely the International Guidelines of the International Association of Pancreatology (IAP), European evidence-based guidelines (EEC) [79], and American Gastroenterological Association guidelines (AGA).

Although they are not uniform regarding indications for surveillance, there is consistent agreement regarding strong indications for surgery. Obstructive jaundice, enhancing MN ≥5 mm and a MPD size ≥10 mm, the so-called high-risk stigmata (HRS) in the IAP guidelines and "absolute indications" (AI) in EEC, are considered indications for surgery [79, 80].

According to IAP guidelines, patients with "worrisome features" (WF) on imaging [cyst ≥3 cm, enhancing MN <5 mm, thickened enhanced cyst walls, MPD size between 5 and 9 mm, abrupt change in the MPD caliber with distal pancreatic atrophy, lymphadenopathy, an elevated serum level of carbohydrate antigen (CA)19-9, and a rapid rate of cyst growth >5 mm/2 years, pancreatitis] should, instead, be

Table 15.2 Main features of PCNs

	IPMN-MD	IPMN-BD	MCN	SCN	SPT
Age (years)	50–70	50–70	40–50	50–70	25–35
Gender	Equal	Equal	90–95% female	70% female	90% female
Pancreatic location	Equal	Equal	Body tail	Equal	Equal
Radiological findings	Dilated MPD	Dilated side branches	Small, unilocular cyst	Multiple cysts separated by septa oriented toward the center of the lesion	Mass >5 cm with solid and cystic areas
Communication w/main pancreatic duct	Yes	Yes	No	No	No
Cystic fluid markers	Glucose <50 mg/dL, CEA >192 ng/mL, Amylase high	Glucose <50 mg/dL, CEA >192 ng/mL, Amylase high	Glucose <50 mg/dL, CEA >192 ng/mL, Amylase variable	Glucose >50 mg/dL CEA <5 ng/mL, Amylase low	
Novel biomarkers	KRAS+, GNAS+, RNF43+,VHL–	KRAS+, GNAS+, RNF43+,VHL–	KRAS+, GNAS–, RNF43+,VHL–	KRAS–, GNAS–, RNF43–, VHL+	
Reasons for misdiagnosis	May mimic MCN, SCN	May mimic MCN, SCN	Plurilocular lesions mimic SCN	Unilocular lesions mimic MCN; solid lesions mimic PanNET	May mimic PanNET or MCN if completely cystic
Malignant potential	60–92%	6–46%	10.9–12%	Negligible	15%

evaluated by EUS, possibly with Doppler or contrast-enhancement. If EUS confirms a MN ≥5 mm, MPD features suspicious for involvement or it obtains cytology suspicious or positive for malignancy, surgery is indicated if clinically appropriate. If these features are not confirmed at EUS, the patient can undergo surveillance with a schedule adjusted to cyst size [80].

The "relative indications" (RI) considered by EEC have different cut-offs as compared to IAP considering growth rate ≥5 mm/year and cyst diameter ≥40 mm. In these guidelines, symptoms such as new-onset diabetes mellitus or acute pancreatitis are also taken into account [79].

The AGA guideline considers only symptomatic cysts. At least two high-risk features, such as a size ≥3 cm, dilated MPD or the presence of an associated solid component should be examined with EUS-FNA. Patients with both a solid component and a dilated MPD and/or concerning features on EUS-FNA have a clear indication for surgery [81].

MN is the only independent predictor of IC and HGD for all types of IPMNs (except for the prediction of HGD in BD-IPMNs) with a sensitivity and a specificity of 62.2% and 75.1%, respectively. For BD-IPMN, the presence of MNs has the highest prognostic factor power for malignancy, followed by MPD dilatation and thick septum/wall. The risk of malignancy is directly proportional to the size of the mural nodule but further studies are needed to provide a dimensional cut-off [44]. If the arterial phase of MRI doesn't clarify the presence of a MN, it is indicated to perform CH-EUS that ensures the best performance in detecting MN and possibly differentiate them from mucin clots. According to EEC guidelines, the hyperenhancement of a mural nodule, solid mass, or septations on CE-EUS represents features at high risk for malignant transformation of the cyst, and EUS-FNA of the lesion should be considered [82, 83].

Some authors reported high rates of malignancy associated with a MPD dilation between 5 and 9 mm [84, 85]. However, malignancy development was shown to be very rare in presence of MPD dilatation alone, as it was associated with a significantly increased incidence of cancer only when associated with other features [86]. Therefore, a dilated MPD in the absence of other clinical and radiological predictors of malignancy may not be used as the sole reason to select patients with presumed IPMNs for surgery. Moreover, these findings reinforce the concept that once a dilated MPD has been detected, further assessment by EUS is necessary, as MPD can appear dilated for other conditions (e.g., chronic pancreatitis) difficult to assess with cross-sectional imaging alone [46, 86, 87].

Regarding the size of the cystic lesion, the cut-offs proposed by the guidelines (cyst size ≥3 cm for IAP and ≥4 cm for EEC) are chosen arbitrarily as a surgical indication. Pergolini et al. showed that small BD-IPMNs (<1.5 cm) without WFs have a significantly lower risk of malignant degeneration compared to larger cysts [88]. In clinical practice, a greater role should be assigned to the rate of growth rather than the cyst size at a single observation; a growth rate ≥2.5 mm/year is the main predictor of malignancy development in presumed BD-IPMN without WF or HRS [89].

Serum CA19-9 is an independent predictor of malignancy in IPMNs, and a CA19-9 value higher than 37 U/L is associated with an increased risk of invasive carcinoma [90, 91].

Further observational studies are needed to better clarify the natural history of PCNs. In an analysis conducted in the US, only 23% of operated IPMNs contained invasive or HGD at final pathology [92]. Therefore, in a multicentric study [93], the role of dynamic variables associated with malignant disease was explored in estimating the presence of HGD and IC at the final pathological examination. In patients with BD-IPMNs, the development of additional WFs and HRS during surveillance was independently associated with the diagnosis of HGD at the final pathological examination but considering the different WFs, no single WF was found to be significantly associated with the presence of HGD at the final pathological examination. Among HRS, only jaundice was associated with the diagnosis of IC.

In a recent surgical series from Heidelberg, the timeliness of resection based on final histology was classified as too early (adenoma and LGD), timely (intermediate-grade dysplasia and in situ carcinoma), and too late (IC). According to the authors, 30.4% of the patients were operated too early and 34.5% too late. The resection was considered timely in 35.1% of cases, but radiological criteria for malignant conditions in this group were detected only in one-third of patients [94]. The low rate of detectable features specific for HGD and the uncertainty about IPMN's biological behavior make it controversial to consider "too early" and "too late" the resections carried out for LGD or IC. In this regard, IPMNs have been compared to the Schrödinger's cat paradox [95]; unless the observer (surgeon) opens the box (patient's belly), the cat (IPMNs) is both alive (low-grade) and dead (high-grade) at the same time [96].

The specific type of surgery is based according to the cyst's location, and major pancreatic resections with standard lymphadenectomy are the goal standard: pancreatoduodenectomy (PD), distal pancreatectomy (DP), or total pancreatectomy (TP) should be performed, either with an open or minimally invasive approach [97]. TP is indicated in cases of diffuse MPD involvement, multifocal disease in patients with a family history positive for PDAC and persistent HGD at the resection margin. When facing a multifocal IPMN, each lesion should be evaluated for surgical resection as a single entity.

It is very important to highlight the role of the frozen section to drive the extent of the resection when performing a partial pancreatectomy [80, 98, 99]; whereas in case of HGD or IC, further resection up to TP is needed, in case of LGD it should be avoided [80]. The frozen section is important also to identify the presence of a denuded epithelium, associated with a poor diagnostic value of the examination; in this case, the need for further resection should be evaluated carefully [100]. To drive the extension of the resection, the direct visualization of the ductal system with pancreatoscopy can be also considered [101, 102].

When considering surgery, it should be always taken into account that pancreatic surgery is still burdened by high rates of major morbidity (defined as Clavien-Dindo ≥3) and mortality [103]. DP with or without splenectomy is burdened by a major morbidity rate ranging from 14 to 38% and mortality from 0 to 2% [103–105]. To personalize the possible surgical indication toward less aggressive management in the absence of features suggestive of malignancy for presumed IPMNs, the risk of major morbidity and postoperative pancreatic insufficiency can be preoperatively established according to the type of surgical intervention. Among PD/TP, age and body mass index (BMI) defined three different classes for predicting postoperative major morbidity (Clavien–Dindo C3), being greater (ranging from 20 to 36%) for older and overweight patients. Two risk classes of major morbidity, with respective probabilities of 5% and 25%, were identified by the preoperative presence of diabetes for DP patients. In this study, long-term outcomes for PD and DP patients were analyzed; new-onset diabetes and worsening of pre-existing diabetes were experienced, respectively, by 25.6 and 66.7% of patients and age, CACI score, history of diabetes, and DP were associated with an increased risk [28].

The role of chemotherapy in IPMNs is not clear. In the postoperative setting, despite the lack of randomized controlled studies, retrospective series suggest that adjuvant chemotherapy improves survival, but only in invasive IPMNs with nodal disease or tubular differentiation [106].

Regarding MCNs, upfront surgery should be considered for lesions with MNs, enhancing walls or cyst size ≥50 mm. In a large surgical series, HGD or IC was never found in lesions smaller than 5 cm [28]. In the absence of these features, the incidence of overt malignancy is negligible and surveillance can be the first option. Cytology might help only when malignant cells are identified. However, no definitive conclusions can be drawn if no malignant cells are observed directly. Radical resection of noninvasive neoplasms (limited to the ovarian stroma) ensures cure, and the recurrence is rare with 5-year disease-specific survival for MCNs around 100% and 58% for patients with noninvasive and invasive tumors, respectively [107]. The radiologic post-resection surveillance depends on final pathology: benign MCNs, after radical resection, do not require a follow-up as the risk for recurrence is absent, while in cases of MCN associated with IC, patients should receive a follow-up similar to patients with PDAC [108].

Surveillance Options for PCNs

The ultimate goal in the surveillance of PCNs is to identify neoplasms which will eventually evolve into malignancy. The decision to initiate a surveillance protocol should consider not only the cyst's characteristics but also the clinical history, the patient's age and comorbidities, familiarity, and above all the patient's will. To date, numerous studies have shown that surveillance can be safe, particularly when facing BD-IPM without WF or HRS [109–111].

Guidelines

According to the IAP guidelines [80], if there are no WFs or HRS on initial observation, it is advisable to re-evaluate with MRI/MRCP or possibly CT after 3–6 months to rule out abrupt changes in cyst features. As mentioned earlier, a surveillance protocol can be initiated if such features are not confirmed. Thereafter, the surveillance protocol may be performed at longer intervals, depending on the size of the cyst. A shorter interval (3–6 months) should be applied for patients with a family history of hereditary PDAC. On the other hand, the EEC guidelines [79] propose the same management of patients with sporadic IPMN.

The AGA guidelines [81] evaluate only symptomatic PCNs. They advise that patients with pancreatic cysts <3 cm without a solid component and dilated pancreatic duct should undergo MRI for surveillance in 1 year and then every 2 years for a total of 5 years if there is no change in size or characteristics. The same protocol is applied for patients undergoing EUS-FNA and lacking the features mentioned.

According to EEC guidelines [79], a surveillance protocol should be considered if there are no relative indications [MPD dilatation between 5 and 9.9 mm, cystic growth rate >5 mm/year, increased level of serum CA 19-9 (>37 U/mL), symptoms, enhancing mural nodules (<5 mm), and/or a cyst diameter ≥40 mm) or absolute indications [jaundice, the presence of an enhancing mural nodule (≥5 mm) or a solid component, positive cytology, or a MPD measuring ≥10 mm] are present. A 6-month follow-up in the first year and yearly thereafter is considered adequate when no risk factors are present. For patients with relative indications for surgery or the "elderly" affected by severe comorbidity, a 6-month follow-up is recommended.

Surveillance Discontinuation

An urgent issue for healthcare systems is the possibility of surveillance discontinuation in selected patients. The extensive use of MRI and CT of thousands of individuals through repeated scans is becoming relevant for healthcare systems. Furthermore, the psychological burden associated with a surveillance program is of no less importance. Indeed, patients under surveillance for presumed IPMN at low risk of malignancy may present with a "sword of Damocles" effect, presenting subclinical symptoms of somatization, depression, anxiety, sleep disorders, and feeling less healthy than patients undergoing surgery [112].

Both IAP and EEC guidelines [79, 80] advise surveillance indefinitely until the patient remains fit for surgery while the AGA guidelines [81] are the only ones to propose a stop of surveillance if the characteristics of the cyst have not changed after 5 years. Marchegiani et al. have identified in "trivial cysts" the potential targets for follow-up discontinuation; trivial BD-IPMNs are those without WF or HRS at baseline and not developing WF or HRS for at least 5 years from baseline. After 5 years of follow-up, the overall cumulative risk of developing WF/HRS and IC was 4.4% and 1.1%, respectively (similar to that of the general population older than 65 years and postoperative mortality due to pancreatic surgery in high-volume centers). In conclusion, a trivial BD-IPMN in patients aged >65 years might not increase the risk of developing PC compared to the age-matched general population [89]. Pergolini et al., on the contrary, suggest that surveillance should not be interrupted in all BD-IPMNs, even in those under surveillance for over 5 years with a stable lesion, and intensification of follow-up might be required after the first 5 years [88]. As a matter of fact, the debate is still ongoing.

Follow-Up Strategy

The follow-up strategy includes dedicated pancreatic protocol CT and pancreatic MRI/MRCP. Pancreatic MRI/MRCP is more sensitive than CT for identifying communication between the cysts and the pancreatic duct system, and the presence of a mural nodule or internal septations [70]. The use of CT should be considered to detect calcification and to exclude malignancy or concomitant PDAC, vascular or peritoneal involvement, metastatic disease, and suspected postoperative recurrence of PDAC [79]. EUS should be reserved for patients with WF. CH-EUS is not used in all centers but is helpful to better evaluate the vascularization of a mural nodule, solid mass, or septations [47]. Fluid markers such as CEA or Ca 19.9 may help with the diagnosis of invasive cancer.

Follow-Up and Outcome of Resected IPMN

A new IPMN or a concomitant PDAC may appear even 10 years after resection, therefore IAP and AGA guidelines advocate life-long surveillance protocol with different intervals depending on the final histology. In particular, if the final histology of an IC is found, then the follow-up does not differ from that of a PDAC. In the case of MD-IPMN or HGD, the reassessment is on a six-month basis in the first 2 years and then annually. IPMN with LGD dysplasia should be followed up in the same manner of non-resected IPMN.

An analysis of 130 patients who underwent resection of noninvasive IPMNs revealed that the 1-, 5-, and 10-year risks of developing a new IPMN are 4%, 25%, and 62%, respectively [113]. The risk of developing an invasive IPMN at 1-, 5-, and 10 years is 0%, 7%, and 38%, respectively [114].

The Verona Policy

From the author's point of view, several subsequent evaluations of the dynamic changes in time of a pancreatic cystic lesion play a more relevant role in the decision-making rather than taking a single "picture." As a matter of fact, a growth rate ≥ 2.5 mm/year is the main predictor of malignancy development in presumed BD-IPMN without WF or HRS. This reinforces the patient-tailored approach based on radiological features, presence of symptoms, and fitness for surgery in order to avoid upfront surgery in patients that potentially could never develop any HRS or WF. The authors recommend surveillance with an MRI/MRCP associating serological tumor markers testing (CEA and CA 19-9) after a short interval (3–6 months) in the first year. In the absence of any suspicious characteristics, surveillance should be continued initially every 12 months and thereafter up to 18 months. If relevant modifications appear, we recommend CH-EUS to advise the decision between surgical resection and surveillance continuation. If relative contraindications are present at the first observation, CH-EUS with FNB or FNA is recommended as the first step.

In case of presumed MCN, <5 cm in size and without MNs, enhancing walls and Ca19-9 in range, non-operative management is recommended, particularly in young patients.

Conclusions

The prevalence of cystic lesions is sharply increasing, due to the more extensive use of CT and MRI. It is essential for the clinician to differentiate between malignant lesions and the ones that may evolve into malignant forms, from those that are not. There are three different guidelines to refer to, namely IAP, AGA, and EEC, in the management of these complex pathologies. These guidelines are mainly based on surgical series and experts' consensus but represent a great tool for the initial diagnostic framework, indications for surgery, and surveillance protocols. A combined approach with MRI, EUS +/− FNA with possible analysis of the cystic fluid and CE-EUS has allowed for improving the diagnostic accuracy even if the misdiagnosis rate is still high. A future perspective is represented by the execution of molecular analyses. As discussed above, several subsequent evaluations of the dynamic changes in time of a pancreatic cystic lesion play a more relevant role in the decision-making of the management rather than taking a single "picture." The overall major postoperative morbidity and mortality of patients undergoing pancreatic resection for PCNs remain relatively high, similar to that for other indications. For this reason, a tailored approach based on the patient's will, age, frailty, and life expectancy is mandatory. Once the patient is considered unfit for surgery for any reason, no further surveillance is required.

References

1. Kromrey ML, Bülow R, Hübner J, et al. Prospective study on the incidence, prevalence and 5-year pancreatic-related mortality of pancreatic cysts in a population-based study. Gut. 2018;67(1):138–45.
2. Chang YR, Park JK, Jang JY, Kwon W, Yoon JH, Kim SW. Incidental pancreatic cystic neoplasms in an asymptomatic healthy population of 21,745 individuals. Medicine. 2016;95(51):e5535.
3. Nagtegaal ID, Odze RD, Klimstra D, et al. The 2019 WHO classification of tumours of the digestive system. Histopathology. 2020;76(2):182–8.
4. Tanaka M, Kobayashi K, Mizumoto K, Yamaguchi K. Clinical aspects of intraductal papillary mucinous neoplasm of the pancreas. J Gastroenterol. 2005;40(7):669–75.

5. Hruban RH, Takaori K, Klimstra DS, et al. An illustrated consensus on the classification of pancreatic intraepithelial neoplasia and intraductal papillary mucinous neoplasms. Am J Surg Pathol. 2004;28(8):977–87.
6. Oyama H, Tada M, Takagi K, et al. Long-term risk of malignancy in branch-duct intraductal papillary mucinous neoplasms. Gastroenterology. 2020;158(1):226–237.e5.
7. Marchegiani G, Andrianello S, Miatello C, et al. The actual prevalence of symptoms in pancreatic cystic neoplasms: a prospective propensity matched cohort analysis. Dig Surg. 2019;36(6):522–9.
8. Attiyeh MA, Fernández-del Castillo C, al Efishat M, et al. Development and validation of a multi-institutional preoperative nomogram for predicting grade of dysplasia in intraductal papillary mucinous neoplasms (IPMNs) of the pancreas. Ann Surg. 2018;267(1):157–63.
9. Tanaka M. Intraductal papillary mucinous neoplasm of the pancreas. Pancreas. 2004;28(3):282–8.
10. Sahora K, del Castillo CF, Dong F, et al. Not all mixed-type intraductal papillary mucinous neoplasms behave like main-duct lesions: implications of minimal involvement of the main pancreatic duct. Surgery. 2014;156(3):611–21.
11. Lévy P, Jouannaud V, O'Toole D, et al. Natural history of intraductal papillary mucinous tumors of the pancreas: actuarial risk of malignancy. Clin Gastroenterol Hepatol. 2006;4(4):460–8.
12. Balduzzi A, Marchegiani G, Pollini T, et al. Systematic review and meta-analysis of observational studies on BD-IPMNS progression to malignancy. Pancreatology. 2021;21(6):1135–45.
13. Adsay V, Mino-Kenudson M, Furukawa T, et al. Pathologic evaluation and reporting of intraductal papillary mucinous neoplasms of the pancreas and other tumoral intraepithelial neoplasms of pancreatobiliary tract: recommendations of Verona consensus meeting. Ann Surg. 2016;263(1):162–77.
14. Distler M, Kersting S, Niedergethmann M, et al. Pathohistological subtype predicts survival in patients with intraductal papillary mucinous neoplasm (IPMN) of the pancreas. Ann Surg. 2013;258(2):324–30.
15. Furukawa T, Hatori T, Fujita I, et al. Prognostic relevance of morphological types of intraductal papillary mucinous neoplasms of the pancreas. Gut. 2011;60(4):509–16.
16. Salvia R, Burelli A, Perri G, Marchegiani G. State-of-the-art surgical treatment of IPMNs. Langenbeck's Arch Surg. 2021;406(8):2633–42.
17. Basturk O, Tan M, Bhanot U, et al. The oncocytic subtype is genetically distinct from other pancreatic intraductal papillary mucinous neoplasm subtypes. Mod Pathol. 2016;29(9):1058–69.
18. Mino-Kenudson M, Fernández-del Castillo C, Baba Y, et al. Prognosis of invasive intraductal papillary mucinous neoplasm depends on histological and precursor epithelial subtypes. Gut. 2011;60(12):1712–20.
19. Mattiolo P, Hong SM, Paolino G, et al. CD117 is a specific marker of intraductal papillary mucinous neoplasms (IPMN) of the pancreas, oncocytic subtype. Int J Mol Sci. 2020;21(16):5794.
20. Hirono S, Kawai M, Okada K, et al. Long-term surveillance is necessary after operative resection for intraductal papillary mucinous neoplasm of the pancreas. Surgery. 2016;160(2):306–17.
21. Wang YZ, Lu J, Jiang BL, Guo JC. Intraductal oncocytic papillary neoplasm of the pancreas: a systematic review. Pancreatology. 2019;19(6):858–65.
22. Remotti HE, Winner M, Saif MW. Intraductal papillary mucinous neoplasms of the pancreas: clinical surveillance and malignant progression, multifocality and implications of a field-defect. JOP. 2012;13(2):135–8.
23. Kamata K, Kitano M, Kudo M, et al. Value of EUS in early detection of pancreatic ductal adenocarcinomas in patients with intraductal papillary mucinous neoplasms. Endoscopy. 2013;46(01):22–9.

24. Sugiyama M, Suzuki Y. Natural history of IPMN: adenoma-carcinoma sequence in IPMN. In: Pancreatic cancer, cystic neoplasms and endocrine tumors. Oxford, UK: John Wiley & Sons; 2015. p. 225–8.
25. Omori Y, Ono Y, Tanino M, et al. Pathways of progression from intraductal papillary mucinous neoplasm to pancreatic ductal adenocarcinoma based on molecular features. Gastroenterology. 2019;156(3):647–661.e2.
26. Karoumpalis I. Cystic lesions of the pancreas. Ann Gastroenterol. 2016;29(2):155.
27. Crippa S, Salvia R, Warshaw AL, et al. Mucinous cystic neoplasm of the pancreas is not an aggressive entity. Ann Surg. 2008 Apr;247(4):571–9.
28. Marchegiani G, Andrianello S, Crippa S, et al. Actual malignancy risk of either operated or non-operated presumed mucinous cystic neoplasms of the pancreas under surveillance. Br J Surg. 2021;108(9):1097–104.
29. Capelli P, Martini PT, D'Onofrio M, et al. Serous neoplasms. In: Imaging and pathology of pancreatic neoplasms. Milano: Springer Milan; 2015. p. 277–310.
30. Reid MD, Choi HJ, Memis B, et al. Serous neoplasms of the pancreas. Am J Surg Pathol. 2015;39(12):1597–610.
31. Malleo G, Bassi C, Rossini R, et al. Growth pattern of serous cystic neoplasms of the pancreas: observational study with long-term magnetic resonance surveillance and recommendations for treatment. Gut. 2012;61(5):746–51.
32. Khashab MA, Shin EJ, Amateau S, et al. Tumor size and location correlate with behavior of pancreatic serous cystic neoplasms. Am J Gastroenterol. 2011;106(8):1521–6.
33. Marchegiani G, Caravati A, Andrianello S, et al. Serous cystic neoplasms of the pancreas management in the real-world: still operating on a benign entity. Ann Surg. 2022;276(6):e868–75.
34. Law JK, Ahmed A, Singh VK, et al. A systematic review of solid-pseudopapillary neoplasms. Pancreas. 2014;43(3):331–7.
35. Yu P, Cheng X, Du Y, et al. Solid pseudopapillary neoplasms of the pancreas: a 19-year multicenter experience in China. J Gastrointest Surg. 2015;19(8):1433–40.
36. Zamboni GA, Ambrosetti MC, Pecori S, Manfredi R, Capelli P. Solid pseudopapillary neoplasms. In: Imaging and pathology of pancreatic neoplasms. Milano: Springer Milan; 2015. p. 349–72.
37. Kang CM, Kim KS, Sub Choi J, Kim H, Jung Lee W, Ro KB. Solid pseudopapillary tumor of the pancreas suggesting malignant potential. Pancreas. 2006;32(3):276–80.
38. Marchegiani G, Andrianello S, Massignani M, et al. Solid pseudopapillary tumors of the pancreas: specific pathological features predict the likelihood of postoperative recurrence. J Surg Oncol. 2016;114(5):597–601.
39. Kang CM, Choi SH, Kim SC, Lee WJ, Choi DW, Kim SW. Predicting recurrence of pancreatic solid pseudopapillary tumors after surgical resection. Ann Surg. 2014;260(2):348–55.
40. Salvia R, Malleo G, Marchegiani G, et al. Pancreatic resections for cystic neoplasms: from the surgeon's presumption to the pathologist's reality. Surgery. 2012;152(3):S135–42.
41. Jones MJ, Buchanan AS, Neal CP, Dennison AR, Metcalfe MS, Garcea G. Imaging of indeterminate pancreatic cystic lesions: a systematic review. Pancreatology. 2013;13(4):436–42.
42. Sainani NI, Saokar A, Deshpande V, del Castillo CF, Hahn P, Sahani DV. Comparative performance of MDCT and MRI with MR cholangiopancreatography in characterizing small pancreatic cysts. Am J Roentgenol. 2009;193(3):722–31.
43. Waters JA, Schmidt CM, Pinchot JW, et al. CT vs MRCP: optimal classification of IPMN type and extent. J Gastrointest Surg. 2008;12(1):101–9.
44. Marchegiani G, Andrianello S, Borin A, et al. Systematic review, meta-analysis, and a high-volume center experience supporting the new role of mural nodules proposed by the updated 2017 international guidelines on IPMN of the pancreas. Surgery. 2018;163(6):1272–9.
45. Harima H. Differential diagnosis of benign and malignant branch duct intraductal papillary mucinous neoplasm using contrast-enhanced endoscopic ultrasonography. World J Gastroenterol. 2015;21(20):6252.

46. Giannone F, Crippa S, Aleotti F, et al. Improving diagnostic accuracy and appropriate indications for surgery in pancreatic cystic neoplasms: the role of EUS. Gastrointest Endosc. 2022;96(4):648–656.e2.

47. Lisotti A, Napoleon B, Facciorusso A, et al. Contrast-enhanced EUS for the characterization of mural nodules within pancreatic cystic neoplasms: systematic review and meta-analysis. Gastrointest Endosc. 2021;94(5):881–889.e5.

48. Michaels PJ, Brachtel EF, Bounds BC, Brugge WR, Bishop Pitman M. Intraductal papillary mucinous neoplasm of the pancreas. Cancer. 2006;108(3):163–73.

49. Emerson RE, Randolph ML, Cramer HM. Endoscopic ultrasound-guided fine-needle aspiration cytology diagnosis of intraductal papillary mucinous neoplasm of the pancreas is highly predictive of pancreatic neoplasia. Diagn Cytopathol. 2006;34(7):457–62.

50. Belsley NA, Pitman MB, Lauwers GY, Brugge WR, Deshpande V. Serous cystadenoma of the pancreas: limitations and pitfalls of endoscopic ultrasound-guided fine-needle aspiration biopsy. Cancer. 2008;114(2):102–10.

51. Konjeti VR, McCarty TR, Rustagi T. Needle-based confocal laser endomicroscopy (nCLE) for evaluation of pancreatic cystic lesions. J Clin Gastroenterol. 2022;56(1):72–80.

52. Boot C. A review of pancreatic cyst fluid analysis in the differential diagnosis of pancreatic cyst lesions. Ann Clin Biochem. 2014;51(2):151–66.

53. McCarty TR, Garg R, Rustagi T. Pancreatic cyst fluid glucose in differentiating mucinous from nonmucinous pancreatic cysts: a systematic review and meta-analysis. Gastrointest Endosc. 2021;94(4):698–712.e6.

54. Singh H, McGrath K, Singhi AD. Novel biomarkers for pancreatic cysts. Dig Dis Sci. 2017;62(7):1796–807.

55. Bailey P, Chang DK, Nones K, et al. Genomic analyses identify molecular subtypes of pancreatic cancer. Nature. 2016;531(7592):47–52.

56. Wu J, Matthaei H, Maitra A, et al. Recurrent *GNAS* mutations define an unexpected pathway for pancreatic cyst development. Sci Transl Med. 2011;3(92):92ra66.

57. Wu J, Jiao Y, Dal Molin M, et al. Whole-exome sequencing of neoplastic cysts of the pancreas reveals recurrent mutations in components of ubiquitin-dependent pathways. Proc Natl Acad Sci USA. 2011;108(52):21188–93.

58. Biankin AV, Biankin SA, Kench JG, et al. Aberrant p16INK4A and DPC4/Smad4 expression in intraductal papillary mucinous tumours of the pancreas is associated with invasive ductal adenocarcinoma. Gut. 2002;50(6):861–8.

59. Garcia-Carracedo D, Chen ZM, Qiu W, et al. PIK3CA mutations in mucinous cystic neoplasms of the pancreas. Pancreas. 2014;43(2):245–9.

60. Sasaki S, Yamamoto H, Kaneto H, et al. Differential roles of alterations of p53, p16, and SMAD4 expression in the progression of intraductal papillary-mucinous tumors of the pancreas. Oncol Rep. 2003;10(1):21–5.

61. Jones M, Zheng Z, Wang J, et al. Impact of next-generation sequencing on the clinical diagnosis of pancreatic cysts. Gastrointest Endosc. 2016;83(1):140–8.

62. Singhi AD, Zeh HJ, Brand RE, et al. American Gastroenterological Association guidelines are inaccurate in detecting pancreatic cysts with advanced neoplasia: a clinicopathologic study of 225 patients with supporting molecular data. Gastrointest Endosc. 2016;83(6):1107–1117.e2.

63. Ryu JK, Matthaei H, dal Molin M, et al. Elevated microRNA miR-21 levels in pancreatic cyst fluid are predictive of mucinous precursor lesions of ductal adenocarcinoma. Pancreatology. 2011;11(3):343–50.

64. Matthaei H, Wylie D, Lloyd MB, et al. miRNA biomarkers in cyst fluid augment the diagnosis and management of pancreatic cysts. Clin Cancer Res. 2012;18(17):4713–24.

65. Haab BB, Porter A, Yue T, et al. Glycosylation variants of mucins and CEACAMs as candidate biomarkers for the diagnosis of pancreatic cystic neoplasms. Ann Surg. 2010;251(5):937–45.

66. Maker AV, Katabi N, Gonen M, et al. Pancreatic cyst fluid and serum mucin levels predict dysplasia in intraductal papillary mucinous neoplasms of the pancreas. Ann Surg Oncol. 2011;18(1):199–206.

67. Räty S, Sand J, Laukkarinen J, et al. Cyst fluid SPINK1 may help to differentiate benign and potentially malignant cystic pancreatic lesions. Pancreatology. 2013;13(5):530–3.
68. Bausch D, Mino-Kenudson M, Fernández-Del Castillo C, Warshaw AL, Kelly KA, Thayer SP. Plectin-1 is a biomarker of malignant pancreatic intraductal papillary mucinous neoplasms. J Gastrointest Surg. 2009;13(11):1948–54; discussion 1954.
69. Das KK, Xiao H, Geng X, et al. mAb Das-1 is specific for high-risk and malignant intraductal papillary mucinous neoplasm (IPMN). Gut. 2014;63(10):1626–34.
70. Berland LL, Silverman SG, Gore RM, et al. Managing incidental findings on abdominal CT: white paper of the ACR incidental findings committee. J Am Coll Radiol. 2010;7(10):754–73.
71. D'Onofrio M, Capelli P, de Robertis R, et al. Mucinous neoplasms. In: Imaging and pathology of pancreatic neoplasms. Milano: Springer Milan; 2015. p. 311–47.
72. D'Onofrio M, Gallotti A, Pozzi Mucelli R. Imaging techniques in pancreatic tumors. Expert Rev Med Devices. 2010;7(2):257–73.
73. Choi JY, Kim MJ, Lee JY, et al. Typical and atypical manifestations of serous cystadenoma of the pancreas: imaging findings with pathologic correlation. Am J Roentgenol. 2009;193(1):136–42.
74. Choi JY, Kim MJ, Kim JH, et al. Solid Pseudopapillary tumor of the pancreas: typical and atypical manifestations. Am J Roentgenol. 2006;187(2):W178–86.
75. Raman SP, Kawamoto S, Law JK, et al. Institutional experience with solid pseudopapillary neoplasms: focus on computed tomography, magnetic resonance imaging, conventional ultrasound, endoscopic ultrasound, and predictors of aggressive histology. J Comput Assist Tomogr. 2013;37(5):824–33.
76. Yu MH, Lee JY, Kim MA, et al. MR imaging features of small solid pseudopapillary tumors: retrospective differentiation from other small solid pancreatic tumors. Am J Roentgenol. 2010;195(6):1324–32.
77. Yao X, Ji Y, Zeng M, Rao S, Yang B. Solid pseudopapillary tumor of the pancreas. Pancreas. 2010;39(4):486–91.
78. Fan Z, Li Y, Yan K, et al. Application of contrast-enhanced ultrasound in the diagnosis of solid pancreatic lesions—a comparison of conventional ultrasound and contrast-enhanced CT. Eur J Radiol. 2013;82(9):1385–90.
79. European evidence-based guidelines on pancreatic cystic neoplasms. Gut. 2018;67(5):789–804.
80. Tanaka M, Fernández-del Castillo C, Kamisawa T, et al. Revisions of international consensus Fukuoka guidelines for the management of IPMN of the pancreas. Pancreatology. 2017;17(5):738–53.
81. Vege SS, Ziring B, Jain R, et al. American Gastroenterological Association Institute guideline on the diagnosis and management of asymptomatic neoplastic pancreatic cysts. Gastroenterology. 2015;148(4):819–22.
82. Muthusamy VR, Chandrasekhara V, Acosta RD, et al. The role of endoscopy in the diagnosis and treatment of cystic pancreatic neoplasms. Gastrointest Endosc. 2016;84(1):1–9.
83. Khashab MA, Kim K, Lennon AM, et al. Should we do EUS/FNA on patients with pancreatic cysts? The incremental diagnostic yield of EUS over CT/MRI for prediction of cystic neoplasms. Pancreas. 2013;42(4):717–21.
84. del Chiaro M, Beckman R, Ateeb Z, et al. Main duct dilatation is the best predictor of high-grade dysplasia or invasion in intraductal papillary mucinous neoplasms of the pancreas. Ann Surg. 2020;272(6):1118–24.
85. Hackert T, Fritz S, Klauss M, et al. Main-duct intraductal papillary mucinous neoplasm: high cancer risk in duct diameter of 5 to 9 mm. Ann Surg. 2015;262(5):875–80; discussion 880–1.
86. Marchegiani G, Andrianello S, Morbin G, et al. Importance of main pancreatic duct dilatation in IPMN undergoing surveillance. Br J Surg. 2018;105(13):1825–34.
87. Dal Borgo C, Perri G, Borin A, Marchegiani G, Salvia R, Bassi C. The clinical management of main duct intraductal papillary mucinous neoplasm of the pancreas. Dig Surg. 2019;36(2):104–10.

88. Pergolini I, Sahora K, Ferrone CR, et al. Long-term risk of pancreatic malignancy in patients with branch duct intraductal papillary mucinous neoplasm in a referral center. Gastroenterology. 2017;153(5):1284–1294.e1.
89. Marchegiani G, Andrianello S, Pollini T, et al. "Trivial" cysts redefine the risk of cancer in presumed branch-duct intraductal papillary mucinous neoplasms of the pancreas: a potential target for follow-up discontinuation? Am J Gastroenterol. 2019;114(10):1678–84.
90. Kim JR, Jang JY, Kang MJ, et al. Clinical implication of serum carcinoembryonic antigen and carbohydrate antigen 19-9 for the prediction of malignancy in intraductal papillary mucinous neoplasm of pancreas. J Hepatobiliary Pancreat Sci. 2015;22(9):699–707.
91. Wang W, Zhang L, Chen L, et al. Serum carcinoembryonic antigen and carbohydrate antigen 19-9 for prediction of malignancy and invasiveness in intraductal papillary mucinous neoplasms of the pancreas: a meta-analysis. Biomed Rep. 2015;3(1):43–50.
92. El Khoury R, Kabir C, Maker VK, Banulescu M, Wasserman M, Maker AV. What is the incidence of malignancy in resected intraductal papillary mucinous neoplasms? An analysis of over 100 US institutions in a single year. Ann Surg Oncol. 2018;25(6):1746–51.
93. Marchegiani G, Pollini T, Andrianello S, et al. Progression vs cyst stability of branch-duct intraductal papillary mucinous neoplasms after observation and surgery. JAMA Surg. 2021;156(7):654.
94. Tjaden C, Sandini M, Mihaljevic AL, et al. Risk of the watch-and-wait concept in surgical treatment of intraductal papillary mucinous neoplasm. JAMA Surg. 2021;156(9):818.
95. Schrödinger E. Die gegenwärtige Situation in der Quantenmechanik. Naturwissenschaften. 1935;23(48):807–12.
96. Marchegiani G, Perri G, Salvia R. The quantum physics of intraductal papillary mucinous neoplasm of the pancreas. BJS Open. 2022;6(3):zrac082.
97. Pollini T, Andrianello S, Caravati A, et al. The management of intraductal papillary mucinous neoplasms of the pancreas. Minerva Chir. 2019;74(5):414–21.
98. Nara S, Shimada K, Sakamoto Y. Clinical significance of frozen section analysis during resection of intraductal papillary mucinous neoplasm: should a positive pancreatic margin for adenoma or borderline lesion be resected additionally? J Am Coll Surg. 2009 Nov;209(5):614–21.
99. Couvelard A, Sauvanet A, Kianmanesh R, et al. Frozen sectioning of the pancreatic cut surface during resection of intraductal papillary mucinous neoplasms of the pancreas is useful and reliable: a prospective evaluation. Ann Surg. 2005;242(6):774–8, discussion 778–80.
100. Falconi M, Salvia R, Bassi C, Zamboni G, Talamini G, Pederzoli P. Clinicopathological features and treatment of intraductal papillary mucinous tumour of the pancreas. Br J Surg. 2002;88(3):376–81.
101. Arnelo U, Siiki A, Swahn F, et al. Single-operator pancreatoscopy is helpful in the evaluation of suspected intraductal papillary mucinous neoplasms (IPMN). Pancreatology. 2014;14(6):510–4.
102. Nagayoshi Y, Aso T, Ohtsuka T, et al. Peroral pancreatoscopy using the SpyGlass system for the assessment of intraductal papillary mucinous neoplasm of the pancreas. J Hepatobiliary Pancreat Sci. 2014;21(6):410–7.
103. Bassi C, Marchegiani G, Giuliani T, et al. Pancreatoduodenectomy at the Verona pancreas institute: the evolution of indications, surgical techniques, and outcomes. Ann Surg. 2022;276(6):1029–38.
104. Björnsson B, Larsson AL, Hjalmarsson C, Gasslander T, Sandström P. Comparison of the duration of hospital stay after laparoscopic or open distal pancreatectomy: randomized controlled trial. Br J Surg. 2020;107(10):1281–8.
105. de Rooij T, van Hilst J, van Santvoort H, et al. Minimally invasive versus open distal pancreatectomy (LEOPARD). Ann Surg. 2019;269(1):2–9.
106. Marchegiani G, Andrianello S, Dal Borgo C, et al. Adjuvant chemotherapy is associated with improved postoperative survival in specific subtypes of invasive intraductal papillary

mucinous neoplasms (IPMN) of the pancreas: it is time for randomized controlled data. HPB. 2019;21(5):596–603.

107. Pulvirenti A, Marchegiani G, Malleo G, et al. Cystic neoplasm of the pancreas. Indian J Surg. 2015;77(5):387–92.

108. Nilsson LN, Keane MG, Shamali A, et al. Nature and management of pancreatic mucinous cystic neoplasm (MCN): a systematic review of the literature. Pancreatology. 2016;16(6):1028–36.

109. del Chiaro M, Ateeb Z, Hansson MR, et al. Survival analysis and risk for progression of intraductal papillary mucinous neoplasia of the pancreas (IPMN) under surveillance: a single-institution experience. Ann Surg Oncol. 2017;24(4):1120–6.

110. Crippa S, Pezzilli R, Bissolati M, et al. Active surveillance beyond 5 years is required for presumed branch-duct intraductal papillary mucinous neoplasms undergoing non-operative management. Am J Gastroenterol. 2017;112(7):1153–61.

111. Malleo G, Marchegiani G, Borin A, et al. Observational study of the incidence of pancreatic and extrapancreatic malignancies during surveillance of patients with branch-duct intraductal papillary mucinous neoplasm. Ann Surg. 2015;261(5):984–90.

112. Marinelli V, Secchettin E, Andrianello S, et al. Psychological distress in patients under surveillance for intraductal papillary mucinous neoplasms of the pancreas: the "Sword of Damocles" effect calls for an integrated medical and psychological approach a prospective analysis. Pancreatology. 2020;20(3):505–10.

113. He J, Cameron JL, Ahuja N, et al. Is it necessary to follow patients after resection of a benign pancreatic intraductal papillary mucinous neoplasm? J Am Coll Surg. 2013;216(4):657–65; discussion 665–7.

114. Kang MJ, Jang JY, Lee KB, Chang YR, Kwon W, Kim SW. Long-term prospective cohort study of patients undergoing pancreatectomy for intraductal papillary mucinous neoplasm of the pancreas: implications for postoperative surveillance. Ann Surg. 2014;260(2):356–63.

Chapter 16
Pancreatic Ductal Adenocarcinoma

Ricardo J. Bello and Callisia N. Clarke

Introduction

It is estimated that over 62,000 people were diagnosed with pancreatic cancer in the United States in 2022. Pancreatic cancer is now the third leading cause of cancer deaths in the United States [1], rising in the mortality ranks as prognosis improves for other cancers. Similarly, the burden of disease caused by pancreatic cancer has significantly increased worldwide over the past three decades [2]. Most pancreatic cancers arise from the exocrine pancreas and are characterized as pancreatic ductal adenocarcinoma (PDAC). Neuroendocrine tumors of the pancreas, the next most prevalent type of pancreatic cancer, represent about 3% of pancreatic cancers. This chapter focuses on work-up and treatment sequencing for PDAC.

Pathophysiology

PDAC most often originates from pancreatic intraepithelial neoplasia (PanIN) lesions. These premalignant lesions gain genetic alterations in a somewhat uniform pattern to ultimately transform into PDAC. Most PanIN lesions will develop early in the KRAS oncogene, with subsequent acquired mutations in CDKN1A and CDKN2A, while TP53 and SMAD4 tend to occur at later stages of malignant transformation. Fewer PDAC cases arise in the setting of intraductal papillary mucinous neoplasms (IPMN) [2]. This limited subset of premalignant lesions arises from proliferation of mucin-secreting neoplastic epithelium and generally carries favorable prognosis at early stages. IPMN offer an opportunity for prophylactic pancreatic

R. J. Bello · C. N. Clarke (✉)
Division of Surgical Oncology, Medical College of Wisconsin, Milwaukee, WI, USA
e-mail: rbello@mcw.edu; cnclarke@mcw.edu

© The Author(s), under exclusive license to Springer Nature
Switzerland AG 2025
E. P. Ceppa et al. (eds.), *The SAGES Manual of Evolving Techniques in
Pancreatic Surgery*, https://doi.org/10.1007/978-3-031-78409-5_16

resection as determined with clinical and radiological surveillance. However, current risk stratification systems imprecisely estimate IPMN malignant potential, resulting in resource-intensive surveillance and overtreatment for some patients with IPMN [3].

Advances in molecular and genomic analyses have led to multiple classifications of PDAC based on molecular signatures of tumor samples. Of these, the classification system that appears to be most clinically relevant distinguishes between basal-like and classical (i.e., pancreatic progenitor) types of PDAC. The basal-like subset has been linked with worse prognosis and decreased response rates to chemotherapy when compared to the classical subset [2].

Work-Up

Computed tomography (CT) is the most frequently used imaging tool for pancreatic cancer diagnosis and staging. Our institutional CT protocol for pancreatic tumors includes multidetector-row CT imaging with thin sections over the upper abdomen and dual phase contrast (late arterial pancreatic and portovenous phases) providing high-resolution images of the primary tumor and its relation to surrounding vascular structures. It also allows detection of metastatic lesions in the lung, liver, and regional lymph nodes and is therefore critical when determining clinical stage [4–6]. From these images, it is possible to render advanced 3D imaging for additional detail on the primary tumor's relationship with surrounding vessels.

There is >90% correlation between high-quality preoperative pancreas protocol CT and intraoperative findings at high-volume pancreas centers [7–9]. It is therefore critical to obtain high-resolution pancreas protocol CT prior to any invasive procedures (e.g., ERCP) which can obscure tissue planes and limit the ability to accurately stage patients due to bleeding, inflammation, or artifact from biliary stents. Similarly, it is critical to obtain updated imaging after completing neoadjuvant treatment and prior to pancreatectomy.

Tissue Diagnosis

A pancreatic mass that is suspicious for PDAC will prompt tissue biopsy to confirm the diagnosis. This is particularly necessary in patients undergoing a neoadjuvant approach to pancreas cancer treatment. Endoscopic ultrasonography (EUS) with fine needle aspiration (FNA) is the preferred approach to obtain tissue samples for diagnosis. Additionally, EUS provides additional information regarding the relationship between the tumor and its surrounding vessels as well as the extent of disease in the regional nodes [10]. EUS needle biopsy avoids the theoretical risk of intra-peritoneal seeding that is described with percutaneous CT-guided biopsies. Moreover, EUS can be done as part of the same anesthesia event as endoscopic retrograde cholangiopancreatography (ERCP), with the option of stenting the bile duct in the common setting of biliary obstruction, to ensure sustainable biliary drainage. The downside of EUS is that it is operator dependent and therefore requires centers to have experienced endoscopists available for reliable, accurate, and safe tissue diagnosis.

Serum Tumor Markers

Serum carbohydrate antigen (CA19-9) should be obtained in all patients with PDAC after serum bilirubin has normalized and before starting any treatment modality. This sialylated Lewis antigen is the most widely validated biomarker for PDAC, and its trends can be informative in more than 70% of patients. However, serum CA19-9 will be non-informative in up to 30% of patients with PDAC. This is because about 5–10% of the population will be CA19-9 "non-producers" because they lack the enzyme to synthesize any level of the antigen. Roughly 20% of patients with PDAC will be CA19-9 non-responders, because their tumor never produces the antigen above the normal range. In these patients, a low CA19-9 does not add any data to inform management. For this reason, it is important to state that a normal CA19-9 in the setting of clinical or imaging findings suggestive of a pancreatic mass does not preclude pancreatic cancer.

For patients who do produce CA19-9, serial measurements of serum levels throughout receipt of multimodal therapies and during surveillance are helpful for prognostic purposes and to guide treatment decisions. Very elevated levels correlate with higher disease burden, lower potential for R0 resection, lower response to therapy, and worse overall survival [11]. After completing neoadjuvant therapy, normalization or CA19-9 or at least a decrease to half of the pre-treatment level is significantly associated with higher rates of surgical resectability and improved survival outcomes [12]. After pancreatectomy, normalization of CA19-9 is also associated with improved survival outcomes, [13] especially for patients with localized PDAC undergoing neoadjuvant treatment who may harbor micrometastatic disease not evident in CT imaging [14]. Sustained elevations of CA19-9 on the other hand will signal tumor recurrence, many times preceding CT or clinical evidence of recurrence for up to 6 months [13, 15–17]. The second most documented tumor marker for PDAC is carcinoembryonic antigen (CEA). Although levels of this glycoprotein have been traditionally associated with colorectal cancer, it is also elevated in other cancer types, including 30–60% of PDAC cases. In patients with PDAC, CEA has been shown to be an independent predictor of worse overall survival and its addition to CA19-9 is more informative than measuring CA19-9 alone [18].

Staging and Classification

Patients with PDAC are classified into four separate categories based on CT findings: resectable, borderline resectable, locally advanced, and metastatic (Table 16.1). This classification allows patients to be stratified on the probability of achieving an R0 (margin-negative) resection while preserving critical visceral blood flow, and guides decision-making on multimodal treatment sequencing. Naturally, oncologic outcomes are significantly superior when R0 resection is achieved compared to R1 (microscopically positive margin) resection. Overall survival ranges between 11 and 15 months for R1 resection achieved in upfront surgery cohorts, compared to 18–23 months among patients with R0 resection [20–22]. Pancreatectomy achieving only a R2 resection offers no survival benefit over systemic therapy alone, demonstrated by similar overall survival when comparing these patients to those undergoing nonoperative treatment for unresectable locally advanced disease or

Table 16.1 Classification of resectable, borderline resectable, and locally advanced pancreatic cancer as determined by the Multidisciplinary Pancreatic Cancer Working Group at the Medical College of Wisconsin

		Resectable	Borderline resectable	Locally advanced A	Locally advanced B
Tumor–arterial interface	SMA	None	≤180° abutment	>180° but ≤270° encasement	>270°
	CA	None	≤180° abutment	>180° without extension to aorta with possibility for celiac resection with or without reconstruction	>180° encasement with extension to aorta
	HA	None	Short segment abutment or encasement without extension to CA or HA bifurcation	>180° with extension to CA but not HA bifurcation and amenable to reconstruction	>180° encasement with extension beyond HA bifurcation
Tumor–venous interface	PV-SMV	None	Tumor-induced narrowing >50% of the SMV, PV or portal confluence with suitable targets above (PV) and below (SMV) for reconstruction	Occlusion of PV/SMV confluence with no targets for reconstruction	
Likely candidate for surgical resection after neoadjuvant therapy		Yes	Yes	Yes	No

Modified from Tsai et al. [19]
SMA superior mesenteric artery, *CA* celiac artery, *HA* hepatic artery, *PV* portal vein

metastatic disease [20, 22, 23]. There is no role for surgical debulking in pancreatic cancer. Resection should only be attempted with the goal of achieving complete tumor extirpation with regional lymphadenectomy or for specific palliative purposes.

Most patients diagnosed with pancreatic cancer will have evidence of metastatic disease on presentation; another 25% will have locally advanced disease with the primary tumor involving surrounding vascular structures. Only about 20% will have truly resectable disease [24]. A subset of patients with limited involvement of surrounding vascular structures will become operable after responding to neoadjuvant multimodality treatment, allowing pancreatectomy with curative intent and with a high probability of R0 resection. These patients are categorized as borderline resectable and they derive significant oncologic benefit from additional treatment modalities such as cytotoxic chemotherapy and external beam radiation prior to pancreatectomy [25, 26]. The classification between resectable and borderline resectable pancreatic cancer is important as it has significant implications for management and prognosis. When compared with patients with resectable pancreatic cancer, patients with borderline resectable disease carry higher risk of occult metastatic disease. They also usually require complex surgical resections with possible vascular reconstruction and have a higher probability of margin-positive resection. These patients benefit the most from neoadjuvant chemotherapy and chemoradiation, increasing rates of R0 resection by tumor downstaging and margin sterilization, as well as from helping to select and only operate on patients who will benefit from pancreatectomy.

Recent improvements in systemic therapy for PDAC with the use of modified FOLFIRINOX and gemcitabine plus nanoparticle albumin-bound paclitaxel have resulted in improved response rates and survival outcomes across all stages of disease. These chemotherapy regimens can be used in the neoadjuvant setting, significantly increasing the proportion of patients who are eligible for resection [26–28], highlighting the importance of accurate staging and early stratification for resectability.

There is a lower likelihood of a margin-negative resection with increasing tumor-vasculature interface [29]. It is now well established that high rates of R0 resection are achievable with acceptable outcomes with resection of the superior mesenteric vein (SMV), portal vein (PV), or portal confluence when there is venous involvement with PDAC primary tumors [30–32]. This is not true for superior mesenteric artery (SMA) and celiac artery involvement. The reason behind this difference is the potential for tumor extension along the periarterial autonomic neural tissue, which acts as a conduit for the tumor along the involved vessel [33]. Patients with PDAC and arterial involvement will often have microscopically positive arterial margins, even away from gross tumor, unless they undergo neoadjuvant treatment with chemotherapy and/or chemoradiation. Logically, there are lower rates of R0 resection as the tumor-artery interface progresses from abutment of the vessel to encasement.

Distinguishing between borderline resectable and locally advanced PDAC depends on careful examination of the relationship between the tumor and arteries (i.e., SMA, celiac trunk, hepatic arteries) to determine abutment (≤180° tumor contact) or encasement (>180° tumor contact) of these structures. Further attention is focused on the tumor's relationship with the SMV or PV, with specific care to identify a proximal and distal target for any reconstruction required for venous involvement with narrowing or occlusion. At our institution, we define borderline resectable disease as that which is limited to tumor abutment at the SMA or celiac axis, or short segment encasement of the hepatic artery. Tumor-associated narrowing of over 50% of the SMV, PV or portal confluence, or occlusion with suitable proximal and distal targets for vascular reconstruction also represents borderline resectable disease (Table 16.1). Locally advanced disease is defined by either encasement of the SMA, celiac artery or long segment of hepatic artery, or SMV-PV occlusion without an option for venous reconstruction.

Most patients with borderline resectable pancreatic cancer can undergo resection with curative intent if there is careful management of multimodal sequencing of neoadjuvant therapy paired with prehabilitation and good patient selection. Katz et al. [25, 26] reported on 160 consecutive patients with borderline resectable pancreatic cancer treated at a single tertiary cancer center over 7 years. All patients underwent neoadjuvant chemotherapy and/or chemoradiation. Chemotherapy included either single-agent gemcitabine or gemcitabine in combination. Chemoradiation included a radio-sensitizing agent such as 5-fluorouracil (FU), paclitaxel, gemcitabine, or capecitabine alongside external beam radiation (most frequently to 50.4 Gy in 28 fractions). Of these 160 patients, 125 (78%) completed neoadjuvant therapy and 66 (41%) proceeded to pancreatectomy, achieving negative margins for 94% of these patients. Median survival for patients who completed all intended therapy was 40 months, compared to 13 months in patients who did not undergo resection ($p < 0.001$).

Contemporary chemotherapy regimens have increased the rates for surgical resectability in patients with locally advanced PDAC. Chatzizacharias et al. [34] described their experience with 96 consecutive patients with locally advanced PDAC treated at a single high-volume tertiary cancer center over a 9-year period. They divided locally advanced disease into two subtypes based on tumor-vascular anatomy (Table 16.1.) In this cohort, 45 patients (47%) had locally advanced type A disease at time of diagnosis while 51 (53%) had locally advanced type B disease. All patients were treated with neoadjuvant induction chemotherapy (FOLFIRINOX and/or Gemcitabine plus nab-paclitaxel) for a minimum of 4 months followed by chemoradiation. Fifty-six patients were not candidates for resection following neoadjuvant therapy due to progression, no improvement, or development of metastasis. Forty patients (42%) underwent pancreatectomy with 80% achieving R0 resection; 28 of these patients were locally advanced type A accounting for 62% of patients initially evaluated, while only 12 patients (24%) of locally advanced type B patients became candidates for resection. These patients underwent complex resections with a major morbidity of 15% (Clavien-Dindo Grade 3 or greater), median length of stay of 9 days, and no perioperative mortality. Patients with locally advanced pancreas cancer who underwent resection had a median overall survival of 37.5 months compared to 15.8 months in those that were not resected. This study demonstrated that with appropriate patient selection and neoadjuvant multimodality sequencing incorporating contemporary chemotherapy regimens, a subset of locally advanced pancreas cancer patients, traditionally deemed unresectable, may undergo complex resections with high probability of complete resection and associated survival benefit when performed at high-volume centers. For this reason, in order to best identify patients at diagnosis with a reasonable chance of proceeding to surgical resection with a survival benefit, our institution has further divided locally advanced pancreas cancer into two subtypes, type A and B, each with an associated probability for resectability of 62% and 24%, respectively. Locally advanced pancreas cancer type A is considered potentially resectable after extensive neoadjuvant treatment while locally advanced type B is generally deemed unresectable.

Multidisciplinary Decision-Making

At the time of diagnosis, there should be consideration of surgical resection for patients with favorable anatomy and good performance status. Treatment plans and appropriate sequencing should be made as part of a multidisciplinary discussion with input from medical oncology, surgery, diagnostic radiology, radiation oncology, and interventional gastroenterology. The decision to approach a patient with the intent to perform curative pancreatectomy should be determined near diagnosis based on patient factors and cross-sectional imaging.

Even in patients with resectable disease at the time of diagnosis, there are significant advantages of pursuing total neoadjuvant therapy (TNT) as the routine approach for PDAC. First, TNT ensures that all intended therapies are completed prior to undergoing pancreatectomy. This increases the proportion of patients receiving all the necessary modalities for optimal survival outcomes after pancreatectomy for PDAC. It is widely accepted that even in the most experienced hand, only about 50–60% of patients will go on to receive adjuvant chemotherapy after pancreatectomy for PDAC. Second, neoadjuvant therapy will often downstage tumors, increasing the likelihood of a margin-negative resection. Finally, a TNT approach helps to identify patients who will develop early distant metastatic disease or tumor progression despite the best available systemic therapy, and who are then spared of the morbidity of a pancreatectomy that would be unlikely to offer any survival benefit.

There has been rapid uptake in the past decade of neoadjuvant chemotherapy for resectable and borderline resectable PDAC. The shift toward neoadjuvant therapies is founded on improved response rates with chemotherapeutic regimens in the adjuvant settings. We will therefore summarize the evidence for adjuvant chemotherapy and radiation therapy before focusing on neoadjuvant therapies.

Adjuvant Trials

Systemic Chemotherapy

Chemotherapy is a key component of treatment for PDAC since it is mainly a systemic disease. The first drug that was studied for advanced pancreatic cancer was fluorouracil (5-FU). Monotherapy with 5-FU produced negligible response rates and did not offer significant palliative or survival benefit [35, 36]. Burris et al. [37] then studied patients with advanced pancreatic cancer treated with gemcitabine, comparing this to patients treated with 5-FU, both as single therapies in a randomized controlled clinical trial. Patients treated with gemcitabine had higher clinical response rates (23.8%) compared to 5-FU (4.8%, $p = 0.002$). Burris et al. also demonstrated a significant increase in median survival by 1 month for these patients (5.7 months vs. 4.4 months, $p = 0.003$). Although these survival outcomes are much lower than those achieved with contemporary chemotherapy regimens, this promising finding led the way to gemcitabine being approved for PDAC as first-line therapy.

Compared to 5-FU, capecitabine (an oral fluoropyrimidine converted in the gastrointestinal tract into 5-FU) results in higher drug concentration in tumor tissue [38]. Capecitabine as monotherapy has been shown to be more efficacious than 5-FU and to have similar response rates (24%) to gemcitabine [39]. Demonstrating effectiveness of both gemcitabine and capecitabine as single agents for PDAC was a key step before developing combination chemotherapy regimens that would later improve response rates and survival outcomes in patients with advanced PDAC. Newer chemotherapy combinations achieved median overall survival approaching 1 year in the setting of unresectable disease [27].

Conroy et al. studied combination chemotherapy using 5-FU/leucovorin, oxaliplatin, and irinotecan (FOLFIRINOX) in a phase II/III randomized controlled clinical trial involving 342 patients with advanced pancreatic cancer and good performance status. Comparing FOLFIRINOX to single-agent gemcitabine, they demonstrated longer overall survival (11.1 months vs. 6.8 months, $p < 0.001$), longer progression-free survival (6.4 months vs. 3.3 months, $p < 0.001$), and higher response rates (31.6% vs. 9.4%, $p < 0.001$) among patients treated with FOLFIRINOX [27]. This study therefore established FOLFIRINOX as first-line therapy for advanced pancreatic cancer in patients with good performance status who can tolerate treatment. Building on this experience, Conroy et al. conducted a more recent randomized controlled, clinical trial using modified FOLFIRINOX (without bolus fluorouracil to decrease toxicity) among patients with PDAC who underwent pancreatectomy with R0 or R1 resection and no evidence of metastatic disease. The PRODIGE-24 trial reported a median follow-up of 33.6 months and established superiority of modified FOLFIRINOX over gemcitabine with longer disease-free survival (21.6 months vs 12.8 months, $p < 0.001$) and longer overall survival (54.4 months vs 35 months, $p = 0.003$). However, there was a higher incidence of toxicity events for patients on the modified FOLFIRINOX arm, as 75.9% of patients developed grade 3 or 4 adverse effects compared to 52.9% of patients on the gemcitabine arm [40].

The development of nanoparticle albumin-bound (nab)-paclitaxel has significantly changed its efficacy in combination therapy. Nab-paclitaxel was developed to make paclitaxel more soluble. Additionally, murine models show that nab-paclitaxel depletes tumor desmoplastic stroma. Nab-paclitaxel, when used in combination with gemcitabine, triples the tumor tissue drug concentration of gemcitabine [41, 42]. In the Metastatic Pancreatic Adenocarcinoma Clinical Trial (MPACT), 861 patients with advanced PDAC and good performance status were randomized to gemcitabine and nab-paclitaxel or gemcitabine alone. Gemcitabine plus nab-paclitaxel showed improved OS (8.5 months vs. 6.7 months $p < 0.001$), longer progression-free survival (5.5 months vs. 3.7 months, $p < 0.001$), and higher response rates (23% vs. 7%, $p < 0.001$) [28]. Like gemcitabine alone, it appears that the toxicity profile of gemcitabine plus nab-paclitaxel therapy is better than that seen in the FOLFIRINOX study. Gemcitabine plus nab-paclitaxel is now another option for first-line chemotherapy for patients with pancreatic cancer.

Chemoradiation

Locoregional recurrence is common even after R0 resection, occurring in up to 20–60% patients. Chemoradiation was initially employed in the adjuvant setting to address this high risk of locoregional recurrence [43–46]. In a cohort of 531 patients who developed recurrence after pancreatectomy, Groot et al. found that 23.7% of patients developed isolated local recurrence while an additional 18.5% of patients had both local and distant sites of recurrence [47]. Similarly, a secondary analysis of the ESPAC-4 trial by Jones et al. showed that 32% of patients who develop recurrence after pancreatectomy develop local-only recurrence [48]. This group of patients would theoretically stand to benefit from chemoradiation as an additional modality of local control for PDAC. Kalser et al. [49] showed that adjuvant chemoradiation improves survival even after R0 resection with a median survival of 20 months vs. 11 months in the observation arm. This study was underpowered but led to increased adoption of chemoradiation as part of the standard of care after pancreatic cancer resection in the United States [50]. Also in the adjuvant setting, a propensity-score-matched study with 1386 patients showed 33% improved overall survival ($p < 0.001$) with the addition of chemoradiation as compared to resection alone [51]. European studies have not reproduced these results and have instead found mixed survival outcomes with the addition of chemoradiation, ranging from statistically significant but small benefit [52] to reduced survival among patients receiving chemoradiation in the ESPAC-1 trial [53]. This has fueled further debate on the use of adjuvant chemoradiation, and it has therefore not been universally adopted. There is consensus, however, that a subset of resected patients may benefit from chemoradiation if carefully selected for high risk of developing locoregional disease recurrence [54].

Neoadjuvant Trials

Chemotherapy

It is now widely accepted that patients with borderline resectable and locally advanced PDAC who are surgical candidates should undergo neoadjuvant chemotherapy prior to pancreatectomy. Precedence is given to induction chemotherapy for these patients, as many reports have demonstrated an increased proportion of borderline resectable patients that will undergo resection with margin-negative resection and consequent improved outcomes after neoadjuvant chemotherapy. In a series of 18 patients with borderline resectable PDAC by Christians et al. [55], patients underwent preoperative FOLFIRINOX (5-FU, oxaliplatin, irinotecan, and leucovorin) followed by chemoradiation with gemcitabine or capecitabine as radiosensitizing agents. Restaging scans prior to chemoradiation showed that none of these patients progressed while on FOLFIRINOX and 12 (67%) of them proceeded to resection, all achieving R0 resection. Ten (83%) of these patients required portal vein resection and reconstruction. All tumors had more than 50% nonviable tumor on final pathology, and only two (17%) patients had positive nodes. This study did not report on median survival for the pancreatectomy group because it has not been reached yet. With 22 months of median follow-up, however, 7 (58%) patients were still alive, and 5 (42%) patients had no evidence of disease. Median survival for the patients who did not undergo resection due to progression of disease was 12.5 months.

There is more room for debate regarding neoadjuvant chemotherapy for patients with resectable PDAC who would be otherwise eligible for upfront resection. The SWOG trial by Sohal et al. randomized 147 patients with localized PDAC to receive either perioperative modified FOLFIRINOX or perioperative Gemcitabine/nab-Paclitaxel. Of the patients enrolled in the study, 72% underwent resection and 85% had R0 resection, demonstrating the feasibility of this treatment approach [56]. They report an 85% completion rate of neoadjuvant chemotherapy in both arms [56], which is substantially higher than the approximately 54% of patients who complete adjuvant therapies after pancreatectomy [57]. The recently published NORPACT-1 trial was a phase 2, randomized, multicenter clinical trial comparing 4 cycles of neoadjuvant FOLFIRINOX to upfront surgery, both followed by adjuvant chemotherapy. This study showed significantly lower survival at 18 months in the intention-to-treat analysis for patients in the neoadjuvant chemotherapy group (60% vs 73%, $p = 0.032$) despite having significantly higher proportions for R0 resection and N0 disease. Per the trial authors, these results were inconclusive as a phase 2 trial. There were significant challenges in implementing neoadjuvant FOLFIRINOX in the trial, as 40% of patients in the neoadjuvant chemotherapy group did not complete all 4 cycles of therapy. Moreover, the proportion of patients in the neoadjuvant chemotherapy group who received modified FOLFIRINOX as adjuvant treatment was lower than in the upfront surgery group (25% vs 43%) [58]. At the author's institution, we favor neoadjuvant chemotherapy for patients with resectable PDAC as a mechanism to administer systemic treatment prior to pancreatectomy for what is primarily a systemic disease. We believe this approach benefits patients by increasing the proportion of patients who complete all intended therapies, as evidenced in the SWOG trial, as well as by selecting patients who will develop early metastatic disease or recurrence, sparing them from the morbidity of a pancreatectomy that would have been unlikely to benefit them. It is necessary to ensure early surgical involvement in treatment decision-making and close follow-up throughout receipt of neoadjuvant therapies to identify and treat any modifiable treatment toxicities and appropriately obtain restaging scans at regular intervals before pancreatectomy.

Chemoradiation

There is emerging evidence for the role of chemoradiation in the neoadjuvant setting, especially for patients with borderline resectable and locally advanced disease. The objective of chemoradiation for these patients, in addition to neoadjuvant chemotherapy, is to downsize the tumor, increase the potential for R0 resection, and decrease regional lymph node positivity.

Neoadjuvant chemoradiation has been demonstrated in some reports to be associated with improved R0 resection rates as well as improved survival for patients with borderline resectable and locally advanced PDAC [26, 34, 59–61]. Recent studies using FOLFIRINOX and chemoradiation have shown margin-negative rates between 80% and 100% [34, 55]. Neoadjuvant chemoradiation is associated with higher rates of negative regional lymph nodes: 73% with chemoradiation compared to 14% in upfront surgery patients ($p < 0.001$) [59]. Conventional chemoradiation has not been shown to significantly reduce tumor size, but when used in combination with contemporary neoadjuvant chemotherapy, approximately 33% of patients with unresectable, locally advanced pancreatic cancer can be downstaged to resectable [62–64]. The PREOPANC study, which failed to demonstrate any significant benefit from neoadjuvant chemoradiation alone in patients undergoing pancreatectomy and adjuvant gemcitabine, recently published long-term results favoring neoadjuvant chemoradiation. For the 119 patients randomized to neoadjuvant chemotherapy, 5-year overall survival was significantly higher than that with upfront surgery (20.5% vs 6.5%, $p = 0.025$) and this benefit was consistent for both resectable and borderline resectable PDAC [65].

Treatment of PDAC with shorter courses of radiation is possible with stereotactic body radiation therapy (SBRT). SBRT delivers higher doses of radiation in fewer fractions, reducing the total length of treatment which is an attractive option in the neoadjuvant setting. There are statistically comparable results for SBRT and conventional fractionation in terms of outcomes in local control and R0 resection [66–68]. In a study by Rajagopalan et al., 12 patients with either borderline resectable or locally advanced pancreatic cancer received between 24 and 36 Gy of neoadjuvant radiation therapy. This was fractionated in between 1 and 3 doses with a median of 3.3 months before surgery. Notably, 11 of these patients had received induction chemotherapy. They reported that R0 resection was achieved in 11 (92%) patients. Furthermore, 3 patients (25%) had complete pathologic response and 2 (17%) had <10% viable tumor in the specimen. Overall survival was 92% at 1 year and 51% at 3 years. Progression-free survival was a median of 27.4 months [68]. In another study by Chuong et al., 73 patients received 35 Gy to the tumor–vascular interface and 25 Gy to the rest of the tumor over five fractions of radiation therapy. Of these, 32 patients (44%) underwent resection with 97% R0 resection and local control rate of 81%. Median overall survival for this cohort was 19.3 months. However, only 20 of these patients (65%) had negative nodes on pathology, a lower node "sterilization" rate than that reported in conventional radiation cohorts [66]. The recent Alliance A021501 trial by Katz et al. randomized patients with borderline resectable PDAC to receive neoadjuvant modified FOLFIRINOX alone or neoadjuvant modified FOLFIRINOX followed by SBRT or hypofractionated image-guided radiotherapy. At the first interim analysis, the radiation therapy arm was closed early due to lower survival rates compared to the neoadjuvant chemotherapy alone arm [69]. It is unclear whether this lack of effectiveness will change with long-term follow-up like the PREOPANC study or if there is a true lower effectiveness in SBRT for this patient population. Another concern for SBRT is development of delayed complications, such as postoperative wound issues and vascular injury [66, 68]. We look forward to results from current clinical trials to add evidence on ideal fractionation of radiation therapy in the neoadjuvant setting for pancreatic cancer.

Pancreatectomy

After completing all intended neoadjuvant therapy, repeat high-resolution CT imaging with a pancreas protocol and serum biomarkers should be obtained prior to pancreatectomy. This allows for assessment of response, and updated surgical planning particularly as it relates to anticipated need for vascular resection and reconstruction. Outcomes are significantly better at high-volume centers for pancreatic resection, in part due to surgeon expertise and also due to institutional-level ability to rescue patients from serious complications and death after developing complications [70]. Timing is also an important determinant of perioperative risk. Since the median age for new pancreatic cancer patients is 70 years [24], pancreatectomy is most often performed in older adults who are at higher risk for deconditioning with chemotherapy and radiation therapy. This highlights the importance of multidisciplinary management of pancreatic cancer patients including an evaluation for surgical candidacy at each stage of neoadjuvant therapy. This should happen at least at the time of diagnosis, at the end of neoadjuvant chemotherapy and, if applicable, at the end of chemoradiation, making it possible to act on any reversible causes of morbidity which could turn a potentially resectable patient into one that is not a surgical candidate anymore. At our institution, we base decisions on surgical resectability for localized pancreatic cancer at each stage of multimodal neoadjuvant therapy, evaluating maintenance of good performance status, improved or stable findings on CT scan, and normalization or improvement of CA19-9 when informative [71]. There has been a move toward implementing enhanced recovery after surgery (ERAS) protocols at large volume centers including prehabilitation interventions before pancreatectomy to optimize patient nutritional status, physical fitness, and education prior to resection. Guidelines for patients undergoing Whipple procedure are available from the Enhanced Recovery After Surgery (ERAS®) Society and aim at reducing deconditioning preoperatively and decreasing postoperative complications [72]. There has been a positive experience with ERAS protocols for pancreatic resection patients. Implementation of these has been associated with shorter hospital length of stay and decreased postoperative complications without a negative impact on oncologic outcomes [73, 74].

Specifically for patients with borderline resectable pancreatic cancer, there should be special attention to the vascular anatomy and presence of encasement of vessels. This is key to maintaining low morbidity and mortality, as well as good oncologic outcomes. Any unanticipated requirement of vascular resection or reconstruction could result in a major vascular injury and major blood loss. There is high correlation between high-quality preoperative CT scans and intraoperative findings, allowing detailed operative plans to be made in advance, including need for vascular resection and reconstruction. Prior to laparotomy, diagnostic laparoscopy should be performed, especially in patients with borderline resectable PDAC as up to 13% will have occult metastatic disease at the time of the operation [60, 62].

Venous Resection and Reconstruction

There has been increasing experience with resecting and reconstructing the PV and SMV in patients with borderline resectable PDAC and venous involvement. Patients with abutment, encasement, and even occlusion of the PV-SMV confluence may still be eligible for resection if there is adequate inflow and outflow targets for reconstruction. R0 resection is still anticipated in these patients. Resection of tumors invading the PV-SMV confluence must be preceded by careful planning due to substantial variation in the anatomy of first order jejunal and ileal branches, as well as variation in drainage of the inferior mesenteric vein (IMV). In general, if the IMV drains into the splenic vein, the splenic vein can be ligated as the IMV will provide enough drainage into the systemic venous circulation for the spleen. Otherwise, if the IMV drains into the SMV or at the SMV-PV confluence, ligation of the splenic vein without reconstruction can lead to sinistral venous hypertension by relying only on the short gastric veins to drain the spleen. Splenorenal shunting is therefore recommended in these cases [75]. Temporary mesocaval shunts can aid in portal dissection for patients with PV occlusion and facilitate exposure of the SMA and root of the mesentery. These can be used in patients with PV-SMV occlusion and patients with SMA involvement [75, 76].

Arterial Resection and Reconstruction

Initial reports of arterial resection during pancreatectomy had shown high complication rates and poor oncologic outcomes. This was related to suboptimal margins and what are now outdated chemotherapeutic regimens [77]. Improvements in chemotherapy and radiation therapy together with advances in surgical technique have rekindled the discussion on optimal patient selection and treatment sequencing to provide benefit from curative pancreatectomy involving arterial resection.

In a series of patients with arterial involvement from PDAC, Christians et al. reported on ten patients undergoing neoadjuvant therapy following curative pancreatectomy with arterial resection. R0 resection was achieved in 85% of the patients and morbidity was acceptable at 20%. There were no perioperative deaths. At an average follow-up of 21 months, 62% of patients were alive and had no evidence of recurrence. None of the remaining patients had locoregional recurrence but instead developed metastatic disease at a median of 33 months from pancreatectomy [76]. Similarly, subsequent studies with larger patient cohorts from other high-volume centers have demonstrated acceptable outcomes and safety profiles for pancreatectomy with arterial resection following extensive courses of neoadjuvant therapy [60, 62]. These reports all emphasized the importance of defining surgical eligibility at the time of diagnosis and reassessing at several stages throughout administration of neoadjuvant therapy.

One of the challenges in managing patients with borderline resectable PDAC is the assessment of radiological response on the tumor–vessel interface after neoadjuvant therapy and prior to pancreatectomy. Ferrone et al. documented significant discordance between CT imaging and pathology results; patients with adequate serological response in CA19-9 levels after receiving FOLFIRINOX, with or without chemoradiation, would often lack radiological response in the form of separation of the tumor from critical vessels on restaging CT scans. Intraoperative pathology would show fibrosis and no viable tumor, indicating a good tumor response. Therefore, Ferrone et al. suggested exploration even in the absence of radiological response on arterial vascular involvement after neoadjuvant therapy. They advocated for proceeding with resection if there is no viable tumor on intraoperative pathologic assessment and aborting if frozen section is positive for malignancy [62]. We consider it crucial to justify the risks of exploration (i.e., risk of vascular complication, delay in resuming chemotherapy, effect of negative laparotomy on tumor immunology) with a clear intent for curative resection, with anticipated vascular resection if required.

Summary

Treatment sequencing is a key component to enhance outcomes in patients undergoing treatment for PDAC, with increased focus on neoadjuvant therapy prior to pancreatectomy even in patients with resectable disease. Decisions regarding treatment modalities, sequencing, and surgical eligibility should be made in a multidisciplinary setting with input from medical oncology, surgery, radiation oncology, diagnostic radiology and ideally also including interventional gastroenterology. Improvements in surgical technique and multimodal neoadjuvant therapy have expanded the pool of patients with PDAC who can undergo potentially curative pancreatic resection. Given the substantial survival benefit that these patients obtain from resection, one of the main goals of PDAC work-up after diagnosis should be to identify patients who are most likely to undergo surgical resection (resectable, borderline resectable, and locally advanced type A) and facilitate sequencing of multimodal therapy. Oncologic outcomes and perioperative safety are optimized with early surgical decision-making as well as careful follow-up throughout the receipt of neoadjuvant therapies. In many cases, pancreatectomy may require complex vascular resection and reconstruction which should be performed only at high-volume pancreatic surgery centers to minimize morbidity and mortality with these high-risk procedures.

References

1. Cancer stat facts: pancreas. 2020; National Cancer Institute. Available from: https://seer.cancer.gov/statfacts/html/pancreas.html
2. Mizrahi JD, Surana R, Valle JW, Shroff RT. Pancreatic cancer. Lancet. 2020;395(10242):2008–20.
3. Tanaka M. Intraductal papillary mucinous neoplasm of the pancreas as the main focus for early detection of pancreatic adenocarcinoma. Pancreas. 2018;47(5):544–50.
4. Brennan DD, Zamboni GA, Raptopoulos VD, Kruskal JB. Comprehensive preoperative assessment of pancreatic adenocarcinoma with 64-section volumetric CT. Radiographics. 2007;27(6):1653–66.
5. Balachandran A, Bhosale PR, Charnsangavej C, Tamm EP. Imaging of pancreatic neoplasms. Surg Oncol Clin N Am. 2014;23(4):751–88.
6. Lee ES, Lee JM. Imaging diagnosis of pancreatic cancer: a state-of-the-art review. World J Gastroenterol. 2014;20(24):7864–77.
7. Lee JK, Kim AY, Kim PN, Lee MG, Ha HK. Prediction of vascular involvement and resectability by multidetector-row CT versus MR imaging with MR angiography in patients who underwent surgery for resection of pancreatic ductal adenocarcinoma. Eur J Radiol. 2010;73(2):310–6.
8. Lu DS, Reber HA, Krasny RM, Kadell BM, Sayre J. Local staging of pancreatic cancer: criteria for unresectability of major vessels as revealed by pancreatic-phase, thin-section helical CT. AJR Am J Roentgenol. 1997;168(6):1439–43.
9. Tamm EP, Loyer EM, Faria S, et al. Staging of pancreatic cancer with multidetector CT in the setting of preoperative chemoradiation therapy. Abdom Imaging. 2006;31(5):568–74.
10. Brugge WR, Van Dam J. Pancreatic and biliary endoscopy. N Engl J Med. 1999;341(24):1808–16.
11. Ballehaninna UK, Chamberlain RS. The clinical utility of serum CA 19-9 in the diagnosis, prognosis and management of pancreatic adenocarcinoma: an evidence based appraisal. J Gastrointest Oncol. 2012;3(2):105–19.
12. Tsai S, Mahmoud A, George B, et al. Association of decline in serum Ca19-9 after neoadjuvant therapy with improved survival among borderline resectable pancreatic cancer patients. J Clin Oncol. 2013;31(15_suppl):e15082.
13. Tian F, Appert HE, Myles J, Howard JM. Prognostic value of serum CA 19-9 levels in pancreatic adenocarcinoma. Ann Surg. 1992;215(4):350–5.

14. Tsai S, George B, Wittmann D, et al. Importance of normalization of CA19-9 levels following neoadjuvant therapy in patients with localized pancreatic cancer. Ann Surg. 2020;271(4):740–7.
15. Hernandez JM, Cowgill SM, Al-Saadi S, et al. CA 19-9 velocity predicts disease-free survival and overall survival after pancreatectomy of curative intent. J Gastrointest Surg. 2009;13(2):349–53.
16. Hata S, Sakamoto Y, Yamamoto Y, et al. Prognostic impact of postoperative serum CA 19-9 levels in patients with resectable pancreatic cancer. Ann Surg Oncol. 2012;19(2):636–41.
17. Montgomery RC, Hoffman JP, Riley LB, Rogatko A, Ridge JA, Eisenberg BL. Prediction of recurrence and survival by postresection CA 19-9 values in patients with adenocarcinoma of the pancreas. Ann Surg Oncol. 1997;4(7):551–6.
18. Meng Q, Shi S, Liang C, et al. Diagnostic and prognostic value of carcinoembryonic antigen in pancreatic cancer: a systematic review and meta-analysis. Onco Targets Ther. 2017;10:4591–8.
19. Tsai S, Christians KK, Ritch PS, et al. Multimodality therapy in patients with borderline resectable or locally advanced pancreatic cancer: importance of locoregional therapies for a systemic disease. J Oncol Pract. 2016;12(10):915–23.
20. Winter JM, Cameron JL, Campbell KA, et al. 1423 pancreaticoduodenectomies for pancreatic cancer: a single-institution experience. J Gastrointest Surg. 2006;10(9):1199–210; discussion 1210–1.
21. Fatima J, Schnelldorfer T, Barton J, et al. Pancreatoduodenectomy for ductal adenocarcinoma: implications of positive margin on survival. Arch Surg. 2010;145(2):167–72.
22. Neoptolemos JP, Stocken DD, Dunn JA, et al. Influence of resection margins on survival for patients with pancreatic cancer treated by adjuvant chemoradiation and/or chemotherapy in the ESPAC-1 randomized controlled trial. Ann Surg. 2001;234(6):758–68.
23. Bilimoria KY, Talamonti MS, Sener SF, et al. Effect of hospital volume on margin status after pancreaticoduodenectomy for cancer. J Am Coll Surg. 2008;207(4):510–9.
24. Noone AM, Howlader N, Krapcho M, et al., editors. SEER cancer statistics review, 1975–2015. Bethesda, MD: National Cancer Institute; 2018 [cited 2018 May 2]. Available from: https://seer.cancer.gov/csr/1975_2015/, based on November 2017 SEER data submission, posted to the SEER web site.
25. Varadhachary GR, Tamm EP, Crane C, Evans DB, Wolff RA. Borderline resectable pancreatic cancer. Curr Treat Options Gastroenterol. 2005;8(5):377–84.
26. Katz MH, Pisters PW, Evans DB, et al. Borderline resectable pancreatic cancer: the importance of this emerging stage of disease. J Am Coll Surg. 2008;206(5):833–46; discussion 846–8.
27. Conroy T, Desseigne F, Ychou M, et al. FOLFIRINOX versus gemcitabine for metastatic pancreatic cancer. N Engl J Med. 2011;364(19):1817–25.
28. Von Hoff DD, Ervin T, Arena FP, et al. Increased survival in pancreatic cancer with nab-paclitaxel plus gemcitabine. N Engl J Med. 2013;369(18):1691–703.
29. Katz MH, Marsh R, Herman JM, et al. Borderline resectable pancreatic cancer: need for standardization and methods for optimal clinical trial design. Ann Surg Oncol. 2013;20(8):2787–95.
30. Tran Cao HS, Balachandran A, Wang H, et al. Radiographic tumor-vein interface as a predictor of intraoperative, pathologic, and oncologic outcomes in resectable and borderline resectable pancreatic cancer. J Gastrointest Surg. 2014;18(2):269–78; discussion 278.
31. Leach SD, Lee JE, Charnsangavej C, et al. Survival following pancreaticoduodenectomy with resection of the superior mesenteric-portal vein confluence for adenocarcinoma of the pancreatic head. Br J Surg. 1998;85(5):611–7.
32. Tseng JF, Raut CP, Lee JE, et al. Pancreaticoduodenectomy with vascular resection: margin status and survival duration. J Gastrointest Surg. 2004;8(8):935–49; discussion 949–50.
33. Nagakawa T, Kayahara M, Ohta T, Ueno K, Konishi I, Miyazaki I. Patterns of neural and plexus invasion of human pancreatic cancer and experimental cancer. Int J Pancreatol. 1991;10(2):113–9.
34. Kharofa J, Tsai S, Kelly T, et al. Neoadjuvant chemoradiation with IMRT in resectable and borderline resectable pancreatic cancer. Radiother Oncol. 2014;113(1):41–6.

35. DeCaprio JA, Mayer RJ, Gonin R, Arbuck SG. Fluorouracil and high-dose leucovorin in previously untreated patients with advanced adenocarcinoma of the pancreas: results of a phase II trial. J Clin Oncol. 1991;9(12):2128–33.
36. Van Rijswijk RE, Jeziorski K, Wagener DJ, et al. Weekly high-dose 5-fluorouracil and folinic acid in metastatic pancreatic carcinoma: a phase II study of the EORTC GastroIntestinal Tract Cancer Cooperative Group. Eur J Cancer. 2004;40(14):2077–81.
37. Burris HA 3rd, Moore MJ, Andersen J, et al. Improvements in survival and clinical benefit with gemcitabine as first-line therapy for patients with advanced pancreas cancer: a randomized trial. J Clin Oncol. 1997;15(6):2403–13.
38. Schüller J, Cassidy J, Dumont E, et al. Preferential activation of capecitabine in tumor following oral administration to colorectal cancer patients. Cancer Chemother Pharmacol. 2000;45(4):291–7.
39. Cartwright TH, Cohn A, Varkey JA, et al. Phase II study of oral capecitabine in patients with advanced or metastatic pancreatic cancer. J Clin Oncol. 2002;20(1):160–4.
40. Conroy T, Hammel P, Hebbar M, et al. FOLFIRINOX or gemcitabine as adjuvant therapy for pancreatic cancer. N Engl J Med. 2018;379(25):2395–406.
41. Von Hoff DD, Ramanathan RK, Borad MJ, et al. Gemcitabine plus nab-paclitaxel is an active regimen in patients with advanced pancreatic cancer: a phase I/II trial. J Clin Oncol. 2011;29(34):4548–54.
42. Frese KK, Neesse A, Cook N, et al. Nab-paclitaxel potentiates gemcitabine activity by reducing cytidine deaminase levels in a mouse model of pancreatic cancer. Cancer Discov. 2012;2(3):260–9.
43. Khawaja MR, Kleyman S, Yu Z, et al. Adjuvant gemcitabine and gemcitabine-based chemoradiotherapy versus gemcitabine alone after pancreatic cancer resection: the Indiana University experience. Am J Clin Oncol. 2017;40(1):42–6.
44. Sohn TA, Yeo CJ, Cameron JL, et al. Resected adenocarcinoma of the pancreas-616 patients: results, outcomes, and prognostic indicators. J Gastrointest Surg. 2000;4(6):567–79.
45. Hishinuma S, Ogata Y, Tomikawa M, Ozawa I, Hirabayashi K, Igarashi S. Patterns of recurrence after curative resection of pancreatic cancer, based on autopsy findings. J Gastrointest Surg. 2006;10(4):511–8.
46. Smeenk HG, van Eijck CH, Hop WC, et al. Long-term survival and metastatic pattern of pancreatic and periampullary cancer after adjuvant chemoradiation or observation: long-term results of EORTC trial 40891. Ann Surg. 2007;246(5):734–40.
47. Groot VP, Rezaee N, Wu W, et al. Patterns, timing, and predictors of recurrence following pancreatectomy for pancreatic ductal adenocarcinoma. Ann Surg. 2018;267(5):936–45.
48. Jones RP, Psarelli EE, Jackson R, et al. Patterns of recurrence after resection of pancreatic ductal adenocarcinoma: a secondary analysis of the ESPAC-4 randomized adjuvant chemotherapy trial. JAMA Surg. 2019;154(11):1038–48. https://doi.org/10.1001/jamasurg.2019.3337.
49. Kalser MH, Ellenberg SS. Pancreatic cancer. Adjuvant combined radiation and chemotherapy following curative resection. Arch Surg. 1985;120(8):899–903.
50. Douglass H, Nava H, Panahon A, et al. Further evidence of effective adjuvant combined radiation and chemotherapy following curative resection of pancreatic cancer. Gastrointestinal Tumor Study Group. Cancer. 1987;59(12):2006–10.
51. Hsu CC, Herman JM, Corsini MM, et al. Adjuvant chemoradiation for pancreatic adenocarcinoma: the Johns Hopkins Hospital-Mayo Clinic collaborative study. Ann Surg Oncol. 2010;17(4):981–90.
52. Klinkenbijl JH, Jeekel J, Sahmoud T, et al. Adjuvant radiotherapy and 5-fluorouracil after curative resection of cancer of the pancreas and periampullary region: phase III trial of the EORTC gastrointestinal tract cancer cooperative group. Ann Surg. 1999;230(6):776–82; discussion 782–4.
53. Neoptolemos JP, Stocken DD, Friess H, et al. A randomized trial of chemoradiotherapy and chemotherapy after resection of pancreatic cancer. N Engl J Med. 2004;350(12):1200–10.
54. Abrams RA, Lowy AM, O'Reilly EM, Wolff RA, Picozzi VJ, Pisters PW. Combined modality treatment of resectable and borderline resectable pancreas cancer: expert consensus statement. Ann Surg Oncol. 2009;16(7):1751–6.

55. Christians KK, Tsai S, Mahmoud A, et al. Neoadjuvant FOLFIRINOX for borderline resectable pancreas cancer: a new treatment paradigm? Oncologist. 2014;19(3):266–74.
56. Sohal DPS, Duong M, Ahmad SA, et al. Efficacy of perioperative chemotherapy for Resectable pancreatic adenocarcinoma: a phase 2 randomized clinical trial. JAMA Oncol. 2021;7(3):421–7. https://doi.org/10.1001/jamaoncol.2020.7328.
57. Wu W, He J, Cameron JL, et al. The impact of postoperative complications on the administration of adjuvant therapy following pancreaticoduodenectomy for adenocarcinoma. Ann Surg Oncol. 2014;21(9):2873–81.
58. Labori KJ, Bratlie SO, Andersson B, et al. Neoadjuvant FOLFIRINOX versus upfront surgery for resectable pancreatic head cancer (NORPACT-1): a multicentre, randomised, phase 2 trial. Lancet Gastroenterol Hepatol. 2024;9(3):205–17.
59. Chun YS, Milestone BN, Watson JC, et al. Defining venous involvement in borderline resectable pancreatic cancer. Ann Surg Oncol. 2010;17(11):2832–8.
60. Chatzizacharias NA, Tsai S, Griffin M, et al. Locally advanced pancreas cancer: staging and goals of therapy. Surgery. 2018;163:1053.
61. Takahashi H, Ogawa H, Ohigashi H, et al. Preoperative chemoradiation reduces the risk of pancreatic fistula after distal pancreatectomy for pancreatic adenocarcinoma. Surgery. 2011;150(3):547–56.
62. Ferrone CR, Marchegiani G, Hong TS, et al. Radiological and surgical implications of neoadjuvant treatment with FOLFIRINOX for locally advanced and borderline resectable pancreatic cancer. Ann Surg. 2015;261(1):12–7.
63. Sadot E, Doussot A, O'Reilly EM, et al. FOLFIRINOX induction therapy for stage 3 pancreatic adenocarcinoma. Ann Surg Oncol. 2015;22(11):3512–21.
64. Gillen S, Schuster T, Meyer Zum Büschenfelde C, Friess H, Kleeff J. Preoperative/neoadjuvant therapy in pancreatic cancer: a systematic review and meta-analysis of response and resection percentages. PLoS Med. 2010;7(4):e1000267.
65. Versteijne E, van Dam JL, Suker M, et al. Neoadjuvant chemoradiotherapy versus upfront surgery for resectable and borderline resectable pancreatic cancer: long-term results of the Dutch randomized PREOPANC trial. J Clin Oncol. 2022;40(11):1220–30.
66. Chuong MD, Springett GM, Freilich JM, et al. Stereotactic body radiation therapy for locally advanced and borderline resectable pancreatic cancer is effective and well tolerated. Int J Radiat Oncol Biol Phys. 2013;86(3):516–22.
67. Mahadevan A, Jain S, Goldstein M, et al. Stereotactic body radiotherapy and gemcitabine for locally advanced pancreatic cancer. Int J Radiat Oncol Biol Phys. 2010;78(3):735–42.
68. Rajagopalan MS, Heron DE, Wegner RE, et al. Pathologic response with neoadjuvant chemotherapy and stereotactic body radiotherapy for borderline resectable and locally-advanced pancreatic cancer. Radiat Oncol. 2013;8:254.
69. Katz MHG, Shi Q, Meyers J, et al. Efficacy of preoperative mFOLFIRINOX vs mFOLFIRINOX plus hypofractionated radiotherapy for borderline resectable adenocarcinoma of the pancreas: the A021501 phase 2 randomized clinical trial. JAMA Oncol. 2022;8(9):1263–70.
70. Finks JF, Osborne NH, Birkmeyer JD. Trends in hospital volume and operative mortality for high-risk surgery. N Engl J Med. 2011;364(22):2128–37.
71. Evans DB, George B, Tsai S. Non-metastatic pancreatic cancer: resectable, borderline resectable, and locally advanced-definitions of increasing importance for the optimal delivery of multimodality therapy. Ann Surg Oncol. 2015;22(11):3409–13.
72. Lassen K, Coolsen MM, Slim K, et al. Guidelines for perioperative care for pancreaticoduodenectomy: Enhanced Recovery After Surgery (ERAS) Society recommendations. World J Surg. 2013;37(2):240–58.
73. Takagi K, Yoshida R, Yagi T, et al. Effect of an enhanced recovery after surgery protocol in patients undergoing pancreaticoduodenectomy: a randomized controlled trial. Clin Nutr. 2019;38(1):174–81.

74. Xiong J, Szatmary P, Huang W, et al. Enhanced recovery after surgery program in patients undergoing pancreaticoduodenectomy: a PRISMA-compliant systematic review and meta-analysis. Medicine (Baltimore). 2016;95(18):e3497.
75. Pilgrim CH, Tsai S, Evans DB, Christians KK. Mesocaval shunting: a novel technique to facilitate venous resection and reconstruction and enhance exposure of the superior mesenteric and celiac arteries during pancreaticoduodenectomy. J Am Coll Surg. 2013;217(3):e17–20.
76. Christians KK, Pilgrim CH, Tsai S, et al. Arterial resection at the time of pancreatectomy for cancer. Surgery. 2014;155(5):919–26.
77. Fortner JG. Regional resection of cancer of the pancreas: a new surgical approach. Surgery. 1973;73(2):307–20.

Chapter 17
Pancreatic Neuroendocrine Neoplasms

Allen A. Razavi, Jaewon Lee, and Alexandra Gangi

Introduction

Pancreatic neuroendocrine neoplasms (PNEN), also previously known as pancreatic neuroendocrine tumors (PNET), originate from islet cells of the pancreas and represent a small percentage of pancreatic malignancies, around 1–3%. Interestingly, their incidence is increasing and attributable to the improved detection with advances in imaging technology [1]. PNEN as a group are quite heterogeneous and can be classified based on functional status, biologic behavior, and risk for development (sporadic vs secondary to inherited syndrome). Ninety percent of PNEN are sporadic but 10% are noted to occur in the setting of hereditary syndromes, most commonly multiple endocrine neoplasia type 1 (MEN1), von-Hippel-Lindau syndrome (VHL), and neurofibromatosis 1 (NF1) [2]. The age of onset for PNEN varies based on hereditary (earlier in life) versus sporadic presentation, but most often occurs between the ages of 40 and 60 years [3]. The etiology of sporadic PNEN is unclear but recently assumed to be secondary to point mutations commonly associated with four main pathways: chromatin remodeling, DNA damage repair, activation of mTOR, and telomere maintenance [2–4].

Diagnosis

PNEN can be classified as functional versus nonfunctional based on clinical manifestation. In general, PNEN typically have an indolent course and are difficult to diagnose with mean time to diagnosis from symptom onset of approximately

A. A. Razavi · J. Lee · A. Gangi (✉)
Department of Surgical Oncology, Cedars-Sinai Medical Center, Los Angeles, CA, USA
e-mail: Armin.Razavi@cshs.org; Jaewon.Lee@cshs.org; Alexandra.Gangi@cshs.org

© The Author(s), under exclusive license to Springer Nature Switzerland AG 2025
E. P. Ceppa et al. (eds.), *The SAGES Manual of Evolving Techniques in Pancreatic Surgery*, https://doi.org/10.1007/978-3-031-78409-5_17

8–10 years, especially for nonfunctional tumors [5]. Patients with functional PNEN present with characteristic syndromes and physiologic derangements based on the hormone(s) they secrete and will be described later in this chapter. Nonfunctional PNEN are generally found incidentally on imaging but can present with symptoms of local disease related to their size: mass effect, pain, bleeding, and/or sequela of biliary obstruction. Once there is suspicion for a PNEN, patients should be thoroughly screened for tumor symptoms with detailed personal and family history to assess for hereditary syndromes. Additionally, patients should have biochemical testing to assist with diagnosis and be appropriately staged with cross-sectional imaging (CT/MRI/Gallium DOTATATE scan) to localize primary tumor and evaluate for metastatic disease [6].

After a thorough history is obtained, if a functional PNEN is suspected, evaluation of elevated hormone or peptide levels is essential for the diagnosis of functional PNEN (Table 17.1). In the absence of symptoms to suggest a functional PNEN, a full hormonal workup is not needed as is unlikely to assist with diagnosis. Chromogranin A (CgA) is one of the most sensitive markers for nonfunctional PNEN [7]. Elevated CgA has been correlated with tumor burden and can be useful for surveillance in the postoperative state. Unfortunately, CgA is a nonspecific test for PNEN as it may be influenced by specific food intake, hepatic/renal insufficiency, cardiac decompensation, as well as use of proton pump inhibitors. Therefore, it is important to corroborate elevated CgA with imaging and not use the CgA level as a diagnostic tool [8].

Table 17.1 Table of functional PNEN and their associated characteristics

Tumor/syndrome	Incidence per 10^6	Biomarker	Symptoms
Insulinoma	1–3	Insulin	Hypoglycemia after fasting with relief of symptoms with glucose
Gastrinoma	0.5–2	Gastrin and gastric pH	Zollinger-Ellison syndrome: GERD, abdominal pain, diarrhea, duodenal ulcers, PUD
VIPoma	0.05–0.02	Vasoactive intestinal peptide	Verner-Morrison syndrome: Watery diarrhea, hypokalemia, achlorhydria
Glucagonoma	0.01–0.1	Glucagon	Necrotic migratory erythema, weight loss, hypoalbuminemia, diabetes/glucose intolerance
Somatostatinoma	Very rare	Somatostatin	Hyperglycemia, cholestasis, diarrhea/steatorrhea
ACTHoma	Very rare	Adrenocorticotropic hormone	Cushing syndrome
GRHoma	Very rare	Gonadotrophin-releasing hormone	Acromegaly
Hypercalcemia	Very rare	Parathyroid hormone-related protein	Hypercalcemia, abdominal pain, constipation, kidney stones, psychiatric disturbances, increased urination

Imaging

Tumor localization is the next step in workup after a thorough history and physical exam and targeted diagnostic studies. As mentioned earlier, PNEN may be incidentally identified on imaging studies. For further imaging workup, a combination of either dual/triple phase CT or MRI and DOTATATE PET/CT, with possible upper endoscopic ultrasound (EUS), may be used to evaluate and diagnose PNEN. CT triple phase with IV contrast is the most common initial imaging study and can provide diagnostic data if obtained correctly. On CT, PNEN are typically well circumscribed and hyperattenuating because of their vascularity. They are best seen in early arterial phases with a bright signal with early portal venous washout. The sensitivity of localizing PNEN with a CT scan is reported to vary between 63% and 83%. MRI is also considered a first-line imaging modality in detecting PNEN. On MRI, PNEN are classically described as low signal intensity on T1-weighted images and high signal intensity on T2-weighted images. The overall sensitivity of MRI for PNEN detection is between 80% and 90% and related to tumor size [9]. If CT or MRI does not yield adequate results, or if a biopsy is required, endoscopy with EUS can be performed. On EUS, PNEN are described as well-defined hypoechoic homogeneous lesions with occasional cystic components. EUS's prime utility is localizing lesions <2 cm, which is where conventional CT and MRI imaging may fall short. In addition, at the time of EUS, tissue acquisition via fine needle aspiration (FNA) can provide a diagnosis and histological grade prior to treatment. EUS limitations include operator skill and occasionally poorly visualized pancreatic masses given the variations in pancreatic parenchyma in patients.

Somatostatin receptor scintigraphy (SRS) is another imaging modality that utilizes the prevalence of somatostatin receptors in most neuroendocrine neoplasms to aid in targeting and visualization. The radiolabeled somatostatin that is administered is picked up by PNEN expressing somatostatin receptors and can theoretically detect lesions with high sensitivity. Unfortunately, SRS is not accurate and may not show the exact location of the tumor or adequately provide size. For these reasons, DOTATATE PET/CT scan has now become the imaging study of choice for detecting PNEN with specificity climbing to 97%. The DOTATATE labeled radioisotope binds with extremely high affinity to the somatostatin receptor and provides superior spatial resolution as compared to the prior modalities, allowing for improved lesion identification [10]. If the aforementioned studies fail to localize the tumor, selective angiography can be used. Angiography utilizes the hypervascular nature of most PNEN, showing a characteristic blush on imaging, though this diagnostic modality is rarely utilized [9, 11, 12].

Biology and Inherited Syndromes

The majority of PNEN occur sporadically but some are associated with genetic syndromes. Patients with genetic syndromes linked to the development of PNEN are generally diagnosed earlier and often develop multiple neoplasms rather than the solitary lesions seen in sporadic disease. In addition, patients with an inherited syndrome tend to have a more prolonged indolent course when compared to sporadic tumors and may benefit from specific treatment targets that are not suitable for the sporadic subtypes [13].

MEN1 is an autosomal dominant disorder and the most common genetic syndrome linked to PNEN. MEN1 is caused by mutations in MENIN (a tumor suppressor on chromosome 11q13 that is key in control of G1 to S phase cell cycle progression) and is characterized by development of parathyroid adenomas/hyperplasia, PNEN, and pituitary adenomas. Malignant PNEN have been reported as the most common cause of death in patients with MEN1. Nonfunctional PNEN are the most prevalent type of neoplasm in patients with MEN1. The most recent Endocrine Society clinical practice guidelines for MEN1 recommend biochemical screening for insulinoma at age 5 and gastrinoma at age 20, with annual imaging (MRI/CT/EUS) for nonfunctional PNEN starting before 10 years old [14].

Von Hippel-Lindau (VHL) is another autosomal dominant syndrome linked to PNEN and characterized by mutations in the VHL gene leading to both malignant and benign tumors and cysts of the central nervous system, retina, kidneys, pancreas, and gastrointestinal tract. The prevalence of PNEN in VHL patients is 5–17%, and diagnosis of a PNEN has a favorable prognosis when compared to sporadic PNEN. Current recommendations from the VHL Alliance guidelines include surveillance MRI of the abdomen starting at age 15 performed every 2 years [15]. Another autosomal dominant condition that may lead to PNEN development is neurofibromatosis-1 (NF-1). NF-1 results in lack of function of neurofibromin, a tumor suppressor protein, leading to increased risk for neurofibromas, pheochromocytomas, and gastrointestinal stromal tumors. Somatostatinomas are the most common type of PNEN in patients with NF-1. Given the rarity of PNEN in NF-1, there are no specific recommendations for surveillance, but clinicians should have a high index of suspicion for symptoms to suggest PNEN in these patients [16].

Functionality

PNEN that are classified as functional are those that secrete a dominant hormone which drives a clinical syndrome. Table 17.1 lists all the types of functional PNEN, the specific biomarker of interest, and related symptoms. Importantly, functional PNEN can secrete more than one hormone and cause additional syndromes. The majority of functional PNEN are well differentiated and diagnosed earlier than nonfunctional tumors given their clinical symptoms. Nonfunctional PNEN can represent three types: PNEN that do not secrete any hormone, PNEN that produce hormones at a low enough level which does not cause symptoms, and PNEN that secrete hormones which do not produce symptoms (CgA, pancreatic polypeptide, neurotensin, and ghrelin). Nonfunctional PNEN are typically found incidentally but can present with nonspecific symptoms secondary to mass effect. Prognostically, tumor grade has a stronger influence on prognosis rather than the functionality of the tumor [2, 8, 17, 18].

Insulinoma

Insulinoma is the most common type of PNEN with a variety of symptoms stemming from hyperactivity of the sympathetic and central nervous system (hunger, tremor, anxiety, irritability, diaphoresis, and weakness). Insulinomas are often sporadic (95%), found in the fourth decade of life and evenly distributed throughout the pancreas. In addition, insulinomas tend to be small, nonmetastatic, thus amenable to surgical resection. Although rare, MEN1 is the most common hereditary syndrome associated with insulinomas and often present with multiple malignant tumors. The gold standard for diagnosis of insulinomas is a 72 h fast with subsequent testing every 6 h for glucose, insulin, C-peptide, proinsulin, and beta-hydroxybutyrate levels. It is important to differentiate an insulinoma from iatrogenic intake of hypoglycemic medications which will yield an elevated plasma insulin level but low C-peptide and proinsulin [19]. The steps required to localize insulinomas are the same for any PNEN with the caveat that SRS is not usually useful as they often lack sufficient somatostatin receptors. As mentioned previously, surgical resection is the mainstay and only curative option for insulinomas. Enucleation is usually the treatment of choice as the majority are benign, typically small (<2 cm) and >2 mm from the pancreatic duct. In the event the insulinoma is identified within 2 mm of the pancreatic duct, formal anatomic resection may be required. Postoperatively, recurrence rates are low (3%) and more likely in patients with associated hereditary syndromes. In patients with metastatic disease, the median survival is approximately 5 years [20, 21].

Gastrinoma

Gastrinomas are the second most common functional PNEN. Unlike insulinomas, >50% of patients diagnosed with a gastrinoma have evidence of metastatic disease at the time of diagnosis [2]. Gastrinomas typically originate within the gastrinoma triangle (90%) and are diagnosed with gastrin levels >1000 and pH < 2 from gastric aspirate. Of note, PPIs must be stopped 2 weeks prior to testing gastrin levels because they can falsely elevate gastrin levels. Gastrinomas may take an aggressive or a benign course. The aggressive form is seen in 20–30% of patients with 90% of tumors found in pancreas. Survival rates for benign and aggressive forms are 90% and 30%, respectively. After diagnosis and localization, PPI is the first-line treatment for symptomatic relief followed by curative surgical resection versus palliative cytoreduction for symptom control [22]. PPI doses can be titrated to higher-than-normal ranges for symptom relief, especially in patients with unresectable metastatic disease. Somatostatin analogues have also been shown to help with symptom control with PPIs. These large doses of PPIs have rendered debulking and acid-reducing procedures exceedingly rare. Given a 50% chance of metastatic disease at time of diagnosis, regional pancreatectomy is preferred. Patients with hereditary syndromes may benefit from pancreatoduodenectomy as most of the recurrent disease in this patient population is in the duodenum [2, 22, 23].

VIPoma

VIPomas are a rare type of PNEN with an incidence of one in ten million. VIPomas secrete vasoactive intestinal peptide (VIP) and associated with the WDHA syndrome causing profuse watery diarrhea, electrolyte disturbances (hypokalemia, hypomagnesemia, hypophosphatemia, and metabolic acidosis), weight loss, abdominal pain, and achlorhydria. Like gastrinomas, the majority of VIPomas are metastatic at time of diagnosis (70%). Diagnosis of VIPoma is suggested with VIP levels >225 pg/mL after an overnight fast. Of note, VIP may be secreted from other tumors including neuroblastomas, ganglioblastomas, and ganglioneuromas; therefore, tumor localization is imperative [24]. Management of VIPomas begins with preoperative resuscitation, electrolyte correction, and administration of somatostatin analogues. As with gastrinomas, anatomic resection with lymphadenectomy is recommended and often warranted in the setting of resectable disease. Resection of liver metastasis can be performed if surgically feasible [25]. In patients with unresectable disease, somatostatin analogues likely prolong progression-free survival with secondary options including peptide receptor radiolabeled SSA, everolimus, sunitinib, chemotherapy, or debulking. If there is evidence of extensive unresectable liver dominant disease, embolization, radioembolization, radiofrequency ablation, or brachytherapy are options to reduce tumor burden. No specific liver-directed therapy has been proven to improve survival, but reduction of liver tumor burden is associated with symptomatic improvement [24–26].

Glucagonoma

Glucagonomas are also exceedingly rare, with an incidence of one in 20 million. They arise from the alpha cells of the pancreas and usually present in the body or tail [27]. Patients can present with dermatitis (necrolytic migrating erythema), depression, DVTs, diabetes, weight loss, and vitamin/amino acid deficiencies. The diagnosis of glucagonoma is confirmed with elevated glucagon levels >1000 pg/mL after a fasting state [28]. Glucagonomas tend to be larger and malignant (50–80%) at the time of diagnosis. Elevated glucagon can place patients in a severe state of catabolism and malnourishment; therefore, treatment begins with optimizing nutrition with enteral supplements. In addition, DVT prophylaxis is imperative in these patients to prevent pulmonary embolism. As with other functional PNEN, anatomic resection is indicated for resectable disease. Postoperatively, patients without evidence of metastasis have an 85% 5-year survival rate, while patients with metastatic disease have a 60% 5-year survival rate [26, 27, 29].

Histology Classifications/Grading

The heterogeneity of PNEN has made it challenging to predict clinical behaviors and prognosis. By this accord, classifying PNEN has also been difficult. In 2010, the WHO released guidelines for stratifying patients with all digestive system neuroendocrine cancers that could be applied to PNEN. This system separated well-differentiated neuroendocrine tumors into low grade (G1) and intermediate grade (G2) depending on Ki67 and mitotic index [9]. High-grade tumors (G3) were considered poorly differentiated then. As expected, this wide application for all neuroendocrine tumors provided some discrepancies for PNEN which resulted in the WHO creating a new classification system specifically for PNEN. Briefly, the WHO 2017 guidelines split PNEN into two broad categories: well-differentiated pancreatic neuroendocrine tumors (PNETs) and poorly differentiated pancreatic neuroendocrine carcinomas (PNECs). PNETs were further classified into grade 1 (G1), grade 2 (G2), and grade 3 (G3) based on Ki-67 proliferation index and mitotic index per high power field (HPF). PNECs are now G3 with poorly differentiated tissue architecture (Table 17.2) [5]. A few key attributes should be noted in the new classification system: (1) the eighth edition system only applies to well-differentiated PNETs G1-G3 while the poorly differentiated G3 PNECs are still classified by the pancreatic adenocarcinoma staging system and (2) there is further emphasis on T stage and location of metastatic site—liver vs extrahepatic vs both liver and extrahepatic [30]. The marked difference in phenotype between PNECs and PNETs is believed to stem from genetic differences, with abnormalities of MEN1, DAXX,

Table 17.2 WHO eighth edition 2017 PNEN classification system

WHO 2017 classification	Mitoses (# per high-powered field)	Ki-67 rate (%)
Well-differentiated PNET, grade 1	<2	<2
Well-differentiated PNET, grade 2	20	3–20
Well-differentiated PNET, grade 3	>20	>20
Poorly differentiated PNEC, grade 3	>20	>20

and ATRX molecular pathways among PNET but not for PNEC. On the other hand, p53 genetic abnormalities have been noted in PNEC but not in PNET. Surgery remains the only curable treatment approach for PNEN and typically recommended when technically feasible. Exceptions to this include patients with widely metastatic disease, small and sporadic nonfunctional PNEN, and in patients with severe comorbidities that would preclude surgery [31].

Staging/Surgical Decision-Making

Nonmetastatic Disease

Primary surgical resection should be offered for all functional or symptomatic PNENs without evidence of distant metastatic spread and irrespective of size. Of note, regional lymph node involvement does not preclude resection despite being a negative prognostic indicator. In patients with locally advanced tumors, extended organ resections with vascular reconstruction can be performed if need be. The management of nonfunctional PNENs has been guided by size >2 cm surgery is recommended and <1 cm observation given low likelihood of lymph node spread. The controversy resides among PNENs 1–2 cm [32]. European Neuroendocrine Tumor Society (ENETS) and National Comprehensive Cancer Network (NCCN) both endorse observation for nonfunctional PNENS <2 cm while the North American Neuroendocrine Tumor Society (NANETS) recommends an individualized approach based on grade, growth rate, age, patient comorbidities/preference, and the extent of surgery required for R0 resection. In lieu of these discrepancies, the decision to watch or operate on a patient with nonfunctional PNENs between 1 and 2 cm should be made on an individualized basis while taking account the tumor grade, growth rate or radiographic progression, and morbidity associated with pancreatic resection [18]. If observation is chosen, guidelines mandate for repeat MRI/CT every 6–12 months with indication to re-evaluate the need for surgery if the lesion increases by 0.5 cm or more.

The goal of PNEN surgery is to resect the primary tumor and associated lymph nodes while preserving as much pancreatic parenchyma as feasible. The surgical approach and extent of resection are dictated by location, degree of local invasion, presence of metastatic disease, grade, and patient factors [33]. Partial pancreatic resection in the form of pancreatoduodenectomy, distal pancreatectomy, or enucleation are all options for resection. In general, PNEN located in the head/uncinate/neck of pancreas require pancreatoduodenectomy and PNEN located in the body or tail of pancreas require distal pancreatectomy with or without splenectomy. Enucleation and central pancreatectomy are options for smaller lesions and have gained wider acceptance to help minimize postoperative pancreatic insufficiency (endocrine/exocrine). Enucleation has the advantage of avoiding complications associated with a pancreatic anastomosis and has been shown to have less severe pancreatic fistulas despite having higher pancreatic leak rates [6, 34]. Importantly, enucleation is not recommended in patients with nodal or metastatic disease, tumors >3 cm in size, or those near the common bile duct or pancreatic duct [6, 18, 32].

Metastatic Disease

At time of diagnosis, 40–80% of PNEN are metastatic. The most frequent site of metastasis is the liver (40–90%) followed by bone (12–20%) and lung (5%). While M1 disease is a negative prognostic indicator, long-term outcomes are significantly more favorable than for pancreatic adenocarcinoma. Metastatic disease is related to several factors including histologic grade, size of primary tumor, mitotic index, and vascular/lymphatic invasion [35]. The treatment of metastatic PNEN is complex and in constant evolution and thus requires multidisciplinary expertise involving surgery, interventional radiology, and medical oncology subspecialists on board. Patients with metastatic PNEN should be presented at multidisciplinary tumor board (MTD) or transferred to a center with high volume PNEN surgeons as there are various treatment modalities for advanced PNEN. Given the indolent nature of PNEN, it is likely that a patient with advanced PNEN will undergo multiple treatments over the course of their disease [36].

Metastatic PNEN should be classified as liver-only disease or those with presence of extrahepatic disease. For liver-only disease, the goal is resection of both primary and hepatic metastatic lesions as it remains the only curative option when the disease is resectable. Hepatic metastases are classified into three patterns: type 1—isolated single lesion, type 2—large focus of metastatic bulk with bilobar small lesions, and type 3 with bilobar disseminated metastatic disease and with minimal normal liver parenchyma. Patients with type 1 and 2 patterns of disease are candidates for resection. Unfortunately, 5-year recurrence rates are as high as 80–94% given the likelihood of microscopic disease that is not visualized on preoperative imaging [37]. Risk factors for recurrence include lymph node involvement and microscopic positive surgical margins in the primary. If a patient's disease pattern after the index operation remains resectable, they may undergo multiple trips to the operating room in combination with other locoregional treatments to obtain long-term disease control [38].

The high hepatic recurrence rate has also allowed liver transplantation to emerge as an option for selected patients with favorable tumor grade. The criteria for liver transplantation are quite strict and include: age <55 years, well-differentiated PNEN with hepatic disease burden <50% of liver, prior resection of primary tumor, absence of extrahepatic disease, and stable disease for 6 months [39]. Frequently, patients eligible for transplant are also eligible for cytoreductive surgery or other liver-directed and systemic treatment options. Outcomes after transplantation in this selected patient population are favorable with 5-year OS between 70% and 90% [40]. For type 3 hepatic metastasis, initial non-surgical management with somatostatin analogue therapy, systemic chemotherapy, or peptide receptor radionucleotide therapy (PRRT) is generally recommended. Patients are followed closely to determine if liver tumor burden downgrades and may qualify for resection. In patients whose tumor does not become resectable, locoregional therapies play a key role as resection of the primary tumor remains controversial given its unclear impact on survival and a potential for increased morbidity and mortality. Transarterial embolization (TAE), transarterial chemoembolization (TACE), and selective internal radiation therapy (SIRT) are among the options to control liver metastasis. The choice among the three should be discussed within a multidisciplinary team as there are no prospective studies yet that directly compare outcomes with the different modalities. TACE and TAE have been shown to improve symptoms in 60–90% of patients with low morbidity and mortality. Overall survival ranges from 12 to 84 months and 14 to 70 months for TAE/TACE and SIRT, respectively [35, 36, 38, 40].

Extrahepatic metastasis has been associated with poor prognosis when compared to liver-only disease. Medical therapies such as SSA, everolimus, and sunitinib have been loosely associated with tumor regression but may not improve symptoms as they are unable to decrease the amount of hormone secretion to provide benefit. The evidence for PRRT is limited to the small bowel, and the ability to improve hormonal burden is questionable. Several systemic therapies are available and discussed later in this chapter. In certain scenarios, based on disease burden, utilization of systemic therapy and cytoreductive surgery has been proposed as an option to directly reduce tumor burden. Studies have shown this option to be beneficial with approximately 70% of patients receiving hormonal response rates in the largest study to date. The authors believe it is necessary to discuss prospective cytoreductive candidates among the multidisciplinary team, particularly considering performance status, hormonal activity, symptomatic burden on life, anatomic location, and volume of extrahepatic tumor. Cytoreductive surgery for asymptomatic disease remains controversial, and more data is needed to provide guidance [41].

Multidisciplinary Decision-Making

Given that most PNEN are nonfunctional and diagnosed in late stages, a multidisciplinary approach to their treatment is essential in improving disease outcome. It is important for clinicians to understand when surgical resection of primary and/or metastatic PNEN is indicated, as well as types and indications of systemic therapies available based on previous trials.

Surgical Resection

Resection of the primary or metastatic PNEN has been associated with improved survival, but surgery may not always be indicated. In patients with PNEN secondary to inherited syndromes such as multiple endocrine neoplasia (MEN) type 1 and von Hippel-Lindau (VHL) syndrome, tumors smaller than 2–3 cm rarely progress or metastasize [42]. Sporadic PNEN under 2 cm may also be observed given their good prognosis [43], unless there are high-risk features such as patients older than 55 years of age, grade 3 tumor, or the presence of distant metastases [44, 45]. However, there is controversy in observing tumors under 2 cm, as there have been other studies showing improved survival in patients who underwent resection of small nonfunctional PNEN [46–48]. Radiofrequency ablation of small PNEN has been described as an alternative based on small series [49, 50].

In patients with liver metastases, both the primary and the metastatic lesions should be resected if technically feasible [51]. However, if the primary tumor is not resectable, the metastatic lesion(s) should not be resected [52]. There is no clear data to suggest whether the primary tumor should be resected if the metastatic disease is unresectable. Even after resection of liver metastasis with curative intent, recurrence rates up to 54% have been reported despite negative margins [53]. Liver-directed regional therapies such as transarterial embolization, chemoembolization, or radioembolization may be an option for those patients with unresectable liver metastases. However, current data demonstrates that surgical resection is superior to intra-arterial therapies in terms of median survival in patients with NEN liver metastases [37, 54]. NANETs and ENETs guidelines suggest that treatment should be individualized based on patient age and comorbidities, distribution of lesions and volume of liver involvement, the presence of symptoms, and rate of progression.

Systemic Treatments

There are multiple systemic therapeutic options for locally advanced and metastatic neuroendocrine neoplasms (NEN) of the gastrointestinal tract including those of the pancreas. The use of somatostatin analog octreotide was shown to extend the time to progression compared to placebo in the PROMID trial [55]. Similarly, the CLARINET demonstrated prolonged progression-free survival in patients treated with lanreotide, another somatostatin analog [56]. The follow-up CLARINET FORTE trial looking at patients with disease progression on standard dosing of lanreotide (every 28 days) who then underwent more frequent dosing (every 14 days) demonstrated some progression-free survival, although this study was single arm [57].

As NEN demonstrate hypervascularity, inhibition of angiogenesis in the treatment of NEN has also been investigated. Sunitinib is a receptor tyrosine kinase inhibitor that targets vascular endothelial growth factor (VEGF) receptors as well as platelet-derived growth factor (PDGF) receptors which have shown to improve both the progression-free survival and the overall survival of patients with advanced well-differentiated PNEN compared to placebo in a phase III trial [58]. This study was terminated early due to more deaths being observed in the placebo group. A follow-up phase IV trial confirmed longer progression-free survival and objective tumor response in PNEN treated with sunitinib [59]. Mammalian target of rapamycin (mTOR) represents another pathway that may be targeted in the treatment of NEN. In the RADIANT-3 trial, patients with advanced PNEN receiving everolimus, an oral mTOR inhibitor, demonstrated significantly longer progression-free survival compared to those receiving placebo [60]. The RADIANT-4 trial broadened the use of everolimus to advanced NEN of the lung or the gastrointestinal tract and confirmed earlier findings of prolonged progression-free survival with everolimus compared to placebo [61].

In recent years, immune checkpoint inhibitors have gained significant clinical interest as they have shown to improve outcomes in many cancer types. In the KEYNOTE-028 trial, 25% of PNEN were positive for programmed death-ligand 1 (PD-L1). Of those, an objective response rate to pembrolizumab was 6.3% at median follow-up of 21 months [62]. Similarly, KEYNOTE-158 showed median progression-free survival of 4.1 months in NEN treated with pembrolizumab [63]. Of the four tumors with partial responses, three were PNEN, and all were PD-L1 negative.

Another study demonstrated a disease control rate of 24.1% in patients with metastatic high-grade NEN who were treated with pembrolizumab, and there was no difference in outcomes between PD-L1-positive and PD-L1-negative tumors [64]. Current evidence shows limited utility of immune therapies in PNEN, but more studies are needed to definitively conclude their utility.

Another option for systemic treatment of NENs is peptide receptor radionuclide therapy using lutetium-177 (^{177}Lu)-Dotatate. The NETTER-1 trial demonstrated improved progression-free survival in patients receiving ^{177}Lu-Dotatate and octreotide compared to those receiving octreotide alone [63], although this trial only included patients with midgut NENs. Despite longer progression-survival, a follow-up analysis did not demonstrate an improved overall survival at 5 years in patients undergoing ^{177}Lu-Dotatate therapy [63].

Open Trials

There are multiple ongoing trials regarding PNEN, especially relating to outcomes with different systemic therapy options. Some of these trials are summarized in Table 17.3.

Table 17.3 Summary of select ongoing trials for systemic therapies for GEP NEN

Trial ID	Phase	Population	Intervention
NCT04234568	1	GEP NEN	Lu 177 with triapine (ribonucleotide reductase inhibitor)
NCT05040360	2	High-risk well-differentiated PNEN	Capecitabine and temozolomide after surgery
NCT02893930	2	Metastatic or refractory PNEN (unresectable)	Sapanisertib (mTOR inhibitor)
NCT02595424	2	Metastatic or unresectable GEP NEN	Temozolomade and capecitabine vs. cisplatin and etoposide
NCT05050942	3	Advanced well-differentiated GEP NEN	CAM2029 (octreotide subcutaneous depot)
NCT04919226	3	Well-differentiated grade 2–3 GEP NEN	Lu 177 and edotreotide (peptide receptor radionuclide therapy)

Surveillance

In a review of 1020 patients who underwent curative-intent resection of PNEN without liver metastasis at time of surgery, 15.1% developed recurrence, with 49.4% of those patients having liver-only recurrence and 22.7% having pancreas-only recurrence [65]. Pancreas-only recurrence decreased with time and was associated with margin status, whereas liver-only recurrence increased with time and was related to cancer characteristics such as Ki-67 index and presence of perineural invasion. Given the heterogeneity of this disease and high recurrence rate, it has been suggested that the surveillance strategies be individualized to each patient [33, 66]. Follow-up should include clinical examination, lab markers, and cross-sectional imaging, and frequency should be based on risk factors based on patient and tumor characteristics. The CommNETS group recommends a follow-up period of at least 10 years [67]. The interim data from the ASPEN trial provides interesting information regarding surveillance for small (<2 cm), sporadic, and asymptomatic nonfunctional PNEN [68]. Among the 406 patients who underwent surveillance over a median follow-up of 2 years, only 2% underwent surgery for increasing main pancreatic duct dilation, tumor size, or patient preference. This suggests that a nonoperative strategy may be a safe option, but long-term follow-up is needed to provide more definitive guidance.

References

1. Lawrence B, Gustafsson BI, Chan A, Svejda B, Kidd M, Modlin IM. The epidemiology of gastroenteropancreatic neuroendocrine tumors. Endocrinol Metab Clin N Am. 2011;40(1):1–18, vii.
2. Batcher E, Madaj P, Gianoukakis AG. Pancreatic neuroendocrine tumors. Endocr Res. 2011;36(1):35–43.

3. Dasari A, Shen C, Halperin D, et al. Trends in the incidence, prevalence, and survival outcomes in patients with neuroendocrine tumors in the United States. JAMA Oncol. 2017;3(10):1335–42.
4. Klimstra DS, Modlin IR, Coppola D, Lloyd RV, Suster S. The pathologic classification of neuroendocrine tumors: a review of nomenclature, grading, and staging systems. Pancreas. 2010;39(6):707–12.
5. Ma ZY, Gong YF, Zhuang HK, et al. Pancreatic neuroendocrine tumors: a review of serum biomarkers, staging, and management. World J Gastroenterol. 2020;26(19):2305–22.
6. Falconi M, Plockinger U, Kwekkeboom DJ, et al. Well-differentiated pancreatic nonfunctioning tumors/carcinoma. Neuroendocrinology. 2006;84(3):196–211.
7. Qiao XW, Qiu L, Chen YJ, et al. Chromogranin A is a reliable serum diagnostic biomarker for pancreatic neuroendocrine tumors but not for insulinomas. BMC Endocr Disord. 2014;14:64.
8. Halfdanarson TR, Rabe KG, Rubin J, Petersen GM. Pancreatic neuroendocrine tumors (PNETs): incidence, prognosis and recent trend toward improved survival. Ann Oncol. 2008;19(10):1727–33.
9. Khanna L, Prasad SR, Sunnapwar A, et al. Pancreatic neuroendocrine neoplasms: 2020 update on pathologic and imaging findings and classification. Radiographics. 2020;40(5):1240–62.
10. Srirajaskanthan R, Kayani I, Quigley AM, Soh J, Caplin ME, Bomanji J. The role of 68Ga-DOTATATE PET in patients with neuroendocrine tumors and negative or equivocal findings on 111In-DTPA-octreotide scintigraphy. J Nucl Med. 2010;51(6):875–82.
11. Kartalis N, Mucelli RM, Sundin A. Recent developments in imaging of pancreatic neuroendocrine tumors. Ann Gastroenterol. 2015;28(2):193–202.
12. Lee L, Ito T, Jensen RT. Imaging of pancreatic neuroendocrine tumors: recent advances, current status, and controversies. Expert Rev Anticancer Ther. 2018;18(9):837–60.
13. Soczomski P, Jurecka-Lubieniecka B, Krzywon A, et al. A direct comparison of patients with hereditary and sporadic pancreatic neuroendocrine tumors: evaluation of clinical course, prognostic factors and genotype-phenotype correlations. Front Endocrinol. 2021;12:681013.
14. Klein Haneveld MJ, van Treijen MJC, Pieterman CRC, et al. Initiating pancreatic neuroendocrine tumor (pNET) screening in young MEN1 patients: results from the DutchMEN Study Group. J Clin Endocrinol Metabol. 2021;106(12):3515–25.
15. Sadowski SM, Triponez F. Management of pancreatic neuroendocrine tumors in patients with MEN 1. Gland Surg. 2015;4(1):63–8.
16. Lodish MB, Stratakis CA. Endocrine tumours in neurofibromatosis type 1, tuberous sclerosis and related syndromes. Best Pract Res Clin Endocrinol Metab. 2010;24(3):439–49.
17. Daskalakis K. Functioning and nonfunctioning PNEN. Curr Opin Endocr Metab Res. 2021;18:284–90.
18. Akirov A, Larouche V, Alshehri S, Asa SL, Ezzat S. Treatment options for pancreatic neuroendocrine tumors. Cancers. 2019;11(6):828.
19. Mathur A, Gorden P, Libutti SK. Insulinoma. Surg Clin North Am. 2009;89(5):1105–21.
20. O'Grady HL, Conlon KC. Pancreatic neuroendocrine tumours. Eur J Surg Oncol. 2008;34(3):324–32.
21. Mathur A, Gorden P, Libutti SK. Insulinoma. Surg Clin. 2009;89(5):1105–21.
22. Metz DC, Cadiot G, Poitras P, Ito T, Jensen RT. Diagnosis of Zollinger-Ellison syndrome in the era of PPIs, faulty gastrin assays, sensitive imaging and limited access to acid secretory testing. Int J Endocr Oncol. 2017;4(4):167–85.
23. Norton JA, Foster DS, Ito T, Jensen RT. Gastrinomas: medical or surgical treatment. Endocrinol Metab Clin N Am. 2018;47(3):577–601.
24. Ghaferi AA, Chojnacki KA, Long WD, Cameron JL, Yeo CJ. Pancreatic VIPomas: subject review and one institutional experience. J Gastrointest Surg. 2008;12(2):382–93.
25. Smith SL, Branton SA, Avino AJ, et al. Vasoactive intestinal polypeptide secreting islet cell tumors: a 15-year experience and review of the literature. Surgery. 1998;124(6):1050–5.
26. Ito T, Igarashi H, Jensen RT. Pancreatic neuroendocrine tumors: clinical features, diagnosis and medical treatment: advances. Best Pract Res Clin Gastroenterol. 2012;26(6):737–53.
27. McGavran MH, Unger RH, Recant L, Polk HC, Kilo C, Levin ME. A glucagon-secreting alpha-cell carcinoma of the pancreas. N Engl J Med. 1966;274(25):1408–13.

28. Ito T, Igarashi H, Jensen RT. Therapy of metastatic pancreatic neuroendocrine tumors (pNETs): recent insights and advances. J Gastroenterol. 2012;47(9):941–60.
29. Kindmark H, Sundin A, Granberg D, et al. Endocrine pancreatic tumors with glucagon hypersecretion: a retrospective study of 23 cases during 20 years. Med Oncol. 2007;24(3):330–7.
30. Perri G, Prakash LR, Katz MHG. Pancreatic neuroendocrine tumors. Curr Opin Gastroenterol. 2019;35(5):468–77.
31. Zhang XF, Xue F, Dong DH, et al. New nodal staging for primary pancreatic neuroendocrine tumors: a multi-institutional and national data analysis. Ann Surg. 2021;274(1):e28–35.
32. Li D, Rock A, Kessler J, et al. Understanding the management and treatment of well-differentiated pancreatic neuroendocrine tumors: a clinician's guide to a complex illness. JCO Oncol Pract. 2020;16(11):720–8.
33. Jeune F, Taibi A, Gaujoux S. Update on the surgical treatment of pancreatic neuroendocrine tumors. Scand J Surg. 2020;109(1):42–52.
34. Fendrich V, Bartsch DK. Surgical treatment of gastrointestinal neuroendocrine tumors. Langenbeck's Arch Surg. 2011;396(3):299–311.
35. Clavien PA, Petrowsky H, DeOliveira ML, Graf R. Strategies for safer liver surgery and partial liver transplantation. N Engl J Med. 2007;356(15):1545–59.
36. Foulfoin M, Graillot E, Adham M, et al. Treatment of metastatic pancreatic neuroendocrine tumors: relevance of ENETS 2016 guidelines. Endocr Relat Cancer. 2017;24(2):71–81.
37. Mayo SC, de Jong MC, Pulitano C, et al. Surgical management of hepatic neuroendocrine tumor metastasis: results from an international multi-institutional analysis. Ann Surg Oncol. 2010;17(12):3129–36.
38. Kulke MH, Anthony LB, Bushnell DL, et al. NANETS treatment guidelines: well-differentiated neuroendocrine tumors of the stomach and pancreas. Pancreas. 2010;39(6):735–52.
39. Mazzaferro V, Pulvirenti A, Coppa J. Neuroendocrine tumors metastatic to the liver: how to select patients for liver transplantation? J Hepatol. 2007;47(4):460–6.
40. Siebenhüner AR, Langheinrich M, Friemel J, Schäfer N, Eshmuminov D, Lehmann K. Orchestrating treatment modalities in metastatic pancreatic neuroendocrine tumors-need for a conductor. Cancers (Basel). 2022;14(6):1478.
41. Chan DL, Dixon M, Law CHL, et al. Outcomes of cytoreductive surgery for metastatic low-grade neuroendocrine tumors in the setting of extrahepatic metastases. Ann Surg Oncol. 2018;25(6):1768–74.
42. Jensen RT, Berna MJ, Bingham DB, Norton JA. Inherited pancreatic endocrine tumor syndromes: advances in molecular pathogenesis, diagnosis, management, and controversies. Cancer. 2008;113(7 Suppl):1807–43.
43. Bettini R, Partelli S, Boninsegna L, et al. Tumor size correlates with malignancy in nonfunctioning pancreatic endocrine tumor. Surgery. 2011;150(1):75–82.
44. Cherenfant J, Stocker SJ, Gage MK, et al. Predicting aggressive behavior in nonfunctioning pancreatic neuroendocrine tumors. Surgery. 2013;154(4):785–91; discussion 91–3.
45. Lee LC, Grant CS, Salomao DR, et al. Small, nonfunctioning, asymptomatic pancreatic neuroendocrine tumors (PNETs): role for nonoperative management. Surgery. 2012;152(6):965–74.
46. Sharpe SM, In H, Winchester DJ, Talamonti MS, Baker MS. Surgical resection provides an overall survival benefit for patients with small pancreatic neuroendocrine tumors. J Gastrointest Surg. 2015;19(1):117–23; discussion 23.
47. Finkelstein P, Sharma R, Picado O, et al. Pancreatic neuroendocrine tumors (panNETs): analysis of overall survival of nonsurgical management versus surgical resection. J Gastrointest Surg. 2017;21(5):855–66.
48. Sun Y, Wang Y, Li R, et al. Surgical resection of primary tumor is associated with prolonged survival in low-grade pancreatic neuroendocrine tumors. Clin Res Hepatol Gastroenterol. 2021;45(1):101432.
49. Barthet M, Giovannini M, Lesavre N, et al. Endoscopic ultrasound-guided radiofrequency ablation for pancreatic neuroendocrine tumors and pancreatic cystic neoplasms: a prospective multicenter study. Endoscopy. 2019;51(9):836–42.

50. Oleinikov K, Dancour A, Epshtein J, et al. Endoscopic ultrasound-guided radiofrequency ablation: a new therapeutic approach for pancreatic neuroendocrine tumors. J Clin Endocrinol Metab. 2019;104(7):2637–47.
51. Sarmiento JM, Heywood G, Rubin J, Ilstrup DM, Nagorney DM, Que FG. Surgical treatment of neuroendocrine metastases to the liver: a plea for resection to increase survival. J Am Coll Surg. 2003;197(1):29–37.
52. Jin M, Roth R, Gayetsky V, Niederberger N, Lehman A, Wakely PE Jr. Grading pancreatic neuroendocrine neoplasms by Ki-67 staining on cytology cell blocks: manual count and digital image analysis of 58 cases. J Am Soc Cytopathol. 2016;5(5):286–95.
53. Bagante F, Spolverato G, Merath K, et al. Neuroendocrine liver metastasis: the chance to be cured after liver surgery. J Surg Oncol. 2017;115(6):687–95.
54. Yuan CH, Wang J, Xiu DR, et al. Meta-analysis of liver resection versus nonsurgical treatments for pancreatic neuroendocrine tumors with liver metastases. Ann Surg Oncol. 2016;23(1):244–9.
55. Rinke A, Müller HH, Schade-Brittinger C, et al. Placebo-controlled, double-blind, prospective, randomized study on the effect of octreotide LAR in the control of tumor growth in patients with metastatic neuroendocrine midgut tumors: a report from the PROMID Study Group. J Clin Oncol Off J Am Soc Clin Oncol. 2009;27(28):4656–63.
56. Caplin ME, Pavel M, Ćwikła JB, et al. Lanreotide in metastatic enteropancreatic neuroendocrine tumors. N Engl J Med. 2014;371(3):224–33.
57. Pavel M, Ćwikła JB, Lombard-Bohas C, et al. Efficacy and safety of high-dose lanreotide autogel in patients with progressive pancreatic or midgut neuroendocrine tumours: CLARINET FORTE phase 2 study results. Eur J Cancer. 2021;157:403–14.
58. Raymond E, Dahan L, Raoul J-L, et al. Sunitinib malate for the treatment of pancreatic neuroendocrine tumors. N Engl J Med. 2011;364(6):501–13.
59. Fazio N, Kulke M, Rosbrook B, Fernandez K, Raymond E. Updated efficacy and safety outcomes for patients with well-differentiated pancreatic neuroendocrine tumors treated with Sunitinib. Target Oncol. 2021;16(1):27–35.
60. Yao JC, Shah MH, Ito T, et al. Everolimus for advanced pancreatic neuroendocrine tumors. N Engl J Med. 2011;364(6):514–23.
61. Yao JC, Pavel M, Lombard-Bohas C, et al. Everolimus for the treatment of advanced pancreatic neuroendocrine tumors: overall survival and circulating biomarkers from the randomized, phase III RADIANT-3 study. J Clin Oncol Off J Am Soc Clin Oncol. 2016;34(32):3906–13.
62. Mehnert JM, Bergsland E, O'Neil BH, et al. Pembrolizumab for the treatment of programmed death-ligand 1-positive advanced carcinoid or pancreatic neuroendocrine tumors: results from the KEYNOTE-028 study. Cancer. 2020;126(13):3021–30.
63. Strosberg J, Leeuwenkamp O, Siddiqui MK. Peptide receptor radiotherapy re-treatment in patients with progressive neuroendocrine tumors: a systematic review and meta-analysis. Cancer Treat Rev. 2021;93:102141.
64. Vijayvergia N, Dasari A. Targeted therapies in the management of well-differentiated digestive and lung neuroendocrine neoplasms. Curr Treat Options in Oncol. 2020;21(12):96.
65. Dong D-H, Zhang X-F, Lopez-Aguiar AG, et al. Surgical outcomes of patients with duodenal vs pancreatic neuroendocrine tumors following pancreatoduodenectomy. J Surg Oncol. 2020;122(3):442–9.
66. Zaidi MY, Lopez-Aguiar AG, Switchenko JM, et al. A novel validated recurrence risk score to guide a pragmatic surveillance strategy after resection of pancreatic neuroendocrine tumors: an international study of 1006 patients. Ann Surg. 2019;270(3):422–33.
67. Singh S, Moody L, Chan DL, et al. Follow-up recommendations for completely resected gastroenteropancreatic neuroendocrine tumors. JAMA Oncol. 2018;4(11):1597–604.
68. Partelli S, Massironi S, Zerbi A, et al. Management of asymptomatic sporadic non-functioning pancreatic neuroendocrine neoplasms no larger than 2 cm: interim analysis of prospective ASPEN trial. Br J Surg. 2022;109(12):1186–90.

Chapter 18
Secondary Malignant Neoplasms

Ross Mudgway ⓘ**, Daniel J. Oliveira, and David Caba Molina** ⓘ

Renal Cell Carcinoma

Introduction/Epidemiology

Metastasis from renal cell carcinoma (RCC) is common and already present during diagnosis in approximately 25% of patients [1]. RCC metastasis is most common to the lung, liver, bone, and adrenal tissue [1–3]. Of the malignant tumors that metastasize to the pancreas, the most common primary tumor site of metastasis is the kidney, accounting for 70.5% [4]. Hematogenous and lymphatic spread have both been considered as the underlying mechanism of RCC metastasis to the pancreas [1, 5, 6]. Studies have found no relation between site of the primary tumor and site of the pancreatic metastasis, supporting a hematogenous spread, whereas a strong correlation between site and pancreatic localization would have suggested a lymphatic spread [1, 5, 6]. Additionally, lymph-node positivity is rare, while a high rate of vascular invasion has been observed during surgery [1, 5, 6]. However, systemic spread would not explain the discrepancy between the relative frequency between multiple pancreatic metastases and the absence of metastasis to other organs, suggesting there is some underlying biochemical mechanism [1, 6]. It has been observed that RCC metastasis to the pancreas is predominantly in males, 62 years old, and is metachronous [3, 7, 8].

R. Mudgway · D. J. Oliveira
Loma Linda University, Loma Linda, CA, USA
e-mail: RMudgway@llu.edu; doliveir@sgu.edu

D. Caba Molina (✉)
Loma Linda University, Loma Linda, CA, USA

Riverside University Health System/University of California-Riverside,
Loma Linda, CA, USA
e-mail: DCabamolina@llu.edu; d.cabamolina@ruhealth.org

E. P. Ceppa et al. (eds.), *The SAGES Manual of Evolving Techniques in Pancreatic Surgery*, https://doi.org/10.1007/978-3-031-78409-5_18

Diagnosis/Radiology/Pathology

Common patient presentations include nonspecific symptoms, such as abdominal pain, anemia, gastrointestinal (GI) bleeding, and jaundice, although 49–55% patients are mostly asymptomatic [6, 7, 9]. There have also been cases of patients presenting with pancreatitis due to pancreatic duct obstruction [6]. Typically, patients will have a median disease-free survival of 6–12 years after nephrectomy [1, 3, 6–8, 10]. However, there have been some reports of disease-free intervals over 30 years suggesting the necessity of long-term follow-up [6].

Tumor size in the pancreas ranges from 1.5 to 12 cm [7]. Grossly, metastatic tumor deposits are well-circumscribed, with bright yellow-orange to red-brown to white-gray masses [7]. The most common location is the head of the pancreas, followed by the tail and then the body [7]. Clear cell renal cell carcinoma is the most common RCC to metastasize to the pancreas; there are also cases of chromophobe RCC and rarely sarcomatoid RCC [7].

Isolated pancreatic metastasis is often found incidentally on routine surveillance, with computed tomography (CT) and magnetic resonance imaging (MRI) being the most used initial diagnostic modality [6, 7, 11]. On CT and MRI, the pancreatic metastasis will show intense enhancement on arterial and venous phase compared to normal tissues (Fig. 18.1) [11]. Pancreatic ductal adenocarcinoma is non-enhancing and can be reliably distinguished, while nonfunctional pancreatic endocrine tumors (PNETs) share the same morphology and enhancement characteristics of RCC [11]. Nuclear medicine testing like fluorodeoxyglucose-positron emission tomography (FDG-PET)/CT is useful for determining the need for surgery because it can exclude distant extrapancreatic metastases [4, 10]. However, it is important to

Fig. 18.1 Contrast-enhanced computed tomography scan of renal cell carcinoma (clear cell type) metastasis to the pancreas. An enhancing soft tissue of the pancreatic neck is demonstrated

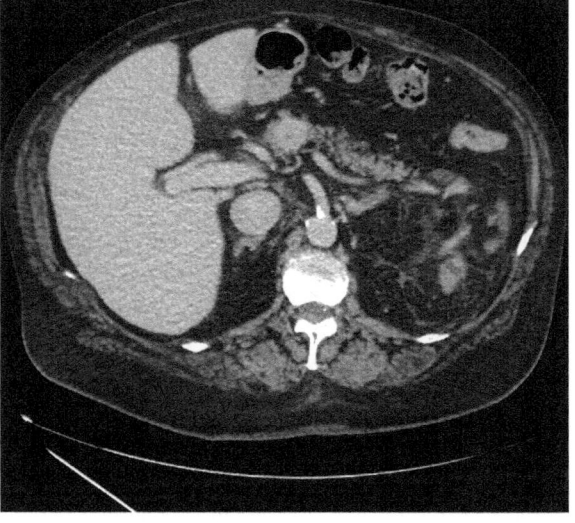

note that the number of actual tumors in the resected pancreatic specimen are generally greater than the number determined by FDG-PET/CT [4].

In general, endoscopic ultrasound-guided fine needle aspiration (EUS-FNA) is to be considered the best and most accurate modality and can be used when CT/MRI cannot make a correct diagnosis [10, 11]. On endoscopic ultrasound (EUS), pancreatic RCC will appear as a hypoechoic, round, well-circumscribed homogeneous lesion [11]. The hypervascularity nature of metastases can be appreciated using Color Doppler imaging [11]. However, on EUS, PNET also has similar morphological features [11]; therefore, biopsy, when possible, allows for comparison to the primary tumor.

Fine needle aspiration (FNA) will show cells in clusters, sheets, and often grow along capillaries [7, 11]. There will be abundant pale and clear cytoplasm with centrally placed nuclei and prominent nucleoli (Fig. 18.2) [11]. Immunochemistry plays an important role in the diagnosis of metastatic RCC to the pancreas [11]. RCC expresses pan-cytokeratin, vimentin, EMA, CD10, and PAX-8 [7, 11]. Also, RCC metastasis to the pancreas is associated with cell clones that have a lower aggressiveness and that can be distinguished from extrapancreatic metastases by a lack of loss of 9p, lower weight genome instability index, low frequency of BAP1 alterations, and a high frequency of PBRM 1 loss [2, 12].

Treatment/Outcome

Current treatment options are surgical resection or biologic-targeted therapies [2, 8]. Surgical treatment includes pylorus-preserving or classic pancreatoduodenectomy, distal pancreatectomy, or total pancreatectomy with or without splenectomy

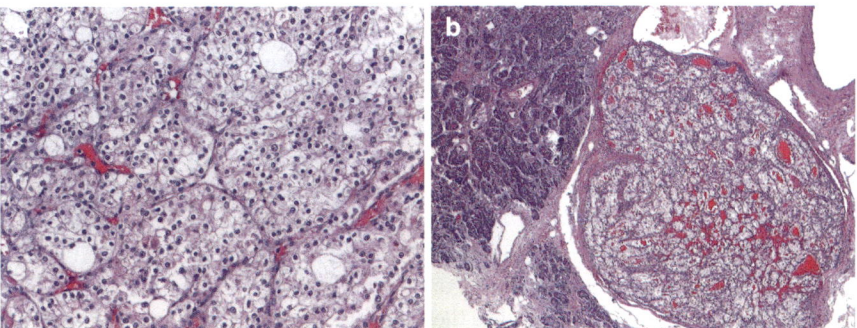

Fig. 18.2 Renal cell carcinoma (clear cell type) involving the pancreas at 4X magnification (**a**) and 20X magnification (**b**). In (**a**), the tumor is composed of malignant cells with prominent cytoplasmic clearing and enlarged nuclei with occasional prominent nucleoli and open chromatin. The clusters of tumor cells are separated by a thin delicate vasculature which contributes to the hemorrhagic appearance of renal cell carcinoma grossly. In (**b**), the tumor is invading the glandular parenchyma composed of acinar cells of the pancreas

and with or without pylorus preservation, and duodenum-preserving total pancreatectomy, depending on the location and number of tumors [4, 10]. Some studies also report that radiofrequency ablation and cytoablative therapy can be performed in addition to surgery as well as IRE (irreversible electroporation) all of which are being currently studied [13].

Targeted therapy includes tyrosine kinase inhibitors (TKI), mTor inhibitors, and immune checkpoint inhibitors such as anti-PD1, anti-PD L1, and anti-CTLA4. These are highly effective for metastatic RCC (mRCC) [8, 12]. However, there is a paucity of data and lack of evidence that shows this to be effective in treatment for mRCC to the pancreas specifically [1, 12].

The 5-year survival rate for untreated mRCC was 13–47% compared to 65–88% after surgical resection [1]. Current data show the 1-, 3-, 5-, and 10-year overall survival after surgical resection to be 88%, 72%, 33–72%, and 32%, respectively [1, 8–10, 14]. The overall survival rate after pancreatectomy for mRCC is longer compared to pancreatectomy for other cancers [4, 11]. The median recurrence-free survival after pancreas metastasectomy was 17.2 months with a median recurrence rate of 44% after 27 months, and a 5-year recurrence-free survival of 43% [2, 10, 12]. In line with the current data, surgical approach in well controlled and resection of isolated mRCC to the pancreas is now an integral part of treatment with good results. Whether synchronous or metachronous, a complete resection can lead to long-term survival [1, 2, 10, 11, 14].

Colorectal Carcinoma

Introduction/Epidemiology

Colorectal carcinoma (CRC) is the third leading cause of cancer-related deaths in the United States, with metastasis most commonly occurring to local lymph nodes (50–70%), the liver (50%), the bones (40%), the lungs (21%), the peritoneum (15%), the ovaries (15%), and the brain (5%) [15, 16]. Though CRC is one of the most common origins for metastatic pancreatic lesions, it is exceedingly rare, accounting for only 1.3–2% of pancreatic metastasis [15–19]. CRC metastasis occurs via direct invasion through the colon, lymphatic channels, and via hematogenous routes [15, 16]. There are two leading theories that explain the metastatic pattern of CRC: the mechanical/hemodynamic theory and the seed-and-soil theory [18]. The mechanical theory is based on anatomical delivery via the venous and lymphatic drainage systems [18]. The theory explains the colonic tumors spread via emboli that drain into the portal venous circulation and metastasize to the liver or by systemic routes to the lung. One study found that pancreatic metastases tend to be from right-sided tumors, which supports the mechanical spread theory where cecal tumors spread directly to the pancreas via the ileocolic and superior mesenteric vessels [18, 20]. The seed-and-soil theory is based on metastasizing tumor cells finding a tissue bed that is compatible for deposit and growth [18]. Given the rarity and unique location of the pancreas not found along normal anatomic drainage routes, seed-and-soil does offer a plausible mechanism [18]. Pancreatic metastases typically occur 3–4 years after initial CRC diagnosis, though some cases have been reported to be more than 5 and even over 10 years later [15–17].

Diagnosis/Radiology/Pathology

The clinical presentation of metastatic CRC) is variable, 45–71% patients with pancreatic metastasis from CRC are asymptomatic [15, 18]. Common presentations of a primary pancreatic tumor are abdominal pain, weight loss, and jaundice. Clinical presentation of patients with pancreatic metastasis from CRC is unique [18, 19]. The incidences of those same symptoms were abdominal pain (20%), weight loss (5%), and jaundice (30%) [19]. A major distinguishing feature is that 55% of patients whose tumor's location was in the head of the pancreas did not present with jaundice, likely related to its location and growth [19].

When symptoms are present or during surveillance, the majority of pancreatic metastases are initially discovered on abdominal CT with a sensitivity of 68–86% and specificity of 65% [15]. Diagnosis with imaging alone is difficult [18, 19, 21]. Enhanced CT of pancreatic metastases from CRC will show a hypodense mass that is occasionally accompanied by the dilation of the distal main pancreatic duct, a similar finding to that of a primary pancreatic cancer which makes it difficult to discern in this context, also taking into account risks for a second primary [21]. Imaging may only be good to differentiate between CRC and RCC origin, which shows an intense enhancement during the arterial phase [18, 21].

In these cases, EUS-FNA has a sensitivity of 75–95%, specificity of 60–100%, and accuracy >91% [15, 21]. EUS typically reports pancreatic metastatic lesions as hypoechoic, heterogeneous masses with well-defined margins, and other findings suggestive of secondary lesions are multiples lesions, lack of a retention cysts, pancreatic duct dilation, and pancreatic atrophy [15]. There is controversy over the necessity of biopsy with EUS-FNA for informed treatment decisions. The opposition argues the risk of tumor cell dissemination, while advocates argue for accurate staging diagnosis with biopsy for the following indications: "(1) all other diagnostic measures failed; (2) pathological examination demonstrates certain markers or gene mutations that are needed for initiation of specific treatments; (3) biopsy results will influence therapy; (4) biopsy results can avoid or minimize surgery; and (5) locoregional staging of pancreatic tumors" [18].

Immunohistochemical findings are helpful in differentiating pancreatic metastasis from primary pancreatic cancer [15, 17, 21]. Immunochemical staining shows a specific pattern (CK20+, CK7-, and CDX2+) [18, 21]. The respective rates of CK20 and CK7 positivity were 100% and 5% in colorectal cancer, and 62% and 92% in pancreatic cancer [21]. CDX2 is expressed positively in the majority of CRC, while in contrast the rate is only 0–50% in pancreatic carcinomas [18, 21]. When performing EUS-FNA, an adequate sample of the specimen is needed [21]. Use of a thicker needle or performing a rapid on-site evaluation to assess the quantity is recommended [21].

Treatment/Prognosis

Treatment for CRC metastasis to the pancreas is primarily chemotherapy and metastasectomy of solitary lesions without extrapancreatic metastasis, as determined on an individual basis [15]. Early pancreatic metastasis could be treated surgically with most of the diagnoses coming at advanced stages with infiltration of local organs, local nodes, or distant metastasis. However, only about 20% of patients are referred for surgery [16]. These surgeries include total pancreatectomy, distal pancreatectomy, pancreatoduodenectomy, and pylorus-preserving pancreatoduodenectomy [16, 19]. Tumor proximity to the SMV or PV in well-selected patients is not a contraindication to resection based on previous reviews of the topic [16]. Palliative surgery is performed to provide adequate biliary or alimentary passage which includes biliary-intestinal anastomoses and gastrointestinal anastomoses [16].

The 5-year survival of CRC with metastasis to the pancreas is 14–50% with mortality and morbidity to be 1.4% and 48.3%, respectively [17]. Patients also have a median survival time of 16.5 months, and a disease-free survival period of 1.5–43 months, with 100% of symptomatic relief until recurrence of death [18]. Though data is scarce for CRC metastasis to the pancreas, and the optimal treatment is yet to be established. Multiple literature reviews and case studies agree that pancreatic resections may provide a definitive diagnosis as well as a survival benefit and should be considered in patients who are well selected, fit for surgery, free of metastasis to other organs, and are discussed properly in multidisciplinary fashion [15–19].

Melanoma

Introduction/Epidemiology

Melanoma is one of the most common malignancies that metastasizes to the gastrointestinal tract and usually affects multiple organ sites [22, 23]. Autopsy data have revealed gastrointestinal tract involvement in 50–60% of patients with melanoma; however, the clinical diagnosis is only made in 1.5–4.4% of melanoma patients [24]. Solitary organ involvement of melanoma to the pancreas is extremely rare, occurring in <1% of metastatic melanoma cases [22, 23, 25]. There are <200 cases of pancreatic metastasis from malignant melanoma found in the literature [22, 23], with the major primary site being cutaneous and ocular [23]. Cases of melanoma metastasis from the nasal cavity to the pancreas have been reported [23]. The primary lesion of melanoma may be difficult to identify. Studies have shown patients with metastatic melanoma to the pancreas who underwent pancreatic resection demonstrate a median time between the treatment of the primary melanoma and the detection of pancreatic metastases of 6 years (range 14 months to 34 years) [22, 26]. A long disease-free interval of more than 2 years after primary melanoma treatment was associated with improved survival in patients with intrapancreatic metastases [26].

Diagnosis/Radiology/Pathology

Obtaining a pre-operative diagnosis of a metastatic pancreatic tumor can be difficult [27]. Positron emission tomography-computed tomography (PET-CT) scan has a high sensitivity and specificity for detection of metastasis from malignant melanoma [28]. On contrast-enhanced CT and MRI imaging, metastatic lesions from malignant melanoma demonstrate hypervascularity and rim enhancement [23, 29]. Metastatic melanoma lesions will demonstrate hyperintensity on T1 MRI, an indication of changes caused by the paramagnetic properties of melanin [30, 31]. Malignant melanoma may or may not show hyperenhancement on contrast-enhanced endoscopic ultrasound (CE-EUS), and the lack of characteristic findings makes diagnosis of malignant melanoma by CE-EUS difficult [23, 32]. EUS reports of malignant melanoma to the pancreas have demonstrated hypoechoic, heterogenous lesions [33].

Pathological examination is necessary to confirm the diagnosis of metastatic melanoma to the pancreas. EUS-FNA with effective sampling and immunohistochemical analysis is important in providing a cytological and histological diagnosis [23]. EUS-FNA with rapid on-site evaluation provides effective sampling and allows a cytopathologist to ensure the samples are adequate for assessment [34]. Aspirate samples of melanoma are cellular and consist of noncohesive malignant-appearing cells with nuclear pleomorphism and prominent nucleoli admixed with malignant, pigmented epithelioid and spindle-shaped cells, and can include the presence of melanin [22]. Pathology reports of melanoma lesions in the pancreas have demonstrated normal pancreatic parenchyma infiltrated with a tumor composed of sheets of heavily pigmented and atypical epithelioid cells with high nuclear-cytoplasmic ratio, eosinophilic cytoplasm, hyperchromatic nuclei with marked pleomorphism, and numerous atypical mitoses [33]. On immunohistochemical analysis, the markers S100, Melan A, and HMB-45 have a reported 97–100%, 75–92%, and 69–93% sensitivity for identifying metastatic melanoma. S100 and

Melan A have a reported 75–87% and 95–100% specificity, respectively [23, 35]. The era of precision medicine has found that approximately 29–66% of melanoma cases are positive for activating mutations in the BRAF gene, with the most common mutation being the V600E substitution [22].

Treatment/Prognosis

Metastatic melanoma has a poor prognosis with a median life expectancy of 6–12 months in cases of gastrointestinal metastasis [33]. The prognosis of metastatic melanoma to the pancreas specifically is unknown. Pancreatic resection for metastatic melanoma is controversial, and there are no guidelines for indications of pancreatic resection for metastatic melanoma cases [23]. As seen for all isolated pancreatic metastases, the benefit of resection on overall and disease-free survival is not clearly established but may provide some benefit in selected patients [36].

For melanoma, some studies have demonstrated prolonged survival after complete surgical resection of localized metastatic melanoma to the pancreas [23, 37, 38]. Pancreas-sparing pancreatectomies are limited due to the limited margins obtained and the exclusion of a formal lymphadenectomy, thus the role of these procedures for isolated pancreatic metastases is not well defined [36]. Standard pancreatic resections, such as pancreatoduodenectomy and distal pancreatectomy, are associated with significant morbidity and may only offer the advantage of improved lymphadenectomy for resection of intrapancreatic metastases, though may provide control of the disease when indicated and adequately performed [36]. However, some authors advocate that non-standard pancreatic resections have an increased risk of early local recurrence and higher morbidity [39, 40]. A retrospective study on survival of patients with isolated pancreatic metastasis from malignant melanoma who underwent complete surgical resection demonstrated a median survival and 5-year disease-free survival of 24 months and 37%, respectively [38]. This was in comparison to patients with incomplete pancreatic resections who had a median survival of 8 months and 5-year disease-free survival of 0% [38]. Cases of pancreatoduodenectomy prolonging survival over 5 years for patients with metastatic melanoma to the pancreas have been reported [23, 36, 41].

The decision to perform pancreatic resection requires exhaustive pre-operative evaluation and staging, with critical assessment of peri-operative risks and the expected survival benefit. Surgical resection should only be considered if complete resection is possible [36], yet surgical therapy may provide palliation in selected cases [42]. Systemic or targeted therapy for melanoma may provide prolonged survival and less morbidity compared to surgical resection for intrapancreatic metastasis and almost always is considered around the planned resection. The role of systemic or targeted therapy in combination with surgical resection is yet to be determined.

Sarcoma

Introduction/Epidemiology

Sarcomas are rare tumors with differentiation toward mesenchymal tissue and account for approximately 1% of all adult cancers [43]. Metastasis of sarcoma to the pancreas is extremely rare. Although limited, cases of sarcoma subtypes metastasizing to the pancreas include those from primary osteosarcoma, Ewing sarcoma, mesenchymal chondrosarcoma, leiomyosarcoma, dermatofibrosarcoma protuberans, synovial sarcoma, myxofibrosarcoma, and solitary fibrous tumors [44–50]. Most sarcomas preferentially metastasize via the vascular system rather than the lymphatic system, and the most frequent sites of metastatic sarcoma are the lung and bone [51]. The connective interspaces and cavities in which tumor cells can become entrapped, such as the peritoneum, provide another possible route of metastatic dissemination of sarcoma [52]. The median overall survival for metastatic sarcoma ranges from 12 to 18 months from time of diagnosis [53]. Unlike other forms of cancer, the prognosis of a sarcoma depends on its grade rather than its specific histological type [51].

Osteosarcoma is the most common primary bone malignancy in all age-groups, and the highest risk period for onset coincides with the adolescent growth spurt (10–14 years old in females, 15–19 years old in males) [45]. Distant metastasis of osteosarcoma occurs in 10–20% of patients [45]. Incidence rates of mesenchymal chondrosarcoma are similar between men and women, with the highest incidence in the second and third decades of life [54]. Approximately 20% of mesenchymal chondrosarcoma cases have metastatic disease at the time of diagnosis [55]. Dermatofibrosarcoma protuberans has a higher incidence in men and commonly occurs between 20 and 50 years of age [48]. Metastasis of dermatofibrosarcoma protuberans occurs in 1–6% of patients, and the fibrosarcomatous variant has a 15% risk of distant metastasis [56, 57]. Synovial sarcoma metastasizes in 50% of patients [58]. Of the three subtypes of synovial sarcoma (monophasic, biphasic, and poorly differentiated), the poorly differentiated subtype is associated with early recurrence and metastasis [59].

Diagnosis/Radiology/Pathology

As is the case with other forms of pancreatic metastases, patients with sarcoma metastasis to the pancreas may be asymptomatic at the time of diagnosis or may present with generalized abdominal pain. Metastatic sarcoma lesions of the pancreas are often incidentally found on imaging. CT (Fig. 18.3) or MRI (Fig. 18.4) is recommended for radiologic evaluation [60]. PET-CT can demonstrate fluorodeoxyglucose (FDG) uptake in the pancreas [48]. Osteosarcoma metastasis to the pancreas may demonstrate the characteristic calcified lesion of osteosarcoma, but some

Fig. 18.3 Contrast-
enhanced CT scan of
osteosarcoma metastasis to
the pancreas. A
retroperitoneal, mixed
cystic and solid mass with
central calcifications
centered on the lesser sac
is demonstrated

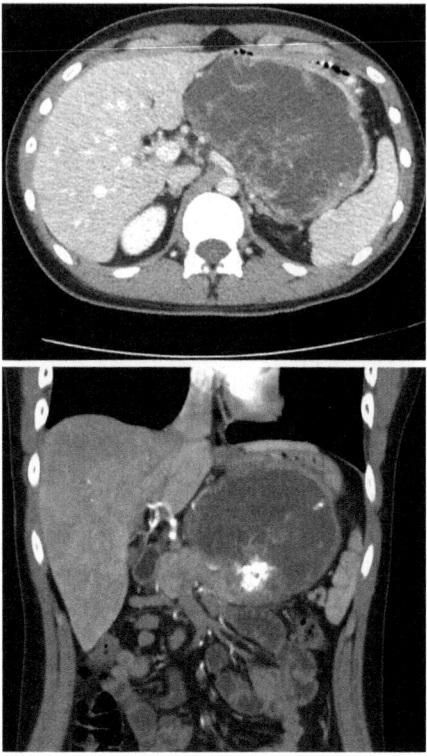

lesions may be indistinguishable from primary pancreatic malignancies and cystic masses have been reported [45]. Mesenchymal chondrosarcoma may demonstrate granular irregular calcifications with a surrounding hypodense tumor on CT scan, and low-intensity calcified areas surrounded by a high-intensity tumor on T2-weighted MRI [46].

Endoscopic ultrasound-guided fine needle biopsy (EUS-FNB) to obtain tissue samples for histological and immunohistochemical analysis (Fig. 18.5) can aid in the diagnosis. Mesenchymal chondrosarcoma is histologically characterized by poorly differentiated small round cells with an abrupt transition to hyaline cartilage [60]. Leiomyosarcoma and synovial sarcoma demonstrate proliferation of spindle-shaped cells with nuclear atypia on histology [47, 49]. Mesenchymal chondrosarcoma is typically positive for NKX2.2, CD99, S100, and SOX9 tumor markers on immunohistochemical stains [61]. CD99 is the most commonly reported marker associated with Ewing sarcoma [50]. Other markers associated with Ewing sarcoma

Fig. 18.4 Magnetic resonance cholangiopancreatography scan of osteosarcoma metastasis to the pancreas. A large, mixed cystic and solid mass lesion originating from the superior aspect of the pancreatic tail and involving the lesser sac with associated edema of the pancreatic tail is demonstrated

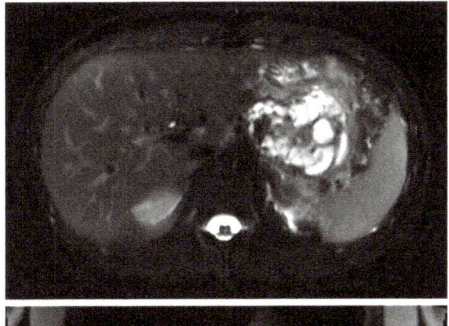

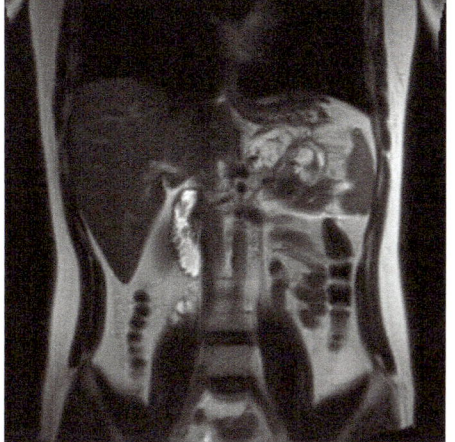

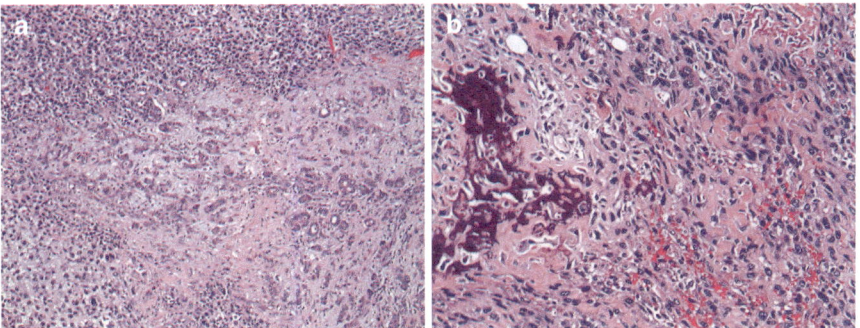

Fig. 18.5 Metastatic, high-grade osteosarcoma involving the pancreas at 10X magnification (**a**) and 20X magnification (**b**). Osteosarcoma extends into the pancreatic parenchyma. There is perineural invasion and perivascular invasion. Figure 18.3b includes the presence of malignant osteoid

include neuron-specific antigen, vimentin, and synaptophysin [50]. Leiomyosarcoma is typically positive for α-smooth muscle actin and vimentin on immunohistochemical analysis [47]. Dermatofibrosarcoma protuberans will be positive for vimentin and platelet-derived growth factor receptor (PDGFR) [48]. Synovial sarcoma has been found to be positive for BCL2, CD99, and cytokeratin on immunohistochemistry and may demonstrate evidence of SS18 gene rearrangement by break-apart fluorescence in situ hybridization [49].

Treatment/Prognosis

The mainstay of treatment for localized sarcoma is complete surgical resection with or without radiation [53]. For metastatic sarcoma, the mainstay of treatment is chemotherapy, and there are an increasing number of systemic therapy options available [62]. Other treatment options for metastatic sarcoma include surgery, radiation, ablation, embolization, and immunotherapy [53]. There is no standard treatment for sarcoma metastasis to the pancreas. Tumor size and extent of tumor invasion to surrounding tissues and structures contribute to treatment approach and survival. The role of surgical resection for sarcoma metastasis to the pancreas is not clearly defined, and treatment regimen should be based on a multidisciplinary approach on an individual basis. For peripancreatic lesions minimally abutting the pancreatic parenchyma, enucleation may be considered [49]. However, involvement of the pancreatic ducts or larger lesion size may warrant pancreatectomy. Formal pancreatic resections, such as distal pancreatectomy with splenectomy, have been reported for resection of osteosarcoma metastasis to the pancreas [45]. Most reports of treatment for mesenchymal chondrosarcoma metastasis to the pancreas consisted of surgical resection followed by adjuvant chemotherapy [46]. The optimal chemotherapy regimen is not well established. Radiation therapy has also been reported [55]. Neoadjuvant chemotherapy followed by pancreatoduodenectomy has been reported for metastatic synovial sarcoma to the pancreas [49]. A single-institution analysis found that factors associated with long-term survival (more than 3 years) included isolated pancreatic metastasis, absence of prior recurrence, >3-year interval between resection of the primary tumor and development of primary metastasis, and if the primary tumor was renal cell carcinoma [63].

For Ewing sarcoma, patients with localized disease have a 5-year overall survival of approximately 70%. On the other hand, metastatic disease has a reported 5-year overall survival between 9% and 41% [64]. Mesenchymal chondrosarcoma has a 5-year overall survival rate of 51% [46]. Synovial sarcoma has a 5-year overall survival rate of 36–76%. Further studies are needed to evaluate the overall survival benefit of pancreatic metastasectomy for sarcoma.

Conclusion

Secondary malignant neoplasms of the pancreas are rare and account for approximately 1–5% of all pancreatic malignancies [2, 3, 7, 10, 65]. The most common primary malignant tumor site is of renal origin, followed by colorectal tumors. Metastasis of melanoma and sarcoma to the pancreas is even less common. Given the rarity of secondary malignant neoplasms to the pancreas, data to provide consensus guidelines for the diagnosis and treatment of these metastatic neoplasms is limited. Most reports of metastases to the pancreas are single patient case reports or single-institution case reviews, yet multi-institutional reviews of published literature have been performed in attempts to summarize these rare diagnoses.

References

1. Ma Y, Yang J, Qin K, et al. Resection of pancreatic metastatic renal cell carcinoma: experience and long-term survival outcome from a large center in China. Int J Clin Oncol. 2019;24(6):686–93.
2. Shin TJ, Song C, Jeong CW, et al. Metastatic renal cell carcinoma to the pancreas: clinical features and treatment outcome. J Surg Oncol. 2021;123(1):204–13.
3. Cheong D, Rho SY, Kim JH, Kang CM, Lee WJ. Laparoscopic pancreaticoduodenectomy for renal cell carcinoma metastasized to ampulla of Vater: a case report and literature review. Ann Hepatobiliary Pancreat Surg. 2018;22(1):83–9.
4. Kitade H, Yanagida H, Yamada M, et al. Pylorus-preserving total pancreatectomy for metastatic renal cell carcinoma: a case report. J Med Case Rep. 2015;9:212.
5. Tosoian JJ, Cameron JL, Allaf ME, et al. Resection of isolated renal cell carcinoma metastases of the pancreas: outcomes from the Johns Hopkins Hospital. J Gastrointest Surg. 2014;18(3):542–8.
6. Ballarin R, Spaggiari M, Cautero N, et al. Pancreatic metastases from renal cell carcinoma: the state of the art. World J Gastroenterol. 2011;17(43):4747–56.
7. Cheng SK, Chuah KL. Metastatic renal cell carcinoma to the pancreas: a review. Arch Pathol Lab Med. 2016;140(6):598–602.
8. Malleo G, Salvia R, Maggino L, et al. Long-term outcomes after surgical resection of pancreatic metastases from renal clear-cell carcinoma. Ann Surg Oncol. 2021;28(6):3100–8.
9. Schwarz L, Sauvanet A, Regenet N, et al. Long-term survival after pancreatic resection for renal cell carcinoma metastasis. Ann Surg Oncol. 2014;21(12):4007–13.
10. Jo S, Yang IJ, Song S. Surgery for metastatic renal cell carcinoma in the pancreatic head: a case report and literature review. Ann Hepatobiliary Pancreat Surg. 2019;23(1):91–5.
11. Pannala R, Hallberg-Wallace KM, Smith AL, et al. Endoscopic ultrasound-guided fine needle aspiration cytology of metastatic renal cell carcinoma to the pancreas: a multi-center experience. Cytojournal. 2016;13:24.
12. Sellner F, Thalhammer S, Klimpfinger M. Isolated pancreatic metastases of renal cell cancer: genetics and epigenetics of an unusual tumour entity. Cancers (Basel). 2022;14(6):1539.
13. Benhaim R, Oussoultzoglou E, Saeedi Y, Mouracade P, Bachellier P, Lang H. Pancreatic metastasis from clear cell renal cell carcinoma: outcome of an aggressive approach. Urology. 2015;85(1):135–40.

14. Brozzetti S, Bini S, De Lio N, Lombardo C, Boggi U. Surgical-only treatment of pancreatic and extra-pancreatic metastases from renal cell carcinoma - quality of life and survival analysis. BMC Surg. 2020;20(1):101.
15. Yoon J, Petrosyan A, Wang T, Ameer A. Colonic adenocarcinoma with synchronous metastasis to the pancreas: a case report and literature review. JGH Open. 2022;6(4):274–6.
16. Olesinski T, Milewska J, Symonides M, Palucki J, Mróz A, Rutkowski A. Pancreatic metastases of rectal cancer-case report and literature review. J Gastrointest Cancer. 2019;50(2):338–41.
17. Tani R, Hori T, Yamada M, et al. Metachronous pancreatic metastasis from rectal cancer that masqueraded as a primary pancreatic cancer: a rare and difficult-to-diagnose metastatic tumor in the pancreas. Am J Case Rep. 2019;20:1781–7.
18. Su L, Wernberg J. Synchronous distal pancreatic metastatic lesion arising from colonic adenocarcinoma: case report and literature review. Clin Med Res. 2014;12(3–4):166–70.
19. Lee CW, Wu RC, Hsu JT, et al. Isolated pancreatic metastasis from rectal cancer: a case report and review of literature. World J Surg Oncol. 2010;8:26.
20. McDaniel KP, Charnsangavej C, DuBrow RA, Varma DG, Granfield CA, Curley SA. Pathways of nodal metastasis in carcinomas of the cecum, ascending colon, and transverse colon: CT demonstration. AJR Am J Roentgenol. 1993;161(1):61–4.
21. Sano I, Katanuma A, Yane K, et al. Pancreatic metastasis from rectal cancer that was diagnosed by endoscopic ultrasonography-guided fine needle aspiration (EUS-FNA). Intern Med. 2017;56(3):301–5.
22. Pang JC, Roh MH. Metastases to the pancreas encountered on endoscopic ultrasound-guided, fine-needle aspiration. Arch Pathol Lab Med. 2015;139(10):1248–52.
23. Nakamura Y, Yamada R, Kaneko M, et al. Isolated pancreatic metastasis from malignant melanoma: a case report and literature review. Clin J Gastroenterol. 2019;12(6):626–36.
24. McLoughlin JM, Zager JS, Sondak VK, Berk LB. Treatment options for limited or symptomatic metastatic melanoma. Cancer Control. 2008;15(3):239–47.
25. Nikfarjam M, Evans P, Christophi C. Pancreatic resection for metastatic melanoma. HPB (Oxford). 2003;5(3):174–9.
26. Sperti C, Polizzi ML, Beltrame V, Moro M, Pedrazzoli S. Pancreatic resection for metastatic melanoma. Case report and review of the literature. J Gastrointest Cancer. 2011;42(4):302–6.
27. Yagi T, Hashimoto D, Taki K, et al. Surgery for metastatic tumors of the pancreas. Surg Case Rep. 2017;3(1):31.
28. Rinne D, Baum RP, Hor G, Kaufmann R. Primary staging and follow-up of high risk melanoma patients with whole-body 18F-fluorodeoxyglucose positron emission tomography: results of a prospective study of 100 patients. Cancer. 1998;82(9):1664–71.
29. Tsitouridis I, Diamantopoulou A, Michaelides M, Arvanity M, Papaioannou S. Pancreatic metastases: CT and MRI findings. Diagn Interv Radiol. 2010;16(1):45–51.
30. Franz D, Esposito I, Kapp AC, Gaa J, Rummeny EJ. Magnetic resonance imaging of less common pancreatic malignancies and pancreatic tumors with malignant potential. Eur J Radiol Open. 2014;1:49–59.
31. Balci NC, Semelka RC. Radiologic features of cystic, endocrine and other pancreatic neoplasms. Eur J Radiol. 2001;38(2):113–9.
32. Fusaroli P, D'Ercole MC, De Giorgio R, Serrani M, Caletti G. Contrast harmonic endoscopic ultrasonography in the characterization of pancreatic metastases (with video). Pancreas. 2014;43(4):584–7.
33. Vargas-Jiménez J, Vargas-Madrigal J, Arias-Mora R, Ulate-Ovares D, Solis-Ugalde B. Pancreatic metastasis from malignant melanoma: not all that glitters is gold. Case Rep Gastroenterol. 2021;15(1):131–6.
34. Yamao K, Sawaki A, Mizuno N, Shimizu Y, Yatabe Y, Koshikawa T. Endoscopic ultrasound-guided fine-needle aspiration biopsy (EUS-FNAB): past, present, and future. J Gastroenterol. 2005;40(11):1013–23.
35. Ohsie SJ, Sarantopoulos GP, Cochran AJ, Binder SW. Immunohistochemical characteristics of melanoma. J Cutan Pathol. 2008;35(5):433–44.

36. Birnbaum DJ, Moutardier V, Turrini O, Gonçalves A, Delpero JR. Isolated pancreatic metastasis from malignant melanoma: is pancreatectomy worthwile? J Surg Tech Case Rep. 2013;5(2):82–4.
37. Goyal J, Lipson EJ, Rezaee N, et al. Surgical resection of malignant melanoma metastatic to the pancreas: case series and review of literature. J Gastrointest Cancer. 2012;43(3):431–6.
38. Wood TF, DiFronzo LA, Rose DM, et al. Does complete resection of melanoma metastatic to solid intra-abdominal organs improve survival? Ann Surg Oncol. 2001;8(8):658–62.
39. Bassi C, Butturini G, Falconi M, Sargenti M, Mantovani W, Pederzoli P. High recurrence rate after atypical resection for pancreatic metastases from renal cell carcinoma. Br J Surg. 2003;90(5):555–9.
40. Reddy S, Wolfgang CL. The role of surgery in the management of isolated metastases to the pancreas. Lancet Oncol. 2009;10(3):287–93.
41. Larsen AK, Krag C, Geertsen P, Jakobsen LP. Isolated malignant melanoma metastasis to the pancreas. Plast Reconstr Surg Glob Open. 2013;1(8):e74.
42. Schuchter LM, Green R, Fraker D. Primary and metastatic diseases in malignant melanoma of the gastrointestinal tract. Curr Opin Oncol. 2000;12(2):181–5.
43. Wibmer C, Leithner A, Zielonke N, Sperl M, Windhager R. Increasing incidence rates of soft tissue sarcomas? A population-based epidemiologic study and literature review. Ann Oncol. 2010;21(5):1106–11.
44. Lee M, Song JS, Hong SM, et al. Sarcoma metastasis to the pancreas: experience at a single institution. J Pathol Transl Med. 2020;54(3):220–7.
45. Cirotski D, Panicker J. Parosteal osteosarcoma with pancreatic metastasis and multiple relapses: a case report and review of the literature. Case Rep Oncol. 2021;2021(2):983–8.
46. Chen JJ, Chou CW. A rare case report of mesenchymal chondrosarcoma with pancreatic metastasis. Medicina (Kaunas). 2022;58(5):639.
47. Ishizaki A, Okuwaki K, Kida M, et al. The first case of metastatic pancreatic leiomyosarcoma derived from the urinary bladder diagnosed using an endoscopic ultrasound-guided fine-needle biopsy. Intern Med. 2021;60(9):1377–81.
48. Chilukuri DS, Premkumar P, Venkitaraman B, Soundararajan JCB. Pancreatic metastasis of dermatofibrosarcoma protuberans: a rare case. BMJ Case Rep. 2020;13(1):e232614.
49. Narayan RR, Charville GW, Delitto D, Ganjoo KN. First recurrence of synovial sarcoma presenting with solitary pancreatic mass. Cureus. 2022;14(6):e26356.
50. Polimera H, Moku P, Abusharar SP, Vasekar M, Chintanaboina J. Metastasis of ewing sarcoma to the pancreas: case report and literature review. Case Rep Oncol Med. 2020;2020:7075048.
51. Leong SP, Cady B, Jablons DM, et al. Clinical patterns of metastasis. Cancer Metastasis Rev. 2006;25(2):221–32.
52. Pennacchioli E, Tosti G, Barberis M, et al. Sarcoma spreads primarily through the vascular system: are there biomarkers associated with vascular spread? Clin Exp Metastasis. 2012;29(7):757–73.
53. Huddy JR, Sodergren MH, Deguara J, Thway K, Jones RL, Mudan SS. Pancreaticoduodenectomy for the management of pancreatic or duodenal metastases from primary sarcoma. Anticancer Res. 2018;38(7):4041–6.
54. Nakashima Y, Unni KK, Shives TC, Swee RG, Dahlin DC. Mesenchymal chondrosarcoma of bone and soft tissue. A review of 111 cases. Cancer. 1986;57(12):2444–53.
55. Cesari M, Bertoni F, Bacchini P, Mercuri M, Palmerini E, Ferrari S. Mesenchymal chondrosarcoma. An analysis of patients treated at a single institution. Tumori. 2007;93(5):423–7.
56. Yokoyama Y, Murakami Y, Sasaki M, et al. Pancreatic metastasis of dermatofibrosarcoma protuberans. J Gastroenterol. 2004;39(8):798–800.
57. Mahajan BB, Sumir K, Singla M. Metastatic dermatofibrosarcoma protuberans: a rare case report from North India. J Cancer Res Ther. 2015;11(3):670.
58. Spurrell EL, Fisher C, Thomas JM, Judson IR. Prognostic factors in advanced synovial sarcoma: an analysis of 104 patients treated at the Royal Marsden Hospital. Ann Oncol. 2005;16(3):437–44.

59. Bakri A, Shinagare AB, Krajewski KM, et al. Synovial sarcoma: imaging features of common and uncommon primary sites, metastatic patterns, and treatment response. AJR Am J Roentgenol. 2012;199(2):W208–15.
60. Fletcher CDM, Unni KK, Mertens F, World Health Organization, International Agency for Research on Cancer. Pathology and genetics of tumours of soft tissue and bone. Lyon: IARC Press; 2002. 427p.
61. Syed M, Mushtaq S, Loya A, Hassan U. NKX3.1 a useful marker for mesenchymal chondrosarcoma: An immunohistochemical study. Ann Diagn Pathol. 2021;50:151660.
62. Noujaim J, Thway K, Sheri A, Keller C, Jones RL. Histology-driven therapy: the importance of diagnostic accuracy in guiding systemic therapy of soft tissue tumors. Int J Surg Pathol. 2016;24(1):5–15.
63. Strobel O, Hackert T, Hartwig W, et al. Survival data justifies resection for pancreatic metastases. Ann Surg Oncol. 2009;16(12):3340–9.
64. Ladenstein R, Potschger U, Le Deley MC, et al. Primary disseminated multifocal Ewing sarcoma: results of the Euro-EWING 99 trial. J Clin Oncol. 2010;28(20):3284–91.
65. Sperti C, Moletta L, Patane G. Metastatic tumors to the pancreas: the role of surgery. World J Gastrointest Oncol. 2014;6(10):381–92.

Chapter 19
Open Whipple

Rachel C. Kim, Jackson A. Baril, and Trang K. Nguyen

Introduction and History

In 1898, Alessandro Codivilla attempted the first documented radical pancreatoduodenectomy for an "epithelioma," or carcinoma of the pancreas, when he was forced to perform an *en bloc* resection rather than the preferred enucleation at that time since the tumor was adherent to duodenum. Codivilla's patient died from cachexia 21 days after the procedure after experiencing wound drainage, "foul diarrhea," and eventually drainage of "milky clots," likely from a pancreatic fistula [1]. Soon after, William Halsted was the first to successfully resect a periampullary cancer, with a transduodenal approach and performing a wedge resection with adjacent segments of the pancreatic and common bile ducts, reimplanting both into the duodenum during the primary closure of the duodenal defect. The patient survived the operation, although still died within a year due to local recurrence of the cancer [2].

In the following decades, there would be several advances in the field of pancreatic surgery. Most notably, in 1935, Allen Oldfather Whipple, Surgeon-in-Chief at Columbia-Presbyterian Medical Center, published his first report on the radical resection of the head of the pancreas and duodenum in three patients. His initial technique was composed of a two-staged procedure, the first consisting of a cholecystogastrostomy and posterior loop gastrojejunostomy, the second composed of the partial duodenal and head of pancreas resection. The pancreatic stump was occluded [3]. Whipple would continue to make advancements in his technique, including condensing the surgery into a one-stage procedure, and in 1946, he

R. C. Kim · J. A. Baril
Department of Surgery, Indiana University School of Medicine, Indianapolis, IN, USA
e-mail: rckim@iu.edu; jbaril@iu.edu

T. K. Nguyen (✉)
Division of Surgical Oncology, Washington University in St. Louis, St. Louis, MO, USA
e-mail: ntrang@wustl.edu

E. P. Ceppa et al. (eds.), *The SAGES Manual of Evolving Techniques in Pancreatic Surgery*, https://doi.org/10.1007/978-3-031-78409-5_19

published his 10-year experience of 37 patients who underwent pancreaticoduodenectomy [4].

The Whipple operation was adapted and advanced outside of its eponym's experience. For instance, Whipple was initially averse to reconstructing the pancreatic duct, believing the anastomosis would place the other anastomoses at risk due to the activation of pancreatic enzymes in the duodenum. However, this approach led to frequent pancreatic fistulas, and in 1941, Verne Hunt successfully incorporated a pancreaticojejunostomy procedure to avoid pancreatic stump leakage [5]. This surgery of the pancreas also show high rates of marginal ulceration until the gastric anastomosis was moved from the most proximal to the most distal of the anastomoses, and adequate gastrectomy was routinely practiced [6]. In 1978, Traverso and Longmire reintroduced the idea of pylorus preservation, first described by Kenneth Watson in 1944, further reducing the frequency of marginal ulcers [7, 8]. The 1980s and beyond saw the dramatic reduction in mortality rates following the Whipple procedure from 20% to 40% to <5%, attributed to the centralization of this complex operation to high-volume centers and pioneered under the leadership of John Cameron at Johns Hopkins Hospital [9–11].

Preoperative Considerations

Preoperative Work-Up and Planning

All patients should undergo cross-sectional imaging prior to scheduled pancreatoduodenectomy, regardless of pathology. A high-quality CT "pancreas protocol" or magnetic resonance imaging (MRI) is recommended to define the anatomy. MRI may be particularly useful in evaluating small (<2 cm) pancreatic tumors and cystic lesions. No data has suggested any advantage in obtaining both CT and MRI.

When reviewing imaging, attention should be directed specifically toward evaluating:

- Relationship of any lesion to surrounding major vascular vessels, including but not limited to the superior mesenteric artery (SMA) and vein (SMV), portal vein (PV), and celiac trunk and its branches, including the common hepatic artery (CHA)
- Soft tissue planes, surfaces, and/or walls of the above major vessels for any distortion or other abnormality which may suggest tumor involvement
- Any anatomical variations, most commonly a replaced right hepatic artery originating from the SMA
- Any regional lymphadenopathy
- Hepatic lesions or other distant metastases

In addition to cross-sectional imaging, endoscopic evaluation is also commonly used in the diagnostic and preoperative work-up for most pancreatic lesions.

Endoscopic ultrasound (EUS) may be used to further characterize any lesion and evaluate any signs of vascular invasion or distortion and may be superior to CT in the detection of venous invasion specifically [12, 13]. Surgeons should also keep in mind that EUS quality and interpretation are operator dependent. Endoscopic retrograde cholangiopancreatography (ERCP) should be performed only if needed for therapeutic purposes (e.g., obstructive jaundice, etc.), due to the risk for post-procedure pancreatitis. Endoscopic ultrasound or a DOTATATE-PET can be considered for patients with pancreatic neuroendocrine tumors to evaluate for additional tumors.

Preoperative Assessment and Management

Patients' baseline functional status and medical comorbidities should be thoroughly assessed and optimized as much as possible prior to surgery. Cardiac risk stratification should be performed if appropriate. Baseline pancreatic endocrine and exocrine insufficiency should also be assessed. It is also important to educate the patient on perioperative expectations due to the high morbidity rate associated with the Whipple operation. Perioperative assessment and postoperative complications after pancreas surgery are discussed further in later chapters.

In the cases of malignancy, venous thromboembolism (VTE) prophylaxis is recommended for all patients with pancreatic cancer prior to surgery according to the American Society of Clinical Oncology (ASCO) 2019 Clinical Practice Guidelines [14]. However, while patients undergoing pancreatic resection for malignancy are certainly at higher risk for VTE, this should be balanced against the risk of perioperative hemorrhage, and the evidence for the benefit of preoperative VTE prophylaxis specific for hepatopancreatobiliary surgery remains inconsistent. The Americas Hepato-Pancreato-Biliary Association (AHPBA) guidelines thus advocate for critical thinking when weighing the potential benefits and risks of preoperative VTE prophylaxis prior to major pancreatic surgery such as the Whipple [15].

Patient Positioning and Set Up

Patients should be assessed in the preoperative area for any recent changes in their medical history. In the operating room, patients should be positioned supine with arms either out or tucked, on an operating table capable of mounting appropriate self-retaining retractors. When positioning the patient's arms, attention should be paid toward ensuring adequate room for the surgeon's desired retractors to be connected to the table. Sequential compression devices or antithrombotic stockings should be placed on the lower extremities. Appropriate preoperative antibiotic prophylaxis such as piperacillin-tazobactam should be administered prior to incision.

We recommend that the entire abdomen be prepped from approximately the nipple line to the level of the pubic symphysis. If a vascular resection with native graft reconstruction is at all anticipated being considered, the relevant donor areas should also be prepped.

Key Steps

Staging Laparoscopy

Whether a staging laparoscopy is performed to assess for small hepatic or peritoneal metastases in patients with malignancy is often dependent surgeon preference, as its yield has decreased as the quality of cross-sectional imaging has improved, but it still has a role in patients who are at increased risk for occult metastasis, such as in those with markedly elevated serum CA 19-9.

Any suspicious lesion should be biopsied and sent for pathologic review to assess for malignancy prior to proceed with the operation. Laparoscopic ultrasonography of the liver can also be considered.

Exposure and Dissection

Typically, an upper midline incision provides adequate exposure to the required operative field. Some surgeons prefer a bi-subcostal incision for patients with wide and short torsos. Once the abdomen is accessed, the falciform ligament is ligated distally and may be preserved to use as a pedicled falciform flap over the pancreaticojejunal anastomosis. Self-retaining retractors are placed until adequate and reliable exposure of the upper abdomen is achieved.

First, the hepatic flexure is mobilized. A wide Kocher maneuver is then performed, mobilizing the duodenum off the retroperitoneal tissue to the ligament of Treitz, exposing the inferior vena cava to the left renal vein. At this time, the SMA can be palpated behind the pancreas to assess for tumor involvement. High-quality cross-sectional imaging that shows no evidence of SMA involvement can render this maneuver unnecessary.

Next, the lesser sac of the peritoneum is accessed. This can be achieved by either dividing the gastrocolic ligament outside of the right gastroepiploic vessels or by freeing the omentum off the transverse colon and mesocolon. The third portion of the duodenum is then dissected free from the colonic mesentery and colon, fully mobilizing the transverse colon inferiorly and off the duodenum until the inferior edge of the pancreas and the SMV are exposed. In cases of pancreatic cancer, the middle colic vein may be involved in the tumor, in which case this vessel can be sacrificed. Interchangeably, entrance to the lesser sac can be done before

Kocherization of the duodenum. At this point, the trunk of Henle can be used as a landmark to trace the right gastroepiploic vein or the middle colic vein down to the superior mesenteric vein (Fig. 19.1a). The caudal edge of the pancreas is then exposed, and a retropancreatic tunnel is developed by blunt dissection between the pancreatic neck and portal vein (PV)-SMV confluence. Dissection directly on top of the middle of the PV-SMV confluence helps to stay in the avascular plane away from the lateral branches on both sides.

Next, attention can be turned to the hepatoduodenal ligament dissection and creating the retropancreatic tunnel from above. A top-down approach is used for the cholecystectomy. Caution should be taken to avoid the right hepatic artery, which most commonly runs posterior to the hepatic duct, but in some patients may run anteriorly. Additionally, as many as 10–15% of patients possess a replaced right hepatic artery, which can be palpated in the hepatoduodenal ligament, and thus preoperative evaluation of the patient's vascular anatomy on cross-sectional imaging is critical (Figs. 19.2 and 19.3) [18, 19].

Next, the portal triad is exposed and dissected. To achieve this, the peritoneal fat over is removed, and in this process, the right gastric artery is divided. The common hepatic artery (CHA) can be identified by the common hepatic artery node (station 8A), also known as "the node of importance." The CHA is traced to the gastroduodenal artery (GDA) and proper hepatic artery. The GDA is then test clamped to

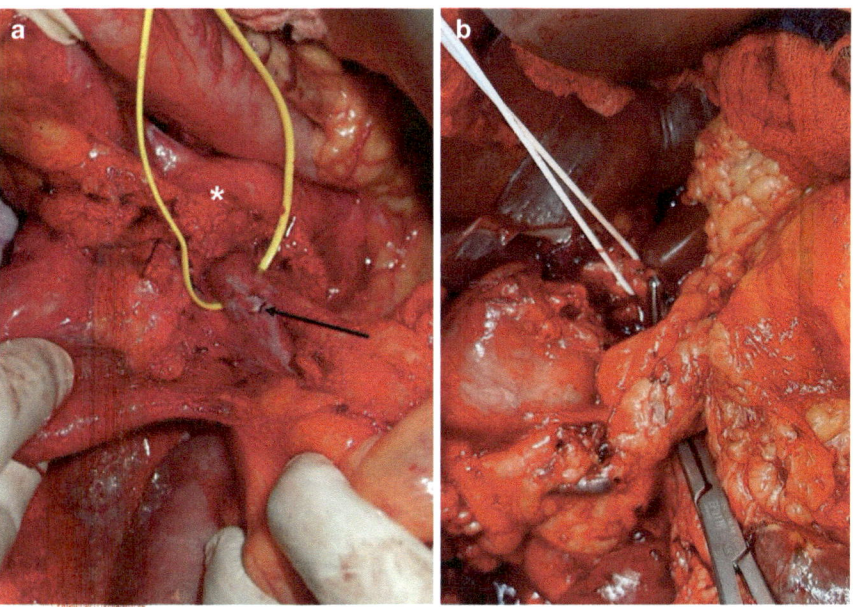

Fig. 19.1 (**a**) The trunk of Henle may be used to identify the SMV. Here, the right gastroepiploic vein has been ligated where it drains into the SMV (black arrow and yellow vessel loop. *marks pancreas) [16]. (**b**) A renal pedicle clamp traversing the retropancreatic tunnel, anterior along the PV/SMV. A vessel loop is around the proper hepatic artery

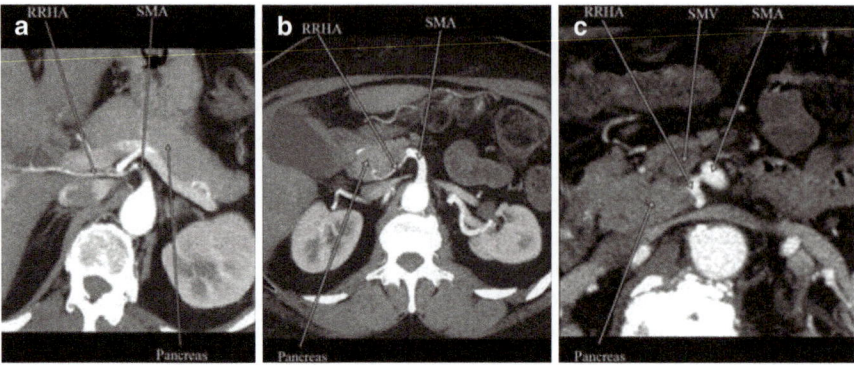

Fig. 19.2 CT imaging demonstrating replaced right hepatic artery (RRHA) anatomic variations, which should be evaluated carefully during preoperative work-up and planning. (**a**) RRHA coursing posterolateral to pancreatic head. (**b**) RRHA traversing the pancreatic head. (**c**) RRHA located within the SMV groove [17]

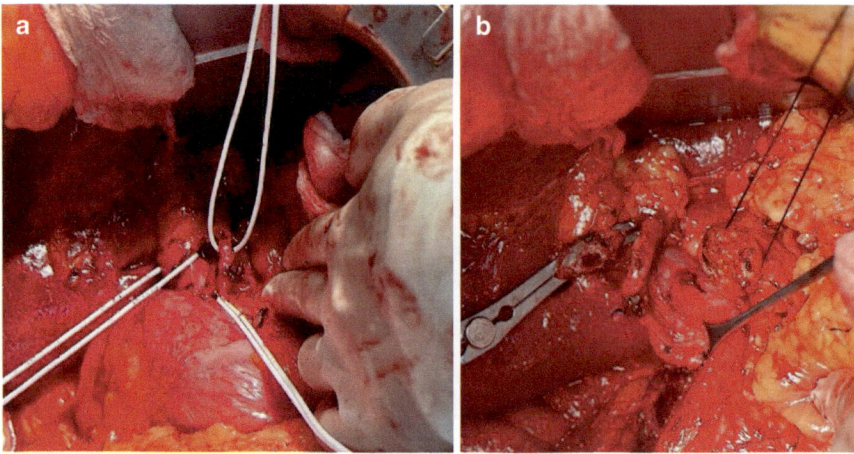

Fig. 19.3 (**a**) Replaced common hepatic artery emerging between the common bile duct (left vessel loop) and portal vein. Top vessel loop—proper hepatic artery, bottom vessel loop—GDA. (**b**) Following resection, the replaced common hepatic artery coming off the SMA and coursing over the SMV/PV. Bulldog—divided hepatic duct. Sutures—pancreatic neck. Vein retractor—SMV

ascertain continued perfusion of the left and right hepatic arteries. At this point, the GDA is ligated and divided. The common hepatic duct (CHD) is then identified and dissected, and finally divided above the insertion of the cystic duct. A bulldog clamp can be placed on the proximal CHD to prevent bile spillage.

The anterior surface of the portal vein should now be exposed posterior to the GDA stump. The tunnel behind the pancreatic neck can now be completed from above along the surface of the PV. Once the tunnel is completed, a vessel loop, umbilical tape, or Penrose drain can be passed through the tunnel for ease of identification and later retraction (Fig. 19.1b).

Specimen Removal

The neck of the pancreas is then transected over the previously developed tunnel over the PV. The superior and inferior pancreatic vessels can be suture ligated to limit bleeding during neck transection. The pancreatic parenchyma may be divided either sharply or with electrocautery; the main pancreatic duct should be identified and the duct itself should be divided sharply.

Attention is then turned to freeing and removing the planned specimen. Proximally, either the antrum of the stomach is divided into the classic Whipple, or the first portion of the duodenum is divided 1 or 2 cm distal to the pylorus in the pylorus-preserving Whipple. Distally, the jejunum is transected distal to the ligament of Treitz. The exact location of jejunal transection is dependent on the planned route for reconstruction and should be chosen such that biliopancreatic limb can reach the planned region for anastomosis in a tension-free manner. The jejunum is mobilized proximally from its mesentery close to the bowel wall until the ligament of Treitz, which is then divided. At this point, the duodenum and proximal jejunum should be completely freed from the remaining intestine and its attachments. Next, the uncinate process and lateral neck of the pancreas are carefully mobilized and dissected from the SMA and SMV/PV, with identification and ligation of the vein of Belcher (posterosuperior pancreaticoduodenal vein). At this point, any remaining attachments to the uncinate and specimen are divided, and the Whipple specimen is removed from the operative field (Fig. 19.4).

Vascular Resection

If a venous resection is needed, first the SMV should be fully dissected, and control of the inferior mesenteric vein (IMV), splenic vein, and left gastric vein should be achieved. Ligation of these veins may be necessary to fully resect the lesion. The PV and/or SMV can then be clamped proximally and distally, and the involved portion of the SMV or PV is then divided and removed with the specimen.

In some cases, the tumor may only just barely involve the lateral wall of the PV-SMV, in which case a tangential or primary repair of the vein may be considered, as long as it does not result in significant narrowing of the vein. However, more commonly a segmental vein resection is needed and thus reconstruction required. If there is adequate length of the portal vein, the PV may be reconstructed in an end-to-end fashion without the need for a graft. The right triangular ligament of the liver may also be divided for mobilization to further advance the reach of the proximal end of the vein.

Fig. 19.4 After the Whipple specimen has been removed, the PV-SMV confluence can be clearly visualized. X marks the transected bile duct [16]

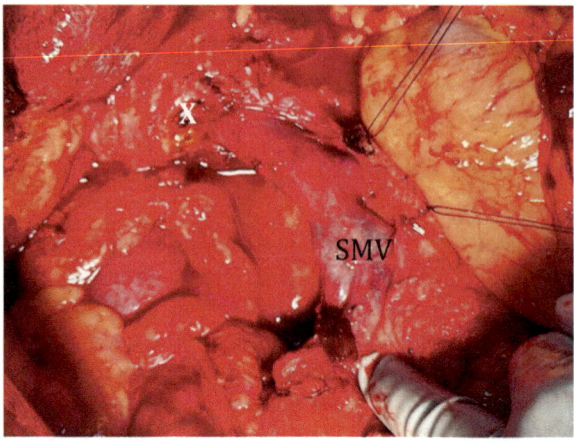

If there is inadequate length for a tension-free, primary end-to-end anastomosis of the resected vein, a conduit may be utilized using another donor vessel. Options include the internal jugular (IJ) vein or the superior femoral vein. The IJ may be harvested via an anterior neck incision along the sternocleidomastoid muscle. The superficial femoral vein may be harvested through a groin incision. If possible, the deep femoral vein should be preserved to avoid inadequate drainage of the lower extremity. The superficial femoral vein is typically narrower than the IJ, and choice of donor site should be dependent on patient-specific anatomy and SMV or PV caliper. Use of the left renal vein and cadaveric or synthetic grafts has also been described.

Reconstruction

In preparation for the reconstruction portion of the operation, the biliopancreatic limb of the jejunum can be brought up the right upper quadrant either retromesenteric via the ligament of Treitz or antimesenteric in the retrocolic space through a defect in the mesocolon to the right of the middle colic vessels.

Pancreaticojejunostomy

There are several variations in techniques and approaches to the pancreaticojejunostomy. To date, there has not been any consistent data supporting the superiority of one approach over others with regard to the rate of pancreatic leak or fistula. The techniques can mainly be categorized into duct-to-mucosa techniques and invagination or "dunking" techniques.

The duct-to-mucosa pancreaticojejunostomy is most commonly performed in a two-layered, end-to-side fashion. The original duct-to-mucosa technique was described by Cattel and Warren in 1956 with variations still in use [20]. The tissue is freed around the pancreatic stump. A posterior layer of interrupted sutures is placed between the posterior pancreatic capsule and seromuscular layer of the jejunum. An enterotomy is made opposite to the pancreatic duct. Interrupted sutures are then placed between the pancreatic duct including some of the surrounding pancreatic parenchyma and full thickness, including the mucosa, of the jejunal enterotomy. An anterior layer of interrupted sutures is then made between the anterior pancreatic capsule and seromuscular layer of the jejunum.

In the Blumgart technique [21], the first layer consists of transpancreatic horizontal mattress-style sutures approximately 2 cm from the cut surface of the pancreas. For each suture, the suture is first passed through and through and perpendicularly (straightening the needle may help to achieve this) to the pancreas from anterior to posterior. A small seromuscular bite is then taken along the jejunum approximately 3 cm away from the transected edge of the bowel. The suture is then passed again perpendicularly through the pancreas posterior to anterior. The needle should kept on the suture later for the final anterior layer. A probe may be placed in the pancreatic duct during the creation of this layer in order to ensure patency. The inner duct-to-mucosa layer is then completed; a small enterotomy is made in the jejunum approximately 1 cm away from the line of horizontal sutures. The pancreatic duct is then sewed to the enterotomy in an interrupted fashion. The posterior wall of the duct is completed first, the tension between the ends removed with the previously made horizontal mattress-type sutures, then the anterior wall. Once this inner layer is tied down and complete, the previously placed horizontal mattress transpancreatic sutures are tied down. The layer is then finished by taking another small seromuscular bite of the jejunum, anterior to the now anastomosed enterotomy, and tied down. The inferior most stitch is completed with two seromuscular jejunal bites, first vertically through the jejunum, with the needle directed anteriorly, then horizontally up toward the pancreas. The superior most stitch is completed in a similar fashion, with first a vertical jejunal bite, then a horizontal bite again directed back toward the pancreas. This allows the jejunum to fold over the anterior surface of the pancreas.

In the invagination pancreaticojejunostomy, all the cut edge of the pancreatic parenchyma is invaginated or "dunked" into the lumen of the jejunum. First, a posterior row of interrupted sutures are made from the pancreatic capsule, 1–2 cm back from the cut surface of the pancreas, to the jejunum using seromuscular bites. Then, a large enough enterotomy is made in the jejunum such that the entire cut surface of the pancreas can be approximated to the jejunal lumen. An inner layer of running locking suture is then made, taking full thickness jejunal bites and large bites of both pancreatic parenchyma and capsule. Finally, an anterior layer of seromuscular sutures are completed similar to the first posterior layer, rolling the jejunum onto the pancreatic capsule and fully "dunking" the pancreas. While the superiority of duct-to-mucosa vs invagination techniques has been debated, the ability to perform both types is useful for adapting to differences in pancreatic duct size and texture [22].

As mentioned earlier, there are many other approaches to the pancreaticojejunostomy, or modifications of the techniques described above. Some surgeons also place a stent or small pediatric feeding tube through the anastomosis as a guide. Leaving an internal stent has fallen out of favor as it has not been shown to decrease pancreatic fistula rates, in fact may increase the risk for them, and postoperative stent complications and migration may occur [23]. However, externalized pancreatic duct stents and omission of prophylactic octreotide have been shown to be effective risk mitigation strategies for situations at high risk for the development of clinically relevant postoperative pancreatic fistulas [24]. Regardless of which method is used, attention should be focused on maintaining good technique and the tenets of any safe anastomosis, including but not limited to careful tissue handling, tension-free layout, adequate perfusion, and no occlusion or distal obstruction.

Hepaticojejunostomy

There are also multiple approaches to the hepaticojejunostomy, although not as numerous as for the pancreaticojejunostomy. The end-to-side anastomosis is made distally along the biliopancreatic limb, is typically single-layered, full thickness, and may be performed in a continuous, interrupted, or mixed fashion. Leaving enough length between the two anastomoses may be useful, particularly in benign cases, in the event future revision to either anastomosis is needed. Theoretically, this may also reduce the risk of activation of the pancreatic enzymes by bile if there is an anastomotic leak.

The "corner" stitches are first placed, at the 3 o'clock and 9 o'clock positions. If done in an interrupted fashion, placing the anterior sutures in the bile duct first can assist with holding the duct open while suturing the posterior wall. Once the anastomosis is completed, the jejunum is tacked to the mesocolon to prevent internal herniation as well as to maintain a tension-free layout to the anastomoses.

Gastro- or Duodeno-Jejunostomy

Whether a classic or pylorus-preserving Whipple is to be performed should depend on the extent of the tumor. There has been no consistent data showing any difference in oncologic outcomes with either procedure, and the rate of delayed gastric emptying and other functional complications are similar in both approaches [25, 26].

In the case of a classic Whipple, a gastrojejunostomy is created in a side-to-side or end-to-side fashion. If a pylorus-preserving Whipple is performed, a duodenojejunostomy is created either in an isoperistaltic side-to-side or end-to-side fashion. This is completed in a standard, handsewn, two-layered intestinal reconstruction approach, with a continuous inner mucosal layer and a seromuscular, interrupted outer layer. The anastomosis is made approximately 30–50 cm downstream of the hepaticojejunostomy. A <30-degree vertical efferent limb flow angle and a gastrojejunal anastomosis are associated with lower delayed gastric emptying rates [27]. The gastro/duodenojejunal anastomosis completes the reconstruction portion of the surgery.

Final Steps

The abdomen is irrigated and inspected for hemostasis. The omentum and/or falciform ligament can be placed between the GDA stump and the pancreatic and biliary anastomoses to help mitigate complications in case of an anastomotic leak.

There has historically been mixed data in the literature regarding routine intraperitoneal drainage after Whipple, with some studies failing to show a clear benefit [28, 29]. However, more recently, a multi-institutional randomized controlled trial demonstrated that intraperitoneal drainage improved both the frequency and severity of postoperative complications. The study itself was also halted early as interval analysis showed a higher risk for mortality in patients without intraperitoneal drains (12% vs 3%) [30]. Routine nasogastric decompression has also not been shown to decrease risk of postoperative complications such as aspiration or anastomotic leak, and thus is not strictly necessary [31]. Intraoperative percutaneous feeding tube placement has also been associated with increased postoperative morbidity in retrospective studies [32, 33]. Ultimately, the decision to place of any of these adjuncts at the end of the surgery should be dependent on patient-specific factors and surgeon's preference.

References

1. Schnelldorfer T, Sarr MG. Alessandro Codivilla and the first pancreatoduodenectomy. Arch Surg. 2009;144(12):1179–84.
2. Halsted WS. Contributions to the surgery of the bile passages, especially of the common bile-duct. Boston Med Surg J. 1899;141(26):645–54.
3. Whipple AO, Parsons WB, Mullins CR. Treatment of carcinoma of the ampulla of Vater. Ann Surg. 1935;102(4):763–79.
4. Whipple AO. Observations on radical surgery for lesions of the pancreas. Surg Gynecol Obstet. 1946;82:623–31.
5. Hunt VC. Surgical management of carcinoma of the ampulla of vater and of the periampullary portion of the duodenum. Ann Surg. 1941;114(4):570–602.
6. Are C, Dhir M, Ravipati L. History of pancreaticoduodenectomy: early misconceptions, initial milestones and the pioneers. HPB (Oxford). 2011;13(6):377–84.
7. Traverso LW, Longmire WP Jr. Preservation of the pylorus in pancreaticoduodenectomy. Surg Gynecol Obstet. 1978;146(6):959–62.
8. Watson K. Carcinoma of ampulla of Vater successful radical resection. Br J Surg. 1944;31(124):368–73.
9. Griffin JF, Poruk KE, Wolfgang CL. Pancreatic cancer surgery: past, present, and future. Chin J Cancer Res. 2015;27(4):332–48.
10. Gordon TA, Bowman HM, Tielsch JM, Bass EB, Burleyson GP, Cameron JL. Statewide regionalization of pancreaticoduodenectomy and its effect on in-hospital mortality. Ann Surg. 1998;228(1):71–8.
11. Winter JM, Cameron JL, Campbell KA, et al. 1423 pancreaticoduodenectomies for pancreatic cancer: a single-institution experience. J Gastrointest Surg. 2006;10(9):1199–210; discussion 210–1.

12. Hunt GC, Faigel DO. Assessment of EUS for diagnosing, staging, and determining resectability of pancreatic cancer: a review. Gastrointest Endosc. 2002;55(2):232–7.
13. Varadarajulu S, Eloubeidi MA. The role of endoscopic ultrasonography in the evaluation of pancreatico-biliary cancer. Surg Clin North Am. 2010;90(2):251–63.
14. Key NS, Khorana AA, Kuderer NM, et al. Venous thromboembolism prophylaxis and treatment in patients with cancer: ASCO clinical practice guideline update. J Clin Oncol. 2020;38(5):496–520.
15. Clancy TE, Baker EH, Maegawa FA, Raoof M, Winslow E, House MG. AHPBA guidelines for managing VTE prophylaxis and anticoagulation for pancreatic surgery. HPB (Oxford). 2022;24(5):575–85.
16. Logarajah SI, Jackson T, Darwish M, et al. Whipple pancreatoduodenectomy: a technical illustration. Surg Open Sci. 2022;7:62–7.
17. Staśkiewicz G, Torres K, Denisow M, Torres A, Czekajska-Chehab E, Drop A. Clinically relevant anatomical parameters of the replaced right hepatic artery (RRHA). Surg Radiol Anat. 2015;37(10):1225–31.
18. Sayyed R, Baig M, Khan A, Niazi IK, Syed AA, Hanif F. Hepatic arterial system anomalies encountered during pancreaticoduodenectomy - our experience. J Pak Med Assoc. 2020;70(2):337–40.
19. Dandekar U, Dandekar K, Chavan S. Right hepatic artery: a cadaver investigation and its clinical significance. Anat Res Int. 2015;2015:412595.
20. Warren KW, Cattell RB. Basic techniques in pancreatic surgery. Surg Clin North Am. 1956;36(3):707–24.
21. Maithel SK, Allen PJ. Techniques of pancreatic resection: pancreaticoduodenectomy, distal pancreatectomy, segmental pancreatectomy, total pancreatectomy, and transduodenal resection of the papilla of Vater. In: Jarnagin WR, Allen PJ, Chapman WC, et al., editors. Blumgart's surgery of the liver, biliary tract and pancreas. 6th ed. Elsevier; 2017. p. 1007–23.
22. Berger AC, Howard TJ, Kennedy EP, et al. Does type of pancreaticojejunostomy after pancreaticoduodenectomy decrease rate of pancreatic fistula? A randomized, prospective, dual-institution trial. J Am Coll Surg. 2009;208(5):738–47; discussion 47–9.
23. Winter JM, Cameron JL, Campbell KA, et al. Does pancreatic duct stenting decrease the rate of pancreatic fistula following pancreaticoduodenectomy? Results of a prospective randomized trial. J Gastrointest Surg. 2006;10(9):1280–90; discussion 90.
24. Ecker BL, McMillan MT, Asbun HJ, et al. Characterization and optimal management of high-risk pancreatic anastomoses during pancreatoduodenectomy. Ann Surg. 2018;267(4):608–16.
25. Horstmann O, Markus PM, Ghadimi MB, Becker H. Pylorus preservation has no impact on delayed gastric emptying after pancreatic head resection. Pancreas. 2004;28(1):69–74.
26. Seiler CA, Wagner M, Sadowski C, Kulli C, Büchler MW. Randomized prospective trial of pylorus-preserving vs. classic duodenopancreatectomy (Whipple procedure): initial clinical results. J Gastrointest Surg. 2000;4(5):443–52.
27. Jung JP, Zenati MS, Dhir M, et al. Use of video review to investigate technical factors that may be associated with delayed gastric emptying after pancreaticoduodenectomy. JAMA Surg. 2018;153(10):918–27.
28. Conlon KC, Labow D, Leung D, et al. Prospective randomized clinical trial of the value of intraperitoneal drainage after pancreatic resection. Ann Surg. 2001;234(4):487–93; discussion 493–4.
29. McMillan MT, Fisher WE, Van Buren G 2nd, et al. The value of drains as a fistula mitigation strategy for pancreatoduodenectomy: something for everyone? Results of a randomized prospective multi-institutional study. J Gastrointest Surg. 2015;19(1):21–30; discussion 30–1.
30. Van Buren G 2nd, Bloomston M, Hughes SJ, et al. A randomized prospective multicenter trial of pancreaticoduodenectomy with and without routine intraperitoneal drainage. Ann Surg. 2014;259(4):605–12.

31. Cheatham ML, Chapman WC, Key SP, Sawyers JL. A meta-analysis of selective versus routine nasogastric decompression after elective laparotomy. Ann Surg. 1995;221(5):469–76; discussion 476–8.
32. Soufi M, Al-Temimi M, Nguyen TK, et al. Friend or foe? Feeding tube placement at the time of pancreatoduodenectomy: propensity score case-matched analysis. Surg Endosc. 2022;36(5):2994–3000.
33. Nussbaum DP, Zani S, Penne K, et al. Feeding jejunostomy tube placement in patients undergoing pancreaticoduodenectomy: an ongoing dilemma. J Gastrointest Surg. 2014;18(10):1752–9.

Chapter 20
Laparoscopic Pancreatoduodenectomy

Núria Lluís, Domenech Asbun, and Horacio J. Asbun

Beginnings of Laparoscopic Pancreatoduodenectomy

On average, 17 years elapsed from conception to application of a clinical novelty [1]. Despite the onset of laparoscopic surgery in the mid-1980s, it would be several decades later before laparoscopic pancreatoduodenectomy (LPD) became an accepted operation by pancreatic surgeons. Its implementation required adequate technological advancements and the courage of pioneering surgeons, whose vision and commitment made LPD a feasible and safe technique (Fig. 20.1). LPD has evolved over the last two decades, as detailed in the historic pearls below.

In 1994, Gagner et al. [2] published the first description of LPD in a patient with chronic pancreatitis. However, early experiences with LPD were discouraging due to the lack of proper minimally invasive equipment and surgical expertise that were still being developed at the time. In 2007, Palanivelu et al. [3] published the first series, including 42 patients with mainly malignant pancreatic diseases, and reported 5-year survival rates ranging from 19.1% to 50%, depending on tumor type and lymph node positivity. In 2010, Kendrick et al. [4] reported 62 patients with different types of malignant and benign diseases and described a median length of hospital stay of 7 days, with 42% of postoperative morbidity events, and one death. In 2012, Asbun et al. [5] compared the outcomes of 215 patients who underwent an open pancreatoduodenectomy (OPD) and 53 patients who underwent a laparoscopic approach, and reported that LPD was feasible, without differences in overall or pancreas-specific complications, and a higher lymph node retrieval rate when compared with the open approach.

N. Lluís · D. Asbun · H. J. Asbun (✉)
Division of Hepatobiliary and Pancreas Surgery, Miami Cancer Institute, Miami, FL, USA
e-mail: horacioa@baptisthealth.net; domenech.asbun@baptisthealth.net

© The Author(s), under exclusive license to Springer Nature Switzerland AG 2025
E. P. Ceppa et al. (eds.), *The SAGES Manual of Evolving Techniques in Pancreatic Surgery*, https://doi.org/10.1007/978-3-031-78409-5_20

343

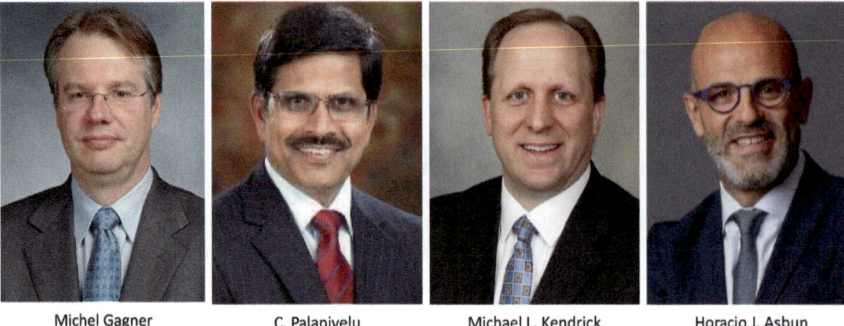

Michel Gagner   C. Palanivelu   Michael L. Kendrick   Horacio J. Asbun

Fig. 20.1 Pioneer surgeons whose vision and commitment made laparoscopic pancreatoduode-nectomy a feasible and safe technique

Comparing Outcomes Between Laparoscopic and Open Approach

Further research has delved into the comparison between the laparoscopic and open approaches to pancreatoduodenectomy. Between 2017 and 2022, 19 studies used propensity score matching analysis to compare outcomes of the two approaches (Table 20.1). The most frequent short-term finding was that the laparoscopic approach resulted in shorter hospital stays. Moreover, some studies noted a decrease in readmission rates, delayed gastric emptying, pain, and use of painkillers. However, there was a mixed result on pancreatic fistula rate, with one study showing a lower rate and another showing an increased rate. In most studies, postoperative morbidity and mortality were similar for both approaches. In terms of oncological outcomes, several studies reported that the laparoscopic approach achieved a comparable negative resection margin rate, with more lymph nodes harvested in one study and fewer in another. Another study found similar tumor progression-free survival, while several studies reported similar overall survival rates. Overall, these findings suggested that LPD achieves non-inferior short- and long-term outcomes when compared to the open procedure.

The findings were further consolidated through subsequent analyses of more comprehensive data. A meta-analysis of eight studies revealed that there was no significant difference in the 5-year overall survival rate between both surgical approaches. Furthermore, laparoscopic surgery was found to have a higher rate of R0 resection and harvested lymph nodes when compared to the open approach [25]. In addition, for elderly patients, another meta-analysis reported no significant differences in blood loss, postoperative pancreatic fistula, and length of hospital stay [26].

Specific benchmark outcomes were provided for LPD in an international multicenter study published in 2019 [27]. The outcomes of low-risk patients undergoing LPD in three centers with expertise in minimally invasive surgery were compared to the benchmark values obtained in low-risk patients undergoing open pancreatoduodenectomy in an international multicenter study. Operative time (benchmark <=7.5 h)

Table 20.1 Retrospective studies using propensity score matching analysis to compare outcomes after laparoscopic versus open pancreatoduodenectomy

Author	Country	Year	Design	Primary outcome	Baseline, n	Outcomes after PSM, lap vs open
Conrad [6]	US	2017	Single-center	Long-term, oncologic, ADC	40 lap, 25 open	• Similar overall and recurrence-free survival
Kutlu [7]	US	2018	Multicenter, NCDB	Short-term according to hospital volume of PDs	430 lap, 4309 open	• The benefits of the lap vs open approach (shorter LOHS, fewer readmissions) were only achieved in hospitals with a high volume of cases (≥25 PDs per year)
Lee [8]	Korea	2018	Single-center	Short-term, benign and borderline disease	31 lap, 76 open	• Less postoperative pain • Shorter LOHS
Nassour [9]	US	2018	Multicenter, ACS-NSQIP	Short-term	334 lap, 4150 open	• Similar morbidity and mortality • Decreased rate of prolonged LOHS • Increased readmission rate
Park [10]	Korea	2018	Single-center	Short-term, acute kidney injury	177 lap, 632 open	• Shorter LOHS • Similar incidence of postoperative acute kidney injury
Shin [11]	Korea	2019	Single-center	Short- and long-term, elderly (≥70 years)	56 lap, 270 open	• Lower pancreatic fistula rate • Less use of painkillers • Similar 3-year overall survival and disease-free survival

(continued)

Table 20.1 (continued)

Author	Country	Year	Design	Primary outcome	Baseline, n	Outcomes after PSM, lap vs open
Zhou [12]	China	2019	Two centers	Short- and long-term, ADC	79 lap, 230 open	• Lower delayed gastric emptying rate • Similar rates of major complications • Similar overall survival
El Nakeeb [13]	Egypt	2020	Single-center	Short- and long-term	37 lap, 74 open	• Shorter LOHS • Similar oncologic outcomes and survival
Han [14]	Korea	2020	Single-center	Short-term	104 lap, 113 open	• Similar morbidity and mortality • Similar negative resection margin rate
Klompmaker [15]	Europe	2020	Multicenter, 14 centers, robotic cases were also included	Short-term	412 lap, 729 open	• Similar LOHS, major morbidity and mortality • Few minimally invasive procedures per center
Yoo [16]	Korea	2020	Single-center	Short- and long-term, ampulla of Vater carcinoma	76 lap, 283 open	• Less use of painkillers • Fewer grade ≥ II complications • Shorter LOHS • Similar overall and recurrence-free survival
Chen [17]	China	2021	Single-center	Short- and long-term, ADC	128 lap, 288 open	• Similar early oncologic and postoperative outcomes • Similar recurrence rate and overall survival
Cheng [18]	China	2021	Single-center, only lap cases	Short- and long-term, liver cirrhosis	28 cirrhotic, 325 control	• Cirrhotic patients had more postoperative complications

(continued)

Table 20.1 (continued)

Author	Country	Year	Design	Primary outcome	Baseline, n	Outcomes after PSM, lap vs open
Dang [19]	China	2021	Single-center	Short- and long-term, non-pancreatic periampullary ADC	172 lap, 316 open	• Less LOHS • Less 30-day and 90-day mortality rate • Similar long-term survival
Ding [20]	China	2021	Single-center	Short-term	114 lap, 140 open	• More harvested lymph nodes • Pancreatic fistula was more common
Katsuki [21]	Japan	2021	Multicenter	Short-term	96 lap, 2004 open	• Similar LOHS and complications • Higher total hospitalization costs
Mazzola [22]	Italy	2021	Single-center	Short-term	52 lap, 125 open	• Shorter LOHS • Similar morbidity and postoperative mortality
Kim [23]	Korea	2022	Two centers	Short- and long-term, distal cholangio-carcinoma	91 lap, 335 open	• Shorter LOHS • Less harvested lymph nodes • Similar R0 resection rate • Similar long-term survival
Zhang [24]	China	2022	Single-center	Long-term, ADC	64 lap, 80 open	• Similar overall survival • Similar adjuvant therapy utilization

ADC adenocarcinoma; *NCDB* National Cancer Data Base; *LOHS* length of hospital stays; *ACS-NSQIP* American College of Surgeons-National Surgical Quality Improvement Program

and readmission rates (benchmark <=21%) exceeded reference values in two of the three centers, whereas other indicators, such as postoperative pancreatic fistula rates, ranged between 0% and 23% (benchmark <=19%). The remaining indicators were within the reference values. More recently, the Miami International Evidence-based Guidelines on Minimally Invasive Pancreas Resection reiterated the need of high-quality prospective data to continuously assess the outcomes of LPD (Table 20.2) [28].

Table 20.2 Recommendations of the Miami international evidence-based guidelines on minimally invasive pancreas resection [28] on the use of minimally invasive (MIPD) vs open pancreatoduodenectomy (OPD)

Recommendation	Grade
• There is insufficient data to recommend MIPD over OPD. Centers performing MIPD should be including all their MIPD outcomes data into national and international registries, and prospectively maintained pancreas databases	2A
• Both MIPD and OPD are valid approaches for selected patients with adenocarcinoma	2B
• No comparative data regarding MIPD vs OPD after neoadjuvant therapy exists and further investigation is warranted	Expert opinion
• Limited comparative data regarding vascular resection in MIPD vs OPD exist and further investigation is warranted. MIPD with vascular resection should only be performed by highly experienced surgeons and in high-volume centers	1C

2A weak recommendation, high quality of evidence; *2B* weak recommendation, moderate quality of evidence; *1C* strong recommendation, weak quality of evidence

Randomized Controlled Trials

To date, four randomized controlled trials comparing short-term outcomes of LPD versus OPD have been published (Table 20.3). Two single-center trials (India [29] and Spain [30]) and two multicenter trials (Netherlands [31] and China [32]) have been performed. These studies focused on length of hospital stay, morbidity, mortality, and time to functional recovery. The Dutch series was terminated early due to concerns regarding complication-related mortality [31]. In the design of this study, participating surgeons were required to have done/participated in only 20 LPD which was since confirmed not to be a sufficient experience to overcome the learning curve and may have played a role in the associated complication-related mortality for the laparoscopic arm. Length of hospital stay was significantly shorter in the laparoscopic arm in the remaining three trials that completed [29, 30, 32] although this was a marginal benefit in one of them [32]. Only one trial [30] showed a reduction in postoperative complications with the laparoscopic approach. Based on these results, the laparoscopic approach has established itself as a solid alternative, in experienced hands, to the open approach in terms of short-term postoperative outcomes. Future randomized controlled trials should determine with a higher level of evidence the long-term and oncologic outcomes of LPD.

Surgical Technique

A detailed explanation of the surgical technique developed and used for over 20 years during LPD is described. The authors preferentially perform pylorus-preserving LPD although the technique can be adjusted in cases where a distal gastrectomy is performed. Surgical instruments and materials commonly used for this procedure are listed in Table 20.4. Advanced laparoscopic skills are required to perform LPD. However, with appropriate commitment and dedication, a surgeon

Table 20.3 Published randomized controlled trials comparing short-term outcomes after laparoscopic versus open pancreatoduodenectomy

Study	Country	Year	Design	Primary outcome	n	Postoperative outcomes
PLOT [29]	India	2017	Single-center, open-label	LOHS	32 lap vs 32 open	• LOHS, median (range): lap 7 (5–52) vs open 13 (6–30), $p = 0.001$ • Similar overall complications and mortality
PADULAP [30]	Spain	2018	Single-center, open-label	LOHS	34 lap vs 32 open	• LOHS, median (range): lap 13.5 (5–54) vs open 17 (6–150), $p = 0.024$ • Clavien-Dindo grade complications ≥3: lap 5 vs open 11, $p = 0.04$ • Similar oncological standards
LEOPARD-2 [31]	Netherlands	2019	Multicenter, patient-blinded, phases 2/3	Safety (phase 2), functional recovery (phase 3)	50 lap vs 49 open	• Complication-related mortality: lap 10% vs open 2%, $p = 0.2$ • Early terminated
MITG-P-CPAM [32]	China	2021	Multicenter, open-label	LOHS	297 lap vs 297 open	• LOHS, median (95% CI): lap 15 (14–16) vs open 16 (15–17), $p = 0.02$ • Similar short-term morbidity and mortality

LOHS, length of hospital stays

can reach the level of expertise needed to perform a safe LPD procedure. Furthermore, several areas of the world do not have access readily available to the robotic platform due to the significant cost involved. In these areas, surgeons have chosen not to be marginalized by the hypothetical idea that one must be an absolute maverick to reach the level of skill necessary. It is in these countries where LPD is being done safely as it is performed in the hands of younger surgeons that have committed to learn the technique as the junior authors in this chapter. Additionally, the authors feel that the magnification and better access to difficult areas offered by the laparoscope ensure a meticulous resection of lesions located in the head of the pancreas and more precise anastomoses than in the open technique, when a small pancreatic duct is present.

1. Patient monitoring devices
   Intravenous access is gained with two large-bore venous catheters and, when needed because of patient comorbidities, a central venous line. An intra-arterial

Table 20.4 Surgical instruments and materials commonly used for laparoscopic pancreatoduodenectomy

• Laparoscopic 5 mm, 0°, camera mounted on an optical insufflating port
• Laparoscopic 10 mm, 45°, 4K camera with ICG capability (resection phase)
• Laparoscopic 10 mm 3D camera (reconstruction phase)
• Smoke evacuator
• Insufflators (x2)
• Laparoscopic liver retractor mounted on an iron intern retractor holder
• Energy devices: Ultrasonic shears, advanced bipolar, and bipolar
• Regular laparoscopic graspers
• Laparoscopic large bowel clamp
• Maryland curved dissector (3 mm and 5 mm)
• Laparoscopic right-angle dissector (3 mm and 5 mm)
• Laparoscopic staplers (vascular and enteric loads)
• Finger retractor
• Laparoscopic curved bulldog and bulldog applicator (10 mm)
• Penrose drain (end cut in long, thin diagonal)
• Endoscopic Kittner
• Vessel loop
• Pediatric 5 Fr pancreatic stent
• Needle driver, 3 mm, mounted in 5 mm shaft
• Sutures: Spiral barbed 3-0 and 4-0; polyglactin 5-0 with a TF (ophthalmologic) needle, and other sutures according to surgeon's preference
• Small, medium, and large-sized clips
• Indocyanine green (ICG)
• Laparoscopic ultrasound with Doppler capability
• Blake 15 Fr drain (x2)
• Laparoscopic 15 cm retrieval bag

catheter, a urinary catheter, and a pulse oximeter are used. General endotracheal anesthesia is induced, and the stomach is decompressed with an orogastric tube. No nasogastric tube is used postoperatively. Pneumatic compression stockings are applied.

2. Patient positioning

The patient is placed in a supine, split-leg position, and carefully secured to the operative table. Proper padding of pressure points is ensured. Table tilting throughout the procedure and the use of gravity will be extremely helpful to achieve proper exposure of the areas of interest and will avoid organ injury due to unnecessary grasping. The proper height of the operative table, position of the screen, as well as the angle of surgeon's shoulders, elbows, and wrists are essential to ensure ergonomics are maintained throughout this long procedure.

3. Position of surgical team members

The surgeon stands between the patient's legs for most of the procedure, except during the biliary reconstruction, when the surgeon moves to the right side of the patient. The first assistant stands on the left side of the patient, and the second assistant on the right. The scrub technician is in between the surgeon and the first assistant.

4. Port placement

A 5 mm, 0°, optical insufflating port, placed in the subxiphoid area and to the left of midline, or in the mid left abdomen depending on body habitus, is used to establish pneumoperitoneum. Its small opening at the tip of the trocar allows for insufflation without requiring the insertion of the entire trocar, avoiding organ injury in case adhesions are present. The layers of the abdominal wall (skin, subcutaneous fat, anterior fascia, rectus abdominis muscle, posterior fascia, and pre-peritoneum) are visually evaluated as CO_2 is insufflated while advancing the trocar. Standard intra-abdominal pressure is initially applied, although it should be modified according to the patient's tolerance of pneumoperitoneum. A total of two 5 mm ports and four 12 mm ports are placed in a semicircular pattern (Fig. 20.2). The trocars are placed under direct visualization, initially keeping the laparoscope in port 6. Ports 1 and 6 are 5 mm; the rest are 12 mm. Usually ports 3, 4, and 5 are about 8 cm apart from each other and at about 16 cm from the xiphoid for all body habitus types. Port 1 should be placed in the subcostal region, high and lateral within the abdomen which will ease biliary reconstruction. The laparoscope is switched to a 10 mm, 45°, inserted through port 4. The hepatic surface and peritoneum are explored to rule out the presence of metastatic deposits.

Fig. 20.2 Port placement (Figure reproduced with permission of Horacio J Asbun)

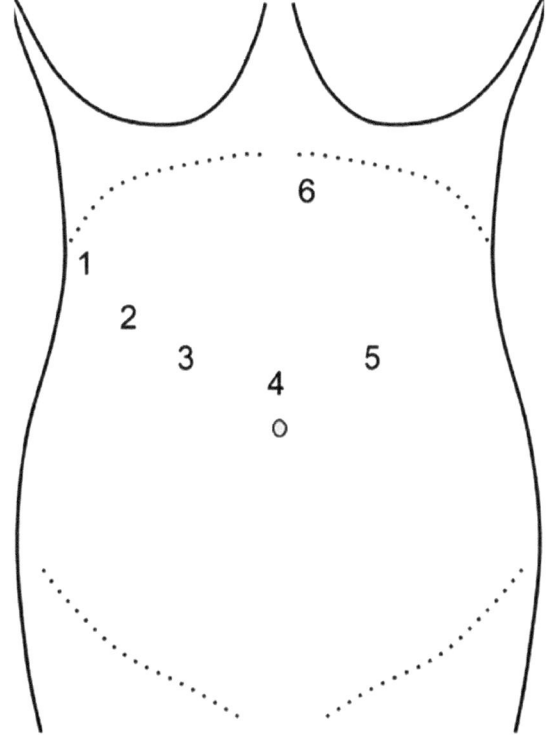

Resection Phase

The procedure starts with two maneuvers that will improve field exposure. First, the ligamentum teres is fixed to the anterior abdominal wall using a nylon suture on a Keith needle passed through the abdominal wall to encircle the structure. Second, a table-mounted liver retractor is placed though port 1 and the liver retracted cephalad/anteriorly.

5. Omental division

   The patient is now placed in a reverse Trendelenburg position. The greater omentum is longitudinally split using ultrasonic shears, starting at the inferior edge left of midline and directed toward the middle of hepatic segment III. The plane of transection should be chosen bearing in mind an estimate of an anticipated location of the eventual antecolic duodenojejunostomy, which is usually about the midpoint of the inferior edge of the left lateral segment of the liver. This maneuver will also facilitate exposure of the area of the ligament of Treitz. Any adhesions here should be taken down now to facilitate jejunal mobilization at a later stage.

6. Lesser sac entry

   The lesser sac is entered through the gastrocolic ligament along the greater curve, preserving the gastroepiploic arcade. Dissection proceeds to the right, extending toward the area of the gallbladder. The first assistant retracts the stomach superiorly with a swiping maneuver using a grasper in port 1. The dissection is extended up to the area of the trunk of Henle. Omental adhesions to the gallbladder or liver are taken down.

7. Colonic hepatic flexure mobilization

   The proximal transverse colon, hepatic flexure, and part of the right colon are mobilized from the retroperitoneum and retracted medially. The dissection is carried through an avascular plane between the right mesocolon and retroperitoneal fat anterior to Gerota's fascia. The duodenum and head of the pancreas will then be exposed, which will later on facilitate the performance of the Kocher maneuver.

8. Tributaries of the trunk of Henle division

   The tributaries of the trunk of Henle are exposed better once the right colon has been mobilized and retracted by gravity away from the upper abdomen. Once identified, the tributaries are isolated using a finger-type retractor which is passed very close to the duodenal wall (Fig. 20.3). These structures are encircled *en bloc* with the surrounding adipose tissue, ligated, and divided using a vascular stapler inserted through port 5. After this division, the near-complete mobilized colon should now fall further because of gravity afforded by the reverse Trendelenburg position and slight left-tilt of the table, giving adequate exposure to the pylorus and duodenum.

9. Duodenum division

   Dissection continues to free the first portion of the duodenum. Small vessels emanating from the head of the pancreas to the first portion of the duodenum

Fig. 20.3 Tributaries of the trunk of Henle are encircled using a finger-type retractor passed very close to the duodenal wall (Figure reproduced with permission of Horacio J Asbun)

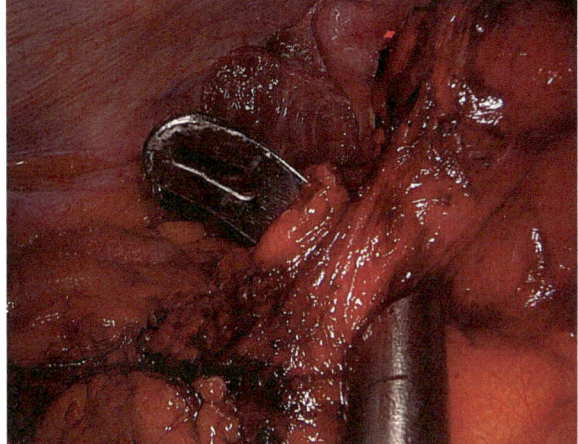

Fig. 20.4 Numerous small vessels emanating from the head of the pancreas to the first portion of the duodenum must be ligated and divided. The use of ultrasonic shears applied in small bites under direct visualization can be helpful to avoid any major vascular injury (Figure reproduced with permission of Horacio J Asbun)

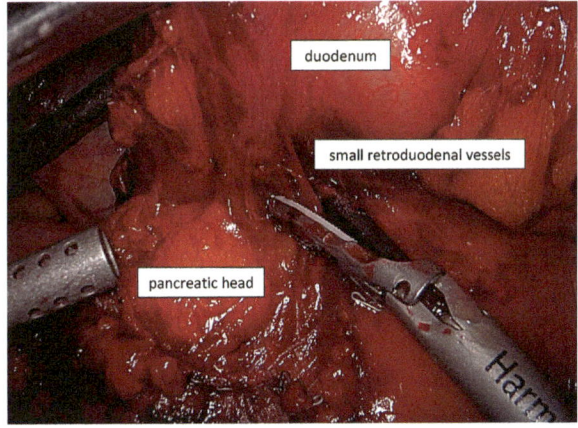

may be encountered and must be ligated and divided (Fig. 20.4). Important vascular structures, such as the common hepatic artery or gastroduodenal artery (GDA), might be encountered in this area as one proceeds posterior to the pylorus, and they should be avoided. The use of ultrasonic shears applied in small bites under direct visualization can be helpful to avoid any vascular injury. The pylorus should be clearly identified. The right gastric artery may be identified and can be isolated and divided before or after division of the duodenum. Care has been taken to preserve the gastroepiploic arcade avoiding entirely devascularizing the pylorus. A finger-type retractor is used to create a tunnel that encircles the first portion of the duodenum. The orogastric tube is partially removed. The duodenum is transversely transected, 2–3 cm distal to the pylorus, using a laparoscopic 60 mm stapler with a blue load, inserted through port 5 (Fig. 20.5). An oblique transection of the bowel should be avoided since it would make the duodenojejunostomy more technically challenging.

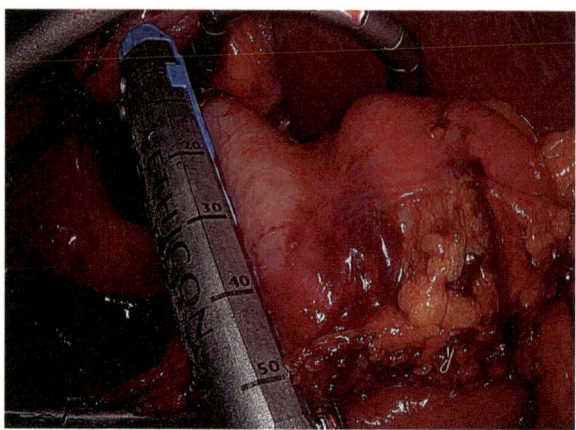

Fig. 20.5 Division of the first portion of the duodenum. The authors preferentially perform pylorus-preserving LPD, although the technique can be adjusted in cases where a distal gastrectomy is performed. The stapler is placed under direct visualization in a manner to optimize the duodenal stump for the future gastrointestinal anastomosis (Figure reproduced with permission of Horacio J Asbun)

10. Pylorus and antrum mobilization

    The hepatogastric ligament is incised at the level of the pylorus, and dissection is progressed through the pars flaccida toward the lesser curvature of the stomach. If still intact, the right gastric artery is ligated and divided. Dissection stops before cutting the hepatic branch of the vagus nerve or nearing the left gastric artery. The pylorus and antrum are now mobilized and are then folded anteriorly and superiorly into the left upper quadrant for the rest of the procedure. This maneuver gives wide exposure of the duodenum, pancreas, and retroperitoneum.

11. Gastroduodenal artery division

    Attention is now turned to the hepatic hilar structures. The peritoneum over the hepatoduodenal ligament is incised. Dissection of the hepatic artery lymph node (station 8a) facilitates exposure of the common hepatic artery (Fig. 20.6). Frozen examination of this lymph node is recommended for staging purposes. In turn, identification of the common hepatic artery serves as a landmark for the GDA takeoff. Intraoperative ultrasound can aid identification of the GDA. If there is any uncertainty a bulldog clamp can be placed across the presumed GDA and Doppler flow assessed in the proper hepatic artery to assure the hepatic artery was not confused for the GDA. The GDA is isolated and divided close to its origin using a vascular stapler. Clips or sutures can be used instead as well. Leaving a 5 mm stump will facilitate endovascular embolization in case of post-pancreatectomy hemorrhage due to pseudoaneurysm formation in this area. Other small accessory branches to the pancreas in this area should be identified and clipped when present, since they are potential sources of pseudoaneurysms.

Fig. 20.6 Hepatic artery lymph node dissection facilitates exposure of the common hepatic artery, which serves as a landmark for the GDA takeoff (Figure reproduced with permission of Horacio J Asbun)

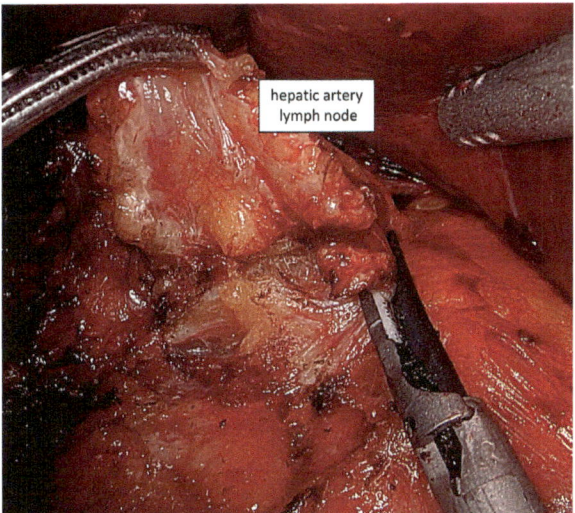

Fig. 20.7 Common bile duct division. A curved bulldog is inserted proximally in the common bile duct, previously encircled by a finger-type retractor (Figure reproduced with permission of Horacio J Asbun)

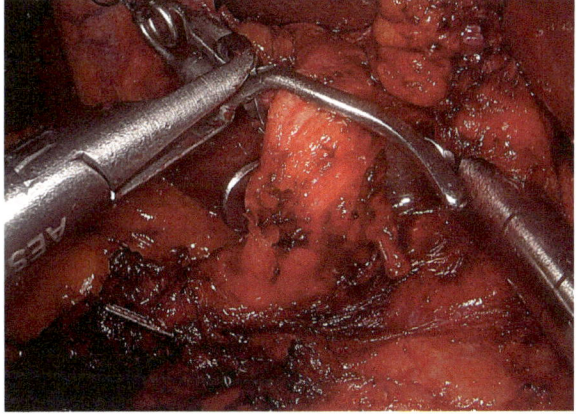

12. Common bile duct division

    Division of the GDA acts as a gateway to the structures of the porta hepatis, and the portal vein is at times visible immediately deep to the GDA. The common bile duct (CBD) is the next structure to be identified. A critical view of safety technique is applied to identify and divide the cystic duct and cystic artery. Completion of the cholecystectomy can be performed at a later stage and after specimen extraction while margins are being evaluated. The cystic duct is followed down to its insertion at the CBD as needed to help delineate the CBD. It is also found anterior and lateral to the portal vein, which may already have been identified. A finger-type retractor is used to safely and individually encircle the CBD (Fig. 20.7).

    Extra attention must be paid to avoid injury to surrounding hepatoduodenal structures located posteriorly (portal vein) or medially (proper and/or right hepatic artery). Other hepatic artery anatomical variations, such as a replaced/accessory right hepatic artery, may run in close proximity to the CBD, usually posterolateral. A thorough inspection of preoperative imaging is key to identify the presence of these variants, especially during this part of the pancreatoduodenectomy. Preoperative biliary stents should be placed low within the CBD. Plastic or fully covered biliary stents are preferred since they are easier to remove intraoperatively, as opposed to uncovered stents where tissue ingrowth makes its removal much more difficult.

Prior to CBD transection, a gauze is placed posteriorly, and a bulldog clamp is passed proximally around the CBD to prevent bile spillage and minimize peritoneal contamination. This is especially important if the patient has a biliary stent in place. The curved bulldog is inserted with a bulldog applier to facilitate manipulation. A silk suture is tied to the back of the bulldog clamp to facilitate removing it from the abdominal cavity. The CBD is transected sharply with scissors, as low as possible, as long as a clear biliary margin is achieved. A lower level of transection will facilitate the angle of the bilioenteric anastomosis, even if it is transected below the junction with the cystic duct. Another useful strategy to facilitate reconstruction is to leave the posterior wall of the bile duct 3–4 mm longer than the anterior wall. Peri-choledochal vessels are coagulated in small bursts using ultrasonic shears. Bile cultures are taken if a stent was present, and the margin is sent for frozen examination to ensure it is not involved by tumor. The distal CBD is closed with a running silk suture to prevent further spillage during the rest of the procedure. If a stent was present, attempts are made to leave it in the specimen. Otherwise, it is removed through the choledochotomy and can be extracted from the abdomen in a retrieval bag.

Once the CBD is clamped, a continuous infusion of indocyanine green (ICG) at a rate of 0.4 mg/min may be started. This allows pancreatic parenchymal impregnation with ICG without significant background uptake by the liver and other organs. Further ICG boluses of 1.25 mg may be given, which help delineate arterial (first) and venous (later) anatomy. Although not always, ICG may be a very useful aid during the resection phase of the pancreatoduodenectomy especially when dissecting the uncinate process of the mesenteric vessels.

13. Retropancreatic window formation

Attention is now paid to the inferior edge of the pancreas. Gentle traction and observation of countermovement of tissues in this area help identify the plane between the pancreas and the adipose tissue of the retroperitoneum/transverse mesocolon. A wide window is created along the inferior edge of the pancreas using ultrasonic shears or a bipolar device. This wide exposure of the area is important to avoid the poor visualization and vascular control, which can happen when "working in a hole." Several tricks may be used to locate the SMV: (1) follow venous tributaries that drain into the SMV, especially the tributaries that form the trunk of Henle; (2) locate the extrahepatic main portal vein above the pancreas and estimate its position caudally; (3) review preoperative imaging to assess, in coronal views, the angle between the main portal vein and the SMV at its confluence; and (4) use of intraoperative ultrasound, including Doppler.

A retropancreatic tunnel is created in a caudad-cephalad fashion, along the avascular plane between the anterior aspect of the SMV and the posterior aspect of the pancreatic neck (Fig. 20.8). Meticulous blunt dissection in small strokes, as well as ultrasonic shears to ligate small veins, is used to create the window. The neck of the pancreas is completely encircled with the aid of a finger-type retractor, and a Penrose drain, or similar, is passed. The tip of the Penrose drain is cut into a long, thin point so that it can be easily introduced through the opening in the finger-type retractor (Fig. 20.9). If necessary, the common hepatic artery is further separated from the superior edge of the pancreas to avoid encircling it with the Penrose drain.

14. Mesenteric-uncinate groove exposure

Venous branches draining from the uncinate process and proximal jejunum into the SMV can be identified by anteriorly retracting the pancreatic neck with the Penrose. Identifying and ligating these veins at their insertion to the SMV can facilitate later separation of the uncinate process from mesentery as they are usually easier to identify here (Fig. 20.10). In case it is not clear whether these vessels drain the uncinate process or the jejunal/colonic mesentery, a Kocher maneuver that swipes the whole mesentery can be useful to identify and divide only those vessels that drain the uncinate process, or those early jejunal branches if they must be sacrificed.

15. Pancreatic neck transection

Preoperative imaging assessment is helpful to identify the location of the main pancreatic duct (MPD) within the pancreas, as well as its size. In sagittal series, the distance from the edge of the pancreas to the MPD, as well as the superior-inferior location, gives an estimate of where the MPD is to be expected during pancreatic transection (Fig. 20.11).

The pancreatic neck is transected in a caudad-cephalad fashion, as follows: the inferior edge of the pancreas is divided by applying a generous bite with ultrasonic shears, and using a gradual compression technique that will divide the inferior pancreatic arcade. Then, the parenchyma is divided using a back-and-forth movement of the active blade of the ultrasonic shears in order to rec-

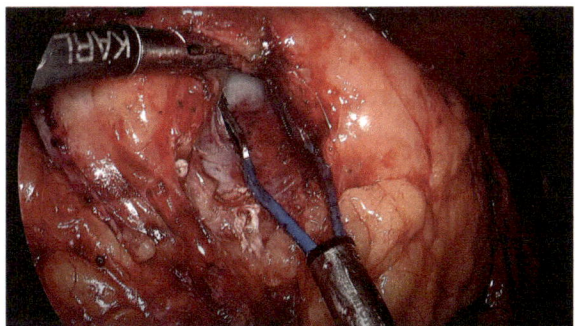

Fig. 20.8 Retropancreatic tunnel. Meticulous blunt dissection is used to create the window between the superior mesenteric vein and the neck of the pancreas (Figure reproduced with permission of Horacio J Asbun)

Fig. 20.9 Pancreatic neck is encircled with a finger-type retractor and a Penrose drain. The tip of the drain is cut in a thin long diagonal to facilitate its insertion through an opening in the finger retractor (Figure reproduced with permission of Horacio J Asbun)

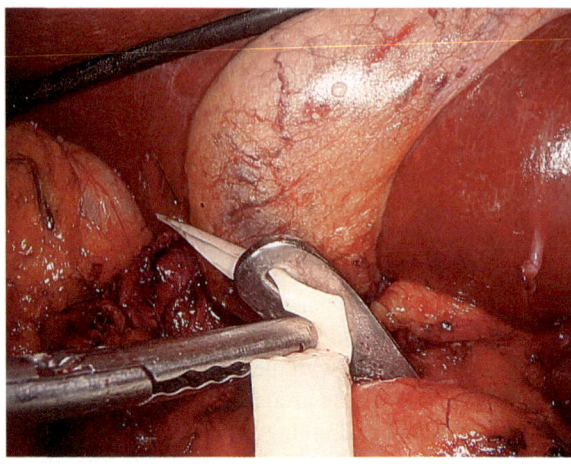

Fig. 20.10 Mesenteric-uncinate groove exposure dissection (Figure reproduced with permission of Horacio J Asbun)

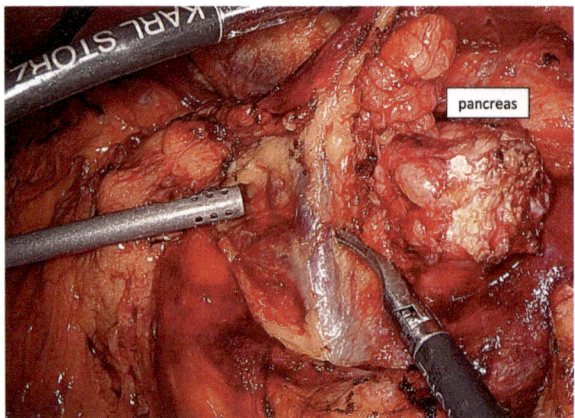

ognize the MPD without thermal injury before its transection (Fig. 20.12). The MPD is divided sharply with scissors, leaving a 2–3 mm protruding stump in preparation for the duct-to-mucosa anastomosis (Fig. 20.13). The distal end of the duct may be stented with a 3.5 or 5 Fr pediatric feeding tube for later identification and manipulation during pancreatic reconstruction. Finally, the remaining parenchyma and the superior pancreatic arcade are transected with ultrasonic shears using gradual compression.

16. Kocher maneuver

    A reverse Trendelenburg position with a left-side down tilt of the operative table is encouraged. The 45-degree laparoscope and camera are moved from port 4 to port 3. The retraction made by the first assistant is crucial to adequately mobilize the duodenum beyond the inferior vena cava (IVC) and to open the ligament of Treitz from the right side. For this, the assistant performs a swiping maneuver toward the midline of the previously mobilized colon with a closed large bowel clamp inserted through port 6. Simultaneously, the divided distal

Fig. 20.11 Preoperative
sagittal MRI series
determine the cephalo-
caudal and antero-posterior
location of the main
pancreatic duct which is
useful to plan for the
pancreatic neck transection
(Figure reproduced with
permission of Horacio J
Asbun)

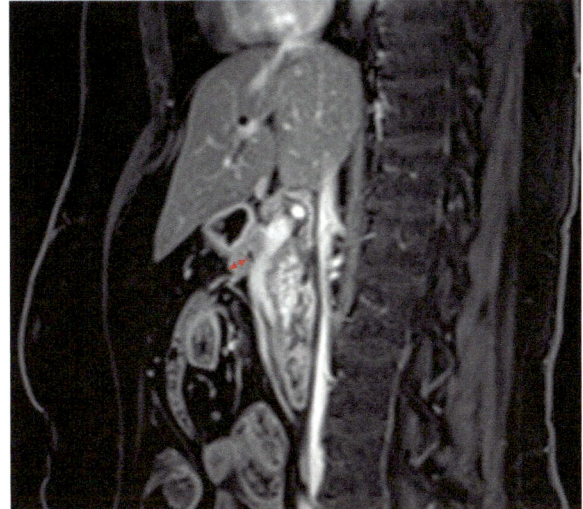

Fig. 20.12 Pancreatic
neck division. The
parenchyma is divided
using a back-and-forth
movement of the active
blade of the ultrasonic
shears in order to
recognize the MPD
without thermal injury
before its transection
(Figure reproduced with
permission of Horacio J
Asbun)

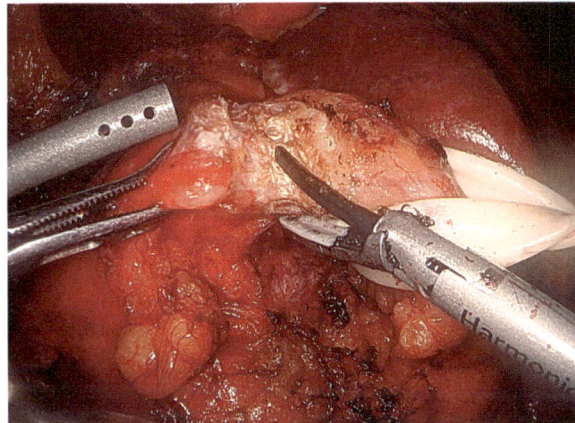

duodenal stump is pulled obliquely toward the left upper quadrant with a grasping forceps through port 5. The IVC and insertion of the left renal vein are
exposed. The duodenum, head of the pancreas, and uncinate process are now
completely mobilized from the retroperitoneum and reflected medially. This
dissection brings the retropancreatic lymph nodes into the specimen.
17. Ligament of Treitz opening and proximal jejunum division
    The ligament of Treitz is accessed and released from the right side of the patient.
    The first jejunal loop is pulled behind the superior mesenteric vessels, tran-
    sected with a laparoscopic 60 mm stapler (blue load), and delivered to the
    supramesocolic compartment. The jejunal mesentery is carefully ligated with a
    vessel sealer to avoid any potential source of post-pancreatectomy hemorrhage.
    Minimizing the amount of jejunum and mesentery that is transected is encour-

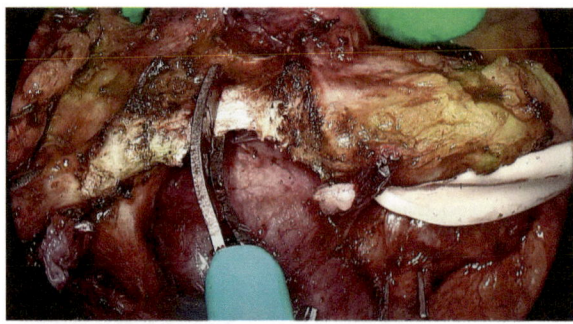

Fig. 20.13 Main pancreatic duct division with scissors. A 2–3 mm protruding stump is left in preparation for the duct-to-mucosa anastomosis (Figure reproduced with permission of Horacio J Asbun)

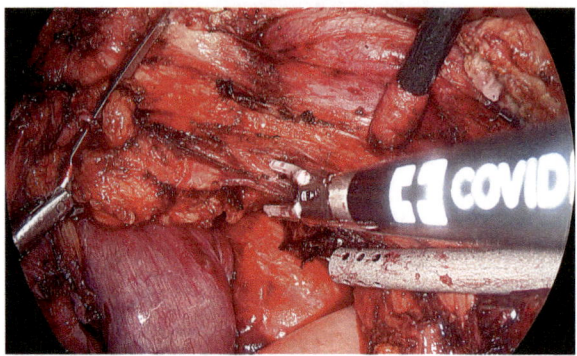

Fig. 20.14 Uncinate process dissection. A partially-opened large bowel grasper retracts the specimen laterally. A 5 mm endo-Kittner retracts the superior mesenteric vein left and cephalad. The parenchyma is dissected with a bipolar vessel sealing device using small bites (Figure reproduced with permission of Horacio J Asbun)

aged, as this decreases the amount of cut mesentery that can bleed postoperatively.

18. Uncinate process dissection

The uncinate process and head of the pancreas are lifted cephalad to the right in the crotch of a partially opened large grasper, such as a bowel clamp. The first assistant is of crucial importance to achieve adequate retraction and exposure, as well as to perform precise hemostasis, if needed. A 5 mm endo-Kittner is used to retract the SMV to the left and cephalad (Fig. 20.14).

Adequate retraction using the above-mentioned method helps identify the plane of dissection between the uncinate process and the superior mesenteric vessels. ICG infusion as mentioned above may aid in achieving complete visualization and resection of the pancreatic parenchyma in this challenging area. The parenchyma is dissected with a bipolar vessel sealing device using small bites. The jaws of the vessel sealer can be continuously opened and closed while active to improve hemostasis. Inferior pancreatoduodenal vessels may be encountered and are ligated and divided. Lymphadenectomy, including tissue lateral to the SMA, is performed en bloc. Extreme caution in this area is needed in case a replaced right hepatic artery off the superior mesenteric artery (SMA) exists (Fig. 20.15). Preoperative imaging review helps assess the origin and trajectory of this anatomic variant. Identification, isolation, and ligation of the inferior pancreatoduodenal artery (IPDA) and other SMA branches to the pancreas are important during this step.

In case of hemorrhage from the SMV or tributaries, the lateral portion of the distal end of the suction shaft is used to apply gentle pressure and achieve temporary control of bleeding; using the tip should be avoided as it may enlarge the hole in the vein. Very short bursts of suction, pressing the suction button only partially allow for clearance of blood and identification of the bleeding site when it occurs. Monofilament sutures are used to control bleeding. Once the stitch is ready to be thrown, the suction shaft is slowly rolled sideways to expose the injured vein and allow the stitch to be placed in the vessel. Advanced laparoscopic skills, such as mounting and passing the needle with one hand, are important, especially in this phase of the procedure. A similar technique can be used to control arterial bleeding, which is less common.

If vascular involvement by the lesion is suspected, the portal confluence should be completely exposed and vessels dissected circumferentially, including the splenic vein. Vessel loops are used to gain proximal and distal vascular control. Depending on anatomic variants, the left gastric vein may also need to be surrounded and looped individually. Heparin is administered prior to clamping the vein, which is resected *en bloc* with the PD specimen when vascular involvement is present.

19. Specimen removal

The specimen is placed in a laparoscopic 15-mm retrieval bag. Orientation of the specimen with the cut jejunal end at the edge of the bag is important to decrease the need to enlarge trocar sites in excess. The jejunum is grasped and pulled outside the abdominal cavity, along with the rest of the specimen, through port 5, which is enlarged only to about 4 cm when the specimen is oriented

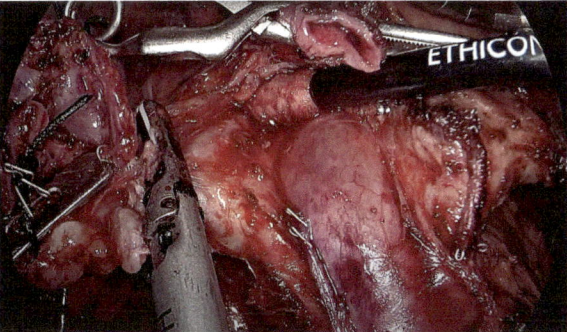

Fig. 20.15 Replaced right hepatic artery off the superior mesenteric artery might be encountered during the uncinate process dissection. Thorough preoperative imaging review is warranted to assess for the presence of vascular variants (Figure reproduced with permission of Horacio J Asbun)

appropriately. A small Pfannenstiel incision may be used instead if the specimen is very large or bulky. Frozen section evaluation of the margins, including the pancreatic neck, uncinate process/SMA margin, and CBD, is performed. Fascia is reapproximated with a monofilament absorbable suture, and pneumoperitoneum is reestablished in preparation for reconstruction. While the resection margins are being evaluated, the cholecystectomy is completed.

Reconstruction Phase

The authors' preference is to use a 3D camera during the reconstruction phase in order to obtain better visualization for stitch placement during the anastomoses.

20. Hepaticojejunostomy

    Once the cholecystectomy is completed, the liver retractor is now placed from the left side. The jejunum is pulled through where the ligament of Treitz was opened. It is positioned in an inverted "J" shape (candy cane) in the right supramesocolic area, where the biliary and pancreatic anastomosis will be performed. Bowel loop kinking or mesenteric torsion should be avoided. The surgeon now moves to the right side of the patient to perform the end-to-side hepaticojejunostomy. This angle facilitates mounting the needle and suturing in a more ergonomic fashion. The camera is placed in port 2 and triangulated with the working ports 1 and 3. A gauze is placed posteriorly to avoid any bile spillage and potential contamination of the abdominal cavity, especially in patients with a previous biliary stent. If possible, the bulldog is left in place until completion of the anastomosis. The first assistant holds suction to avoid bile spillage after enterotomy and holds the jejunum in place using a grasper through port 5. An enterotomy slightly smaller than the size of the cut common bile/hepatic duct is preferred. The posterior wall is sutured with a 4-0 or 5-0 barbed spiral suture mounted on a TF or RB-1 needle, in a running method from patient left to right. The previously cut longer posterior wall of the bile duct provides space that facilitates adequate placement of stitches in this area (Fig. 20.16). The anterior wall is then sutured similarly. A 15 Fr Blake drain is inserted through port 1 and will serve to drain the posterior aspect of both the biliary and pancreatic anastomosis. Placing the drain before the pancreaticojejunostomy avoids the need to place traction on that anastomosis once completed. The jejunal loop is fixed to the Gerota's fascia with a silk to avoid its kinking, prevent the drain from being in direct contact with the bilioenteric anastomoses, and decrease tension on the anastomosis.

21. Pancreaticojejunostomy

    The surgeon now stands between the legs of the patient. The camera is placed in port 4 and triangulated with the working ports 3 and 5. Precise stitching and maneuvering of the needle during this part of the procedure are facilitated by

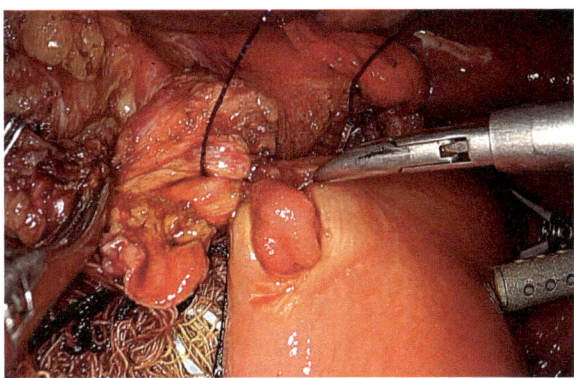

Fig. 20.16 Hepaticojejunostomy. The previously cut longer posterior wall of the bile duct (3–4 mm longer than the anterior wall) provides space that facilitates adequate placement of stitches in this area (Figure reproduced with permission of Horacio J Asbun)

3D visualization, as well as instruments (needle driver, grasper) with a 3 mm tip mounted on a 5 mm shaft.

The anastomosis is constructed in four layers in a duct-to-mucosa fashion. A first posterior outer layer will propel the duct stump anteriorly. For this, a running 4-0 absorbable barbed spiral suture mounted on an RB1 needle is performed between the posterior surface of the pancreas and the posterior seromuscular layer of the jejunum, near the mesenteric border and well into the posterior aspect of the pancreas. This suture is started cranially and left untied caudally. Each stitch is placed at the same level and spaced equally in the bowel wall. This creates a ledge of seromuscular layer behind the pancreas creating a patch of bowel wall behind the future duct-to-mucosa layer.

An enterotomy is created using ultrasonic shears. The enterotomy is tailored to be a little larger than the size of the MPD opening. A pediatric feeding tube may be placed in the MPD during reconstruction to facilitate manipulation, retraction, and stitch placement, and removed prior to finishing the anastomosis. If the MPD is very small, a very small anterior slit can be used to gently dilate its opening. The pediatric feeding tube or the tip of a 3 mm Maryland retractor may also be used for this purpose. However, one should not risk damaging the duct opening. A duct-to-mucosa anastomosis is performed. A first suture in the posterior layer, including both the duct and jejunum, is placed at 6 o'clock (most posterior aspect) and left untied. A 5-0 or 6-0 polyglactin suture mounted on a TF needle is used. This suture, as well as the MPD stent, is manipulated in different directions exposing the edge of the duct to be stitched. The next interrupted suture is placed cranially, and then one caudally. These are tied and cut immediately after being placed, and the 6 o'clock suture is generally tied at the end of the posterior wall. The number of stitches to be placed will depend on the size of the MPD but the minimum used is usually three posterior stitches even for a 1 mm duct.

The anterior layer is constructed. A first stay suture at 12 o'clock is passed only in the MPD opening and left untied (Fig. 20.17). This will open the duct and allow for continuous visualization of the duct lumen. The rest of the interrupted stitches are passed from cephalad to caudad and left untied until all stitches are passed (Fig. 20.18). When placing each stitch, care is taken not to cross the sutures. After all anterior sutures are placed, the initial 12 o'clock stitch is completed by passing it through the jejunum, and all are tied. Caution to ensure the suture tails are also not crossed when tying. At least four anterior stitches are usually placed even for the very small ducts. Since the size of the enterotomy is a little larger than the MPD opening, the stitches are placed in a radial fashion on the side of the enterotomy, taking a good purchase of the bowel, almost with the intent of inserting the MPD opening well inside the bowel opening.

An anterior outer layer is created in a running fashion between the anterior aspect of the pancreas and the anterior seromuscular layer of the jejunum (Fig. 20.19). The same 4-0 absorbable barbed suture on an RB1 needle is used. Caution is advised when placing these sutures on a soft pancreas. In order to avoid tearing of the pancreas and increasing the risk of a postoperative pancreatic fistula, the knot should be tied by pushing on the jejunal side of the knot. A falciform flap may be wrapped around the anastomosis if desired and if it reaches easily.

22. Duodenojejunostomy

The gastrointestinal reconstruction is done using the same jejunal loop as for the other two anastomoses, but using a segment distally, approximately 20–30 cm distal to the ligament of Treitz. The area of the ligament of Treitz is identified by retracting the transverse colon mesentery superiorly and looking in the area between the two pedicles of omentum that were created at the initial part of the operation. The anastomoses will end up sitting between these two

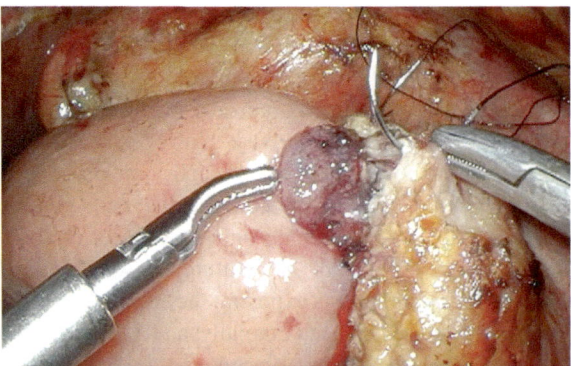

Fig. 20.17 Pancreatojejunostomy. A first stay suture at 12 o'clock is passed only in the main pancreatic duct and left untied. This allows for continuous visualization of the duct lumen while placing the remaining stitches of the anterior layer of the duct-to-mucosa anastomosis (Figure reproduced with permission of Horacio J Asbun)

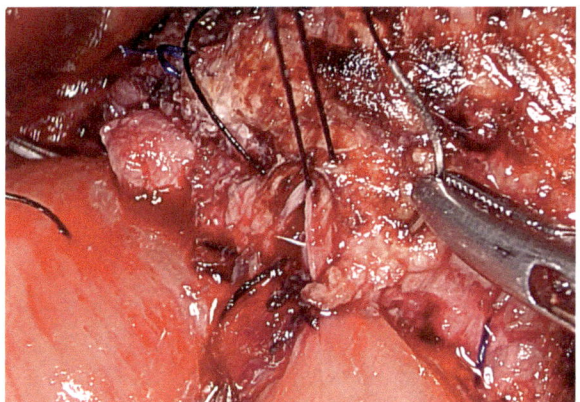

Fig. 20.18 The stitches of the posterior layer of the duct-to-mucosa anastomosis are already tied. The suture at 12 o'clock in the anterior layer is manipulated in different directions exposing the edge of the duct to be stitched. The rest of the interrupted stitches are passed superiorly and inferiorly (Figure reproduced with permission of Horacio J Asbun)

Fig. 20.19 An anterior outer layer is created in a running fashion between the anterior aspect of the pancreas and the anterior seromuscular layer of the jejunum. A 4-0 or 5-0 absorbable barbed suture on a RB1 needle is used (Figure reproduced with permission of Horacio J Asbun)

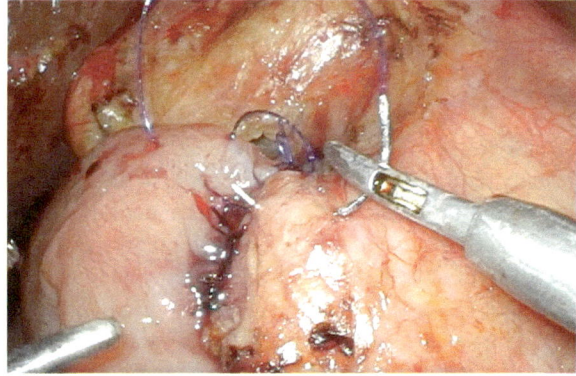

omental pedicles. An end-to-side duodenojejunostomy is constructed in four layers, with barbed sutures, and in an antecolic fashion (Fig. 20.20). The first seromuscular posterior layer is created in a running fashion. The first stitch is placed approximating the right aspect of the jejunum to the greater curvature end of the divided post-pyloric duodenum. A 3-0 polydioxanone absorbable barbed suture is used for all layers. The duodenum and jejunum are opened after the outer posterior layer is run. The duodenal staple line is kept when opening the bowel parallel to it. This facilitates the anastomoses. The inner posterior and anterior layers are done. Since the duodenal staple line potentially may have decreased blood supply, the authors encourage its inclusion in the inner posterior layer of the anastomosis. The anastomosis ends with an outer anterior seromuscular layer. If needed, a second 15 Fr Blake drain is inserted through port 6 and will serve to drain the anterior aspect of the pancreatojeju-

Fig. 20.20 An end-to-side duodenojejunostomy is constructed in four layers, with running barbed sutures, and in an antecolic fashion (Figure reproduced with permission of Horacio J Asbun)

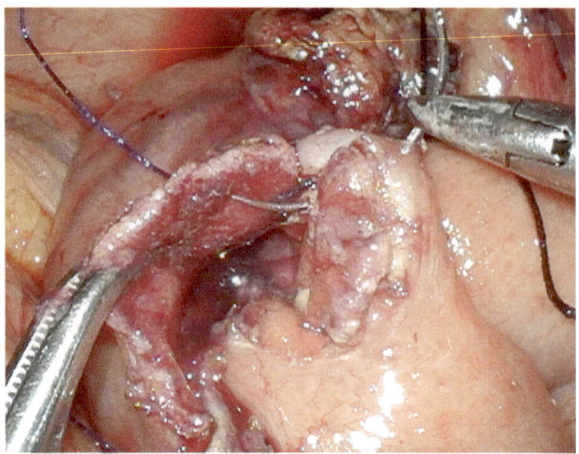

nostomy as well the duodenojejunostomy. It is positioned into the left upper quadrant up behind the tip of the spleen and run under the left lobe of the liver.

Postoperative Course

A nasogastric tube is not left in place postoperatively, and the urinary catheter is usually removed on the first postoperative day. The patient is started on a clear liquid diet in the immediate postoperative period. Early ambulation is enforced, as is avoidance of narcotics if possible. Drain amylase is checked regularly and prior to removal. Length of stay ranges between 4 and 6 days if no complications arise.

Conclusions

This minimally invasive approach for PD is reproducible, yet advanced laparoscopic skills are required. Although there are variations in technique, this chapter summarizes the authors' experience with the goal of maximizing the safety, reproducibility, and efficiency of this complex operation.

Conflict of Interest   The authors have no conflict of interest to declare.

References

1. Morris ZS, wooding S, Grant J. The answer is 17 years, what is the question: understanding time lags in translational research. J R Soc Med. 2011;104(12):510–20. https://doi.org/10.1258/jrsm.2011.110180.
2. Gagner M, Pomp A. Laparoscopic pylorus-preserving pancreatoduodenectomy. Surg Endosc. 1994;8(5):408–10. https://doi.org/10.1007/BF00642443.
3. Palanivelu C, Jani K, Senthilnathan P, Parthasarathi R, Rajapandian S, Madhankumar MV. Laparoscopic pancreaticoduodenectomy: technique and outcomes. J Am Coll Surg. 2007;205(2):222–30. https://doi.org/10.1016/j.jamcollsurg.2007.04.004.
4. Kendrick ML, Cusati D. Total laparoscopic pancreaticoduodenectomy: feasibility and outcome in an early experience. Arch Surg. 2010;145(1):19–23. https://doi.org/10.1001/archsurg.2009.243.
5. Asbun HJ, Stauffer JA. Laparoscopic vs open pancreaticoduodenectomy: overall outcomes and severity of complications using the accordion severity grading system. J Am Coll Surg. 2012;215(6):810–9. https://doi.org/10.1016/j.jamcollsurg.2012.08.006.
6. Conrad C, Basso V, Passot G, et al. Comparable long-term oncologic outcomes of laparoscopic versus open pancreaticoduodenectomy for adenocarcinoma: a propensity score weighting analysis. Surg Endosc. 2017;31(10):3970–8. https://doi.org/10.1007/s00464-017-5430-3.
7. Kutlu OC, Lee JE, Katz MH, et al. Open pancreaticoduodenectomy case volume predicts outcome of laparoscopic approach: a population-based analysis. Ann Surg. 2018;267(3):552–60. https://doi.org/10.1097/SLA.0000000000002111.
8. Lee CS, Kim EY, You YK, Hong TH. Perioperative outcomes of laparoscopic pancreaticoduodenectomy for benign and borderline malignant periampullary disease compared to open pancreaticoduodenectomy. Langenbeck's Arch Surg. 2018;403(5):591–7. https://doi.org/10.1007/s00423-018-1691-0.
9. Nassour I, Wang SC, Christie A, et al. Minimally invasive versus open pancreaticoduodenectomy. Ann Surg. 2018;268(1):151–7. https://doi.org/10.1097/SLA.0000000000002259.
10. Park YS, Jun IG, Go Y, Song JG, Hwang GS. Comparison of acute kidney injury between open and laparoscopic pylorus-preserving pancreaticoduodenectomy: propensity score analysis. PLoS One. 2018;13(8):1–12. https://doi.org/10.1371/journal.pone.0202980.
11. Shin H, Song KB, Kim YI, et al. Propensity score-matching analysis comparing laparoscopic and open pancreaticoduodenectomy in elderly patients. Sci Rep. 2019;9(1):1–9. https://doi.org/10.1038/s41598-019-49455-9.
12. Zhou W, Jin W, Wang D, et al. Laparoscopic versus open pancreaticoduodenectomy for pancreatic ductal adenocarcinoma: a propensity score matching analysis. Cancer Commun. 2019;39(1):1–11. https://doi.org/10.1186/s40880-019-0410-8.
13. El Nakeeb A, Attia M, El Sorogy M, et al. Laparoscopic pancreaticodudenectomy for periampullary tumor: should it be a routine? A propensity score-matched study. Surg Laparosc Endosc Percutan Tech. 2020;30(1):7–13. https://doi.org/10.1097/SLE.0000000000000715.
14. Han SH, Kang CM, Hwang HK, Yoon DS, Lee WJ. The Yonsei experience of 104 laparoscopic pancreaticoduodenectomies: a propensity score-matched analysis with open pancreaticoduodenectomy. Surg Endosc. 2020;34(4):1658–64. https://doi.org/10.1007/s00464-019-06942-4.
15. Klompmaker S, Van Hilst J, Wellner UF, et al. Outcomes after minimally-invasive versus open pancreatoduodenectomy: a pan-European propensity score matched study. Ann Surg. 2020;271(2):356–63. https://doi.org/10.1097/SLA.0000000000002850.
16. Yoo D, Song KB, Lee JW, et al. A comparative study of laparoscopic versus open pancreaticoduodenectomy for ampulla of Vater carcinoma. J Clin Med. 2020;9(7):2214. https://doi.org/10.3390/jcm9072214.
17. Chen K, Pan Y, Huang C-J, et al. Laparoscopic versus open pancreatic resection for ductal adenocarcinoma: separate propensity score matching analyses of distal pancreatectomy and pancreaticoduodenectomy. BMC Cancer. 2021;21(1):1–12. https://doi.org/10.1186/s12885-021-08117-8.

N. Lluís et al.

18. Cheng K, Liu W, You J, et al. Safety of laparoscopic pancreaticoduodenectomy in patients with liver cirrhosis using propensity score matching. PLoS One. 2021;16(1 January):1–13. https://doi.org/10.1371/journal.pone.0246364.
19. Dang C, Wang M, Zhu F, Qin T, Qin R. Comparison of laparoscopic and open pancreaticoduodenectomy for the treatment of nonpancreatic periampullary adenocarcinomas: a propensity score matching analysis. Am J Surg. 2021;222(2):377–82. https://doi.org/10.1016/j.amjsurg.2020.12.023.
20. Ding W, Wu W, Tan Y, et al. The comparison of short-term outcome between laparoscopic and open pancreaticoduodenectomy: a propensity score matching analysis. Updat Surg. 2021;73(2):419–27. https://doi.org/10.1007/s13304-021-00997-6.
21. Katsuki R, Jo T, Yasunaga H, Kumazawa R, Uda K. Outcomes of laparoscopic versus open pancreatoduodenectomy: a nationwide retrospective cohort study. Surgery. 2021;169(6):1427–33. https://doi.org/10.1016/j.surg.2020.12.018.
22. Mazzola M, Giani A, Crippa J, et al. Totally laparoscopic versus open pancreaticoduodenectomy: a propensity score matching analysis of short-term outcomes. Eur J Surg Oncol. 2021;47(3):674–80. https://doi.org/10.1016/j.ejso.2020.10.036.
23. Kim SH, Lee B, Hwang HK, et al. Comparison of postoperative complications and long-term oncological outcomes in minimally invasive versus open pancreatoduodenectomy for distal cholangiocarcinoma: a propensity score-matched analysis. J Hepatobiliary Pancreat Sci. 2022;29(3):329–37. https://doi.org/10.1002/jhbp.1067.
24. Zhang Z, Yin T, Qin T, et al. Comparison of laparoscopic versus open pancreaticoduodenectomy in patients with resectable pancreatic ductal adenocarcinoma: a propensity score-matching analysis of long-term survival. Pancreatology. 2022;22(2):317–24. https://doi.org/10.1016/j.pan.2021.12.005.
25. Jiang Y-L, Zhang R-C, Zhou Y-C. Comparison of overall survival and perioperative outcomes of laparoscopic pancreaticoduodenectomy and open pancreaticoduodenectomy for pancreatic ductal adenocarcinoma: a systematic review and meta-analysis. BMC Cancer. 2019;19(1):781. https://doi.org/10.1186/s12885-019-6001-x.
26. van der Heijde N, Balduzzi A, Alseidi A, et al. The role of older age and obesity in minimally invasive and open pancreatic surgery: a systematic review and meta-analysis. Pancreatology. 2020;20(6):1234–42. https://doi.org/10.1016/j.pan.2020.06.013.
27. Sánchez-Velázquez P, Muller X, Malleo G, et al. Benchmarks in pancreatic surgery: a novel tool for unbiased outcome comparisons. Ann Surg. 2019;270(2):211–8. https://doi.org/10.1097/SLA.0000000000003223.
28. Asbun HJ, Moekotte AL, Vissers FL, et al. The Miami international evidence-based guidelines on minimally invasive pancreas resection. Ann Surg. 2020;271(1):1–14. https://doi.org/10.1097/SLA.0000000000003590.
29. Palanivelu C, Senthilnathan P, Sabnis SC, et al. Randomized clinical trial of laparoscopic versus open pancreatoduodenectomy for periampullary tumours. Br J Surg. 2017;104(11):1443–50. https://doi.org/10.1002/bjs.10662.
30. Poves I, Burdío F, Morató O, et al. Comparison of perioperative outcomes between laparoscopic and open approach for pancreatoduodenectomy: the Padulap randomized controlled trial. Ann Surg. 2018;268(5):731–9. https://doi.org/10.1097/SLA.0000000000002893.
31. van Hilst J, De Rooij T, Bosscha K, et al. Laparoscopic versus open pancreatoduodenectomy for pancreatic or periampullary tumours (LEOPARD-2): a multicentre, patient-blinded, randomised controlled phase 2/3 trial. Lancet Gastroenterol Hepatol. 2019;4(3):199–207. https://doi.org/10.1016/S2468-1253(19)30004-4.
32. Wang M, Li D, Chen R, et al. Laparoscopic versus open pancreatoduodenectomy for pancreatic or periampullary tumours: a multicentre, open-label, randomised controlled trial. Lancet Gastroenterol Hepatol. 2021;6(6):438–47. https://doi.org/10.1016/S2468-1253(21)00054-6.

Chapter 21
Robotic Pancreatoduodenectomy

Sharona Ross, Harel Jacoby, Cameron Syblis, Iswanto Sucandy, and Alexander Rosemurgy

Introduction

Pancreaticoduodenectomy is one of the most complex and challenging abdominal operations. It requires high surgical skill with meticulous precision and excellent anatomic knowledge. Ever since Whipple reported his experience with three patients who underwent a two-stage pancreaticoduodenectomy, this operation has evolved tremendously [1]. With experience gained over the years, along with the improvement of surgical tools, the pancreatoduodenectomy has become a common operation with acceptable morbidity and mortality [2, 3].

Minimally invasive surgery has gained popularity in many surgical fields including pancreatic surgery. The first laparoscopic pancreaticoduodenectomy was performed in 1994 and ever since the laparoscopic approach gradually increased but eventually plateaued [4–6]. This approach was criticized by many surgeons stating it required a long learning curve and had the potential for high morbidity and mortality [7, 8].

The robotic platform transformed pancreatic surgery and led to a new era of minimally invasive surgery. The robotic platform has several advantages compared

S. Ross (✉) · I. Sucandy · A. Rosemurgy
Department of Surgery, University of Central Florida, Orlando, FL, USA

Advent Health Tampa Digestive Health Institute, Tampa, FL, USA

H. Jacoby
Advent Health Tampa Digestive Health Institute, Tampa, FL, USA

Sheba Medical Center, Tel-Aviv, Israel

C. Syblis
University of South Florida Morsani College of Medicine, Tampa, FL, USA

Advent Health Tampa Digestive Health Institute, Tampa, FL, USA

E. P. Ceppa et al. (eds.), *The SAGES Manual of Evolving Techniques in Pancreatic Surgery*, https://doi.org/10.1007/978-3-031-78409-5_21

to conventional laparoscopy including elimination of hand tremor, seven degrees of freedom, high resolution three-dimensional visualization, stable camera, ambidextrous suturing, and excellent ergonomics [9–13]. These advantages enable surgeons to overcome the limitations of traditional laparoscopy to perform complex operations safely and meticulously without compromising oncologic outcomes. RPD has already been implemented in several centers worldwide with promising results [14–18]. The purpose of this chapter is to describe the key steps for performing a RPD. As this technology continues to evolve and become widely adopted, we believe that the robotic platform will become the preferred approach among pancreatic surgeons.

Preoperative Workup

Preoperative Planning

- Following diagnosis of pancreatic malignancies or high-risk neoplastic lesions, all patients should complete a preoperative assessment including overall performance status, medical comorbidities, and clinical staging when indicated.
- All patients with pancreatic cancer should be discussed in a multidisciplinary tumor board, with a special focus on those with borderline resectable/locally advanced lesions or patients with significant comorbidities [19].
- Multidisciplinary review should consider involving expertise from diagnostic imaging, interventional endoscopy, medical oncology, radiation oncology, hepato-pancreatico-biliary (HPB) surgery, pathology, geriatric medicine, genetic counseling, and palliative care [20].
- Cardiac assessment is recommended for patients with a presumably higher risk for perioperative cardiac events [21].
- Age and frailty may predict a difficult postoperative course and should be considered preoperatively [22, 23].
- Preoperative counseling for Enhanced Recovery After Surgery (ERAS) protocol is recommended to achieve early recovery and improved outcomes [24].
- Malnourished patients should be given special attention and may need preoperative nutritional optimization by a nutritionist.

Imaging and Additional Diagnostic Studies

- In most institutions, computed tomography (CT) is the initial modality for staging. We use triphasic pancreatic protocol CT scan with 1 mm cuts with reconstruction for all patients during the month preceding their operation.
- Magnetic resonance imaging (MRI) with magnetic resonance cholangiopancreatography (MRCP) offers additional information to equivocal CT findings regard-

ing localized disease description and providing additional information regarding hepatic lesions. However, it does not add superior sensitivity or specificity and therefore should be used in selected cases [25].

- F-fluorodeoxyglucose-positron emission tomography (FDG-PET)/CT is a controversial modality in the staging of pancreatic cancer. We use it to rule out metastatic disease in high-risk patients.
- Endoscopic ultrasound (EUS) with EUS-guided biopsy is the preferred method of obtaining histologic confirmation. While it is not recommended as a routine staging stool as it is highly operator dependent, we find it to be a very useful tool and use it in most patients [26].
- Endoscopic retrograde cholangiopancreatography (ERCP) with stent placement is recommended for patients with active infection (cholangitis), patients planned for neoadjuvant chemotherapy, or patients with long-standing jaundice with high bilirubin.

Surgical Management

Patient Preparation

- Patient lies supine with their legs secured to the table using a belt around the pelvis, and both arms are extended and secured to the arm board.
- A single shot of intra-thecal morphine sulfate is injected prior to induction.
- Following endotracheal intubation, a urinary catheter, nasogastric tube, and arterial line are inserted.
- Perioperative measures are taken which include IV Zosyn within 30 min prior to the initial skin incision and sequential compression devices to prevent deep vein thrombosis (DVT).

Diagnostic Laparoscopy and Port Placement

- We begin the operation with a small incision at the umbilicus and insertion of an 8 mm robotic trocar.
- Once pneumoperitoneum is established, diagnostic laparoscopy is undertaken to exclude liver metastasis and peritoneal carcinomatosis. After ruling out distant metastases, additional trocars are placed under videoscopic visualization.
- An 8-mm trocar is inserted at the level of the umbilicus just to the right of the right midclavicular line. A 12-mm trocar, to accommodate the 45 mm EndoWrist® Stapler (Intuitive Surgical Inc., Sunnyvale, CA), is placed at the level of the umbilicus in the left midclavicular line. An 8-mm trocar is placed along the left anterior axillary line slightly cephalad to the umbilicus.

- An additional 3–5 cm incision is made, between and slightly caudal to the umbilical trocar and the right midclavicular line trocar, for a multi-trocar port, and an Applied GelPoint® (Applied Medical, Rancho Santa Margarita, CA) (Fig. 21.1). AirSeal® Access Port (Conmed Corporation, Utica, NY) is placed through the multi-trocar port.
- The bed is placed in 15–22° (depending on BMI) reverse Trendelenburg and 5° tilted to the left.
- The Da Vinci Xi™ robot (Intuitive Surgical Inc., Sunnyvale, CA) is then docked from the right side of the patient. The scrub tech stands on the left and the first assistant on the right side of the patient (Fig. 21.2).
- We use integrated table motion that enables dynamical positioning of the patient while the surgeon operates.

Fig. 21.1 Port placement

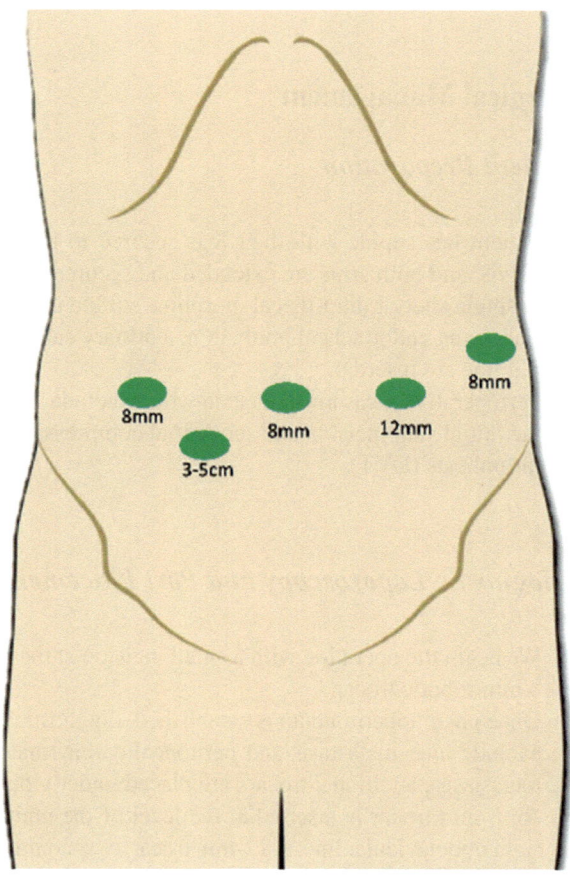

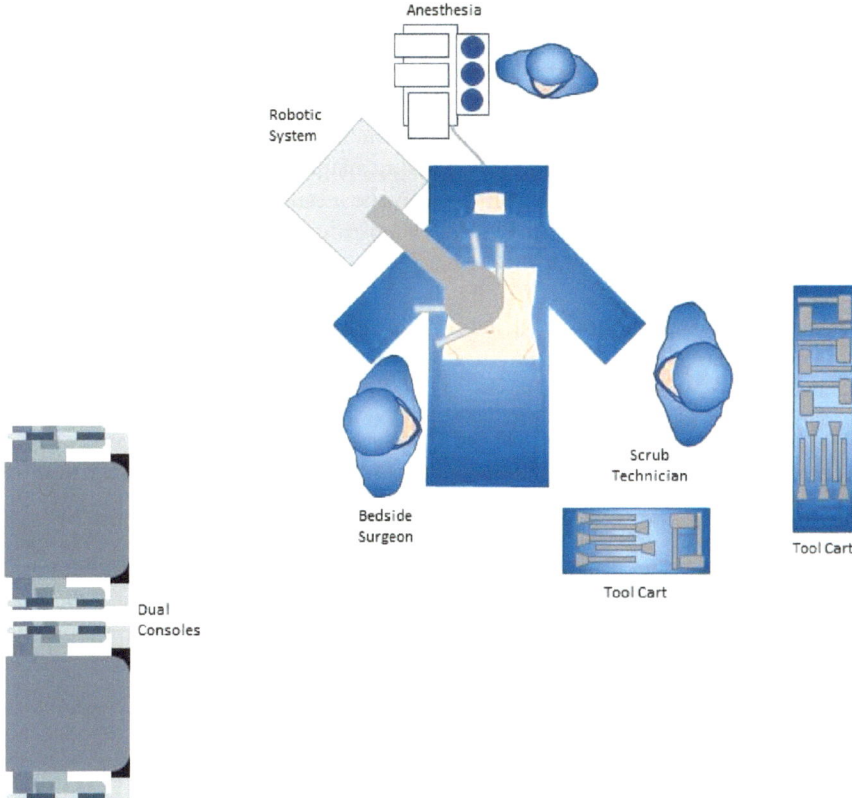

Fig. 21.2   Operation room setup

Surgical Steps

Step 1: Kocher Maneuver

- Arms setup:
    - Arm #1: Fenestrated bipolar
    - Arm #2: Camera
    - Arm #3: Monopolar scissors
    - Arm #4: Small grasping retractor (Bowel Grasper)
    - Bedside assistant: laparoscopic bowel grasper and suctioning device
- The operation begins with retraction of the right lobe of the liver utilizing a 12-inch, 3-0 V-Loc™ wound closure device (Medtronic™, Minneapolis, MN, USA), the hepatic flexure is partially mobilized until the duodenum is well exposed.
- The duodenum is medially mobilized starting by freeing the lateral attachments of D2 using the monopolar scissors and the fenestrated bipolar. The dissection is carried superiorly to the border of D1 and D2 and then toward to D3 and D4

while Arm #4 is used for medial retraction of the duodenum to facilitate full exposure (Fig. 21.3).

- An important landmark for sufficient mobilization is identifying the left renal vein entering the inferior vena cava (IVC).
- The bedside assistant has an important role in this step, retracting the transverse colon toward the right lower quadrant using a laparoscopic bowel grasper while using the suction device to retract medially the mesocolon to enable access to the ligament of Treitz. (Using single incision laparoscopic principals for instruments placement through the multi-trocar ports.)
- After dividing the ligament of Treitz, the jejunum is pulled back enough to enable transection using a robotic blue load da Vinci® Xi EndoWrist Stapler 45 mm with SmartClamp™ technology (Intuitive Surgical, Sunnyvale, CA, USA) (Figs. 21.4 and 21.5).
- Tips and Key points:
    - Retracting medially the duodenum using arm #4, improves the retraction for better exposure after sufficient dissection is completed.
    - Medial retraction of the transverse mesocolon using the suction device by the bedside surgeon is needed to expose and dissect the ligament of Treitz.
    - Replace as needed arm #1 and arm #3 to bowel graspers to pull back the jejunum behind the mesenteric root.

Step 2: Gastrohepatic and Hepatoduodenal Dissection

- Arms setup:
    - Arm #1: Fenestrated bipolar
    - Arm #2: Camera

Fig. 21.3 Kocher Maneuver. *IVC* inferior vena cava

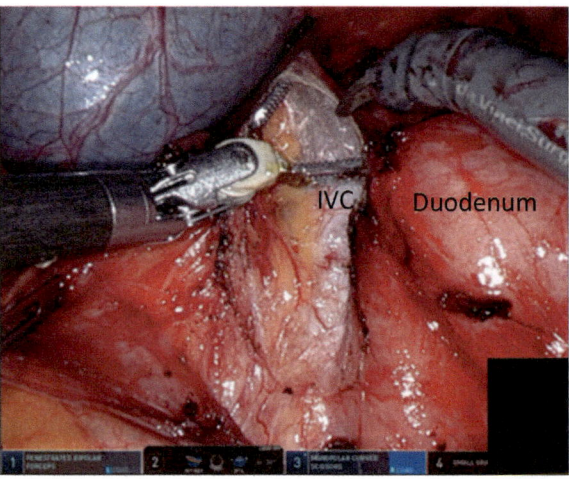

Fig. 21.4 Pulling back the proximal jejunum behind the mesenteric root

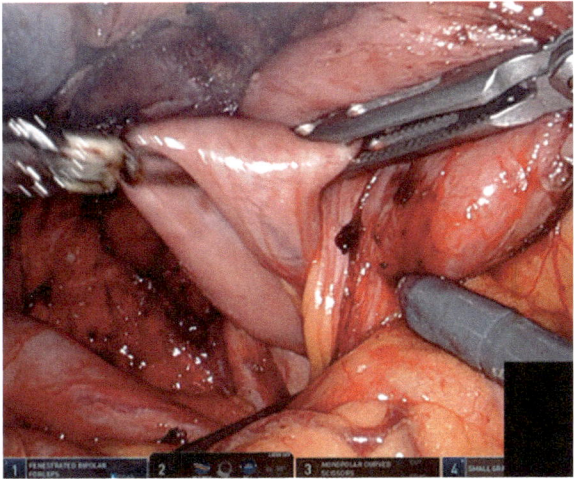

Fig. 21.5 Transection of the proximal jejunum

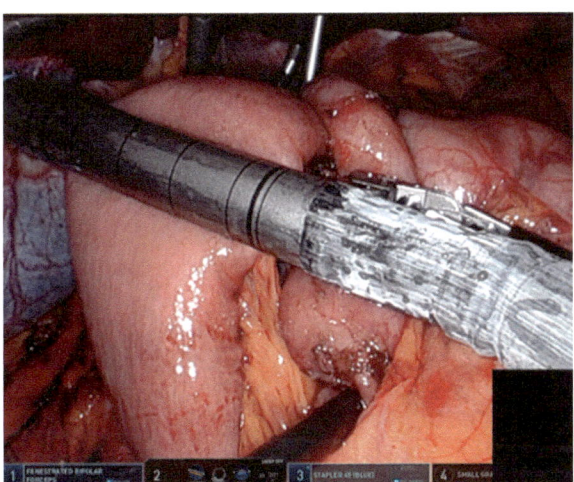

- – Arm #3: Monopolar scissors, hook cautery, and medium-size clip
- – Arm #4: Small grasping retractor (bowel grasper)
- – Bedside assistant: suctioning device
- Using the monopolar scissors, the lesser sac is entered at the gastrohepatic ligament, and the common hepatic artery is identified (Fig. 21.6).
- The right gastric vessels are identified, ligated, and divided using the fenestrated bipolar and monopolar scissors.
- Lymphadenectomy is completed starting at the common hepatic artery lymph node and continuing toward the celiac trunk. Lymph nodes along the celiac trunk, gastric vessels, splenic artery, and portal vein are all excised.

Fig. 21.6 Gastrohepatic ligament dissection. *CHA* common hepatic artery

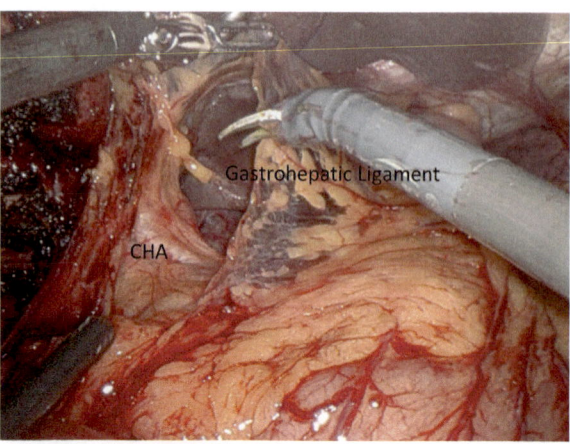

Fig. 21.7 Hepatoduodenal dissection. *IVC* inferior vena cava, *PHA* proper hepatic artery, *CHA* common hepatic artery, *GDA* gastroduodenal artery

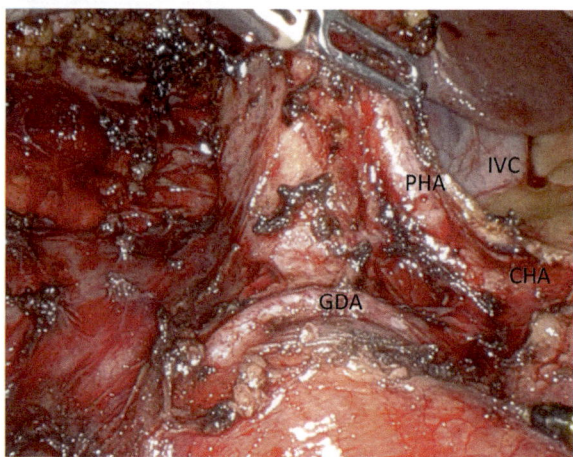

- The proper hepatic artery and gastroduodenal artery (GDA) are next identified, and lymph node dissection is ensued along the porta hepatis (Fig. 21.7).
- The GDA is clipped and divided following a test-clamp that verifies pulsation along the proper hepatic artery (Fig. 21.8). A silk suture is placed to secure the clips to the GDA stump.
- Tips and key points:
  - Retraction of the pancreas caudally using arm #4 for better exposure.
  - Intraoperative viewing the coronal section of the CT scan arterial phase is useful to anticipate the course of the CHA, the GDA, the hepatic artery proper, and any other aberrant vasculature.
  - Meticulous dissection of the GDA using the hook cautery is key.

Fig. 21.8 Division of gastroduodenal artery (GDA)

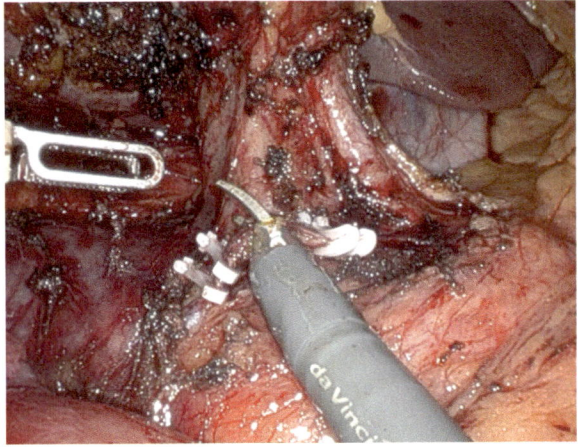

Step 3: Gastrocolic Ligament Dissection and Duodenal Transection

- Arms setup:
  - Arm #1: Fenestrated bipolar
  - Arm #2: Camera
  - Arm #3: Monopolar scissors, vessel sealer
  - Arm #4: Small grasping retractor (bowel grasper)
  - Bedside assistant: bowel grasper, suctioning device
- The stomach is retracted cephalad by the bedside surgeon using a bowel grasper while the transverse colon is retracted caudally using arm #4. The gastrocolic ligament is dissected and the dissection is carried on along the greater curvature of the stomach while preserving the gastroepiploic arcades.
- The dissection continues toward the duodenum while gastro-pancreatic attachments are being divided. The right gastroepiploic artery and vein are identified and divided using the vessel sealer.
- When the duodenum is fully exposed, it is transected 2–3 cm post pyloric using a robotic blue load EndoWrist Stapler 45 mm with SmartClamp™ technology (Intuitive Surgical, Sunnyvale, CA, USA) (Fig. 21.9). The stomach is then retracted toward the left upper quadrant to fully expose the head and neck of the pancreas.

Step 4: Pancreatic Transection

- Arms setup:

Fig. 21.9 Duodenal
transection

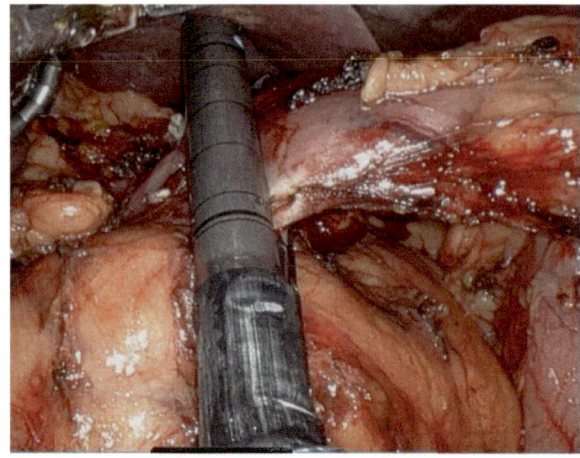

Fig. 21.10 Pancreatic
transection. *SMV* superior
mesenteric vein

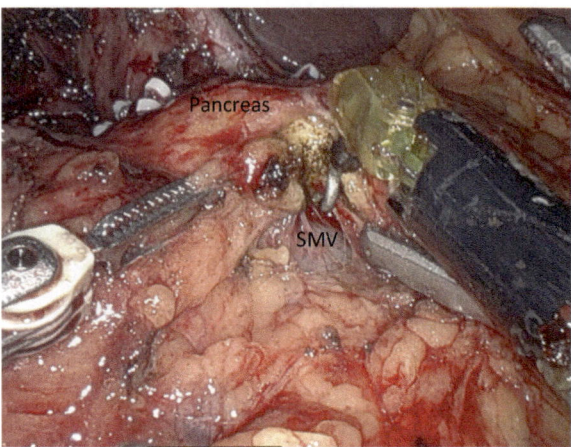

- Arm #1: Fenestrated bipolar
- Arm #2: Camera
- Arm #3: Hook cautery
- Arm #4: Small grasping retractor (bowel grasper)
- Bedside assistant: suctioning device

- Dissection is carried along the inferior edge of the pancreatic neck using a hook cautery and the superior mesenteric vein (SMV) is identified.
- A gentle blunt dissection using the fenestrated bipolar separates the SMV from the pancreatic neck. This is followed by hook cautery to transect the pancreatic neck (Figs. 21.10 and 21.11).
- The transection of the pancreas begins at the inferior border and carried along in the cephalad direction and parallel to the SMV while arm #4 retracts the mesocolon caudally.

Fig. 21.11 Pancreatic transection, completed. *PV* portal vein, *SV* splenic vein, *SMV* superior mesenteric vein

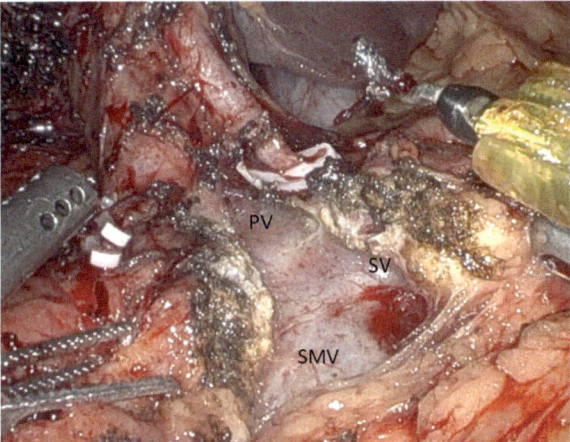

- The bedside surgeon may use the suctioning device to carefully retract and protect the SMV and portal vein (PV) during the transection.
- Tips and key points:
  - Try to identify the pancreatic duct during the transection. Typically, when the PD is blocked, a sudden outflow of clear fluid is seen when entering the duct.
  - During pancreatic transection, make sure to identify the common hepatic artery and the GDA stump to avoid inadvertent injury to these structures.

Step 5: PV/SMV and Uncinate Process Dissection

- Arms Setup:
  - Arm #1: Vessel sealer, fenestrated bipolar (needle driver as needed)
  - Arm #2: Camera
  - Arm #3: Hook cautery, vessel sealer, medium size clip (needle driver and scissors as needed)
  - Arm #4: Small grasping retractor (bowel grasper)
  - Bedside assistant: bowel grasper and suctioning device
- Retract the mesenteric vessels medially using arm #4 to further expose the attachments between the head of the pancreas and the PV/SMV. Dissect these attachments using the hook cautery (Fig. 21.12)
- While the bedside surgeon lifts cranially the proximal jejunum, use the vessel sealer with arm #1 to divide the jejunal mesentery toward the SMV/SMA (Fig. 21.13)
- Continue dissection along the PV/SMV in a caudal to cephalad direction. Use the vessel sealer or hook cautery in arm #3 to separate the uncinate process from

Fig. 21.12 Uncinate
process dissection

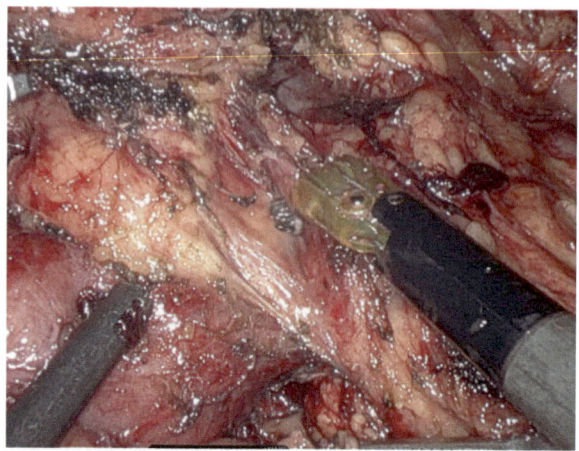

Fig. 21.13 Jejunal
mesentery dissection

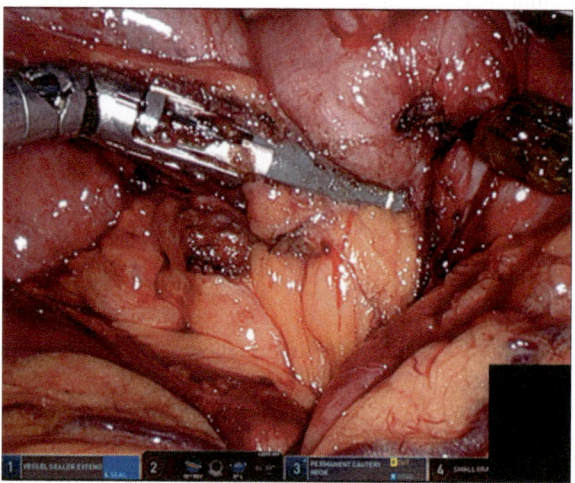

the PV/SMV. Use clips to divide large pancreaticoduodenal vessels or suture
ligation (Fig. 21.14)

- Tips and key points:

    - This is the hardest part of the dissection. It should be done with great caution.
      Depending on the location of the tumor and the level of the inflammatory
      process, this step may be completed in a different order.
    - View the CT scan intra-op to anticipate the course of the major blood vessels
      and their branches as well as to rule out aberrant blood supply.
    - During the dissection of the uncinate process along the PV/SMV, identify the
      SMA and make sure it is not over-retracted laterally. An injury to this vessel
      can result in major bleeding or unnecessary conversion.

Fig. 21.14 Uncinate
process dissection

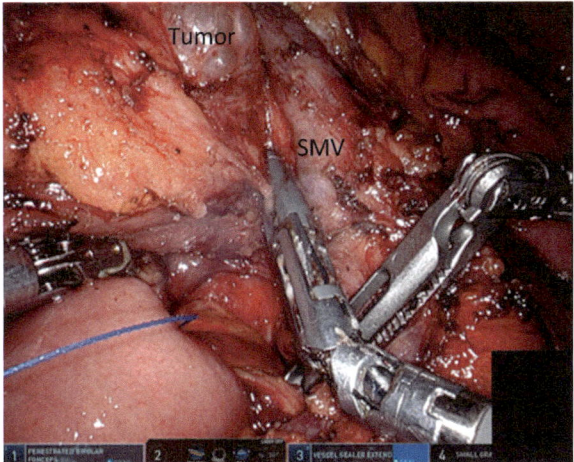

- In a case of a replaced right hepatic artery, it is crucial to identify and preserve it.
- When the dissection between the SMV/PV and the uncinate process is challenging, you may use the back side of the robotic hook to gently dissect these structures.

Step 6: CHD Transection and Cholecystectomy

- Arms setup:
  - Arm #1: Fenestrated bipolar
  - Arm #2: Camera
  - Arm #3: Vessel sealer, hook cautery
  - Arm #4: Small grasping retractor (bowel grasper)
  - Bedside assistant: Suctioning device
- Identify the common bile duct and continue dissection toward the common hepatic duct (CHD).
- Complete lymphadenectomy next to the bile duct and the portal vein.
- Transect the hepatic duct, remove biliary stent if present (Fig. 21.15).
- Expose the cystic artery and cystic duct and complete cholecystectomy.
- Once the hepatic duct is transected, the specimen is completely disconnected. It is removed through a laparoscopic EndoCatch Bag (Applied Medical, Rancho Santa Margarita, CA) inserted through the gel port.
- All specimen margins are marked and sent for pathological evaluation.
- Resection margins of pancreatic neck, distal CHD, and duodenum are sent for frozen sections which may dictate further resection.

Fig. 21.15 CHD
transection

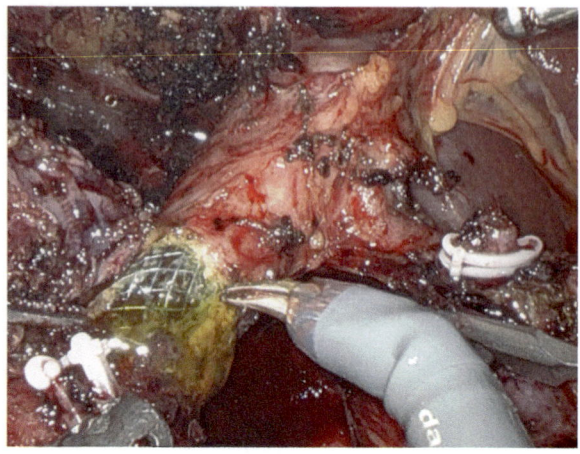

Reconstruction

All anastomoses are done using a jejunal loop in a retro-mesenteric approach. The
first anastomosis is the hepaticojejunostomy, followed by the pancreaticojejunostomy and the duodenojejunostomy. Arm setup for all anastomoses is the same.

- Arm #1: Needle driver
- Arm #2: Camera
- Arm #3: Monopolar scissors/megacut/needle driver
- Arm #4: Small grasping retractor (bowel grasper)
- Bedside surgeon: Needle driver, suction device

Hepaticojejunostomy

- Place the jejunal limb at the right direction where the stapler line is next to the
  pancreatic neck and the bowel courses along the pancreas to the hepatic duct.
- Approximately 10–12 cm distal to the staple line, make a 5–10 mm incision on
  the anti-mesenterial side of the bowel using monopolar scissors.
- We use two 3-0 absorbable V-loc™ sutures (Medtronic™, Minneapolis, MN,
  USA), 6–9 inches in length, starting at the 9 o'clock position (lateral side) to the
  3 o'clock position (medial side)
- Begin with the posterior aspect of the anastomosis by passing full-thickness
  sutures from the extra-luminal to the intra-luminal surface of the bowel and from
  the intra-luminal to the extra-luminal surface of the transected CHD (out-in,
  in-out).

- Using additional 3-0 or 4-0 absorbable V-Loc™ sutures, the anterior surface is sutured in a similar technique.
- In cases where the CHD is not dilated, a longitudinal ventral incision of the duct may increase the surface area of the anastomosis (Fig. 21.16).
- Once reaching the 3 o'clock position, both sutures are tied (Fig. 21.17).

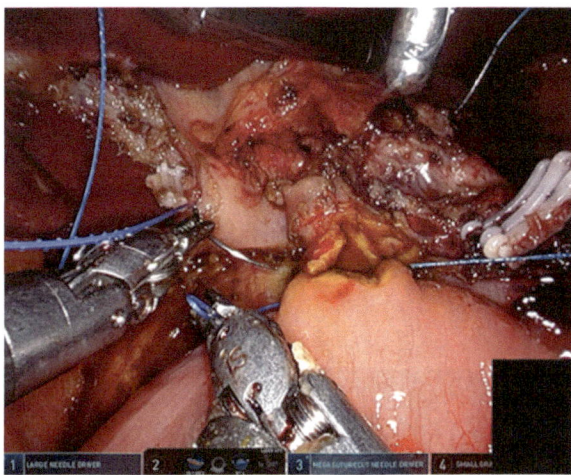

Fig. 21.16 Hepaticojejunostomy using a longitudinal ventral incision

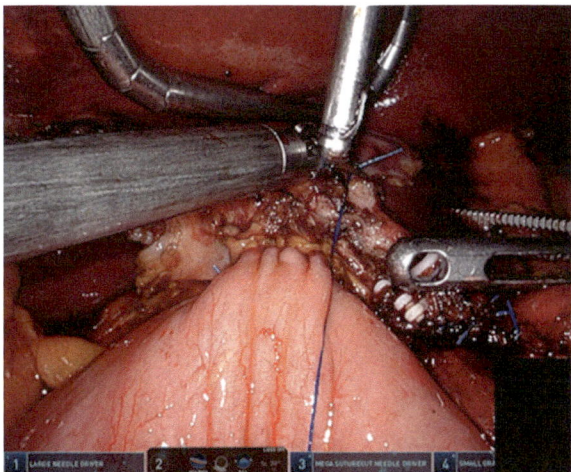

Fig. 21.17 Hepaticojejunostomy, completed

Pancreaticojejunostomy

- The jejunal limb is approximated to the pancreatic neck, the pancreatic duct is identified and accordingly, a small enterotomy is made for the anastomosis.
- The first layer is done using a running non-absorbable 3-0 V-lock™ starting on the superior part of the pancreas (Fig. 21.18).
- The first stitches are full thickness of the pancreatic substance. When reaching the pancreatic duct, we continue suturing the posterior wall only to avoid compressing the pancreatic duct.
- The inner layer includes interrupted 4-0 absorbable V-Loc™ sutures starting at the posterior side of the pancreatic duct. Four to five sutures are placed to complete the duct-to-mucosa layer (Fig. 21.19).
- A second running 3-0 non-absorbable V-Loc™ suture is then used to form the anterior-outer layer between the pancreatic parenchyma capsule and the seromuscular layer of the jejunal limb when the anterior and posterior outer-layer sutures are eventually tied together (Fig. 21.20).

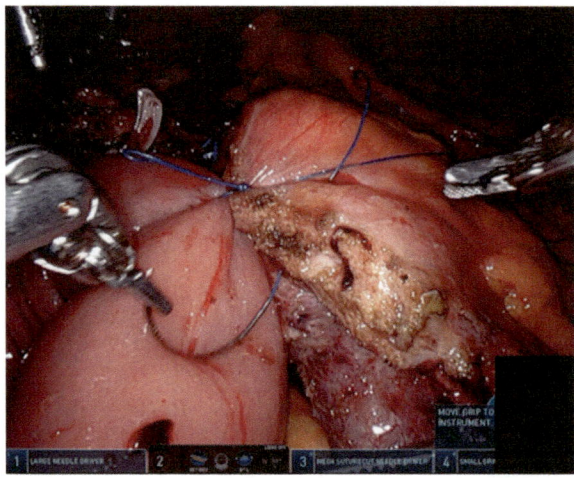

Fig. 21.18 Pancreaticojejunostomy

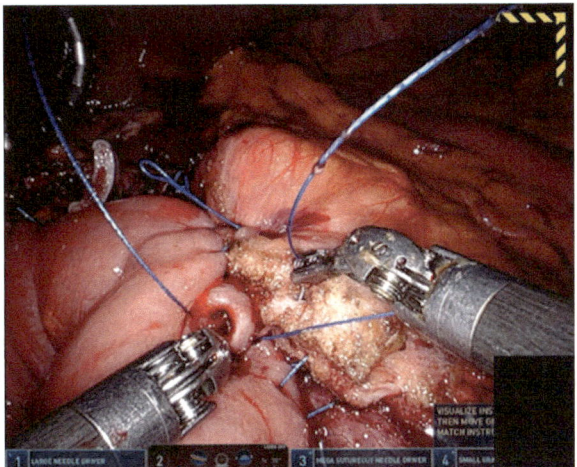

Fig. 21.19 Pancreaticojejunostomy, inner layer

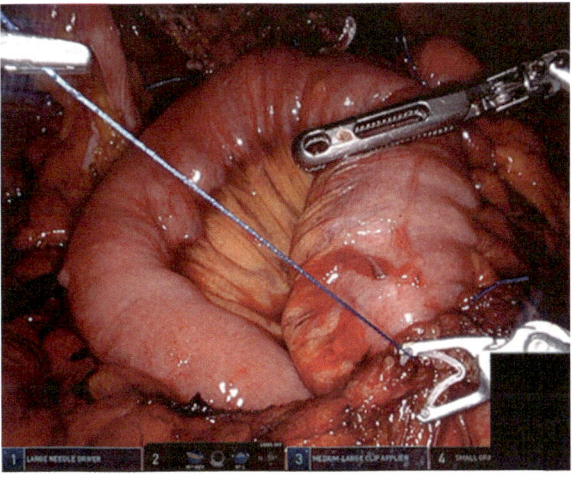

Fig. 21.20 Pancreaticojejunostomy, completed

Ligament of Treitz Restoration

- A 3-0 non-absorbable V-Loc™ suture is used to adhere the small bowel to a superficial layer of the transverse mesocolon, thus closing the Treitz-mesentery defect and preventing internal herniation of the small bowel.
- This suture is placed superficially to prevent injury to the bowel mesentery.

Duodenojejunostomy

- The jejunum distal to the hepaticojejunostomy is brought up in an antecolic fashion to the duodenal staple line.
- Using the scissors, we remove the duodenal staple line to expose the lumen. A generous incision is made with scissors on the anti-mesenteric aspect of the jejunal limb to expose the lumen.
- The duodenojejunostomy is undertaken in a similar fashion to the hepaticojejunostomy, this time using two running 3-0 non-absorbable V-Loc™ sutures (Figs. 21.21, 21.22, 21.23, and 21.24).
- Arm #4 is used to retract the stomach in the cephalad and ventral direction by grasping the stapler line.
- We run the dorsal and ventral layers of the anastomosis from the 9-o'clock to 3-o'clock positions, with knots tied on the extra-luminal surface at the 3-o' clock position. On the ventral layer, a Gambee technique allows inversion of the serosal surfaces and prevents mucosal perturbance.

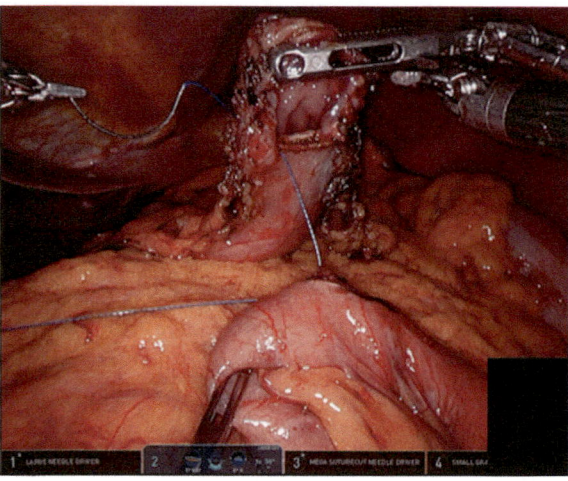

Fig. 21.21 Duodenojejunostomy

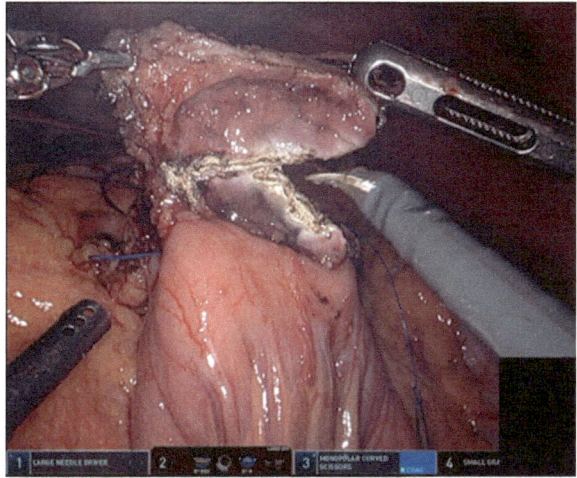

Fig. 21.22 Duodenojejunostomy

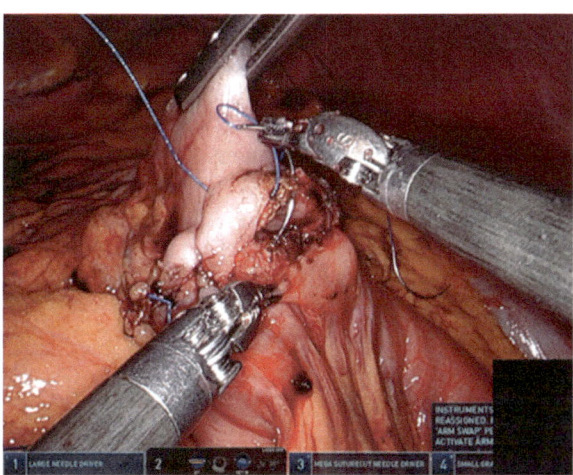

Fig. 21.23 Duodenojejunostomy

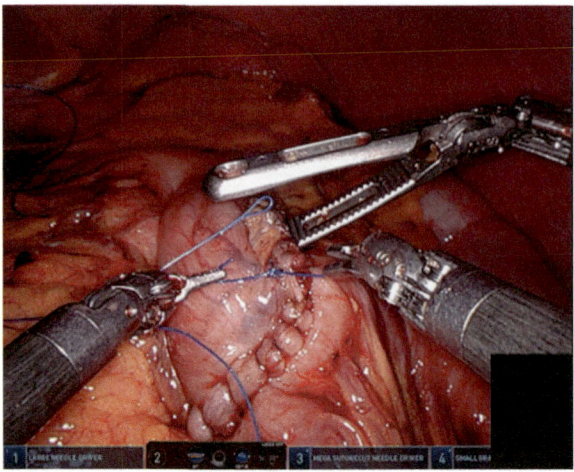

Fig. 21.24 Duodenojejunostomy, completed

Drainage and Closure

- Using the energized scissors, a falciform ligament flap is developed and placed over the hepaticojejunostomy and the GDA stump for reinforcement.
- An omental flap is placed over the pancreatojejunostomy and duodenojejunostomy to minimize leaks.
- A closed suction Jackson-Pratt drain is placed next to the hepaticojejunostomy and pancreatojejunostomy anastomosis.
- The robot is undocked, and the diaphragm is irrigated with bupivacaine to minimize postoperative pain.
- The fascia for all working ports is closed using an absorbable monofilament suture. The skin is closed with 4-0 Vicryl® sutures (Johnson & Johnson, New Brunswick, NJ, USA).

References

1. Whipple AO, Parsons WB, Mullins CR. Treatment of carcinoma of the ampulla of Vater. Ann Surg. 1935;102:763–79.
2. Newhook TE, LaPar DJ, Lindberg JM, Bauer TW, Adams RB, Zaydfudim VM. Morbidity and mortality of pancreatoduodenectomy for benign and premalignant pancreatic neoplasms. J Gastrointest Surg. 2015;19:1072–7.
3. Luu AM, Braumann C, Belyaev O, et al. Long-term survival after pancreatoduodenectomy in patients with ductal adenocarcinoma of the pancreatic head. Hepatobiliary Pancreat Dis Int. 2021;20:271–8.
4. Gagner M, Pomp A. Laparoscopic pylorus-preserving pancreatoduodenectomy. Surg Endosc. 1994;8:408–10.

5. Wang M, Peng B, Liu J, et al. Practice patterns and perioperative outcomes of laparoscopic pancreatoduodenectomy in China: a retrospective multicenter analysis of 1029 patients. Ann Surg. 2021;273(1):145–53.
6. Kuroki T, Fujioka H. Training for laparoscopic pancreatoduodenectomy. Surg Today. 2019;49(2):103–7.
7. Nickel F, Haney CM, Kowalewski KF, et al. Laparoscopic versus open pancreatoduodenectomy: a systematic review and meta-analysis of randomized controlled trials. Ann Surg. 2020;271:54–66.
8. van Hilst J, de Rooij T, Bosscha K, et al. Laparoscopic versus open pancreatoduodenectomy for pancreatic or periampullary tumours (LEOPARD-2): a multicentre, patient-blinded, randomised controlled phase 2/3 trial. Lancet Gastroenterol Hepatol. 2019;4:199–207.
9. Leal Ghezzi T, Campos Corleta O. 30 years of robotic surgery. World J Surg. 2016;40(10):2550–7.
10. Ross SB, Downs D, Sucandy I, Rosemurgy AS. Robotic pylorus-preserving pancreatoduodenectomy. In: Fong Y, Woo Y, Hyung W, Lau C, Strong V, editors. The SAGES atlas of robotic surgery. Cham: Springer; 2018. p. 319–34.
11. Rosemurgy A, Ross S, Luberice K, Browning H, Sucandy I. Robotic pancreatic surgery for solid, cystic, and mixed lesions. Surg Clin North Am. 2020;100:303–36.
12. Ross S, Rosemurgy A, Wecowski J, Bourdeau T, Sucandy I. Robotic pylorus-preserving pancreatoduodenectomy and cholecystectomy. Robotic general surgery. In: Atlas of robotic general surgery. Elsevier; 2021. p. 309–22.
13. Ross S, Rayman S, Sucandy I, Syblis C, Rosemurgy A. Whipple's operation and distal pancreatectomy. In: Costello T, editor. Principles and practice of robotic surgery. Elsevier; 2023.
14. Rosemurgy A, Ross S, Bourdeau T, et al. Cost analysis of pancreatoduodenectomy at a high-volume robotic hepatopancreaticobiliary surgery program. J Am Coll Surg. 2021;232:461–9.
15. Rosemurgy A, Ross S, Espeut A, et al. Survival and robotic approach for pancreatoduodenectomy: a propensity score-match study. J Am Coll Surg. 2022;234:677–84.
16. Rice MK, Hodges JC, Bellon J, et al. Association of mentorship and a formal robotic proficiency skills curriculum with subsequent generations' learning curve and safety for robotic pancreatoduodenectomy. JAMA Surg. 2020;155:607–15.
17. Rosemurgy A, Ross S, Bourdeau T, et al. Robotic pancreatoduodenectomy is the future: here and now. J Am Coll Surg. 2019;228(4):613–24.
18. Ouyang L, Zhang J, Feng Q, Zhang Z, Ma H, Zhang G. Robotic versus laparoscopic pancreatoduodenectomy: an up-to-date system review and meta-analysis. Front Oncol. 2022;12:834382.
19. Fogel EL, Shahda S, Sandrasegaran K, et al. A multidisciplinary approach to pancreas cancer in 2016: a review. Am J Gastroenterol. 2017;112(4):537–54.
20. National Comprehensive Cancer Network. Pancreatic adenocarcinoma (version 1.2022). Available from: https://www.nccn.org/professionals/physician_gls/pdf/pancreatic.pdf
21. Wiltberger G, Muhl B, Benzing C, et al. Preoperative risk stratification for major complications following pancreatoduodenectomy: identification of high-risk patients. Int J Surg. 2016;31:33–9.
22. Liang Y, Zhao L, Jiang C, et al. Laparoscopic pancreatoduodenectomy in elderly patients. Surg Endosc. 2020;34:2028–34.
23. Mogal H, Vermilion SA, Dodson R, et al. Modified frailty index predicts morbidity and mortality after pancreatoduodenectomy. Ann Surg Oncol. 2017;24(6):1714–21.
24. Melloul E, Lassen K, Roulin D, et al. Guidelines for perioperative care for pancreatoduodenectomy: enhanced recovery after surgery (ERAS) recommendations 2019. World J Surg. 2020;44(7):2056–84.
25. Zhang L, Sanagapalli S, Stoita A. Challenges in diagnosis of pancreatic cancer. World J Gastroenterol. 2018;24(19):2047–60.
26. Bispo M, Marques S, Rio-Tinto R, Fidalgo P, Devière J. The role of endoscopic ultrasound in pancreatic cancer staging in the era of neoadjuvant therapy and personalised medicine. GE Port J Gastroenterol. 2021;28(2):111–20.

Part VI
Surgical Technique—Distal Pancreatectomy

Chapter 22
Open Distal Pancreatectomy

Andrew J. Sinnamon and Pamela J. Hodul

Introduction

First reported attempts at open distal pancreatectomy date back to the 1880s, with Trendelenburg's resection of a pancreatic tail sarcoma in 1882, and Billroth performing resections of both the pancreatic head and tail in 1884 [1]. Sadly, Trendelenburg's initial foray into a distal pancreatic resection did not end well, as the patient reportedly died on postoperative day 1. Distal pancreatic resection was subsequently accomplished by the likes of Finney and Mayo at the turn of the century, but in general, significant gains in pancreatic resection were limited due to the three observations made by Mickulicz: (1) the pancreas being "exceedingly difficult to reach," (2) the notoriously difficult diagnosis of pancreatic disease, and (3) the "overwhelming physiological pitfalls" of surgery itself [1–3]. However, with the discovery of tumors of the endocrine pancreas in the late 1920s, enthusiasm for attempts at pancreatic resection returned, with a burst of activity by pancreatic surgeons including Mayo, Roscoe, and Whipple, during which time the technique for the distal pancreatectomy was refined [1, 4].

Following the establishment of pancreatic resection by these founders of surgery, modern surgical methodology generally favored a retrograde approach to distal pancreatectomy. This has classically been described and taught utilizing a lateral-to-medial operative flow. In this way, the spleen is mobilized first and retracted medially to gain exposure to the distal pancreas and lift it from the retroperitoneum. The popularity of this method is perhaps related to the ease of controlling the pancreas once the spleen is mobilized and manipulated with the left hand of the operating surgeon. However, this maneuver poses obvious risk of bleeding and may not place due focus on lymphadenectomy or resection margins in cases of malignancy.

A. J. Sinnamon (✉) · P. J. Hodul
Moffitt Cancer Center, Tampa, FL, USA
e-mail: Andrew.Sinnamon@moffitt.org; Pamela.Hodul@moffitt.org

© The Author(s), under exclusive license to Springer Nature Switzerland AG 2025
E. P. Ceppa et al. (eds.), *The SAGES Manual of Evolving Techniques in Pancreatic Surgery*, https://doi.org/10.1007/978-3-031-78409-5_22

393

As emphasis on oncologic principles over trauma principles grew for elective resections, a transition to an antegrade approach gradually took hold in the surgical school of thought. The most referenced technique for an antegrade operative approach was described by Strasberg, Drebin, and Linehan in 2003 and termed the radical antegrade modular pancreatosplenectomy (RAMPS) [5]. The rationale for the RAMPS approach was to utilize a medial-to-lateral dissection to provide early vascular control and optimize lymphadenectomy (the "antegrade" aspect of RAMPS) and to achieve negative tangential margins by tailoring dissection to the appropriate retroperitoneal fascial plane by adjusting as needed ("modular"). By "modulating" the dissection, one may perform an *anterior* RAMPS by removing the anterior renal fascia while preserving the left adrenal gland or, alternatively, perform a *posterior* RAMPS by removing the adrenal en bloc with the retroperitoneal dissection. Modern high-quality cross-sectional imaging allows for careful preoperative planning to plan between the two. Initial experience with RAMPS showed good lymph node retrieval rate with median of 15 nodes removed as well as over 90% negative tangential margins in cases of adenocarcinoma, which was confirmed in a subsequent follow-up study [6, 7]. While prospective comparison of RAMPS to standard retrograde distal pancreatectomy is limited, growing retrospective data suggests a higher lymph node retrieval rate and more frequent R0 resection for oncologic resections [8–11]. Differences in intraoperative blood loss and operative time remain unclear [8, 11].

Since lymphadenectomy and clear retroperitoneal margins were the intended goals of the RAMPS technique, it is most appropriate for oncologic resections. However, because of the advantages of early vascular control with an antegrade approach, the technique has been applied to other indications for distal pancreatic resection as well. As a result, RAMPS has steadily become a preferred approach among many surgeons for open distal pancreatectomy and splenectomy and has subsequently been adapted for minimally invasive approaches, not to be discussed in this chapter.

With the rise of laparoscopy and robotic platforms, minimally invasive approaches have become preferable for many distal pancreatic resections using either antegrade or retrograde approach. However, open distal pancreatectomy remains the safest option in many cases. This is particularly so for patients with significant past surgical history, pancreatitis, and locally invasive malignancy. Borderline resectable pancreatic adenocarcinoma is often best approached in an open manner for vascular involvement or need for en bloc resection of adjacent organs. When approaching these cases, the surgeon should be comfortable with both retrograde and antegrade approach so they may adapt to the case at hand. As such, both will be described in this chapter.

Preoperative Planning

Appropriate preoperative imaging to guide operative planning is critical. Pancreatic protocol CT scan is the preferred imaging modality in most cases, including thin section cuts at least <3 mm in thickness and preferably 0.5–1 mm [12]. Intravenous contrast should be used with imaging acquisition to include pancreatic parenchymal and arterial phase as well as delayed portal venous phase. If a specific pancreatic protocol is not available, a CT of the abdomen and pelvis with as thin as cuts as possible with arterial and venous phase may be an acceptable alternative. MRI with MRCP may be additionally helpful in cases with pancreatic cystic neoplasms where the relationship between cyst and pancreatic duct is of importance.

Open distal pancreatectomy is often performed for the specific reason that vascular involvement by a pathologic process makes a minimally invasive approach unsafe. For this reason, preoperative planning must include careful review of pancreas-dedicated imaging with attention to vascular anatomy. A potential site to divide the splenic artery must be identified that is free of disease pathology. This includes the absence of tumor encasement or abutment, but also in vasculopathic patients, this site must also be free of significant calcifications to be compliant for safe ligation. If there is no site for margin-negative division of the splenic artery due to tumor involvement up to and including the celiac trunk, en bloc resection of the celiac trunk (Appleby procedure) may be required. En bloc celiac resection with distal pancreatectomy will be thoroughly discussed in a subsequent chapter. In addition to identifying a suitable site for division, the course of the splenic artery should also be noted preoperatively to minimize any possibility of disastrously mistaking the common hepatic artery for the splenic during the operation.

An understanding of the portal venous anatomy is also mandatory for preoperative planning. It should be known if the inferior mesenteric vein (IMV) drains into the splenic vein as this would be necessarily divided during the resection. Similarly, the drainage of the left gastric vein should be noted as it may be preferable to leave this intact for improved gastric venous outflow. Identification of a proper site for ligation and division of the splenic vein is critical. For pancreatic cancer cases, thrombosis of the splenic vein is relatively common and may propagate to the level of the junction with the superior mesenteric vein (SMV). Occlusion of the splenic vein due to thrombosis or tumor encasement may result in left-sided portal hypertension. The presence of large varices, collaterals, or splenomegaly should be noted to prepare for safe resection while avoiding hemorrhage.

Based on preoperative imaging review, a general operative strategy may be planned. Depending on the site of disease, one may decide whether to divide the pancreas at the surgical neck (i.e., a subtotal pancreatectomy) versus transection at a point more distally. A more distal resection spares exocrine and endocrine function but also typically involves dividing a thicker pancreas. Transection of the body appears to result in a higher rate of postoperative pancreatic fistula but no difference in clinically significant fistulae [13–15]. Operative planning must also consider the possibility of resection of adjacent structures, most commonly the splenic flexure of colon, posterior stomach, or left adrenal gland. The possibility of splenic preservation will be discussed in detail in a subsequent chapter. If partial colectomy is planned, appropriate bowel preparation is warranted if not routinely performed for pancreatectomy. Surgical planning should consider whether an antegrade or retrograde approach is most suitable given the anatomy. Lastly, the retroperitoneal margin should be examined for an oncologic resection; if the posterior margin appears threatened with a standard resection plane, an anterior or posterior RAMPS (en bloc adrenalectomy) should be considered depending on the depth of invasion.

Other preoperative planning to consider for open distal pancreatectomy includes splenic immunization, thromboprophylaxis, consideration of bowel preparation, preoperative antibiotics, and relevant medications for an Enhanced Recovery After Surgery (ERAS) protocol. For planned splenectomy, vaccination against *S. pneumoniae, N. meningitidis,* and *H. influenzae* should ideally be started 10–12 weeks preoperatively, if possible, for completion of all vaccines 2 weeks prior to surgery. If not possible, vaccine series may be safely resumed 14 days postoperatively [16, 17]. Thromboprophylaxis should be considered according to a patient's calculated risk for venous thromboembolism. Bowel preparation should be performed if considering partial colectomy as noted above. However, the use of routine preparation for distal pancreatectomy is not standard; among 23 surveyed European centers performing distal pancreatectomy, routine bowel preparation was standard in only 8 [18]. Antibiotic prophylaxis should be administered within 1 h of incision and redosed accordingly during surgery. The use of ERAS protocols for pancreatectomy, potentially utilizing epidural anesthesia, will be discussed in a subsequent chapter, but may be an important piece of preoperative planning for open distal pancreatectomy.

Operative Setup and Steps

After induction of general anesthesia and placement of appropriate monitoring lines and urinary catheter, the patient is placed in the supine position with arms out. The abdomen is shaved, and sterile skin prep is applied. Open distal pancreatectomy may be performed using a variety of incisions, most commonly either a midline or transverse subcostal incision, and is per the operating surgeon's preference. Appropriate incision may be tailored according to patient body habitus and intraabdominal anatomy based on imaging review. A transverse incision is more beneficial than midline for distal pancreatectomy according to one survey of pancreatic surgeons [18]. Furthermore, a Cochrane review pooling data from different operations to compare midline versus transverse incision concluded that there is no difference in infection rate for elective operations and a lower rate of incisional hernia for transverse incision, and possibly less pain [19]. A left subcostal incision approximately two fingerbreadths inferior to and in a parallel orientation with the costal margin is most appropriate and may be extended across the midline as needed. It is our preference in many cases to use a bilateral subcostal incision for optimal exposure, providing ample visualization of both the medial aspect of vascular dissection and the lateral peri-splenic dissection, both sites of potential unwanted nuisance bleeding. We prefer to use the Thompson retractor system for open distal pancreatectomy.

Diagnostic Laparoscopy

Regardless of the preferred open incision, diagnostic laparoscopy is valuable prior to entering the abdomen as it may spare a considerable proportion of patients a nontherapeutic laparotomy. This is particularly the case when operating for pancreatic adenocarcinoma. Older data suggests that diagnostic laparoscopy at the outset of a planned pancreatic resection for adenocarcinoma may change management in up to 44% of cases [20]. More contemporary data from the Dutch PREOPANC trial found that staging laparoscopy identified occult peritoneal metastatic disease in 11–12% of cases [21]. Laparoscopy may be rapidly performed using a single camera port, with placement of additional ports as needed for visualization and/or biopsy of suspicious lesions. Ports may be placed that will be incorporated into the open incision, but this is not mandatory; a supraumbilical camera port is typically most appropriate for staging purposes and will obviously not lie in a subcostal incision. When operating for malignancy, laparoscopy should include thorough examination of the liver surface, omentum, peritoneal surface, and pelvis. Any suspicious lesions are biopsied and sent for frozen pathologic examination.

Open Exposure of the Pancreas

Once the decision is made to proceed with laparotomy, the abdomen is entered via the preferred incision. Care should be taken during this step to spare the falciform ligament so that it may be used later for flap coverage of the transected pancreas. Exposure of the pancreas may be first obtained by dividing the gastrocolic ligament to enter the lesser sac. Dissection is continued up the greater curvature of the stomach dividing the gastrocolic and gastrosplenic ligaments containing the short gastric vessels all the way to the left crura. Bipolar energy devices are useful for efficient hemostasis at this step. The gastroepiploic pedicle should be spared for gastric perfusion. Once the superior-most short gastric vessels are divided, it can be helpful to turn laterally to dissect just superior to the spleen in order to simplify completion of the dissection at a later point. Division of the gastrocolic ligament is then continued medially toward the pylorus. Dissection in this direction can proceed as far toward the patient's right as necessary to provide adequate exposure. In cases with a history of pancreatitis, the gastrocolic ligament may be found to be fused to the transverse mesocolon, or the posterior stomach may be densely adhered to the anterior pancreatic body. Careful dissection at this time should be undertaken to avoid entering the transverse mesocolon unnecessarily. Similarly, judgment should be exercised to distinguish adhesions to be divided as opposed to tumor to be resected en bloc. The stomach may now be reflected cranially and supported with a mounted retractor, providing complete exposure of the pancreatic neck and body.

Mobilization of the distal transverse colon and splenic flexure is typically required to complete exposure of the inferior border of the pancreas, although the amount of mobilization needed is variable. To mobilize the splenic flexure, dissection can be performed in two directions which converge at the spleen. Laterally, electrocautery dissection along the white line of Toldt while gently retracting the colon medially will separate the mesocolon from retroperitoneum. This may proceed in an inferior-to-superior direction. Medially, the distal transverse colon may be mobilized inferiorly by continuing division of the gastrocolic ligament toward the splenocolic ligamentous attachments. These attachments are typically well-vascularized; we generally use a bipolar energy device for hemostatic division. These two paths of dissection will meet near the spleen and then the fully mobilized splenic flexure may be safely retracted with a mounted retractor, gently placed to avoid traction injury.

Radical Antegrade Modular Pancreatosplenectomy (RAMPS)

If electing to proceed with a RAMPS approach, attention is next paid to the patient's midline. The root of the splenic artery is typically identified superior and posterior to the superior border of the pancreas, although there is significant variability, and this may be more posterior to the body. The left gastric vein will often drain at the level of the portosplenic confluence and may require ligation and division to clearly identify the splenic artery, but this is not necessary in all cases. Great care should be taken to delineate the root of the splenic artery from the root of the common hepatic artery, as these may be easily mistaken, particularly if both are running in a horizontal fashion. Identification and removal of the hepatic artery lymph node will expose the underlying common hepatic artery. Longitudinal dissection along the hepatic artery will identify the gastroduodenal artery; careful dissection just medial to this and above the superior border of the pancreas will expose the portal vein. To identify the SMV at the inferior neck of the pancreas, the right gastroepiploic and middle colic veins are identified and followed along their course to lead to their drainage into the SMV. This is best achieved by retracting the distal stomach anteriorly and toward the liver while simultaneously retracting the transverse colon inferiorly. These branches may be ligated and divided as needed to provide exposure.

Now that the portal vein has been identified superiorly and the SMV inferiorly, a retropancreatic tunnel may be developed to isolate the pancreas if planning to transect it at the surgical neck. This is achieved by carefully dissecting along the avascular plane posterior to the pancreatic neck at the level of the SMV until the tunnel meets the exposed portal vein superiorly. This dissection may be performed with a blunt dissector of the surgeon's preference, with deliberate, downward strokes to separate the vein away from the pancreas. Once this dissector has reached the level of the previously exposed portal vein, the pancreatic neck may be circled with a vessel loop or umbilical tape, if preferred, for division.

Once the pancreas has been circled, the splenic artery may be ligated and divided using clips, ties, or a vascular stapler. The pancreatic parenchyma may be subsequently divided. It is our preference to divide the pancreas using a triple-height linear stapler. Judgment must be exercised to use the appropriate thickness stapler load. Alternatively, if the pancreas is to be transected sharply, which may be necessary for an excessively thick pancreas, the pancreatic duct should be identified and directly closed with a U-stitch. The remainder of the gland may be closed in a running or U-stitch pattern. While initial prospective trial data showed no difference in rate of postoperative leak between staple and suture method for pancreatic transection, meta-analysis of the accumulated available data suggests that stapled transection is associated with a lower leak rate [22, 23].

Once the pancreas is transected, the distal aspect may be retracted laterally exposing the splenic vein, which may be ligated and divided. It should be noted that transection of the pancreas may be performed before division of the splenic artery if it is positioned posterior to the pancreatic body and therefore not easily accessed. In general, it is preferable to divide the artery before the vein to minimize hypertension within the spleen and allow for autotransfusion as the spleen drains. At this point, there remains no arterial flow to the spleen with division of the short gastric vessels and splenic artery so risk of hemorrhage is minimized.

After the splenic vein is divided, the root of the SMA should lie directly posteriorly allowing removal of the overlying lymph nodes en bloc with the specimen. Dissection along the inferior and superior borders of the pancreas allows for further retraction of the pancreatic body laterally. It is critical to remain cognizant of the fourth portion of the duodenum at this location to avoid injury. Dissection then continues just to the patient left of the SMA and proceeds posteriorly, deep to the anterior renal fascia to obtain a negative retroperitoneal margin. If an anterior RAMPS is planned, dissection continues laterally, staying just superficial to the adrenal gland and kidney. If a posterior RAMPS is planned for a more invasive tumor, dissection continues laterally, staying *deep* to the left adrenal and removing this en bloc. During this lateral dissection, any remaining attachments between the splenic flexure and inferior pancreas and spleen are divided using bipolar energy as they are commonly vascularized. Eventually the only remaining attachments to the specimen to be freed are the ligamentous attachments of the spleen to the left diaphragm. These are divided, taking care not to cause a full thickness injury to the diaphragm that would need repair. The specimen is then removed from the field.

Retrograde Distal Pancreatectomy and Splenectomy

The initial steps of a standard retrograde approach include division of the gastro-colic and gastrosplenic ligaments to expose the anterior aspect of the pancreas as described above.

A retrograde approach begins with takedown of the splenic flexure to expose the inferior border of the pancreas. The inferior and superior borders of the pancreas are mobilized by incising the overlying peritoneum allowing the pancreas to be lifted from the retroperitoneum. The splenic artery may then be identified superior to pancreas and subsequently ligated and divided. Early ligation of the short gastric vessels and splenic artery in this way now allows for relatively safe lateral-to-medial dissection beginning by dividing the attachments of the spleen to the diaphragm laterally. The spleen is then rotated medially, and the pancreas is dissected free from the anterior renal fascia in a lateral-to-medial manner. A deeper retroperitoneal margin may be taken as needed. This approach to dissection leaves the pancreas and spleen in the air ready for transection at the end. The splenic vein may be safely ligated and divided with the same fire of a linear stapler as the pancreas, or it may be taken separately. The specimen is then removed from the field. A retrograde approach may be preferable for cases when a more limited distal pancreatectomy is to be performed, as dissection at the level of the pancreatic neck may not be necessary.

Regardless of whether performing an antegrade or retrograde dissection, the resection bed is copiously irrigated and examined for hemostasis after removal of the specimen. The adjacent colon is examined for possible injury. The transection margin may be examined by frozen pathologic analysis during this time. A surgical drain is placed taking a long, looping course under the diaphragm with the end at the pancreatic resection line for management of possible postoperative leak. The looping course under the diaphragm helps to prevent dislodgement of the drain to a site where it is no longer effectively draining the pancreas. It is our preference to routinely harvest a falciform pedicle flap for coverage of the transection line, as discussed below. This may be secured in place with one or two sutures to the tissue adjacent to the pancreas.

Technical Pearls and Pitfalls

Early Ligation of Splenic Arterial Supply

If it is technically feasible to ligate the splenic artery early in the operation after committing to resection, this should help to significantly reduce the risk of significant splenic bleeding later. As the short gastric vessels are divided during initial exposure of the pancreas, ligation of the splenic artery leaves the spleen with no arterial supply and reduces pressure in the system. If it is still undetermined whether the surgeon will be committing to resection, a vessel loop or loose silk tie may be placed around the splenic artery early in the operation for urgent ligation at a later point for uncontrolled bleeding. This may even be performed before opening of the gastrocolic ligament, as the root of the splenic artery may alternatively be accessed by entering the lesser sac by opening the pars flaccida along the lesser curve of the stomach. As noted above, arterial ligation should be performed before division of the splenic vein to allow drainage of the spleen.

Splenic Artery Calcification

As discussed above, it should be re-emphasized that review of preoperative imaging should be very mindful of significant calcifications in the splenic artery. This might be overlooked while focusing on pancreatic pathology. A heavily calcified splenic artery will be noncompliant with a vascular stapler and may result in catastrophic hemorrhage. Intraoperative palpation for a soft segment of artery when there is known calcific disease is critical.

Splenic Vein Stump Length

If performing a distal pancreatectomy with transection of the pancreas at the surgical neck, it is preferable to divide the splenic vein flush with the SMV, if possible. There is evidence that the length of the residual splenic vein stump is a risk factor for postoperative thrombosis. This is presumably due to stagnant flow causing a nidus for thrombus formation. While thrombosis of the SMV stump is itself not problematic, forward propagation into the portal vein is potentially problematic.

Ligamentum Teres/Falciform Pedicle Flap

Care should be taken to preserve the falciform ligament/ligamentum teres during initial laparotomy so that it may be used as a vascularized flap to cover the transected pancreatic stump. A sizeable flap may be obtained by dissecting the ligament down to the umbilicus distally before dividing it and freeing the ligament from its membranous hepatic attachments to gain length. Leaving some preperitoneal fat on the distal aspect allows for an appreciable flap for coverage. Prospective data has shown the ligamentum teres flap to be associated with reduced rate of clinically relevant postoperative pancreatic fistula [24].

Reinforced Staple Line for Transection

Several products include reinforced stapler loads with the goal to reduce the rate of leak at the transection margin. While initial trial results were promising for reducing the rate of clinically relevant postoperative leak, more recent trial data has shown no difference in leak rate between reinforced and standard staplers [25–27]. There is evidence that reinforced staplers may be effective in the subset of patients with a thin pancreas [26]. We do not routinely use a reinforced stapler load for transection of the pancreatic parenchyma, but will selectively do so for cases with particularly soft pancreas.

References

1. McClusky DA 3rd, Skandalakis LJ, Colborn GL, Skandalakis JE. Harbinger or hermit? Pancreatic anatomy and surgery through the ages--part 2. World J Surg. 2002;26(11):1370–81.
2. Link GV. The treatment of chronic pancreatitis by pancreatostomy: a new operation. Ann Surg. 1911;53(6):768–82.
3. Mayo WJ. I. The surgery of the pancreas: I. Injuries to the pancreas in the course of operations on the stomach. II. Injuries to the pancreas in the course of operations on the spleen. III. Resection of half the pancreas for tumor. Ann Surg. 1913;58(2):145–50.
4. Whipple AO. Islet cell tumors of the pancreas. Can Med Assoc J. 1952;66(4):334–42.
5. Strasberg SM, Drebin JA, Linehan D. Radical antegrade modular pancreatosplenectomy. Surgery. 2003;133(5):521–7.
6. Mitchem JB, Hamilton N, Gao F, Hawkins WG, Linehan DC, Strasberg SM. Long-term results of resection of adenocarcinoma of the body and tail of the pancreas using radical antegrade modular pancreatosplenectomy procedure. J Am Coll Surg. 2012;214(1):46–52.
7. Strasberg SM, Linehan DC, Hawkins WG. Radical antegrade modular pancreatosplenectomy procedure for adenocarcinoma of the body and tail of the pancreas: ability to obtain negative tangential margins. J Am Coll Surg. 2007;204(2):244–9.
8. Latorre M, Ziparo V, Nigri G, Balducci G, Cavallini M, Ramacciato G. Standard retrograde pancreatosplenectomy versus radical antegrade modular pancreatosplenectomy for body and tail pancreatic adenocarcinoma. Am Surg. 2013;79(11):1154–8.
9. Park HJ, You DD, Choi DW, Heo JS, Choi SH. Role of radical antegrade modular pancreatosplenectomy for adenocarcinoma of the body and tail of the pancreas. World J Surg. 2014;38(1):186–93.
10. Trottman P, Swett K, Shen P, Sirintrapun J. Comparison of standard distal pancreatectomy and splenectomy with radical antegrade modular pancreatosplenectomy. Am Surg. 2014;80(3):295–300.
11. Abe T, Ohuchida K, Miyasaka Y, Ohtsuka T, Oda Y, Nakamura M. Comparison of surgical outcomes between radical antegrade modular pancreatosplenectomy (RAMPS) and standard retrograde pancreatosplenectomy (SPRS) for left-sided pancreatic cancer. World J Surg. 2016;40(9):2267–75.
12. Al-Hawary MM, Francis IR, Chari ST, et al. Pancreatic ductal adenocarcinoma radiology reporting template: consensus statement of the Society of Abdominal Radiology and the American Pancreatic Association. Radiology. 2014;270(1):248–60.
13. Pannegeon V, Pessaux P, Sauvanet A, Vullierme MP, Kianmanesh R, Belghiti J. Pancreatic fistula after distal pancreatectomy: predictive risk factors and value of conservative treatment. Arch Surg. 2006;141(11):1071–6; discussion 1076.

14. Sell NM, Pucci MJ, Gabale S, et al. The influence of transection site on the development of pancreatic fistula in patients undergoing distal pancreatectomy: a review of 294 consecutive cases. Surgery. 2015;157(6):1080–7.
15. Silvestri M, Coignac A, Delicque J, et al. Level of pancreatic division and postoperative pancreatic fistula after distal pancreatectomy: a retrospective case-control study of 157 patients with non-pancreatic ductal adenocarcinoma lesions. Int J Surg. 2019;65:128–33.
16. Shatz DV, Schinsky MF, Pais LB, Romero-Steiner S, Kirton OC, Carlone GM. Immune responses of splenectomized trauma patients to the 23-valent pneumococcal polysaccharide vaccine at 1 versus 7 versus 14 days after splenectomy. J Trauma. 1998;44(5):760–5; discussion 765–6.
17. Shatz DV, Romero-Steiner S, Elie CM, Holder PF, Carlone GM. Antibody responses in postsplenectomy trauma patients receiving the 23-valent pneumococcal polysaccharide vaccine at 14 versus 28 days postoperatively. J Trauma. 2002;53(6):1037–42.
18. Bruns H, Rahbari NN, Loffler T, et al. Perioperative management in distal pancreatectomy: results of a survey in 23 European participating centres of the DISPACT trial and a review of literature. Trials. 2009;10:58.
19. Brown SR, Goodfellow PB. Transverse verses midline incisions for abdominal surgery. Cochrane Database Syst Rev. 2005;(4):CD005199.
20. Doucas H, Sutton CD, Zimmerman A, Dennison AR, Berry DP. Assessment of pancreatic malignancy with laparoscopy and intraoperative ultrasound. Surg Endosc. 2007;21(7):1147–52.
21. Versteijne E, Suker M, Groothuis K, et al. Preoperative chemoradiotherapy versus immediate surgery for resectable and borderline resectable pancreatic cancer: results of the Dutch randomized phase III PREOPANC trial. J Clin Oncol. 2020;38(16):1763–73.
22. Diener MK, Seiler CM, Rossion I, et al. Efficacy of stapler versus hand-sewn closure after distal pancreatectomy (DISPACT): a randomised, controlled multicentre trial. Lancet. 2011;377(9776):1514–22.
23. Zhang H, Zhu F, Shen M, et al. Systematic review and meta-analysis comparing three techniques for pancreatic remnant closure following distal pancreatectomy. Br J Surg. 2015;102(1):4–15.
24. Hassenpflug M, Hinz U, Strobel O, et al. Teres ligament patch reduces relevant morbidity after distal pancreatectomy (the DISCOVER randomized controlled trial). Ann Surg. 2016;264(5):723–30.
25. Hamilton NA, Porembka MR, Johnston FM, et al. Mesh reinforcement of pancreatic transection decreases incidence of pancreatic occlusion failure for left pancreatectomy: a single-blinded, randomized controlled trial. Ann Surg. 2012;255(6):1037–42.
26. Kondo N, Uemura K, Nakagawa N, et al. A multicenter, randomized, controlled trial comparing reinforced staplers with bare staplers during distal pancreatectomy (HiSCO-07 trial). Ann Surg Oncol. 2019;26(5):1519–27.
27. Wennerblom J, Ateeb Z, Jonsson C, et al. Reinforced versus standard stapler transection on postoperative pancreatic fistula in distal pancreatectomy: multicentre randomized clinical trial. Br J Surg. 2021;108(3):265–70.

Chapter 23
Laparoscopic Distal Pancreatectomy

Elena Panettieri, Eduardo A. Vega, Ariana Chirban, and Claudius Conrad

History

Early Exploration

The location of the pancreas in the retroperitoneum and its complex anatomical relationships led to a late adoption of laparoscopic distal pancreatectomy (LDP). Initially, LDP was only considered for patients with benign conditions such as cystic lesions or neuroendocrine tumors [1–3]. There were concerns about the ability to

E. Panettieri
Department of Surgery, St. Elizabeth's Medical Center, Boston University School of Medicine, Boston, MA, USA

Hepatobiliary Surgery, Fondazione "Policlinico Universitario A. Gemelli", IRCCS, Università Cattolica del Sacro Cuore, Rome, Italy
e-mail: elena.panettieri@unicatt.it

E. A. Vega
Department of Surgery, St. Elizabeth's Medical Center, Boston University School of Medicine, Boston, MA, USA
e-mail: eduardo.vega@steward.org

A. Chirban
Department of Surgery, St. Elizabeth's Medical Center, Boston University School of Medicine, Boston, MA, USA

University of California, San Diego, School of Medicine, La Jolla, CA, USA
e-mail: achirban@health.ucsd.edu

C. Conrad (✉)
Department of Surgery, St. Elizabeth's Medical Center, Boston University School of Medicine, Boston, MA, USA

Carle Cancer Institute, Carle Illinois College of Medicine, Urbana, IL, USA
e-mail: cc@claudiusconrad.com

© The Author(s), under exclusive license to Springer Nature Switzerland AG 2025
E. P. Ceppa et al. (eds.), *The SAGES Manual of Evolving Techniques in Pancreatic Surgery*, https://doi.org/10.1007/978-3-031-78409-5_23

obtain safe oncological surgical margins or an adequate lymphadenectomy for pancreatic ductal adenocarcinoma (PDAC). Further, there were concerns regarding port-site tumor seeding [4]. In the early period, PDAC was an incidental postoperative pathological finding and not identified preoperatively [1–3].

The first cases of laparoscopic distal pancreatectomy (LDP) were described in 1994 by Sir Alfred Cuschieri [5, 6]. In his case-series of 5 patients, LDP of 70% of the gland with associated splenectomy was performed. The team used a 5-port technique, and the indication was intractable chronic pain from pancreatitis [7].

In 2006, D'Angelica et al. [8] reported their experience with minimally invasive distal pancreatectomy using a hand-assisted technique. The hand port enabled the surgeon to palpate the tumor and critical anatomic structures. Alternatively, the surgical assistant could use the hand port, allowing the surgeon to operate with two laparoscopic instruments while providing retraction. In their series of 17 cases, this approach demonstrated feasibility.

Trends Over Time

In 2010, a 7-year experience with LDP was reported. At the beginning of the period (2003), pure LDP was performed in 29% of cases, which increased to 40% in 2008, and 38% in 2009, with a rise in conversion rate [9]. Over the same time, there was a significant decrease in utilization of the hand-assisted technique from 80% to 17%. Regarding pancreatic remnant stump closure, there was a shift toward greater use of staplers and staples with a bioabsorbable staple line reinforcement (Seamguard®), corresponding with a decrease in sutured stump closure in both LDP and open distal pancreatectomy (ODP).

In 2012, an 11-year experience with LDP was reported, whereby the cohort was divided in an "early experience" (2000–2007) and a "recent experience" (2008–2011) group [10]. The most common indication was a cystic tumor (50.8%). It was observed that centrally located tumors of the pancreatic body (23% vs. 66.1%) and neck (3.3% vs. 8.1%) were increasingly resected using LDP, whereas the rate of tail neoplasm resection decreased (73.7% vs. 25.8%) ($p < 0.001$). The rate of patients with a Charlson's Comorbidity Score [11] ≥3 rose from 16.7% to 40.9% ($p = 0.003$). The medial-to-lateral dissection (described in detail later) became more popular in the recent period (39.4% vs. 53%, $p = 0.12$), as well as stapler reinforcement with the Seamguard® (4.7% vs. 28.8%, $p < 0.001$). Despite the growing complexity of cases, the hand-assisted technique was less commonly performed (68.1% vs. 25.6%, $p < 0.001$) and operative time reduced from 172 ± 69.1 to 141 ± 60.3 min ($p = 0.007$). Despite an increase in complexity over time, there were no differences in overall complications, postoperative pancreatic fistula (POPF), length of stay (LOS), or mortality.

Morbidity

Since these first reports, LDP has consistently been reported to lead to improved short-term outcomes when compared to ODP. For example, the Central Pancreas Consortium performed a matched comparison of 200 ODPs and 142 LDPs in 2008 [12]. Their results demonstrated lower average blood loss (BL) (357 vs. 588 mL, $p < 0.01$), fewer complications (40% vs. 57%, $p < 0.01$), and shorter LOS (5.9 vs. 9.0 days, $p < 0.01$) in patients undergoing LDP. There were no differences detected in terms of positive margin status (8% vs. 7%, $p = 0.8$), operative time (216 vs. 230 min, $p = 0.3$), or POPF rates (18% vs. 11%, $p = 0.1$). A later review and meta-analysis by Venkat et al. [13] confirmed lower BL by 355 mL ($p < 0.001$), decreased LOS by 4 days ($p < 0.001$), and a lower incidence of postoperative complications (33.9% vs. 44.2%, $p = 0.02$) in patients undergoing LDP vs. ODP. There were no significant differences between operative time, margin status, POPF, or postoperative mortality.

Safety

An overview of seven meta-analyses on LDP reported on outcomes and safety of published data between 2011 and 2016 [14]. The report demonstrated with a level of evidence 3a (recommendation grade B) that mortality of LDP is not inferior to ODP. This is particularly true for cases of benign/low-grade malignant tumors of the body/tail (six meta-analyses). LOS has been consistently reported to be shorter after LDP, but given the heterogeneity of studies analyzed, the authors concluded that LDP is only associated with a slightly shorter LOS than ODP (three meta-analyses—grade B recommendation). The rate of overall complications is lower after LDP for benign/low-grade malignant tumors (three meta-analyses with a 3a level of evidence, grade B recommendation). Regarding POPF, LDP is not inferior to ODP (seven meta-analysis—grade B recommendation). Only one meta-analysis by the same authors [15] described no differences in terms of overall survival (OS) and number of harvested lymph nodes for PDAC.

At the 2016 International Hepato-Pancreato-Biliary Association (IHPBA) conference, a panel of experts discussed the evidence and outcomes of minimally invasive distal pancreatectomy (MIDP) [16], suggesting that despite the high number of papers available, the superior efficacy of LDP vs. ODP remains controversial.

Further randomized controlled prospective data comparing MIDP to ODP is available. The important multicenter patient-blinded randomized controlled superiority trial [17] by the Dutch Pancreatic Cancer Group compared ODP with MIDP. Despite the latter also including robotic procedures, results notably demonstrated faster recovery and reduced BL for MIDP. While no differences were reported in terms of overall complications, and delayed gastric emptying. An improved quality of life was also shown without increased hospital costs among MIDP patients.

Notably, results from two clinical trials were recently published.

The prospective single-center, superiority, parallel, open-label, randomized control trial "*Laparoscopic* versus *open distal pancreatectomy* (LAPOP)" [18] focused on quality of life after ODP vs. LDP after a 1:1 randomization. Twenty-six patients in the open group and 28 in the laparoscopic group were included in the quality of life analysis and received the QLQ-C30 and PAN26 questionnaires at 5–6 weeks, 6 months, 1 year, and 2 years after surgery. The two questionnaires were developed to assess emotional and social well-being and physical symptoms among cancer and PDAC patients, respectively. LDP patients' answers demonstrated better results in terms of emotional functioning, pain, insomnia, pancreatic pain, future worries, and indigestion. Some of these differences persisted up to 2 years after surgery. In particular, social functioning, insomnia, and pancreatic pain were significantly worse after ODP at that time point.

The "*Minimally invasive versus open distal pancreatectomy for pancreatic ductal adenocarcinoma* (DIPLOMA)" [19] multicenter, randomized, non-inferiority trial aimed to compare MIDP with ODP to assess radical resection rate for potentially resectable PDAC located in the pancreatic body or tail. Surgical margins included the posterior and transection margins. LDP rate in the MIDP group was 73.5%. An R0 resection was achieved in 83 (72.8%) patients in the MIDP group and in 76 (69.1%) patients in the ODP group (difference 3.7%, 90% CI −6.2% to 13.6%; $p_{non-inferiority} = 0.039$). Median lymph node yield was comparable (22.0 [16.0–30.0] vs 23.0 [14.0–32.0] nodes, $p = 0.86$). Other postoperative outcomes were comparable, including median time to functional recovery and OS. It is important to note that patients receiving neoadjuvant treatment were well balanced between the two groups and that sensitivity analysis showed no impact of the inclusion of these patients on outcomes.

Finally, the Miami International Evidence-based Guidelines on Minimally Invasive Pancreas Resection [20] concluded that MIDP for benign and low-grade malignant tumors should be considered over ODP (grade 1B, expert agreement 95%, quality score 85%, audience agreement 100%). MIDP for PDAC is thought to be feasible, safe, and equivalent in experienced hands when performed for PDAC (grade 2B, expert agreement 95%, quality score 87%, audience agreement 96%).

Oncologic Safety

Upon confirming the safety and reduction in morbidity of LDP in selected patients, LDP for PDAC was explored by the Central Pancreas Consortium [21]. Of 212 patients undergoing distal pancreatectomy, 23 (11%) underwent LDP. Comparing LDP to ODP, before matching, only BL >500 mL was independently associated with a positive margin resection. After matching, a significantly higher body mass index (BMI) was found in patients undergoing LDP vs. ODP (28.5 ± 5.7 vs. 25.8 ± 4.6, $p = 0.03$). Operative BL was 329 mL higher ($p = 0.08$), and LOS was 2 days longer (9.4 ± 4.7 vs. 7.4 ± 3.4, $p = 0.006$) in the ODP group. OS was similar in the two groups (16 months each, $p = 0.71$), as well as the number of lymph nodes retrieved (ODP 12.3 ± 8.3 vs. LDP 14.0 ± 8.0, $p = 0.41$).

The Miami International Evidence-based Guidelines on Minimally Invasive Pancreas Resection [20] previously mentioned and concluded that MIDP for PDAC is feasible, safe, and equivalent to ODP in experienced hands when performed for PDAC (grade 2B, expert agreement 95%, quality score 87%, audience agreement 96%).

A National Cancer Database-based study by our group [22] showed that LDP for PDAC is not only safe, but it is also associated with oncological benefits such as lower margin positivity (odds ratio [OR] 0.581, $p = 0.005$), increased adjuvant chemotherapy use (third quartile: OR 1.844, $p = 0.026$; fourth quartile; OR 2.144, $p = 0.045$), and fewer delays in administration of adjuvant chemotherapy (fourth quartile: OR 0.786, $p = 0.045$) in higher-volume centers.

Preoperative Planning

Several clinical and anatomical variables need to be evaluated before planning a LDP. The IHPBA expert panel [16] identified five categories of factors to assess: surgeon related (individual and team experience), patient related (general health, previous abdominal surgery, BMI, and preoperative diagnosis), procedure related (visualization, wound issues, and adequate surgical equipment), tumor related (benign vs. malignant, anatomy, local advancement, and multivisceral resection), and society related (cost-effectiveness).

Clinical Considerations

Age alone should not be considered an absolute contraindication for LDP. It was demonstrated that LDP may be safe and feasible for patients >70 years old [23–25]. Sahakyan et al. [26] discussed how poor physical status, identified with how poor physical status, identified with American Society of Anesthesiology (ASA) grade 3–4, is associated with medical complications after LDP, but not with overall/major morbidity, surgical complications, or mortality.

The same authors [27] reported that obesity independently predicted prolonged operative time and was significantly associated with an increased intraoperative BL after LDP, while conversion, LOS, and major morbidity did not differ significantly between normal weight, overweight, and obese patients. Most notably, multivariate logistic regression analyses did not demonstrate an association between obesity and postoperative morbidity ($p = 0.09$), confirming results from previous reports [28,

29]. Others advocate that LDP may be particularly advantageous for obese patients as it increases accessibility to the deep abdomen, reduces wound complications, and is associated with the fastest recovery [30].

A study showed how LDP after previous upper abdominal surgery did not affect intraoperative course, postoperative morbidity, mortality, or LOS [31]. According to a global survey, surgeons routinely performing MIDP considered advanced age (2% vs. 11%; $p = 0.001$), ASA score >3 (16% vs. 28%; $p = 0.01$), and a prior laparotomy (11% vs. 19%; $p = 0.04$) less often a contraindication for choosing this approach in comparison to surgeons who did not have familiarity with the technique [32]. Similarly, a pan-European survey confirmed how patient selection is highly influenced by personal preference and team expertise [33].

Anatomical Considerations

Regarding tumor and anatomical factors, most surgeons consider both multivisceral and vascular involvement as critical contraindications for LDP, while a minority of them believe there are no absolute contraindications [33]. Two papers offered an insightful perspective on preoperative planning. The first [34] identified three factors associated with open conversion at univariate analyses: site of the tumor, extent of the resection, and adjacent organ involvement. Only extension into adjacent organs remained significant after multivariate analyses. The second [35] provided a difficulty scoring system, which reported five significant factors: type of resection, resection line (i.e., transection near the portal vein that requires tunneling under the pancreatic neck or more distal resection with no need for tunneling), proximity of tumor to major vessels, tumor extension to peripancreatic tissue, and left-sided portal hypertension/splenomegaly. The authors also suggested to look for the following on preoperative imaging: parenchymal thickness at the expected resection line, preoperative indicators of pancreatic texture (obstructive pancreatitis with a dilated distal pancreatic duct and parenchymal atrophy, loss of lobulated parenchymal structure, and calcifications), and presence of a circumportal pancreas.

Similarly, Partelli et al. [36] demonstrated how a thick parenchyma at the resection line ($p = 0.014$) and tumor proximity to major vessels ($p = 0.002$) were significant risk factors for the presence of ≥ 1 outcomes of surgical difficulty.

An International Expert Consensus on Precision Anatomy for MIDP [37] recommended caution regarding celiac artery (CA) variations, origin, and course of the splenic artery (SA) and dorsal pancreatic arteries (DPAs), as well as drainage pattern of the left gastric (LGV) and inferior mesenteric (IMV) veins. In this setting, preoperative three-dimensional (3D) reconstruction can help to visualize the anatomy and is correlated with better depth perception, decreased physical demand [38], BL, and operative time in small series [38, 39]. Nakata et al. [40] described two variants based on the relationship between the root of the SA and the pancreatic parenchyma: the buried type (60%) where the root of the SA was in close proximity behind the pancreatic parenchyma, and the non-buried type (40%) where the root of the SA is separated from the pancreatic parenchyma by a wide space. Using

Table 23.1 A summary of radiologic features to look for when planning a laparoscopic distal pancreatectomy

Location and size of the tumor
Proximity to major vessels
Extension to peripancreatic tissue
Multivisceral involvement
Distance of the expected resection line from the main portal vein
Parenchymal thickness at the expected resection line
Left sided portal hypertension/splenomegaly
Circumportal pancreas
Obstructive pancreatitis
Parenchymal atrophy
Loss of lobulated parenchymal texture
Calcifications

preoperative 3D computed tomography (CT) for anatomical reconstruction, the buried type was associated with a significantly longer median operative time, a higher mean BL, and prolonged overall operative time.

Table 23.1 summarizes radiologic factors to consider when planning a LDP. Figure 23.1 shows a CT image of a mucinous cystadenoma of the tail of the pancreas amenable to LDP. Figure 23.2 presents an example of preoperative CT-based 3D reconstruction.

Surgical Technique

1. *Patient position and placement of trocars*:

    In the author's practice, the patient is placed in the French position, with arms tucked and legs in stirrups. It can be helpful to rotate the patient 45° to the right and have the patient in the reversed Trendelenburg position. A 12-mm optical trocar is placed in the left paramedian location below the left costal margin. Pneumoperitoneum is established with a pressure of 12–15 mmHg. Three additional operative trocars are placed to the left of the midline as follows:

    - A 12 mm midline mid-epigastric camera port
    - A 5 mm subxiphoid assistant port
    - A 5 mm left anterior axillary port

2. *Lateral-to-medial vs. medial-to-lateral approach*

    There are two approaches to expose the pancreas and allow for pancreatic transection. The dissection can be carried out from lateral-to-medial or medial-to-lateral [41–43].

    (a) *Lateral to medial*

        For the lateral-to-medial technique, the inferior border of the pancreas is exposed by deflecting the transverse mesocolon inferiorly. The splenic flexure of the colon is grasped, and the gastrosplenic and splenocolic ligaments, both avascular, are divided with help of an energy device using ultrasonic

Fig. 23.1 A computed tomography image (arterial phase) of a mucinous cystadenoma at the tail of the pancreas in a 68-year-old man. There is no abnormal enhancement, solid component, or septation of the lesion. No parenchymal atrophy of ductal dilation is detected

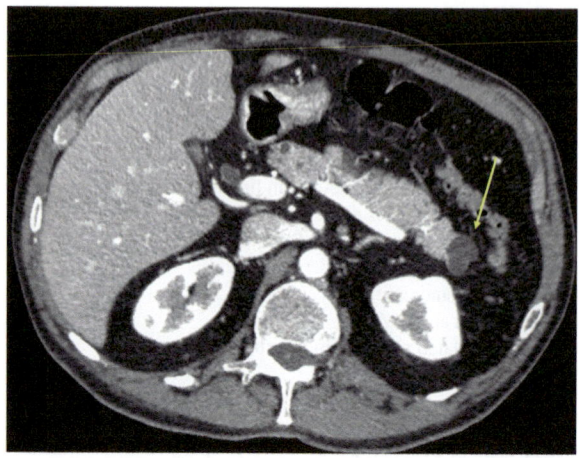

Fig. 23.2 A computed tomography based three-dimensional pancreatic vascular reconstruction

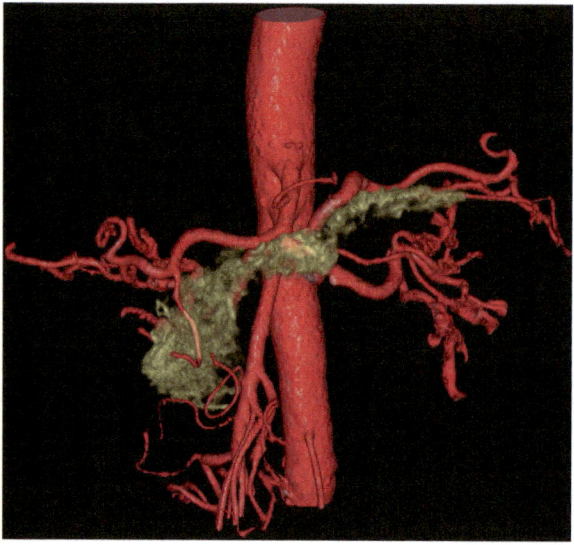

and bipolar energy. The left colon distal to the splenic flexure is partially mobilized along the white line of Toldt and deflected medially. It is critical to not accidently enter Gerota's fascia or dissect the interspace between the lateral abdominal wall and kidney. The greater omentum is incised to enter the lesser sac. The splenic flexure is peeled down off Gerota's fascia, revealing the tail of the pancreas.

The dissection continues medially along the transverse colon, dividing the attachments of the greater omentum to the greater curvature of the stomach near the origin of the right gastroepiploic artery. The greater omentum is swept medially, gaining access to the lesser sac, and allowing access to the body of the pancreas medial to the tail. The stomach is retracted superomedially using a transfixing free-eyed needle placed through the abdominal wall [44].

In case of splenic vessel preservation, the splenic artery and vein are carefully dissected off the posterior surface of the pancreas starting at the splenic hilum. The dissection is carried out past the target lesion in the pancreas and then the pancreas transected. In case of splenic resection, the short gastric arteries and lienorenal ligament are divided early, and the spleen is resected "en bloc" with the specimen.

(b) *Medial-to-lateral*

For the medial-to-lateral dissection, the portal venous confluence is dissected out early by following the SMV and its branches to its drainage to the portal vein. Working underneath the pancreas, the capsule is carefully detached from the underlying SMV/splenic vein (SV) confluence. When the tunnel is created, care must be taken to prevent injury to the celiac trunk. A tunnel behind the neck of the pancreas is formed. An umbilical tape is passed around the body of the pancreas, medial to the site of the tumor, through the retro-pancreatic tunnel. Prior to stapling, one has to confirm that neither the common hepatic artery nor celiac trunk are caught in the stapler. The neck of the pancreas is transected using a stapler. The dissection continues to the left toward the splenic hilum. Gentle traction on the spleen is applied medially to divide the splenorenal and splenophrenic ligaments. The short gastric vessels are ligated.

3. *Splenic vessel dissection*

In case of splenic vessel preservation, the pancreas is detached from the splenic artery and vein with careful dissection using a vessel sealer and bipolar cautery. We have previously reported a detailed instructional video on successful splenic vessel preservation [44]. Minimizing splenic vein manipulation is critical in reducing postoperative thrombosis.

4. *Pancreatic transection and mobilization*

According to the Miami guidelines [20], both stapler and non-stapler closure can be used in LDP, with similar outcomes, and no evidence suggests a benefit of reinforcing the staple line (recommendation grade 2C).

5. *Specimen retrieval and drain placement*

The specimen is retrieved using an endoscopic retrieval bag through a midline incision. Based on surgeons' preference, a #19 Blake drain is left in the resection zone and secured in the upper left quadrant, followed by closure of port sites in a standard fashion.

Tips and tricks are summarized in Table 23.2.

Table 23.2 Tips and tricks

Port placement high in the right upper quadrant
Wide colonic mobilization to facilitate exposure of the inferior border of the pancreas
Gastric retraction transfixion needle to save ports
Careful division of splenic ligaments to avoid capsular tearing
Slow stapler closure and transection to reduce leaks

Lymphadenectomy and Radical Anterograde Modular Pancreatosplenectomy

According to the Japanese Pancreas Society [45], a standard lymphadenectomy for PDAC should include lymph node stations 10, 11, and 18 for tumors located in the body and tail of the pancreas. To increase the probability of achieving negative margins and harvesting an appropriate number of lymph nodes, Strasberg et al. [46] introduced the radical anterograde modular pancreatosplenectomy (RAMPS). This approach aims to perform a complete N1 lymph node dissection and to minimize a positive retroperitoneal margin. During RAMPS, the division of the neck of the pancreas and splenic vessels with celiac node dissection is performed first. The dissection proceeds to the left of the CA and SMA to their origin. The posterior plane of dissection can be carried out superior to the left adrenal gland and Gerota's fascia (anterior RAMPS) or can be posterior to the adrenal and Gerota's fascia (posterior RAMPS). The dissection then continues from right-to-left in two possible posterior dissection planes based on the depth of invasion of the PDAC [47, 48]. According to this technique, the N1 lymphadenectomy includes lymph nodes along the superior and inferior borders of the left-sided pancreas (10, 11, and 18), the celiac lymph nodes (9), and the lymph nodes along the front and left side of superior mesenteric artery (14p and 14d).

Distal Pancreatectomy with En Bloc Celiac Axis Resection

In the case of advanced body/tail PDAC involving the CA or the CHA, the distal pancreas can be resected "en-bloc" with the surrounding structures: CA (with CHA and SA), the left adrenal gland, and the celiac plexus [49]. This can be achieved through a right retroperitoneal, left retroperitoneal, ventral, or median approach [50].

Training and Learning Curve

With the rising popularity of LDP, the learning curve of LDP has been investigated. The Dutch Pancreatic Cancer Group proposed a nationwide training program (LEALAPS-1) [51] including following a detailed technique outline and video training (2 hrs combined), followed by on-site or off-site proctoring by MIDP experts. The surgeon could then start practicing MIDP independently after the proctor's approval. Comparing results before and after training, improvement in conversion rate, estimated BL, and LOS were evident. According to different authors, a single surgeon learning curve is achieved after 17 LDPs [52] and a reduction in morbidity and LOS is achieved after 30 LDPs [53]. While surgeons should be familiar with different MIDP approaches, it is recommended to standardize their proper technique [37].

Conclusion

In this chapter, the advantages and safety of LDP vs. ODP are detailed. Today, LDP can be considered an appropriate approach for malignant disease by experienced surgeons for selected patients and may improve morbidity and oncologic outcomes. While the benefits regarding morbidity include reduced operative time, BL, margins, and subsequently hospital costs, the oncologic benefits may include faster return to and fewer delays in initiating adjuvant chemotherapy.

References

1. Gagner M, Pomp A. Laparoscopic pancreatic resection: is it worthwhile? J Gastrointest Surg. 1997;1(1):20–5; discussion 25–6. https://doi.org/10.1007/s11605-006-0005-y.
2. Cuschieri SA, Jakimowicz JJ. Laparoscopic pancreatic resections. Semin Laparosc Surg. 1998;5(3):168–79. https://doi.org/10.1177/155335069800500303.
3. Patterson EJ, Gagner M, Salky B, Inabmet WB, Brower S, Edye M, et al. Laparoscopic pancreatic resection: single-institution experience of 19 patients. J Am Coll Surg. 2001;193(3):281–7. https://doi.org/10.1016/s1072-7515(01)01018-3.
4. Johnstone PA, Rohde DC, Swartz SE, Fetter JE, Wexner SD. Port site recurrences after laparoscopic and thoracoscopic procedures in malignancy. J Clin Oncol. 1996;14(6):1950–6. https://doi.org/10.1200/JCO.1996.14.6.1950.
5. Cuschieri A. Laparoscopic surgery of the pancreas. J R Coll Surg Edinb. 1994;39(3):178–84.
6. Morris K. Alfred Cuschieri: pioneer of minimal access therapies. Lancet. 1999;353(9151):474. https://doi.org/10.1016/S0140-6736(05)75151-5.
7. Cuschieri A, Jakimowicz JJ, van Spreewuel J. Laparoscopic distal 70% pancreatectomy and splenectomy for chronic pancreatitis. Ann Surg. 1996;223(3):280–5. https://doi.org/10.1097/00000658-199603000-00008.
8. D'Angelica M, Are C, Jarnagin W, DeGregoris G, Coit D, Jaques D, et al. Initial experience with hand-assisted laparoscopic distal pancreatectomy. Surg Endosc. 2006;20(1):142–8. https://doi.org/10.1007/s00464-005-0209-3.
9. Jayaraman S, Gonen M, Brennan MF, D'Angelica M, DeMatteo RP, Fong Y, et al. Laparoscopic distal pancreatectomy: evolution of a technique at a single institution. J Am Coll Surg. 2010;211(4):503–9. https://doi.org/10.1016/j.jamcollsurg.2010.06.010.
10. Kneuertz PJ, Patel SH, Chu CK, Fisher SB, Maithel SK, Sarmiento JM, et al. Laparoscopic distal pancreatectomy: trends and lessons learned through an 11-year experience. J Am Coll Surg. 2012;215(2):167–76. https://doi.org/10.1016/j.jamcollsurg.2012.03.023.
11. Charlson ME, Pompei P, Ales KL, MacKenzie CR. A new method of classifying prognostic comorbidity in longitudinal studies: development and validation. J Chronic Dis. 1987;40(5):373–83. https://doi.org/10.1016/0021-9681(87)90171-8.
12. Kooby DA, Gillespie T, Bentrem D, Nakeeb A, Schmidt MC, Merchant NB, et al. Left-sided pancreatectomy: a multicenter comparison of laparoscopic and open approaches. Ann Surg. 2008;248(3):438–46. https://doi.org/10.1097/SLA.0b013e318185a990.

13. Venkat R, Edil BH, Schulick RD, Lidor AO, Makary MA, Wolfgang CL. Laparoscopic distal pancreatectomy is associated with significantly less overall morbidity compared to the open technique: a systematic review and meta-analysis. Ann Surg. 2012;255(6):1048–59. https://doi.org/10.1097/SLA.0b013e318251ee09.

14. Ricci C, Casadei R, Taffurelli G, Pacilio CA, Minni F. Laparoscopic distal pancreatectomy: many meta-analyses, few certainties. Updat Surg. 2016;68(3):225–34. https://doi.org/10.1007/s13304-016-0389-5.

15. Ricci C, Casadei R, Taffurelli G, Toscano F, Pacilio CA, Bogoni S, et al. Laparoscopic versus open distal pancreatectomy for ductal adenocarcinoma: a systematic review and meta-analysis. J Gastrointest Surg. 2015;19(4):770–81. https://doi.org/10.1007/s11605-014-2721-z.

16. Røsok BI, de Rooij T, van Hilst J, Kiener MK, Allen PJ, Vollmer CM, et al. Minimally invasive distal pancreatectomy. HPB (Oxford). 2017;19(3):205–14. https://doi.org/10.1016/j.hpb.2017.01.009.

17. De Rooij T, van Hilst J, van Santvoort H, Boerma D, van den Boezem P, Daams F, et al. Minimally invasive versus open distal pancreatectomy (LEOPARD): a multicenter patient-blinded randomized controlled trial. Ann Surg. 2019;269(1):2–9. https://doi.org/10.1097/SLA.0000000000002979.

18. Johansen K, Lindhoff Larsson A, Lundgren L, Gasslander T, Hjalmarsson C, Sandström P, Björnsson B. Quality of life after open versus laparoscopic distal pancreatectomy: long-term results from a randomized clinical trial. BJS Open. 2023;7(2):zrad002. https://doi.org/10.1093/bjsopen/zrad002.

19. Korrel M, Jones LR, van Hilst J, Balzano G, Björnsson B, Boggi U, Bratlie SO, et al., European Consortium on Minimally Invasive Pancreatic Surgery (E-MIPS). Minimally invasive versus open distal pancreatectomy for resectable pancreatic cancer (DIPLOMA): an international randomised non-inferiority trial. Lancet Reg Health Eur. 2023;31:100673. https://doi.org/10.1016/j.lanepe.2023.100673.

20. Asbun HJ, Moekotte AL, Vissers FL, Kunzler F, Cipriani F, Alseidi A, et al. The Miami international evidence-based guidelines on minimally invasive pancreas resection. Ann Surg. 2020;271(1):1–14. https://doi.org/10.1097/SLA.0000000000003590.

21. Kooby DA, Hawkins WG, Schmidt MC, Weber SM, Bentrem DJ, Gillepsie TW, et al. A multicenter analysis of distal pancreatectomy for adenocarcinoma: is laparoscopic resection appropriate? J Am Coll Surg. 2010;210(5):779–87. https://doi.org/10.1016/j.jamcollsurg.2009.12.033.

22. Salehi O, Vega EA, Kutlu OC, Krishnan S, Sleeman D, De La Cruz MN, et al. Does a laparoscopic approach to distal pancreatectomy for cancer contribute to optimal adjuvant chemotherapy utilization? Ann Surg Oncol. 2021;28(13):8273–80. https://doi.org/10.1245/s10434-021-10241-5.

23. Giuliani A, Ceccarelli G, Rocca A. The role of laparoscopic distal pancreatectomy in elderly patients. Minerva Chir. 2018;73(2):179–87. https://doi.org/10.23736/S0026-4733.18.07594-6.

24. Chen K, Pan Y, Mou YP, Yan JF, Zhang RC, Zhang MZ, et al. Surgical outcomes of laparoscopic distal pancreatectomy in elderly and octogenarian patients: a single-center, comparative study. Surg Endosc. 2019;33(7):2142–51. https://doi.org/10.1007/s00464-018-6489-1.

25. van der Heijde N, Balduzzi A, Alseidi A, Dokmak S, Polanco PM, Sandford D, et al. The role of older age and obesity in minimally invasive and open pancreatic surgery: a systematic review and meta-analysis. Pancreatology. 2020;20(6):1234–42. https://doi.org/10.1016/j.pan.2020.06.013.

26. Sahakyan MA, Tholfsen T, Kleive D, Waage A, Buanes T, Labon KJ, et al. Laparoscopic distal pancreatectomy in patients with poor physical status. HPB (Oxford). 2021;23(6):877–81. https://doi.org/10.1016/j.hpb.2020.10.004.

27. Sahakyan MA, Røsok BI, Kazaryan AM, Barkhatov L, Lai X, Kleive D, et al. Impact of obesity on surgical outcomes of laparoscopic distal pancreatectomy: a Norwegian single-center study. Surgery. 2016;160(5):1271–8. https://doi.org/10.1016/j.surg.2016.05.046.

28. Malleo G, Salvia R, Mascetta G, Esposito A, Landoni L, Casetti L, et al. Assessment of a complication risk score and study of complication profile in laparoscopic distal pancreatectomy. J Gastrointest Surg. 2014;18(11):2009–15. https://doi.org/10.1007/s11605-014-2651-9.

29. de Rooij T, Jilesen AP, Boerma J, Bonsing BA, Bosscha K, van Dam RM, et al. A nationwide comparison of laparoscopic and open distal pancreatectomy for benign and malignant disease. J Am Coll Surg. 2015;220(3):263–270.e1. https://doi.org/10.1016/j.jamcollsurg.2014.11.010.

30. Liang S, Hameed U, Jayaraman S. Laparoscopic pancreatectomy: indications and outcomes. World J Gastroenterol. 2014;20(39):14246–54. https://doi.org/10.3748/wjg.v20.i39.14246.

31. Sahakyan MA, Tholfsen T, Kleive D, Yaqub S, Kazaryan AM, Buanes T, et al. Laparoscopic distal pancreatectomy following prior upper abdominal surgery (pancreatectomy and prior surgery). J Gastrointest Surg. 2021;25(7):1787–94. https://doi.org/10.1007/s11605-020-04858-2.

32. van Hilst J, de Rooij T, Abu Hilal M, Asbun HJ, Barkun J, Boggi U, et al. Worldwide survey on opinions and use of minimally invasive pancreatic resection. HPB (Oxford). 2017;19(3):190–204. https://doi.org/10.1016/j.hpb.2017.01.011.

33. de Rooij T, Besselink MG, Shamali A, Butturini G, Busch OR, Edwin B, et al. Pan-European survey on the implementation of minimally invasive pancreatic surgery with emphasis on cancer. HPB (Oxford). 2016;18(2):170–6. https://doi.org/10.1016/j.hpb.2015.08.005.

34. Casadei R, Ricci C, Pacilio CA, Ingaldi C, Taffurelli G, Minni F. Laparoscopic distal pancreatectomy: which factors are related to open conversion? Lessons learned from 68 consecutive procedures in a high-volume pancreatic center. Surg Endosc. 2018;32(9):3839–45. https://doi.org/10.1007/s00464-018-6113-4.

35. Ohtsuka T, Ban D, Nakamura Y, Nagakawa Y, Tanabe M, Gotoh Y, et al. Difficulty scoring system in laparoscopic distal pancreatectomy. J Hepatobiliary Pancreat Sci. 2018;25(11):489–97. https://doi.org/10.1002/jhbp.578.

36. Partelli S, Ricci C, Rancoita PMV, Montorsi R, Andreasi V, Ingaldi C, et al. Preoperative predictive factors of laparoscopic distal pancreatectomy difficulty. HPB (Oxford). 2020;22(12):1766–74. https://doi.org/10.1016/j.hpb.2020.04.002.

37. Ban D, Nishino H, Ohtsuka T, Nagakawa Y, Abu Hilal M, Asbun HJ, et al. International Expert Consensus on Precision Anatomy for minimally invasive distal pancreatectomy: PAM-HBP Surgery Project. J Hepatobiliary Pancreat Sci. 2022;29(1):161–73. https://doi.org/10.1002/jhbp.1071.

38. Jun E, Alshahrani AA, Song KB, Hwang DW, Lee JH, Shin SH, et al. Validation and verification of three-dimensional systems in laparoscopic distal pancreatectomy. Anticancer Res. 2019;39(2):867–74. https://doi.org/10.21873/anticanres.13187.

39. Aoki T, Koizumi T, Mansour DA, Fujimori A, Kusano T, Matsuda K, et al. Virtual reality with three-dimensional image guidance of individual patients' vessel anatomy in laparoscopic distal pancreatectomy. Langenbecks Arch Surg. 2020;405(3):381–9. https://doi.org/10.1007/s00423-020-01871-6.

40. Nakata K, Ohtsuka T, Miyasaka Y, Watanabe Y, Ideno N, Mori Y, et al. Evaluation of relationship between splenic artery and pancreatic parenchyma using three-dimensional computed tomography for laparoscopic distal pancreatectomy. Langenbecks Arch Surg. 2021;406(6):1885–92. https://doi.org/10.1007/s00423-021-02101-3.

41. Dokmak S, Aussilhou B, Ftériche FS, Soubrane O, Sauvanet A. Laparoscopic central pancreatectomy: surgical technique. J Visc Surg. 2020;157(3):249–53. https://doi.org/10.1016/j.jviscsurg.2020.04.009.

42. Werner J, Büchler MW. Chapter 62A: Resectional techniques: pancreaticoduodenectomy, distal pancreatectomy, segmental pancreatectomy, total pancreatectomy, and transduodenal resection of the papilla of Vater. In: Blumgart's surgery of the liver, biliary tract, and pancreas. 5th ed. Elsevier Saunders; 2012.

43. Strickland M, Hallet J, Abramowitz D, Liang S, Law CHL, Jayaraman S. Lateral approach in laparoscopic distal pancreatectomy is safe and potentially beneficial compared to the traditional medial approach. Surg Endosc. 2015;29(9):2825–31. https://doi.org/10.1007/s00464-014-3997-5.

E. Panettieri et al.

44. Goumard C, Ogiso S, Okuno M, Fleming JB, Kim M, Tzeng CD, et al. Tips and tricks of splenic vessel preservation during laparoscopic distal pancreatectomy. Surg Endosc. 2018;32(4):2149–50. https://doi.org/10.1007/s00464-017-5744-1.
45. Isaji S, Murata Y, Kishiwada M. New Japanese classification of pancreatic cancer. In: Neoptolemos J, Urrutia R, Abbruzzese J, Büchler M, editors. Pancreatic cancer. New York: Springer; 2018. https://doi.org/10.1007/978-1-4939-7193-0_84.
46. Strasberg SM, Drebin JA, Linehan D. Radical antegrade modular pancreatosplenectomy. Surgery. 2003;133(5):521–7. https://doi.org/10.1067/msy.2003.146.
47. Strasberg SM, Linehan DC, Hawkins WG. Radical antegrade modular pancreatosplenectomy procedure for adenocarcinoma of the body and tail of the pancreas: ability to obtain negative tangential margins. J Am Coll Surg. 2007;204(2):244–9. https://doi.org/10.1016/j.jamcollsurg.2006.11.002.
48. Zhou Y, Shi B, Wu L, Si X. A systematic review of radical antegrade modular pancreatosplenectomy for adenocarcinoma of the body and tail of the pancreas. HPB (Oxford). 2017;19(1):10–5. https://doi.org/10.1016/j.hpb.2016.07.014.
49. Addeo P, Guerra M, Bachellier P. Distal pancreatectomy with en bloc celiac axis resection (DP-CAR) and arterial reconstruction: techniques and outcomes. J Surg Oncol. 2021;123(7):1592–8. https://doi.org/10.1002/jso.26424.
50. Hirashi S. Distal pancreatectomy with celiac axis resection. In: Japanese mastery in hepato-pancreato-biliary surgery. 1st ed. Gakken; 2021.
51. de Rooij T, van Hilst J, Boerma D, Bonsing BA, Daams F, van Dam RM, et al. Impact of a nationwide training program in minimally invasive distal pancreatectomy (LAELAPS). Ann Surg. 2016;264(5):754–62. https://doi.org/10.1097/SLA.0000000000001888.
52. Ricci C, Casadei R, Buscemi S, Taffurelli G, D'Ambra M, Pacillo CA, et al. Laparoscopic distal pancreatectomy: what factors are related to the learning curve? Surg Today. 2015;45(1):50–6. https://doi.org/10.1007/s00595-014-0872-x.
53. de Rooij T, Cipriani F, Rawashdeh M, van Dieren S, Barbaro S, Abuawwad M, et al. Single-surgeon learning curve in 111 laparoscopic distal pancreatectomies: does operative time tell the whole story? J Am Coll Surg. 2017;224(5):826–832.e1. https://doi.org/10.1016/j.jamcollsurg.2017.01.023.

Chapter 24
Robotic-Assisted Approach to Minimally Invasive Distal Pancreatectomy

Chelsea F. Cardell and Gerard J. Abood

Introduction

Robotic surgical platforms are rapidly gaining popularity across all avenues of surgery with improved visualization and enhanced dexterity. Complex pancreatic surgery is no exception to this evolution in surgical technique. Minimally invasive pancreatic surgery, especially distal pancreatectomy, has helped decrease incision size and hasten patient recovery, and the extension from laparoscopic to robotic surgery is a natural progression. In this chapter, we will describe our technique to robotic distal pancreatomy, as well as review existing literature evaluating the safety and efficacy of a robotic approach.

Indications

Both benign and malignant pancreatic diseases are indications for robotic distal pancreatectomy. Benign indications include cystic neoplasms, acute and chronic pancreatitis, and trauma with pancreatic ductal disruption. Malignant etiologies include adenocarcinoma, pancreatic neuroendocrine tumors, as well as malignant disease from other primary cancers that have metastasized to the pancreas.

C. F. Cardell · G. J. Abood (✉)
Department of Surgery, Loyola University Medical Center, Maywood, IL, USA
e-mail: Chelsea.cardell@lumc.edu; Gabood@lumc.edu

© The Author(s), under exclusive license to Springer Nature
Switzerland AG 2025
E. P. Ceppa et al. (eds.), *The SAGES Manual of Evolving Techniques in Pancreatic Surgery*, https://doi.org/10.1007/978-3-031-78409-5_24

419

Preoperative Testing

Patients are initially evaluated with a detailed history and physical and pertinent lab values, including tumor markers. High-quality cross-sectional imaging is utilized for surgical planning, in our practice commonly a pancreatic protocol CT with triple phase contrast and thin cuts. Additional imaging in the form of MRI/MRCP and EUS is utilized where necessary and appropriate for diagnosis of pancreatic lesions.

Once diagnosis of a pancreatic lesion has been made and surgical resection determined to be appropriate management, patients are assessed for tolerance of general anesthesia needed for surgery. Focus is given to cardiopulmonary status and assessment of tolerance to pneumoperitoneum. We frequently collaborate with anesthesia colleagues in optimization of our patients prior to surgery. In the case of adenocarcinomas of the pancreas and planned splenectomy, appropriate splenic vaccines are administered in the preoperative setting.

Patient Positioning and Preparation

The patient is brought to the operating room and placed in supine position, with extremities appropriately padded, secured, and a footboard added to allow steep Trendelenburg positioning. Additional intravenous access and arterial lines are placed at the discretion of anesthesia before padding and tucking both arms at the sides. A urinary catheter is placed; central lines are inserted when determined necessary by the surgeon and anesthesia team. Upper and lower forced air warming devices are placed over the patient to ensure normothermia throughout the procedure. The patient's bed is rotated 45° to the patient right to allow for docking of the robot (Fig. 24.1). Preoperative antibiotics and DVT prophylaxis are administered, and the patient is prepped and draped in the usual standard fashion.

Operative Approach

Peritoneal Access

The peritoneum is accessed using a 5 mm optical port in the left upper quadrant using a 0° laparoscopic camera. The abdomen is insufflated to 15 mmHg. The abdominal cavity is then inspected for injury and evidence of metastatic disease or anatomic features that may alter operative approach. Three additional 8 mm ports, and one 12 mm (to accommodate a stapler and intraoperative ultrasound) robotic ports are inserted to triangulate on the dissection field in the configuration shown in Fig. 24.2. An 8 mm assistant port is placed in the right lower quadrant, and a 5 mm incision made to accommodate a liver retractor. The patient is placed in a steep

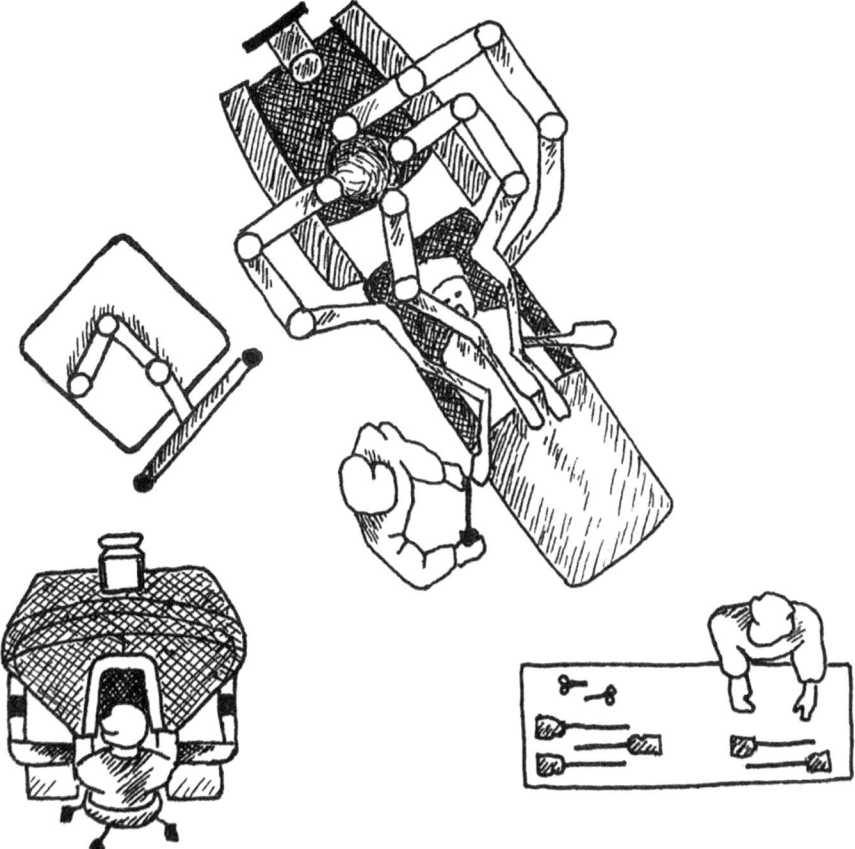

Fig. 24.1 Robotic configuration and patient positioning

reverse Trendelenburg position and rotated to the patient's right. A Nathanson liver retractor is inserted to retract the left lateral lobe of the liver. At this point, the DaVinci system is brought into the field and docked. Arm 1 is docked to the right of the camera, and arms 3 and 4 are docked to the left of the camera. A 30° robotic camera is inserted into arm 2 with a 30° downward orientation. Instruments are subsequently inserted under direct visualization, typically a fenestrated bipolar grasper in arm 1, a vessel sealer into arm 3, and a Cadiere grasper in arm 4. A long laparoscopic suction device is used in through the assistant port to assist with retraction and field visualization.

Fig. 24.2 Port placement

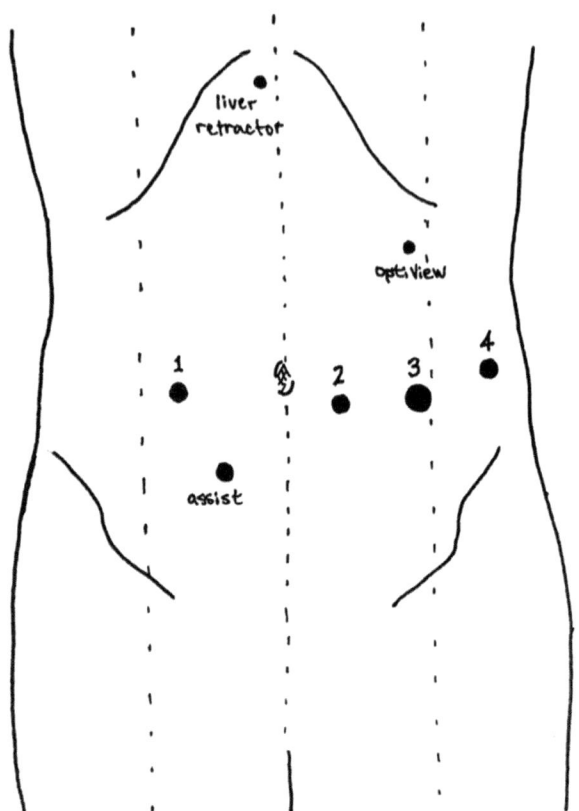

Access to the Lesser Sac

The anterior surface of the pancreas is exposed by dividing the gastrocolic ligament just outside of the gastroepiploic arcade using a robotic vessel sealer. Graspers in arms 1 and 4 are used to facilitate retraction and identification of the dissection plane. This dissection plane is carried up along the stomach, taking down the short gastric vessels to the left crus of the diaphragm. With the stomach fully mobilized, it is placed behind the Nathanson liver retractor with the left lobe of the liver to maintain visualization of the retroperitoneum. Mobilization is continued medially toward the neck and head of the pancreas until there is a clear view of the retroperitoneum.

Mobilization of Pancreatic Body and Isolation of Splenic Artery

The robotic vessel sealer is exchanged for a monopolar hook cautery to continue the dissection of the pancreatic body. The superior border of the pancreas is identified and dissected. The proximal splenic artery, at its origin from the celiac trunk, is typically identified at this point in the dissection and carefully isolated with blunt dissection and use of the hook cautery. Additionally, a robotic Maryland dissector can be useful to dissect circumferentially around the artery. It is then encircled with a vessel loop to provide gentle traction and divided with a single fire of a 45 mm vascular load through the assistant port (Fig. 24.3). Depending on the patient anatomy, a vessel loop placed around the pancreatic body may aid in retraction and identification and dissection of the splenic artery on the superior edge of the pancreas. We routinely use intraoperative pancreatic ultrasound, typically through the 12 mm left working port, to identify the resection margin. Pancreatic cancers are typically divided at the neck to ensure adequate lymph node harvest; benign tumors can be divided 1–2 cm to the right of the lesion as determined by intraoperative ultrasound.

Isolation of the Splenic Vein

After the resection point on the pancreatic body has been identified, attention is turned to dissection of the inferior border of the pancreas. Dissection is typically carried out using hook cautery and robotic vessel sealer, starting at the inferior border of the pancreas and extending posteriorly along the avascular plane between the pancreas and retroperitoneum. The superior mesenteric vein (SMV) is identified and marks the proximal extent of dissection. A vessel loop passed around the pancreatic body aids in retraction and identification of vessels. Care is also taken to

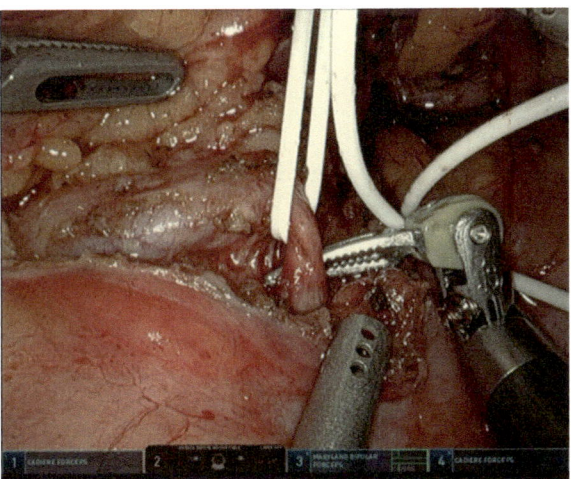

Fig. 24.3 Isolation and division of splenic artery

identify the inferior mesenteric vein (IMV) at its insertion into the splenic vein or SMV to avoid injury. Along the course of the dissection of pancreas, the splenic vein is identified and isolated. The pancreatic body is then divided with a 60 mm stapler through the assistant port (Fig. 24.4). We find that a stapler is an effective method to divide the gland in the majority of cases. Following division of the gland, any remaining dissection of the splenic vein is completed, and the vessel divided with a 45 mm vascular staple load through the assistant port (Fig. 24.5).

Fig. 24.4 Dissection of pancreatic body and neck just prior to gland division

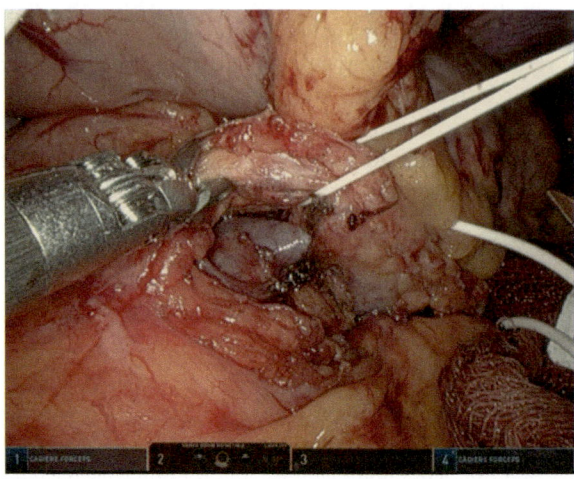

Fig. 24.5 Isolation of splenic vein

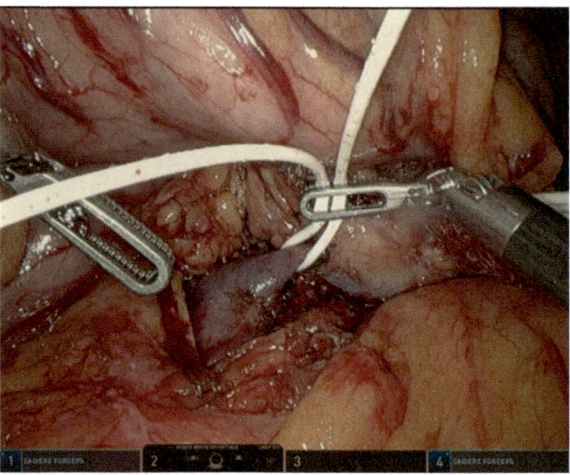

Mobilization from the Retroperitoneum and Splenic Mobilization

At this point, all major vascular tributaries to the spleen have been controlled. The pancreas is gently retracted toward the anterior abdominal wall using arm 4 and dissected from the retroperitoneum using a combination of hook cautery and robotic vessel sealer. The assistant uses suction to retract and keep the field clear of blood and smoke. Continuing this dissection plane laterally leads the surgeon to the spleen. The interior, superior, and posterior splenic ligaments are divided using the robotic vessel sealer for complete mobilization of the specimen.

Specimen Extraction

The specimen is placed en bloc in a retrieval bag and to be extracted through a small upper midline incision. A drain is left in the resection bed only in the circumstances of high intraoperative blood loss (>1 L), prolonged operative time greater than 4 h, or a thick gland requiring oversewing of the pancreatic duct. At this point, the robotic system is undocked and the patient returned to a supine position to allow for incision closure.

Closure

The upper midline port is closed with 2-0 PDS sutures in a figure-of-eight fashion, the 12 mm left working port is closed with a figure-of-eight using a Vicryl suture on a Carter-Thomason device. Skin incisions of all ports are closed with running subcuticular 4-0 Monocryl sutures and skin glue.

Clinical Outcomes

Introducing Robotic Technology to Pancreatic Surgery

Although robotic surgery had gained traction in other surgical specialties after introduction of the DaVinci system, it was not widely applied to complex pancreatic surgery. Initial reports regarding the use of the robotic platform to perform distal pancreatectomy focused on establishing feasibility of the new technology. Giulianotti et al. helped introduce robotic technology to complex pancreatic surgery in a descriptive series. They described the use of robotics in a small series of pancreatic operations from 2007 to 2010, including one distal pancreatectomy, two

Appleby procedures, and two pancreatoduodenectomies with portal vein resection [1]. No procedures required conversion to open, mean operative time was 392 min, and there were no mortalities [1]. This early description of robotic distal pancreatectomy was limited in number but allowed introduction of the technique to the surgical community.

This initial series was followed by multiple larger, single-institution studies establishing the safety and feasibility of robotic distal pancreatectomy. Suman et al. reported a series of 49 robotic distal pancreatectomies, including splenic preservation. In their patients, the rate of major morbidity (Clavien-Dindo grade III/IV) was 5%, with 5% of patients developing a grade B/C pancreatic fistula. However, the patients described in their series required a conversion to open in 18.4% of cases [2]. Zureikat et al. published a slightly larger series of 250 robotic pancreatic resections, 83 of which were distal pancreatectomy [3]. They observed a 13% Clavien-Dindo grade III morbidity rate, a 17% rate of grade B/C pancreatic fistula, and only a 2% rate of conversion-to-open procedures [3]. Several other small, single-institution studies demonstrated similar rates of morbidity, pancreatic fistula, and conversion-to-open procedures [4, 5]. While still limited by small numbers and lacking comparison control groups, these studies introduced cases to potentially compare to historic controls and helped solidify the safety and feasibility of robotic distal pancreatectomies.

Introduction of any new technology, even to familiar procedures, is associated with a significant operator learning curve. Shakir et al. examined this learning curve using cumulative sum analysis (CUSUM) in 100 robotic distal pancreatectomies. They noted significant reductions in operative time after 20 and 40 cases to 266 and 210 min, respectively, from an initial average operative time of 331 min [6]. Reductions in readmissions (40–20%) and grade B/C fistulas (27.5–11.7%) were also noted after 40 cases [6]. Similar cumulative sum analysis in another 55 patients found the learning curve to be only 10 cases to achieve similar operative times as Shakir et al., although both studies were conducted at high volume institutions with considerable support and mentorship from experienced robotic surgeons [7].

Comparison with Open and Laparoscopic Approaches

After demonstration that the robotic approach is both a feasible and safe approach to distal pancreatectomy, comparison to existing approaches is necessary prior to justification of widespread adoption. Existing literature has compared clinical outcomes between both open and laparoscopic approaches to the robotic approach.

The largest study comparing operative approaches in distal pancreatectomy by Lee et al. examined 805 distal pancreatectomies in a well-matched cohort: 37 robotic, 131 laparoscopic, and 637 open procedures. Compared to robotic and minimally invasive approaches, open procedures had a significantly higher blood loss ($p < 0.001$) and trended toward a longer hospital stay [8]. Rates of R0 oncologic resections were similar among all three groups. Clinical outcomes between laparoscopic and robotic approaches were comparable, with no clear advantage of one over the other [8].

Much of the existing literature comparing robotic and laparoscopic distal pancreatectomy has been conducted in single-institution series. However, Guerrini et al. conducted a systematic review and meta-analysis which included ten studies with 813 patients [9]. Among 267 robotic and 546 laparoscopic distal pancreatectomies, pancreatic fistula formation, bleeding rate, and Clavien-Dindo complications grade III were equivalent between the groups. However, the robotic approach demonstrated lower rates of conversion-to-open (OR 0.33 95% CI 0.12–0.92) and shorter hospital stay (mean difference −0.74 95% CI −1.31 to 0.15) [9].

A more contemporary propensity matched analysis compared 102 robotic distal pancreatectomies to 102 laparoscopic distal pancreatectomies and found that there were no significant differences in operative time, estimated blood loss, transfusion rate, pancreatic fistula, and overall morbidity between the groups [10]. The robotic approach reduced the conversion-to-open rate (2.9% vs 9.8%, $p = 0.045$), especially in large tumors and improved splenic preservation rates in patients without malignancy (95.5% vs 52.4%, $p = 0.001$). Decreased length of hospital stay was also associated with the robotic approach (7.67 vs 8.58 days, $p = 0.032$) [10].

Cost may present a practical limitation to widespread adoption of the robotic approach to distal pancreatectomy, especially as a robotic system requires significant upfront investment from hospitals. Waters et al. explored this possible limitation by studying cost-effectiveness between robotic, laparoscopic, and open distal pancreatectomy. In their series of 77 patients (32 open, 28 laparoscopic, and 17 robotic), ASA class and patient characteristics were similar, although both minimally invasive approaches were performed less frequently for malignancy than open pancreatectomy in that era (29% vs 47%) [11]. Operative time was longer in robotic cases, 298 min vs 245 in laparoscopic cases vs 222 min in open cases ($p < 0.05$) [11]. Length of stay was notably shorter in robotic cases (4 vs 8 days [open] vs 6 days [laparoscopic]). Total cost was lowest among the robotic cases, with an average total cost of $10,588 compared to $16,059 in open cases and $12,986 in laparoscopic cases, with total cost including operative time, supplies, anesthesia, nursing, laboratory, and overall hospital costs as recording in hospital accounting records [11].

Magge et al. also examined comparative cost data between robotic, laparoscopic, and open distal pancreatectomy. In their cohort of 374 total patients, open surgery included the most malignant pathologies (48% vs 20% in the laparoscopic group, and 31% in the robotic group, $p < 0.0001$) [12]. Analysis of postoperative outcomes in multivariate analysis adjusting for patient factors demonstrated that the robotic approach had statistically significant lower rates of any Clavien complication ($p = 0.012$), 30-day mortality (0.016), and shorter length of stay ($p = 0.0001$) compared to laparoscopic and open approaches [12]. The authors similarly found robotic distal pancreatectomy to have the lowest total cost ($15,440, $p = 0.002$), compared to laparoscopic ($16,733) and open ($23,228). Cost in this study was defined as direct costs of admission, including operating room time, instruments, medications, tests, personnel, capital investments of operating room purchases with amortization over time, and salaries of operating personnel [12].

While encouraging, it is important to interpret the existing literature with knowledge that much of the early described literature is lacking in rigorous methodology such as randomized clinical trials. Some effort has been made to examine minimally invasive techniques in a randomized fashion in the DIPLOMA trial, a trial which demonstrated non-inferior oncologic outcomes of minimally invasive distal pancreatectomy compared to open surgery, but did not distinguish between laparoscopic and robotic techniques [13]. The majority of the studies discussed here were carried out in highly specialized tertiary referral centers with existing expertise in robotic surgery and significant resources. Additionally, none of the studies randomized patients to operation approach, leaving the choice to surgeon discretion. As evidenced by several studies having higher proportions of benign disease in the robotic group, it is likely that surgeons elected more straightforward cases to be performed robotically, especially early on in their experience with the robotic approach to distal pancreatectomy. This has potential to underestimate rates of complications, length of stay, and ultimately cost. It is critical to continue to evaluate the role of emerging technology as it becomes more commonplace in complex surgery.

Conclusions

In this chapter, we present our approach utilizing a robotic platform to perform a distal pancreatectomy. Our robotic approach maintains the same principles of dissection planes and careful vessel identification as in laparoscopic or open surgery, yet, we feel the robotic platform offers superior visualization and versatility in dissection that cannot be as easily achieved in open or laparoscopic approaches. Existing literature has established that use of a robotic platform is feasible, safe, and results in non-inferior clinical outcomes compared to more traditional approaches. Additionally, patients undergoing a robotic approach may benefit from decreased conversion rates and shorter hospital stays. Cost-effectiveness analysis suggests that despite the common assumption that robotic surgery may be more expensive, it is actually more cost effective than other surgical approaches. Although existing literature is lacking in randomized controlled trials and may be subject to selection bias, we believe the benefits of robotic distal pancreatectomy will continue to be evident as more surgeons familiarize themselves with the technique and will be applied to increasingly complex cases. Future efforts should focus on robotic training and proctoring to spread this technology outside of specialized centers.

References

1. Giulianotti PC, Addeo P, Buchs NC, Ayloo SM, Bianco FM. Robotic extended pancreatectomy with vascular resection for locally advanced pancreatic tumors. Pancreas. 2011;40(8):1264–70.
2. Suman P, Rutledge J, Yiengpruksawan A. Robotic distal pancreatectomy. JSLS. 2013;17(4):627–35.
3. Zureikat AH, Moser AJ, Boone BA, Bartlett DL, Zenati M, Zeh HJ 3rd. 250 robotic pancreatic resections: safety and feasibility. Ann Surg. 2013;258(4):554–9; discussion 559–62.
4. Hwang HK, Kang CM, Chung YE, Kim KA, Choi SH, Lee WJ. Robot-assisted spleen-preserving distal pancreatectomy: a single surgeon's experiences and proposal of clinical application. Surg Endosc. 2013;27(3):774–81.
5. Zhan Q, Deng XX, Han B, Liu Q, Shen BY, Peng CH, et al. Robotic-assisted pancreatic resection: a report of 47 cases. Int J Med Robot Comput Assist Surg. 2013;9(1):44–51.
6. Shakir M, Boone BA, Polanco PM, Zenati MS, Hogg ME, Tsung A, et al. The learning curve for robotic distal pancreatectomy: an analysis of the first 100 consecutive cases at a high-volume pancreatic centre. HPB. 2015;17(7):580–6.
7. Napoli N, Kauffmann EF, Perrone VG, Miccoli M, Brozzetti S, Boggi U. The learning curve in robotic distal pancreatectomy. Updat Surg. 2015;67(3):257–64.
8. Lee SY, Allen PJ, Sadot E, D'Angelica MI, DeMatteo RP, Fong Y, et al. Distal pancreatectomy: a single institution's experience in open, laparoscopic, and robotic approaches. J Am Coll Surg. 2015;220(1):18–27.
9. Guerrini GP, Lauretta A, Belluco C, Olivieri M, Forlin M, Basso S, et al. Robotic versus laparoscopic distal pancreatectomy: an up-to-date meta-analysis. BMC Surg. 2017;17(1):105.
10. Liu R, Liu Q, Zhao ZM, Tan XL, Gao YX, Zhao GD. Robotic versus laparoscopic distal pancreatectomy: a propensity score-matched study. J Surg Oncol. 2017;116(4):461–9.
11. Waters JA, Canal DF, Wiebke EA, Dumas RP, Beane JD, Aguilar-Saavedra JR, et al. Robotic distal pancreatectomy: cost effective? Surgery. 2010;148(4):814–23.
12. Magge DR, Zenati MS, Hamad A, Rieser C, Zureikat AH, Zeh HJ, et al. Comprehensive comparative analysis of cost-effectiveness and perioperative outcomes between open, laparoscopic, and robotic distal pancreatectomy. HPB. 2018;20(12):1172–80.
13. Korrel M, Jones LR, van Hilst J, et al. Minimally invasive versus open distal pancreatectomy for resectable pancreatic cancer (DIPLOMA): an international randomised non-inferiority trial. Lancet Reg Health Eur. 2023;31:100673.

Chapter 25
Spleen-Preserving Distal Pancreatectomy

Jane Wang, Camilla Gomes, Zaim Chaudhary, and Adnan Alseidi

Introduction

Multiple surgical approaches exist for distal pancreas pathology and include options such as radical antegrade modular pancreatosplenectomy (RAMPS), distal pancreatectomy-splenectomy (DPS), vessel-resecting, spleen-preserving distal pancreatectomy (VR-SPDP) or Warshaw technique, and vessel-preserving, spleen-preserving distal pancreatectomy (VP-SPDP) or Kimura technique. These procedures can be accomplished in a minimally invasive fashion [1], and surgeons should choose the procedure based on experience, patient factors, and specific pathology.

Proper oncologic resections are essential for malignant neoplasms to ensure the best outcomes. For such an indication, the RAMPS procedure remains the best option [1]. However, distal pancreatectomy alone is acceptable for benign disease, premalignant lesions such as cystic neoplasms, and early neuroendocrine tumors. In these instances, a less aggressive approach should be considered, including splenic preservation. This is important, as resecting the spleen can lead to complications such as overwhelming post-splenectomy infections (OPSI), portal vein thrombosis, and even increased cancer risk [2].

Supplementary Information The online version contains supplementary material available at https://doi.org/10.1007/978-3-031-78409-5_25.

J. Wang (✉) · C. Gomes · A. Alseidi
Department of Surgery, University of California, San Francisco, San Francisco, CA, USA
e-mail: jaeyunjane.wang@ucsf.edu; camilla.gomes@ucsf.edu; adnan.alseidi@ucsf.edu

Z. Chaudhary
University of California, Berkeley, Berkeley, CA, USA

E. P. Ceppa et al. (eds.), *The SAGES Manual of Evolving Techniques in Pancreatic Surgery*, https://doi.org/10.1007/978-3-031-78409-5_25

431

Existing literature supports the superiority of SPDP, which has been associated with improved short- and long-term outcomes and decreased cost when compared to DPS. A meta-analysis conducted by Nakata et al. analyzed 404 patients with regard to SPDP vs DPS [3]. They found that the former had fewer infectious complications, clinically significant pancreatic fistulas, and abdominal abscesses [3]. They also found that SPDP was associated with significantly shorter operative times and less intraoperative blood loss [3]. Similar findings were reported in another meta-analysis by Shi et al. which analyzed 448 patients from 16 studies, although they reported no difference in operative time or hospital length of stay [4]. Finally, a study conducted by Lopez et al. demonstrated that SPDP was associated with lower cost compared to DPS at \$52,951 vs \$45,123, respectively [5].

Thus, we believe that splenic resection should be reserved only for cases with clear indications, such as for malignancies, and when technically necessary, like in the setting of splenic vein thrombosis. Within the realm of splenic preservation, one can pursue either VR-SPDP or VP-SPDP, both with their own risks and benefits. The remainder of this chapter will focus on key pre- and intraoperative steps for both procedures, as well as our recommendations and preferences.

Preoperative Preparation

A contrast-enhanced CT scan is an important tool to not only assess the pancreatic pathology in question, but also to evaluate the key vasculature and anatomy. Appropriate workup, such as endoscopic ultrasound with or without fine needle aspiration, should be pursued based on the suspected pathology. Patients who ultimately undergo a DPS should receive vaccinations 14 days after surgery [6].

Key Shared Operative Steps

SPDP can be performed in either a vessel-preserving or vessel-resecting manner. Both approaches share the same patient set-up and key fundamental steps, which will be described in this section. We place the patient in the supine position with both arms out. A urinary catheter and nasogastric tube should be placed.

Trocar Placement

After the abdomen is entered and pneumoperitoneum achieved via either Veress needle or open Hasson technique, the authors place four trocars. The goal is to triangulate around the body and tail of the pancreas while maintaining an adequate working distance for sufficient range of motion. We use a 12 mm trocar for the camera port and place it approximately 15–20 cm away from the target anatomy (typically supraumbilical or to the left of midline for non-obese patients). We then place a second 12 mm trocar at the left mid-clavicular line, approximately 10–12 cm from the target anatomy and more cephalad than the camera port. This port is often used for the stapler as well as ultrasound. We typically place an assistant 5 mm trocar at the left anterior axillary line at about the same height as the second 12 mm trocar; this port site can eventually be used for a drain if needed. Finally, the last 5 mm trocar is placed approximately 5 cm below the xiphoid either in the midline or to the right of the midline (depending on the location of the pathology). An optional, additional 5 mm trocar can be placed in the right anterior axillary line (a mirror image of the port on the left) to assist with liver/stomach retraction. Figure 25.1 illustrates the final trocar placement.

Pearls and Pitfalls

In general, we avoid placing the camera port at a fixed location relative to the umbilicus as patient habitus can alter optimal placement. Instead, we think about trocar placement relative to the target anatomy. For example, if the tumor is in the pancreas neck and very close to midline, the trocar should be placed to the right of midline to allow for optimal angles for dissection.

Fig. 25.1 This diagram illustrates port placement, with the larger circles representing 12 mm trocars and the smaller circles representing 5 mm trocars

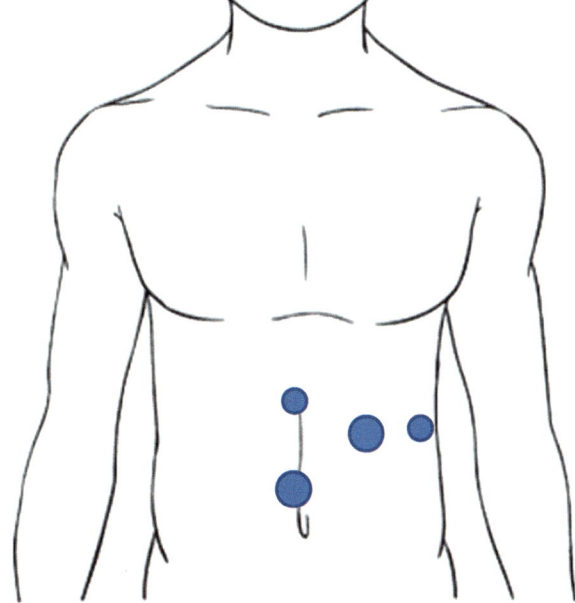

Entry into the Lesser Sac

The next step is to enter the lesser sac. If the liver obscures the surgical field, a liver retractor can be placed to retract the left lobe. The stomach should be retracted in the cephalad direction toward the diaphragm, and the transverse colon identified. The lesser sac is entered through the gastrocolic ligament approximately 1 cm inferior to the gastroepiploic vessels. Video 25.1 illustrates this step.

Pearls and Pitfalls

Care must be taken to avoid entering and otherwise injuring the transverse mesocolon. This can be avoided by elevating the stomach sufficiently, staying in a plane parallel to the posterior surface of the stomach, and keeping the tip of the energy device pointed toward the diaphragm. In addition, this step may be particularly challenging in patients with a history of chronic pancreatitis, as the planes may be fused. If the surgeon is not able to enter the lesser sac from a specific area, we recommend moving to another location.

Division of the Short Gastric Vessels

The aforementioned dissection is carried along the greater curvature of the stomach, and an energy device is used to divide the short gastric vessels to release the stomach from the spleen. The surgeon should maintain a distance of 1 cm inferior to the gastroepiploic artery. This dissection should be continued even after the gastric fundus is released from the left crus until the left gastric artery and vein are reached, staying inferior to these vessels. The peritoneal fold between the anterior pancreas and posterior stomach should also be divided. Finally, the dissection should be carried medially enough to visualize the pancreatic neck. Video 25.1 illustrates this step.

Pearls and Pitfalls

The surgeon should avoid veering too far from the inferior border of the stomach, as one may inadvertently take down the omentum or even injure a high splenic flexure. One should also avoid pulling too hard as this may avulse the vessels.

Splenic Flexure Mobilization

Although there are multiple ways to approach splenic flexure mobilization, we recommend starting with a lateral approach. The surgeon should start by developing a plane between the mesocolon and Gerota's fascia and continuing the dissection superiorly until the inferior pole of the spleen is visualized. We then recommend starting the medial dissection by first incising the peritoneum at the inferior border of the pancreatic body and then continuing this dissection laterally while gently retracting the pancreas up. Finally, the medial dissection should be connected to the previous lateral dissection plane and the splenocolic ligament transected. This approach to splenic flexure mobilization is particularly helpful in obese patients. Video 25.2 illustrates this step.

Pearls and Pitfalls

During the lateral dissection, the surgeon should be wary of carrying the dissection too deep and ending up retrorenal. In addition, especially in patients with thick omentum, one must be cautious not to injure the pancreas or colon as these structures are in close proximity and can easily get mistaken for or pulled up into omental tissue.

Pancreas Mobilization

The inferior border of the pancreas should already be mobilized after completion of the previous step. The surgeon should then proceed with retropancreatic dissection. Specifically, the pancreas should be gently lifted up and the retropancreatic tissue distal to the anticipated transection plane pushed down. Once this is complete, the superior border of the pancreas should be mobilized as well. This results in complete mobilization of the pancreas. Video 25.3 illustrates this step.

Pearls and Pitfalls

Elevation of the pancreas should be done gently as to not avulse the vessels. To help differentiate between the splenic artery and the left gastric artery, both of which can be encountered with pancreas mobilization, one can gently move the pancreas back and forth; the splenic artery will move in unison with the pancreas, whereas the left gastric artery will not.

Identify Pancreatic Pathology

This step can be done at any point after adequate exposure of the pancreas is achieved. If the pathology of interest is not clearly visualized, one can consider using intraoperative ultrasound as an adjunct. This allows for identification of an appropriate transection plane.

The next key steps involve the splenic vessels. These will be discussed in the context of VP and VR-SPDP, as outlined in the sections "Steps Unique to Vessel-Preserving, Spleen-Preserving Distal Pancreatectomy" and "Steps Unique to Vessel-Resecting, Spleen-Preserving Distal Pancreatectomy." The remaining shared steps are detailed below.

Pancreatic Transection

Pancreatic transection should be performed with a linear stapler. The exact load depends on the thickness of the tissue, although the authors typically use a black load. Buttressing technology has not proven helpful and the authors no longer use it in their practice. The decision to place a drain depends on the appearance of the transection line; if it appears uncrushed and intact, we do not leave a drain.

Pearls and Pitfalls

The key to successful, non-traumatic transection is gentle and slow compression of the tissue and careful firing of the stapler. In fact, the authors slowly compress the pancreas over a 3–5 min period and then pause for 1–2 min prior to transection. In addition, the authors are careful to minimize any rotational movement during this process. One must also take care to visualize the tip of the stapler prior to firing to avoid injury to other structures. On occasion, the pancreas is too thick for the stapler, in which case the surgeon has a few options. First, the surgeon can transect the pancreas at a more proximal location (i.e., at the neck) where the tissue is thinner. Another option is to use advanced bipolar energy to thin the pancreas anteriorly before stapling. Finally, one can also transect the pancreas with a bipolar energy device and then place buttressing U-stitch sutures on the remnant pancreas.

Specimen Removal and Closure

The specimen is removed via a large retrieval bag through the 12 mm camera port site. The incision should be extended as needed to allow for specimen extraction. This is a notable advantage to the spleen-preserving approach, as resecting the spleen often requires specimen extraction through a larger incision such as a separate Pfannenstiel incision. The surgical field is then examined for hemostasis, pneumoperitoneum released, all trocars removed under direct visualization, and the fascia and incisions closed. This concludes the operation.

Steps Unique to Vessel-Preserving, Spleen-Preserving Distal Pancreatectomy

VP-SPDP is thought to be more technically challenging but is also accompanied by fewer splenectomy-related complications [7]. The key to success is adequate dissection and extensive mobilization of the splenic flexure and pancreas. This approach involves dissecting the vessels off the pancreas.

Splenic Vein Dissection

The splenic vein is situated fairly deep in the pancreatic parenchyma and is typically visualized during the retropancreatic dissection as described above. The vein should be carefully dissected from the pancreas using a hook electrocautery from a medial to lateral approach; this step must be approached with caution given the thin vessel wall as well as the numerous branches. These smaller vessels should be carefully isolated and divided with an energy device.

Splenic Artery Dissection

The splenic artery can typically be found in an anterior and cephalad location and can be identified either via a posterior retropancreatic approach or anterior-superior approach, though the latter approach has a higher risk of misidentification of the hepatic artery. Upon successful dissection of the splenic artery, the pancreas body and tail should be fully mobilized. This step is followed by stapled pancreatic transection, which is detailed above in "Key Shared Operative Steps." Of note, one can also choose to transect the pancreas parenchyma as the first step (after carefully developing a plane at the proposed transection line between the splenic vessels and pancreas), and then free the pancreas from the splenic vein and artery starting at the point of parenchymal transection and progressing laterally toward the spleen. The surgeon can use umbilical tape as a handle assist with this step. Video 25.4 illustrates this step.

Pearls and Pitfalls

Bleeding is a feared complication of the vessel-preserving approach. If one encounters bleeding from arterial branches, we recommend placing a clip on the bleeding branch and then using an energy device (i.e., advanced bipolar) to divide the vessel on the specimen side. If the bleeding is more profuse, one can consider placing a Bulldog clamp on the splenic artery to allow for visualization of the injury and vessel repair. For suspected venous bleeding, small pancreatic vein branches are easily coagulated, and clips are rarely necessary for veins with a luminal diameter ≤5 mm. Significant uncontrolled bleeding from the splenic vein, however, may require conversion to a vessel-resecting, spleen-preserving distal pancreatectomy. Finally, one should be gentle while dissecting the splenic vein to prevent vessel thrombosis.

Steps Unique to Vessel-Resecting, Spleen-Preserving Distal Pancreatectomy

VR-SPDP was first described by Warshaw in 1988 and relies on collateral circulation from the short gastric vessels [8].

Dissection and Division of Splenic Vessels

After mobilization of the pancreas, a tunnel is created at the tip of the pancreatic tail, after which the splenic vessels are divided (typically with a linear stapling device). The next step is division of the pancreas parenchyma and splenic vessels proximally at the proposed transection line. Although some will divide the parenchyma and vessels together, we recommend dividing the splenic vein, artery, and parenchyma with three separate stapler loads. If unable to take them individually, we recommend taking the artery first and then the vein and parenchyma together. Finally, the spleen should be inspected prior to and after vessel division to assess for color and viability.

Recommendations and Preferences

There is currently no consensus on whether VR or VP-SPDP is superior. In general, those in favor of the former quote significantly shorter operative times, less intraoperative blood loss, and overall shorter hospital length of stay [3]. This may also be the preferred technique in cases when the splenic artery and vein are significantly inflamed, thrombosed, fibrosed, or otherwise involved in the pancreas pathology.

The vessel-preserving method is significantly more technically demanding as it requires meticulous dissection of the splenic vessels. However, it is associated with fewer spleen-related complications such as splenic infarction, secondary splenectomy, and overall morbidity [3]. Thus, we ultimately recommend pursuing VP-SPDP, with VR-SPDP serving as a contingency if the surgeon encounters significant bleeding or if tumor involvement or degree of inflammation poses a high risk of morbidity and mortality.

Conclusion

In summary, we have described the benefits of splenic preservation when indicated and have also reviewed the two main methods of SPDP. While there is no formal consensus on the superiority of one method versus another, there is literature describing increased morbidity with vessel-resection, and we thus recommend vessel-preservation as the first-line approach, followed by vessel-resection as a bail-out maneuver.

References

1. Asbun HJ, Moekotte AL, Vissers FL, Kunzler F, Cipriani F, Alseidi A, D'Angelica MI, Balduzzi A, Bassi C, Björnsson B, Boggi U, Callery MP, Del Chiaro M, Coimbra FJ, Conrad C, Cook A, Coppola A, Dervenis C, Dokmak S, et al. The Miami international evidence-based guidelines on minimally invasive pancreas resection. Ann Surg. 2020;271(1):1–14.
2. Di Sabatino A, Carsetti R, Corazza GR. Post-splenectomy and hyposplenic states. Lancet. 2011;378:86–97.
3. Nakata K, Shikata S, Ohtsuka T, Ukai T, Miyasaka Y, Mori Y, Velasquez VVD, Gotoh Y, Ban D, Nakamura Y, Nagakawa Y, Tanabe M, Sahara Y, Takaori K, Honda G, Misawa T, Kawai M, Yamaue H, Morikawa T, et al. Minimally invasive preservation versus splenectomy during distal pancreatectomy: a systematic review and meta-analysis. J Hepatobiliary Pancreat Sci. 2018;25(11):476–88. https://doi.org/10.1002/jhbp.569.
4. Shi N, Liu S-L, Li Y-T, You L, Dai M-H, Zhao Y-P. Splenic preservation versus splenectomy during distal pancreatectomy: a systematic review and meta-analysis. Ann Surg Oncol. 2016;23(2):365–74.
5. Lopez N, Strassle PD, Laks S, Meyers MO, Kim HJ, Yeh JJ. Take only what You need? A nationwide analysis revealing the cost of splenectomy in distal pancreatectomy. J Am Coll Surg. 2016;223(4):S80. https://doi.org/10.1016/j.jamcollsurg.2016.06.154.
6. Bonanni P, Grazzini M, Niccolai G, Paolini D, Varone O, Bartoloni A, Bartalesi F, Santini MG, Baretti S, Bonito C, Zini P, Mechi MT, Niccolini F, Magistri L, Pulci MB, Boccalini S, Bechini A. Recommended vaccinations for asplenic and hyposplenic adult patients. Hum Vaccin Immunother. 2017;13(2):359–68.

7. Jain G, Chakravartty S, Patel AG. Spleen-preserving distal pancreatectomy with and without splenic vessel ligation: a systematic review. HPB (Oxford). 2013;15(6):403–10. https://doi.org/10.1111/hpb.12003. Epub 2012 Dec 2.
8. Ferrone CR, Konstantinidis IT, Sahani DV, Wargo JA, Fernandez-del Castillo C, Warshaw AL. Twenty-three years of the Warshaw operation for distal pancreatectomy with preservation of the spleen. Ann Surg. 2011;253(6):1136–9. https://doi.org/10.1097/SLA.0b013e318212c1e2.

Chapter 26
Minimally Invasive Distal Pancreatectomy with Celiac Artery Resection

Gilbert Murimwa and Patricio M. Polanco

Introduction

Locally advanced tumors with involvement of the celiac axis (CA) were tradition-ally considered unresectable. Yet, with the advancement of perioperative systemic chemotherapy and improvements in surgical techniques and perioperative care, dis-tal pancreatectomy (DP) with CA resection (DP-CAR) has become a feasible surgi-cal option for selected patients that meet strict criteria. In fact, the most recent versions of the National Comprehensive Cancer Network (NCCN) guidelines des-ignate pancreatic neck/body tumors with invasion of the CA as borderline resect-able tumors when managed at high-volume centers with expertise in these types of resections [1]. With the advancement of minimally invasive techniques, this proce-dure is now performed laparoscopically and robotically in many high-volume cen-ters. This chapter will cover general considerations, perioperative adjuncts, surgical technique, and outcomes of minimally invasive DP-CAR, also known as a *modified Appleby procedure*.

G. Murimwa
Department of Surgery, University of Texas Southwestern Medical Center, Dallas, TX, USA

P. M. Polanco (✉)
Division of Surgical Oncology, Department of Surgery, University of Texas Southwestern Medical Center, Dallas, TX, USA
e-mail: Patricio.Polanco@UTSouthwestern.edu

© The Author(s), under exclusive license to Springer Nature Switzerland AG 2025
E. P. Ceppa et al. (eds.), *The SAGES Manual of Evolving Techniques in Pancreatic Surgery*, https://doi.org/10.1007/978-3-031-78409-5_26

Historical Evolution

Lyon Appleby initially proposed the eponymous "Appleby" procedure in 1953 when he described an en bloc total gastrectomy with DP and celiac trunk resection for locally advanced gastric cancer [2]. Nimura et al. then went on to describe a modified Appleby procedure for pancreatic adenocarcinoma of the body and tail in 1976 [3]. The initial case reports for the procedure all came out of Japan, with multiple surgeons reporting their experience performing DP with en bloc resection of the celiac artery during the 1970s and 1980s [4–6]. Mayumi and collaborators reported the first case series of six patients receiving DP-CAR in 1997, a procedure they referred to as an "extended DP" and compared this cohort to 19 patients who received "standard" DP [7]. Notably, they reported no difference in operative time, postoperative elevation of liver enzymes, or length of stay, while seeing a survival benefit of DP-CAR over the outcomes of unresectable patients. Since these initial reports, several other groups have reported larger series of DP-CAR operations that showed improved perioperative and oncologic outcomes (Table 26.1) [8, 9]. Cho and collaborators reported one of the first experiences with and feasibility of a purely laparoscopic DP-CAR for pancreatic cancer in 2011 [10]. Subsequently, Zureikat et al. at the University of Pittsburgh reported the first series of robotic-assisted DP-CAR operations with comparable results to the open approach [11]. Over the last decade, several other experienced groups have adopted the minimally invasive approach for this complex operation.

Table 26.1 Selected relevant series and outcomes of distal pancreatectomy with celiac artery resection (DP-CAR)

Study	Study design	Population	# of Patients	R0 margin rate (%)	Mortality (%)	Morbidity (%)	Median survival (months)
Beane et al. 2015 [13]	Multicenter retrospective	DP/ DP-CAR	172/20	NR	1/10	10/15	NR
Nakamura et al. 2016 [9]	Single institution retrospective	DP-CAR	80	92	5	41	31
Ocuin et al. 2016 [11]	Single institution retrospective	DP-CAR	30	80	14	35	35
Yamamoto et al. 2018 [8]	Multicenter retrospective	DP/ DP-CAR	323/72	80/67	1/4	28/42	29/18
Klompmaker et al. 2019 [14]	Multicenter retrospective	DP-CAR	191	60	9.5	27	19
Truty et al. 2020 [15]	Single institution retrospective	DP-CAR	90	88	10	53	36.2

DP distal pancreatectomy, *DP-CAR* distal pancreatectomy with celiac artery resection

Perioperative and Oncologic Outcomes

Perioperative Outcomes

Morbidity and mortality unique to the DP-CAR procedure center around the altered perfusion of the hepatic parenchyma and stomach that postoperatively rely on reversed, collateral flow through the gastroduodenal artery (GDA) and right gastric arteries from the superior mesenteric artery (SMA). As such, avoiding hepatic and gastric ischemia through pre- and intraoperative assessment of these vessels and their adequacy is essential. In addition to pancreatectomy-specific complications, early and delayed hemorrhage, particularly from the CA stump or proximal common hepatic artery (CHA) stump, are feared complications driving patient deaths within the first 90 days. These complications are far more likely in the setting of postoperative pancreatic fistula, and they encourage surgeons to leave drains [12].

In 2015, Beane et al. sought to characterize the perioperative outcomes for DP-CAR in the US using the National Surgical Quality Improvement Program database from the American College of Surgeons [13]. Of 822 distal pancreatectomies performed at 43 US hospitals over a 14-month period, only 2.4% of patients received a CA resection. Operative time for DP-CAR was 70 min longer (207 vs. 276 min; $p < 0.01$), with a higher rate of postoperative acute kidney injury (1% vs. 10%; $p < 0.03$) and 30-day mortality (1% vs. 10%; $p < 0.03$) when compared with DP. At high-volume centers, mortality following pancreatic head resections as well as distal pancreatectomies has fallen to below 2% from historical peaks. However, mortality remains high at experienced, high-volume centers for DP-CAR.

In the largest single-center Japanese series reported by Nakamura et al. involving 80 patients receiving DP-CAR over a 17-year period, the incidence of pancreatic fistula, delayed gastric emptying, and ischemic gastropathy was 58%, 25%, and 29%, respectively. Clavien-Dindo grade 3 complications occurred in 41% of patients, and 4 of them (5%) experienced in-hospital mortality. The 90-day mortality rate was not reported for this series [9].

In a large, international study that included 20 European centers, one Japanese center, and two American centers (Johns Hopkins Hospital and at the University of Pittsburgh), 90-day mortality at high-volume centers (performing a median of 70 pancreatoduodenectomies annually) was 16%. When defining high-volume for DP-CAR as being a single operation performed a year over a 3-year period, Klompmaker et al. found that 18% of patients who underwent DP-CAR at low-volume centers died within 90 days after surgery, compared with only 5.5% of patients at one of the five high-volume DP-CAR centers. The authors also found significant differences in mortality rates across European, Japanese, and American institutions (16% vs. 8% vs. 4%), likely related to different patient selection criteria and more aggressive interventions [14].

Truty et al. reported the largest single-center series of DP-CAR, which included 90 patients over 14 years with pancreatic ductal adenocarcinoma treated at the Mayo Clinic [15]. In this series, 45% of patients had celiac-only arterial involvement while the remaining 55% of cases required additional arterial resection and reconstruction. Only 4% of patients received preoperative arterial embolization, and 13% of operations were completed laparoscopically. In all, 53% of patients had grade IIIA or higher complications, and 20% suffered from hepatic ischemia and 18% from gastric ischemia, with 10% requiring emergent gastrectomy. In addition, 18% of patients required reoperation. Grade B/C delayed gastric emptying and grade B/C postoperative pancreatic fistula occurred in roughly one-third of patients while 20% suffered from grade B/C post-pancreatectomy hemorrhage. The 90-day mortality in the Mayo Clinic series was 10%, with a decrease to 4% in the last 50 cases. Most of the deaths were associated with liver failure, gastric necrosis, or bleeding. This highlights the significant morbidity associated with performing DP-CAR, even in high-volume centers by experienced hands.

Oncologic Outcomes

The oncologic outcomes of DP-CAR for pancreatic adenocarcinoma in the largest reported series are summarized in Table 26.1. Across this aggregate of heterogeneous populations, institutions, and approaches, R0 resection margins ranged from 60% to 92%, while median overall survival varied from 19 to 35 months [9, 13–16]. These R0 resection rates and survival outcomes are comparable to the ones for cephalic and distal pancreatectomies without vascular resection. In Nakamura's series, the R0 resection rate was 92% and the median overall survival was 31%. Strikingly, 21% of patients were alive at 5 years postoperatively, which is an impressive result for pancreatic cancer with borderline resectable/locally advanced features [9].

In a multicenter international study by Klompmaker et al., median overall survival for the resection was 19 months with some differences across the Japanese, European, and American cohorts, whose median overall survival was 20, 16, and 24 months, respectively. Some of these differences were likely related to variations in perioperative and multimodality management, including longer neoadjuvant therapy regimens at the American centers [14].

In the Mayo Clinic series, the rate of R0 margins was 88% with a median overall survival of 36 months. Survival was significantly better for patients who received neoadjuvant chemotherapy (44 vs. 8 months). Neoadjuvant chemotherapy use rose from 13% before 2011 to 96% afterward. Ten percent of patients had a local recurrence of disease, 18% had recurrence in the peritoneum, 25% in distant sites, and 14% in multiple sites. In all, 42% of patients remained alive with no evidence of disease at the time of analysis [15].

Given the wide timeframe in which patients were treated in the aforementioned studies, significant variation in the management of pancreatic cancer would be expected across early and later periods. These mainly include the increased utilization of adjuvant chemotherapy (single-agent first and then multi-agent) as well as the use of neoadjuvant chemotherapy and or chemoradiation, among other treatments. Similarly, advances in imaging modalities, the optimization of surgical technique, the completion of learning curves, and improvements in perioperative care have most likely played a role in the improvement of perioperative and long-term oncologic outcomes over time.

Minimally Invasive and Robotic DP-CAR

Minimally invasive surgery (MIS) approaches have now been routinely adopted for pancreatic resections. Several multi-institutional series, prospective trials, and society guidelines support the use of MIS in pancreatic cancer resections which appears to have equivalent outcomes to the open approach [17–19]. Moreover, two recent randomized trials have shown that MIS distal pancreatectomies result in shorter time to functional recovery, less pain, and less blood loss when compared to the open approach [20, 21]. It has also been shown that in high-volume centers with experienced surgeons, MIS pancreatectomies with vascular resections and reconstructions can be performed utilizing the robotic platform [22].

Zureikat et al. reported a 30-case series of their experience with robotic DP-CAR, comparing 19 open to 11 robotic cases [11]. This University of Pittsburgh group found no significant differences in morbidity but saw improvements in operative time, blood loss, and transfusion requirements in the robotic cohort. Median overall survival approached 3 years for both cohorts. In the large international series mentioned above, 15% of DP-CAR procedures were performed using an MIS approach.

Although laparoscopic DP and splenectomy have been increasingly adopted as the standard of care for left-sided pancreatic body and tail tumors, the technical complexity of DP with celiac artery resection demands a higher level of expertise and skill. The technical limitations of the laparoscopic approach for some complex pancreatic resections have been highlighted, with vascular resections resulting in a much higher level of conversions [23, 24]. In robotic surgery, the added benefits of three-dimensional stereotactic vision, tremor attenuation, optical magnification, a higher degree of articulation, and improved ergonomics make it the approach of choice for high-volume hepatobiliary surgeons with robotic experience who seek to perform DP-CAR and other complex pancreas operations in a minimally invasive way.

The ultimate decision on what approach to use in a complex operation like DP-CAR relies on the experience of the surgeon and the surgical team. We strongly advise against attempting complex pancreas operations robotically if the surgeon is in the early phases of their pancreas surgery experience or have not achieved robotic skills proficiency. Having disclosed that and for the purpose of the current SAGES-HPB Surgery Manual, the following sections describe our perioperative management, preoperative planning, and technique considerations for robotic-assisted DP-CAR.

Neoadjuvant Therapy

"Biology is the king, case selection is the queen, and the technical maneuvers undertaken are the princes and princesses of the realm" [25]. Due to the high morbidity, increased perioperative mortality, and limited chance of durable cure, patient selection is paramount before proceeding with DP-CAR. Patients with pancreatic cancer should be managed in a multidisciplinary fashion and their cases discussed by tumor boards, ensuring the use of guideline-concordant treatments [1]. To select for patient "biology," most centers utilize extended courses of neoadjuvant chemotherapy with or without radiation therapy. There are compelling data regarding the use of neoadjuvant treatments for pancreatic adenocarcinoma of all stages [26, 27]. This is particularly true for patients with locally advanced tumors where the chances of early systemic disease and locoregional recurrence are higher than for localized pancreatic cancer [28, 29]. In the USA, most institutions recommend multi-agent therapy with FOLFIRINOX (5-fluoracil, irinotecan, and oxaliplatin) or gemcitabine and nab-paclitaxel for 3–6 months (or more) before committing the patient to a DP-CAR. Treatment response is monitored by a drop in CA 19-9 levels and evidence of stable disease or response on imaging and a lack of systemic progression. Different thresholds for CA 19-9 declines (30–50%) and even the normalization of CA 19-9 levels have been proposed as prerequisites before proceeding with an intervention [14, 30]. In our institution, we favor a 50% drop of CA 19-9 and normalization. It is important to acknowledge that 6–22% of patients with pancreatic cancer could have normal levels or are non-secretors of CA 19-9 [31]. Some of these patients may have elevation of serum CEA levels; therefore, baseline serum testing is recommended [1].

Preoperative Assessment for DP-CAR

In addition to the standard preoperative assessment, careful patient selection criteria and anatomic delineation are necessary for surgical planning [16, 32, 33].

Our patient selection criteria include:

- Adequate performance status (ECOG 0–1)
- No major atherosclerotic vascular disease (predominantly in the SMA territory)
- Adequate nutritional status
- No current use of high dose of steroids
- Absence of distant metastatic lesions
- Absence of other prohibitive chronic medical conditions (e.g., Child-Pugh C cirrhosis, severe chronic pulmonary disease with high oxygen needs, major cardiomyopathy with low ejection fraction, etc.)
- Good response to neoadjuvant therapy defined as a decline in CA 19-9 levels or stable or improved tumor involvement in cross-sectional imaging

For anatomic delineation and surgical planning, high-quality CT chest images are obtained (to rule out lung metastases) as CT or MRI images of the abdomen and pelvis with a multiphasic pancreas protocol (arterial and portal venous phase). A dedicated CT arteriogram is rarely needed but sometimes can be useful to better characterize abnormal anatomic variants.

With this imaging we specifically assess for:

- The presence of variant vascular anatomy such as an accessory right hepatic artery, replaced right hepatic artery, totally replaced CHA, and accessory left hepatic arteries, among other anatomic variations. The presence of accessory or replaced hepatic vessels could favor feasibility of celiac artery resection without compromising liver perfusion.
- Tumor involvement of the aorta and the most proximal aspect of the celiac artery.
- Tumor involvement of the GDA or proper hepatic artery (PHA).
- Tumor involvement of the portal vein, superior mesenteric vein (SMV), and splenic vein.
- Overall tumor extension to peripancreatic structures besides the vascular structures.

In our experience, tumor involvement of the GDA, PHA, and aorta are contraindications for DP-CAR unless arterial revascularization (an aorto-hepatic bypass) is planned for PHA involvement.

Preoperative Adjuncts

Preoperative Coiling

Preoperative coiling of the CHA and at times the CA is performed at some centers prior to DP-CAR [14]. This procedure is thought to improve collateral flow to the liver and stomach, reducing rates of postoperative ischemia [14]. Proponents of this approach argue this also allows preoperative assessment of collateral flow and avoids futile operations [34–36]. There is no clear evidence for the effectiveness of preoperative embolization of the CHA for DP-CAR. When coiling is performed, the coils should be placed by an experienced interventional radiologist, making sure to leave sufficient space between coil in the CHA and the takeoff of the GDA.

Aortic Stenting

Trabulsi et al. have proposed a novel method, performed in two patients, in which an endovascular aortic stent is placed to cover the CA at 3 weeks prior to definitive DP-CAR [37]. They hypothesize that this allows the formation of adequate collaterals preoperatively, minimizing the risk of hepatic or gastric ischemia. While fascinating, this approach has yet to be widely adopted.

Robotic DP-CAR Surgical Technique

This section will describe our standard approach for robotic DP-CAR procedures. Variations in set-up, technique, and approach are expected based on the surgeon's preferences and expertise. While different types of combined arterial and venous resections/reconstructions (primary anastomosis, grafts, or others) are occasionally necessary in cases with more advanced disease, these will not be discussed in this chapter, since we recommend the open surgical approach for them.

Positioning

After general endotracheal intubation, the patient is placed in a supine French position on a split-leg table over an anti-slip pad that has adequate cushioning for all pressure points of the back and extremities. Straps or tape across the chest and legs are placed to prevent sliding of the patient during position changes. The abdomen is widely prepped and draped using sterile technique. After the ports are inserted, the patient is placed in 14–16° in a reverse Trendelenburg position with 6–7° of right-sided tilt (see Fig. 26.1).

Fig. 26.1 Patient in supine position with split-leg table and both arms tucked. After trocar placement the patient is positioned in 14° of reverse Trendelenburg and 6–7° of right tilt

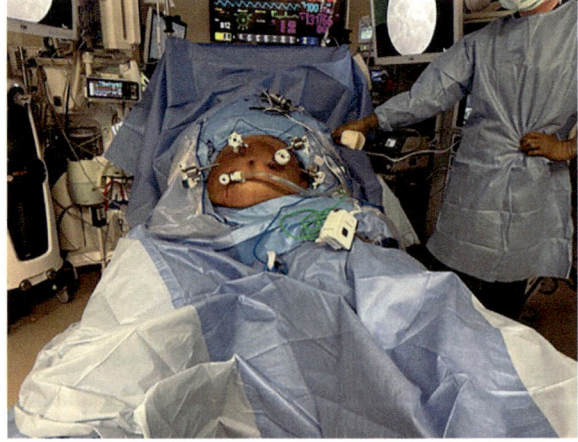

Port Placement

We start by placing a 5 mm optical trocar in the left upper quadrant. This is later exchanged for an 8 mm robotic trocar. We complete a thorough diagnostic laparoscopy to rule out peritoneal metastasis. A second trocar (8 mm robotic) can be placed to assist with diagnostic laparoscopy or to perform peritoneal biopsies.

Once peritoneal disease is ruled out, we place the remainder of our trocars. Our standard approach is to place four robotic trocars of 8 mm across the upper abdomen, two assistant ports in the lower abdomen (8 mm for the AirSeal insufflation system and 15 mm for a utility port), and a right-sided 5-mm port for the "snake" liver retractor. Figure 26.2 depicts our preferred approach for trocar placement. Once trocars are in place, we position the patient as described above and dock the robotic arms. For our standard DP-CAR using the da Vinci Xi system (Intuitive Surgical), we use the following instruments: fenestrated bipolar forceps (arm 1, right abdomen), a camera (arm 2, umbilicus), a robotic hook cautery/vessel sealer (arm 3, mid-left abdomen), and Cadiere forceps (arm 4, left lateral abdomen).

Surgical Steps

1. *Division of gastrocolic ligament and mobilization of the greater curvature of the stomach*

    We start the procedure by dividing the gastrocolic ligament (bursa) and exposing the lesser sac. This is followed by division of the short gastric vessels with the laparoscopic or robotic vessel sealer and cephalad traction of the stomach and left liver with a snake/auto-static liver retractor. Special attention is given to preserving the right gastroepiploic artery and right gastric arteries to minimize the chances of gastric ischemia. If invasion of the portal vein by tumor is anticipated, mobilization of the hepatic flexure of the colon and the Kocher

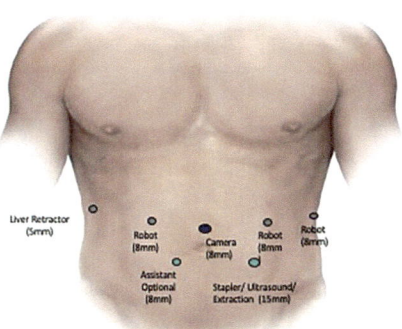
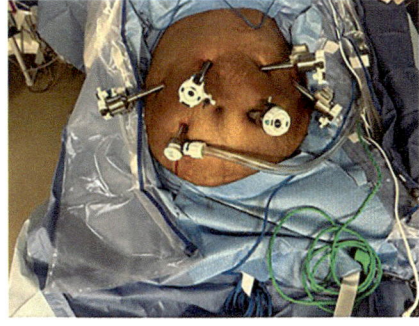

Fig. 26.2 Trocar placement for robotic distal pancreatectomy with celiac axis resection

maneuver is recommended, which is particularly useful if portal vein or SMV resection and repair is anticipated (Fig. 26.3).

2. *Dissection of the hepatic artery node, CHA, PHA, and GDA, and the "clamping test"*

The dissection of the anterior hepatic artery node (station 8A) allows for easier identification and dissection of the CHA. Once the CHA is identified, we extend dissection toward the PHA, carefully preserving the right gastric artery if possible. The GDA is then dissected at the superior border of the pancreas. These vessels are encircled with vessel loops for gentle traction. At this point, we perform a "clamping test" on the CHA to confirm adequate retrograde flow from the SMA, pancreatoduodenal arch, and GDA toward the PHA. Pulsatile triphasic duplex/Doppler signal confirmation of the PHA and liver arterial blood supply is recommended via intraoperative ultrasound. If adequate liver arterial flow is confirmed, we proceed with the DP-CAR (Fig. 26.4a, b).

3. *Dissection of the pancreas neck, retropancreatic tunnel creation, and pancreas division*

The inferior border of the pancreas is dissected. The anterior aspect of the SMV is identified and dissected cranially under the pancreas neck. Once a retropancreatic tunnel is completed, we proceed with the division of the pancreas neck with a linear laparoscopic or robotic stapler load. The stapler size (color) will vary based on pancreas parenchyma thickness. If thick tissue is found, we recommend staplers ranging from 2.5 to 4 mm (green, purple, or black loads). If there is concern for distance to the tumor or margin involvement, ultrasound can be used. If there is limited space between the GDA and the tumor margin to fit in a linear stapler, the pancreas is divided with scissors and then oversewn with 4-0 barbed sutures in continuous fashion (Fig. 26.5a–c).

4. *Dissection of the left gastric artery and vein (LGA, LGV), splenic vein, CA, and diaphragm crus*

Division of the pancreas neck facilitates the exposure and dissection of the LGV (also known as coronary vein) and splenoportal confluence. This is performed with hook monopolar dissection and vessel sealer dissection. If the splenoportal confluence is not compromised by tumor, early division of the LGV (with a vessel sealer) and splenic vein (with a linear vascular stapler) allows

Fig. 26.3 Division of gastrocolic ligament and mobilization of the greater curvature of the stomach

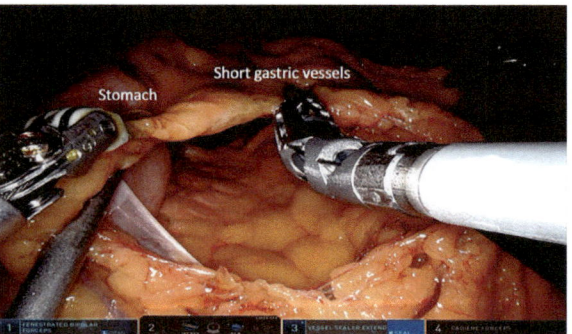

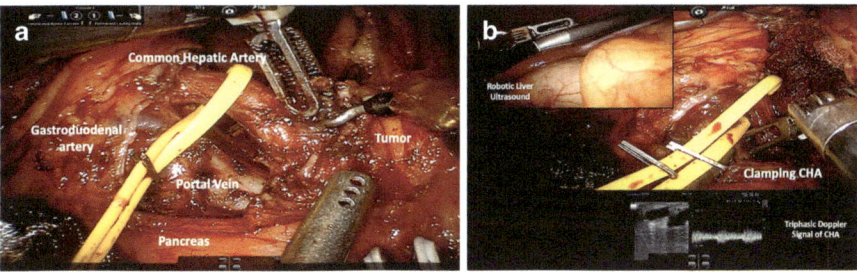

Fig. 26.4 (**a**) Dissection of the hepatic artery node, common hepatic artery (CHA), proper hepatic artery (PHA), and gastroduodenal artery (GDA). (**b**) Clamping of common hepatic artery (CHA) with robotic ultrasound confirming adequate pulsatile arterial blood supply (with triphasic doppler signal) to the liver by reverse flow from gastroduodenal artery

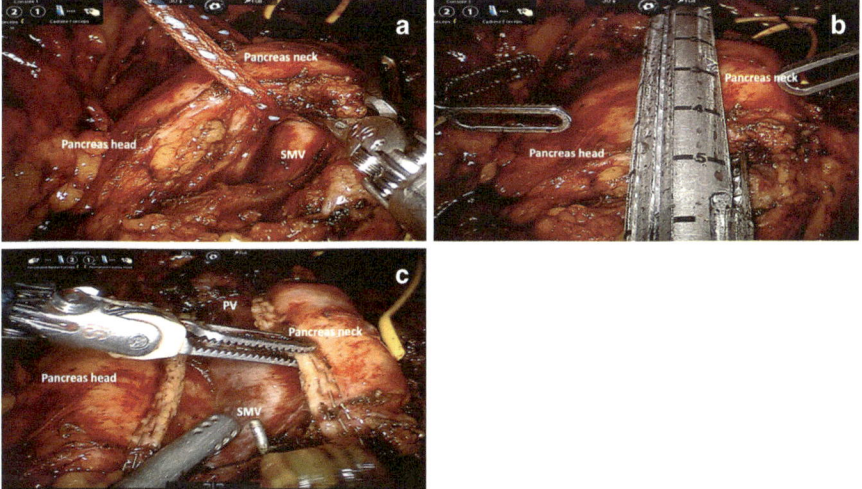

Fig. 26.5 (**a**) Pancreas neck and superior mesenteric vein (SMV) dissection with creation of retropancreatic tunnel. (**b**) Division of pancreas neck with linear gastrointestinal stapler. (**c**) Divided pancreas neck. *SMV* superior mesenteric vein

better exposure of the arterial anatomy, including the LGA, splenic artery, and cranial aspect of the CA. After the LGA is circumferentially dissected, a vessel loop is placed around it for traction. This allows exposure and dissection of the diaphragmatic crus. Division of the median arcuate ligament is recommended to expose the anterior and proximal aspect of the CA and aorta (Fig. 26.6a, b).

5. *Division of the CHA and LGA and dissection of the SMA and aorta*

The CHA and LGA are now divided with linear vascular staplers. The left lateral aspect of the SMV and the root of the mesentery is dissected to expose the anterior aspect of the SMA. The SMA is dissected cranially. All the periadventitial lymphatic and nerve tissue is dissected and divided until the anterior wall of

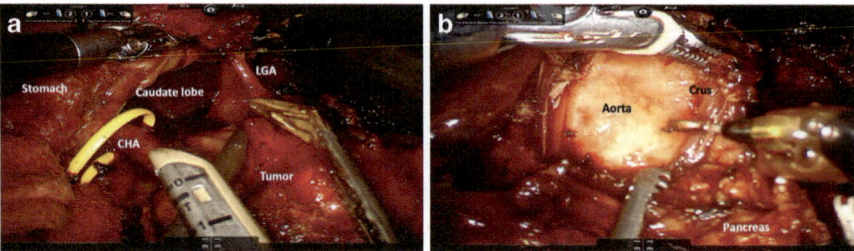

Fig. 26.6 (**a**) Dissection and division of left gastric artery (LGA). (**b**) Division of median arcuate ligament and diaphragm crus

Fig. 26.7 Division of common hepatic artery (CHA). Dissected gastroduodenal artery (GDA) and proper hepatic artery (PHA) shown

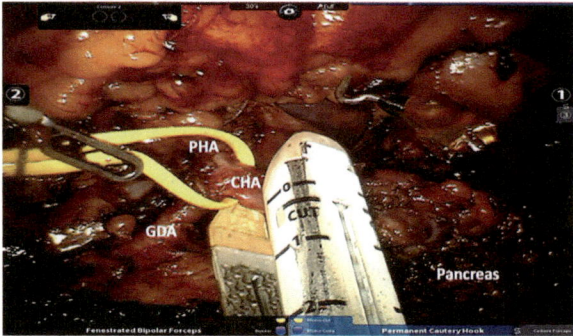

the aorta is exposed. Dissection is continued cranially with monopolar dissection and vessel sealer until the emergence of the CA is identified. Lateral muscle fibers of the diaphragm crus need to be divided for adequate exposure of the celiac trunk. During this step, lymph node stations 7, 9, 14, 16, and 18 are dissected toward surgical specimens (Fig. 26.7).

6. *Dissection and division of the CA and completion of radical antegrade modular pancreatosplenectomy (RAMPS) medial-to-lateral **or** lateral-to-medial RAMPS with a final dissection and division of the CA*

    At this point of the procedure, we often contemplate two options.

    (a) If dissection of the anterior aspect of the aorta and CA appears feasible, we continue the dissection until circumferential dissection is obtained. The dissection of the body of the pancreas with complete dissection of periaortic lymphatic and neural tissue with anterior traction is necessary to clearly identify and dissect the CA. The CA is divided with a vascular linear stapler. The surgery is completed via principles of conventional anterior RAMPS, with resection of anterior renal fascia or posterior RAMPS if the adrenal gland is involved. Nodal stations 10 and 11 are dissected during this portion of the procedure (Fig. 26.8a–c).

    (b) If exposure or dissection of the anterior aspect of the SMA, aorta, or CA is challenging due to an extension of mass fibrotic post-radiation tissue or excess retroperitoneal fat and lymphatic tissue, we recommend turning the

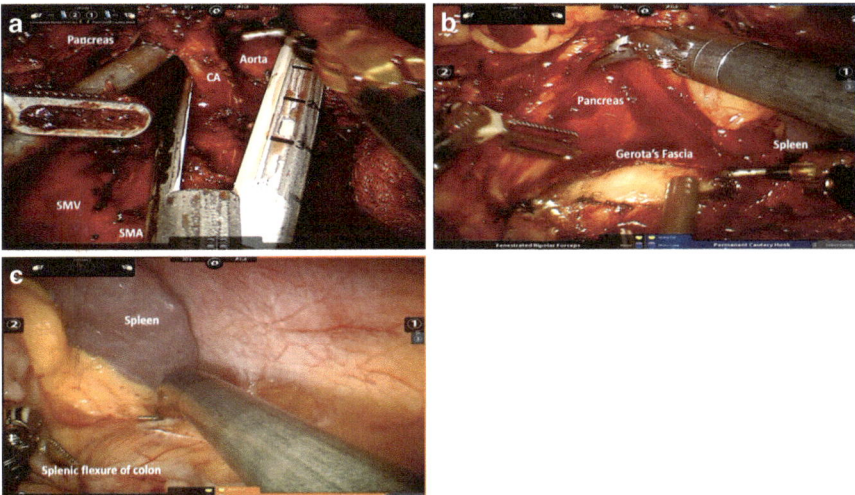

Fig. 26.8 (**a**) Dissection of superior mesenteric artery (SMA), aorta and circumferential dissection and division of celiac axis (CA). (**b**) Completion of anterior radical antegrade modular pancreatosplenectomy (RAMPS) with dissection of Gerota's fascia. (**c**) Dissection of splenocolic attachments and spleen mobilization

attention to the distal pancreas and spleen. Dissection of the distal pancreas and spleen is performed by mobilizing the splenic flexure of colon and lateral attachments of the spleen. The splenic hilum is circumferentially dissected and divided with vascular linear stapling. Separating the spleen from the pancreas permits easier manipulation and anterior traction of the pancreas while performing a lateral-to-medial RAMPS. This allows easier identification of the left crus, dissection of the anterolateral aspect of the aorta, and an easier dissection of the CA. Once the CA is circumferentially dissected, it is divided with a vascular stapler.

(c) If the portal vein, SMV, or portal confluence has any involvement with tumor, dissection of this area should be carried out last after the CA is divided. In these scenarios, partial resection and repair, a vein patch, or resection and primary anastomosis are needed (Fig. 26.9a, b). While all these could be performed robotically in very qualified hands, the decision to continue robotically or convert to open relies on the surgeon's judgment and experience.

7. *Placement of specimens in a bag, revision of hemostasis, drain placement, retrieval of specimens, and closure*

 After placement of the specimens in an endoscopic bag, we perform thorough hemostasis revision of all blood vessel stumps. We routinely create a falciform flap to place around the PHA, GDA, and the CA stump to protect these vessels from potential pancreatic leaks. A round Blake drain is left in the resection bed connected to closed bulb suction. The specimens are removed through an extended incision of our 15-mm utility port

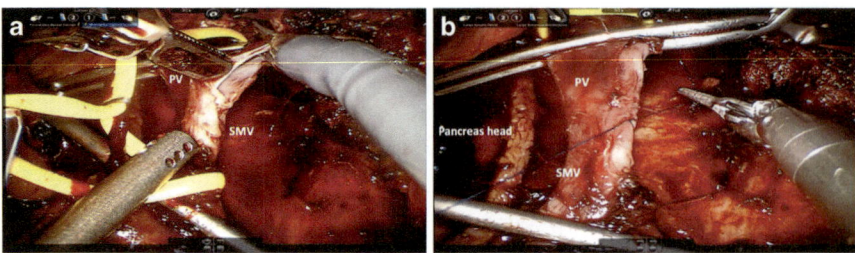

Fig. 26.9 (**a**) Proximal and distal control of portal vein (PV) and superior mesenteric vein (SMV) with laparoscopic "bulldog" clamps and resection PV wall due to tumor involvement. (**b**) Robotic repair of portal vein with running 5-0 prolene suture

Fig. 26.10 Retrieval of specimen with an endoscopic bag

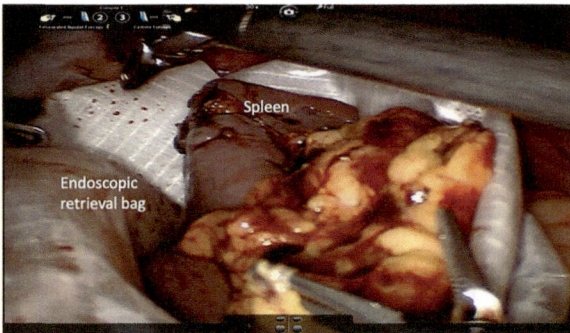

(Fig. 26.10). Alternatively, a small Pfannenstiel incision is created to remove the specimens. Incisions and trocar sites are closed in a standard fashion.

Perioperative Care

While we selectively admit patients to the intensive care unit, such admission is recommended if major blood loss or any critical occurrence is encountered during the operation or if liver and gastric ischemia are present. Standard management under enhanced recovery after surgery (ERAS) protocols is recommended. Diet progression starts on postoperative day 1 with a liquid diet. Bloodwork during the early postoperative days should include a liver panel. We routinely check amylase levels in drain fluid on day 1 and 3 and advocate for early drain removal if there is no evidence of a leak. If a chyle leak is suspected due to a "milky" appearance in the drain output, triglyceride levels are tested to confirm the leak. Medium-chain triglyceride diet is recommended if this complication occurs. If the patient develops delayed gastric emptying, nasogastric decompression could be needed. If this issue doesn't resolve within a week, the patient may require transient total parenteral nutrition or post-pyloric enteric feeding.

Conclusion

DP-CAR is an aggressive and challenging surgical intervention with a higher risk of morbidity and mortality than standard pancreatic operations. Yet minimally invasive DP-CAR, when performed at high-volume and experienced centers, is safe and feasible and could provide improved long-term survival for a selected group of pancreatic cancer patients in combination with multimodality therapy.

References

1. Tempero MA, Malafa MP, Al-Hawary M, Behrman SW, Benson AB, Cardin DB, et al. Pancreatic adenocarcinoma, version 2.2021, NCCN clinical practice guidelines in oncology. J Natl Compr Cancer Netw. 2021;19(4):439–57.
2. Appleby LH. The coeliac axis in the expansion of the operation for gastric carcinoma. Cancer. 1953;6(4):704–7.
3. Nimura Y, Hattori T, Miura K, Nakashima N, Hibi M. Resection of advanced pancreatic body-tail carcinoma by Appleby's operation. Shujutu. 1976;30:885–9.
4. Fujita T, Imaizumi T, Yoshikawa T, Miyagawa S, Hanyu H. A resected pancreatic body and tail carcinoma by Appleby's operation with portal vein resection. Pancreas. 1987;2:122–8.
5. Imaizumi T, Nakamura M, Takada T, Fukushima Y, Kanayama S, Hanyu F. Appleby operation on carcinoma of the body and tail of the pancreas: a case report. Surgery. 1979;41:532–7.
6. Wada T, Konishi T. Appleby operation in double carcinomas of the stomach and pancreas. Surg Diagn Treatm. 1977;10:155–7.
7. Mayumi T, Nimura Y, Kamiya J, Kondo S, Nagino M, Kanai M, et al. Distal pancreatectomy with en bloc resection of the celiac artery for carcinoma of the body and tail of the pancreas. Int J Pancreatol. 1997;22(1):15–21.
8. Yamamoto T, Satoi S, Kawai M, Motoi F, Sho M, Uemura KI, et al. Is distal pancreatectomy with en-bloc celiac axis resection effective for patients with locally advanced pancreatic ductal adenocarcinoma? Multicenter surgical group study. Pancreatology. 2018;18(1):106–13.
9. Nakamura T, Hirano S, Noji T, Asano T, Okamura K, Tsuchikawa T, et al. Distal pancreatectomy with en bloc celiac axis resection (modified Appleby procedure) for locally advanced pancreatic body cancer: a single-center review of 80 consecutive patients. Ann Surg Oncol. 2016;23(5):969–75.
10. Cho A, Yamamoto H, Kainuma O, Ota T, Park S, Ikeda A, et al. Pure laparoscopic distal pancreatectomy with en bloc celiac axis resection. J Laparoendosc Adv Surg Tech A. 2011;21(10):957–9.
11. Ocuin LM, Miller-Ocuin JL, Novak SM, Bartlett DL, Marsh JW, Tsung A, et al. Robotic and open distal pancreatectomy with celiac axis resection for locally advanced pancreatic body tumors: a single institutional assessment of perioperative outcomes and survival. HPB (Oxford). 2016;18(10):835–42.
12. Nigri G, Petrucciani N, Belloni E, Lucarini A, Aurello P, D'Angelo F, et al. Distal pancreatectomy with celiac axis resection: systematic review and meta-analysis. Cancers (Basel). 2021;13(8):1967.
13. Beane JD, House MG, Pitt SC, Kilbane EM, Hall BL, Parmar AD, et al. Distal pancreatectomy with celiac axis resection: what are the added risks? HPB (Oxford). 2015;17(9):777–84.
14. Klompmaker S, Peters NA, van Hilst J, Bassi C, Boggi U, Busch OR, et al. Outcomes and risk score for distal pancreatectomy with celiac axis resection (DP-CAR): an international multicenter analysis. Ann Surg Oncol. 2019;26(3):772–81.

15. Truty MJ, Colglazier JJ, Mendes BC, Nagorney DM, Bower TC, Smoot RL, et al. En bloc celiac axis resection for pancreatic cancer: classification of anatomical variants based on tumor extent. J Am Coll Surg. 2020;231(1):8–29.
16. Klompmaker S, Boggi U, Hackert T, Salvia R, Weiss M, Yamaue H, et al. Distal pancreatectomy with celiac axis resection (DP-CAR) for pancreatic cancer. How I do it. J Gastrointest Surg. 2018;22(10):1804–10.
17. Asbun HJ, Moekotte AL, Vissers FL, Kunzler F, Cipriani F, Alseidi A, et al. The Miami international evidence-based guidelines on minimally invasive pancreas resection. Ann Surg. 2020;271(1):1–14.
18. Shakir M, Boone BA, Polanco PM, Zenati MS, Hogg ME, Tsung A, et al. The learning curve for robotic distal pancreatectomy: an analysis of outcomes of the first 100 consecutive cases at a high-volume pancreatic centre. HPB (Oxford). 2015;17(7):580–6.
19. Zureikat AH, Moser AJ, Boone BA, Bartlett DL, Zenati M, Zeh HJ 3rd. 250 robotic pancreatic resections: safety and feasibility. Ann Surg. 2013;258(4):554–9; discussion 559–62.
20. Bjornsson B, Larsson AL, Hjalmarsson C, Gasslander T, Sandstrom P. Comparison of the duration of hospital stay after laparoscopic or open distal pancreatectomy: randomized controlled trial. Br J Surg. 2020;107(10):1281–8.
21. de Rooij T, van Hilst J, van Santvoort H, Boerma D, van den Boezem P, Daams F, et al. Minimally invasive versus open distal pancreatectomy (LEOPARD): a multicenter patient-blinded randomized controlled trial. Ann Surg. 2019;269(1):2–9.
22. Beane JD, Zenati M, Hamad A, Hogg ME, Zeh HJ 3rd, Zureikat AH. Robotic pancreatoduodenectomy with vascular resection: outcomes and learning curve. Surgery. 2019;166(1):8–14.
23. Nassour I, Wang SC, Porembka MR, Augustine MM, Yopp AC, Mansour JC, et al. Conversion of minimally invasive distal pancreatectomy: predictors and outcomes. Ann Surg Oncol. 2017;24(12):3725–31.
24. Hester CA, Nassour I, Christie A, Augustine MM, Mansour JC, Polanco PM, et al. Predictors and outcomes of converted minimally invasive pancreaticoduodenectomy: a propensity score matched analysis. Surg Endosc. 2020;34(2):544–50.
25. Cady B. Presidential address to the Society of Surgical Oncology. 1988.
26. Mokdad AA, Minter RM, Zhu H, Augustine MM, Porembka MR, Wang SC, et al. Neoadjuvant therapy followed by resection versus upfront resection for resectable pancreatic cancer: a propensity score matched analysis. J Clin Oncol. 2017;35(5):515–22.
27. Versteijne E, van Dam JL, Suker M, Janssen QP, Groothuis K, Akkermans-Vogelaar JM, et al. Neoadjuvant chemoradiotherapy versus upfront surgery for resectable and borderline resectable pancreatic cancer: long-term results of the dutch randomized PREOPANC trial. J Clin Oncol. 2022;40(11):1220–30.
28. Hackert T, Sachsenmaier M, Hinz U, Schneider L, Michalski CW, Springfeld C, et al. Locally advanced pancreatic cancer: neoadjuvant therapy with folfirinox results in resectability in 60% of the patients. Ann Surg. 2016;264(3):457–63.
29. Gemenetzis G, Groot VP, Blair AB, Laheru DA, Zheng L, Narang AK, et al. Survival in locally advanced pancreatic cancer after neoadjuvant therapy and surgical resection. Ann Surg. 2019;270(2):340–7.
30. Boone BA, Steve J, Zenati MS, Hogg ME, Singhi AD, Bartlett DL, et al. Serum CA 19-9 response to neoadjuvant therapy is associated with outcome in pancreatic adenocarcinoma. Ann Surg Oncol. 2014;21(13):4351–8.
31. Bergquist JR, Puig CA, Shubert CR, Groeschl RT, Habermann EB, Kendrick ML, et al. Carbohydrate antigen 19-9 elevation in anatomically resectable, early stage pancreatic cancer is independently associated with decreased overall survival and an indication for neoadjuvant therapy: a national cancer database study. J Am Coll Surg. 2016;223(1):52–65.
32. Greer J, Zureikat AH. Robotic distal pancreatectomy combined with celiac axis resection. J Vis Surg. 2017;3:145.

33. Cannella R, Borhani AA, Zureikat AH, Tublin ME. Appleby procedure (distal pancreatectomy with celiac artery resection) for locally advanced pancreatic carcinoma: indications, outcomes, and imaging. AJR Am J Roentgenol. 2019;213(1):35–44.
34. Ueda A, Sakai N, Yoshitomi H, Furukawa K, Takayashiki T, Kuboki S, et al. Is hepatic artery coil embolization useful in distal pancreatectomy with en bloc celiac axis resection for locally advanced pancreatic cancer? World J Surg Oncol. 2019;17(1):124.
35. Zimmermann M, Liebl M, Schulze-Hagen M, Pedersoli F, Pfeffer J, Schmeding M, et al. Preoperative embolization of the celiac axis or common hepatic artery before distal pancreatectomy with resection of the celiac axis. J Vasc Interv Radiol. 2017;28(1):60–3.
36. Ramia JM, de Vicente E, Pardo F, Sabater L, Lopez-Ben S, Quijano MY, et al. Preoperative hepatic artery embolization before distal pancreatectomy plus celiac axis resection does not improve surgical results: a Spanish multicentre study. Surgeon. 2021;19(5):e117–24.
37. Trabulsi N, Pelletier JS, Abraham C, Vanounou T. Preoperative diagnostic angiogram and endovascular aortic stent placement for Appleby resection candidates: a novel surgical technique in the management of locally advanced pancreatic cancer. HPB Surg. 2015;2015:523273.

Chapter 27
Enucleation

Luca Milone, Mei Zhen Cao, Andrew Gumbs, and Romulo Genato

Introduction

The conventional approach for most pancreatic neoplasms is to perform formal anatomic resections such as pancreatoduodenectomy for lesions found in the head or the uncinate process (right side of the superior mesenteric vein) and distal or subtotal pancreatectomy for body or tail lesions (left sided). These surgeries offer the advantage of regional lymph node clearance but are technically demanding and carry significant postoperative morbidity often requiring extensive postoperative management. Postoperative complications of anatomic resections include not only postoperative pancreatic fistula, but also exocrine or endocrine insufficiency as a considerable amount of pancreatic parenchyma is removed. To prevent these complications, in case of benign and low-grade lesions of the pancreas, enucleation has been proposed as an atypical, parenchymal sparing procedure. Enucleation consists in shelling out the lesion while preserving the surrounding tissue. It is a safe and feasible technique that can be performed in minimally invasive fashion and provides advantages over anatomical resections due to lower complication rate, higher parenchymal preservation, shorter hospital stay, and lower cost of treatment [1–3].

L. Milone (✉)
Division of Robotic Surgery, Department of General Surgery, The Brooklyn Hospital Center, Icahn School of Medicine at Mount Sinai, New York, NY, USA
e-mail: lmilone@tbh.org

M. Z. Cao · A. Gumbs · R. Genato
Department of General Surgery, The Brooklyn Hospital Center, Icahn School of Medicine at Mount Sinai, New York, NY, USA

© The Author(s), under exclusive license to Springer Nature Switzerland AG 2025
E. P. Ceppa et al. (eds.), *The SAGES Manual of Evolving Techniques in Pancreatic Surgery*, https://doi.org/10.1007/978-3-031-78409-5_27

459

Preoperative Considerations

Preoperative patient selection is the most important aspect when considering enucleation. Neoplasms that are likely to be low-grade, solitary, and not involving the main pancreatic or common bile duct are appropriate for enucleation. Indications include small low-grade non-functioning or functioning pancreatic neuroendocrine tumors (NET) (i.e., insulinoma or gastrinoma). The lesion should be less than 2 cm in diameter and have a low Ki-67 mitotic index (<3%) [4]. Larger NETs (>2 cm) or lesions that involve major structures, such as the main pancreatic duct, bile duct, gastroduodenal artery, or portal vein should proceed with standard surgical resection for oncological adequacy. Enucleation has also been proposed for low-grade pancreatic cysts such as small solid pseudo-papillary neoplasms and branch-duct IPMNs. As non-operative management (mostly surveillance) represents the most common approach for small, asymptomatic BD-IPMNs, enucleation remains indicated in much selected cases [3].

Perioperative identification of the target pancreatic lesion(s) is critical for the overall outcome of enucleation. Cross-sectional imaging, such as contrast-enhanced abdominal CT scan or MRI, can identify the lesion in most cases, and provide preoperative staging to rule out local invasion or metastasis. MRCP can also provide crucial information on the lesion relationship with the pancreatic ductal system. Well-differentiated NETs express a high level of somatostatin receptors and thus somatostatin receptor scans such as Indium-DTPA-pentetreotide (Octreoscan) have been used to confirm the nature of the lesion and complete staging. Recently a more sensitive imaging modality, gallium-DOTA-D-Phe1-Tyr3-Thr8-octreotide positron emission tomography/computed tomography (DOTATATE PET/CT) has replaced Octreoscan as it increases accuracy in the detection of pancreatic NETs and distant metastatic lesions (Fig. 27.1). Endoscopic ultrasound (EUS) has a very high sensitivity for small lesions and is indicated to identify occult insulinomas as well as allowing cytological confirmation. It can also provide useful information regarding depth of tumor invasion, involvement of nearby major organs or neuro-vasculature

Fig. 27.1 Magnetic resonance imaging of a 9 mm pancreatic lesion of the body (circle in red)

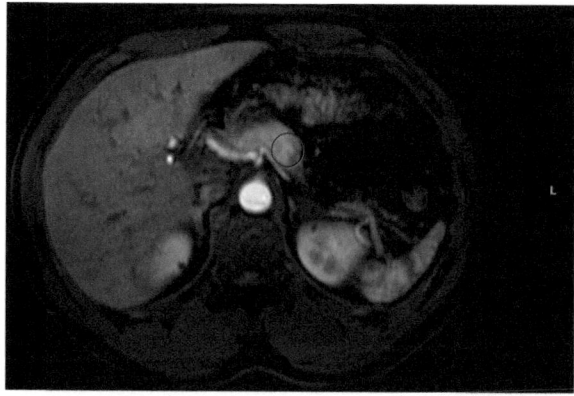

Fig. 27.2 Intraoperative ultrasound of a pancreatic tumor. The pancreatic duct (depicted by small arrow) is identified running posterior and superior to the tumor (a large arrow). (Courtesy from Gumbs, AA and Inabnet, WB. Laparoscopic Pancreatic Enucleation/ Resection for Neuroendocrine Tumor)

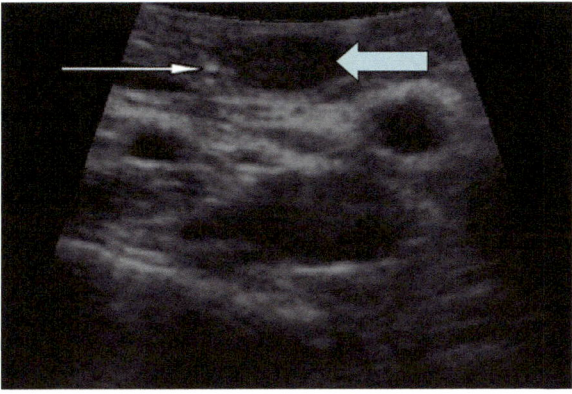

and distance between the lesion and the main pancreatic duct (MPD) for operative planning, as shown in Fig. 27.2. Prior studies have reported that the distance between the tumor and MPD of 3 mm or less as independent risk factors for postoperative pancreatic fistula following enucleation [5]. If preoperative imaging shows involvement of the duct or less than 3 mm distance, it should discourage an enucleation attempt, as MPD injury can lead to persistent postoperative pancreatic fistula.

Specialized studies including selective angiography with arterial calcium stimulation and portal venous sampling are now used only sporadically to localize functioning tumors that cannot be identified on imaging studies.

Patients with small isolated pancreatic lesions and planned for MIS enucleation, a diagnostic laparoscopy can be considered to evaluate for any peritoneal lesions and a suspicious lesion should be sent for frozen section examination prior to enucleation. For pancreatic lesions proximal to the pancreatic duct, sometimes a preoperative pancreatic stent can be used to for better localization during the operation and hormonally active NETs should be evaluated and medicated appropriately prior to surgery.

Laparoscopic Enucleation

Patient Positioning

The patient should be placed in a supine position in a low lithotomy position (on split table or stirrups) as shown in Fig. 27.3. Both nasogastric tube and Foley should be placed prior to operation. Two large bore IVs should be available during the procedure and the patient should be on both chemical and mechanical prophylaxis prior to surgery. The operating surgeon operates between the stirrups, while the surgical technician is on the patient's right and the assistant is on the patient's left side. Alternative positioning includes placing the patient in supine position with the surgeon on the patient's right side and assistant on the left.

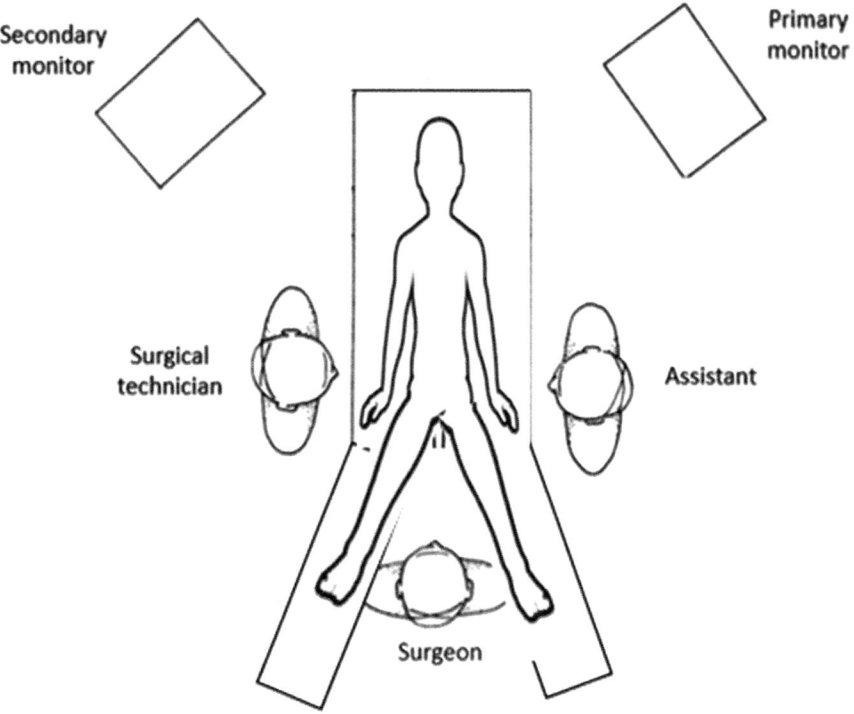

Fig. 27.3 Patient position for laparoscopic enucleation of small PNETs

Procedure

For laparoscopic enucleation, commonly used instruments include a monopolar laparoscopic spatula (Storz, Tuttlingen, Germany, Fig. 27.4), laparoscopic bipolar cautery forceps (LigaSure, COVIDIEN, USA), and ultrasonic shears (Thunderbeat, Olypmus, USA). Large vessels and pancreatic parenchymal transection can be done with laparoscopic endo-GIA staplers (COVIDIEN, USA). Pneumoperitoneum is obtained by either using a Veress needle at the Palmer point or Hassen cut down along the midline approximately 2–5 cm above and to the left of the umbilicus. After obtaining abdominal pressure of 15 mmHg, one to two 12 mm working ports (to accommodate the laparoscopic ultrasound probe) are placed on either side of the camera port. Two 5 mm assistant ports are placed in the right upper quadrant (along the mid-axillary line) and subxiphoid for retraction, respectively (Fig. 27.5). Once entered the abdomen, using a bowel grasper to raise both the stomach and transverse colon, the ultrasonic shear is used to open the gastrocolic ligament to enter the lesser sac. Once the anterior surface of the pancreas is exposed, a flexible laparoscopic ultrasound probe with color-flow Doppler (7.5 MHz) is used to identify the lesion of interest, other lesions, and evaluate the relative distance from the pancreatic duct. Sometimes, an extended Kocher maneuver to the aorta is necessarily performed to

Fig. 27.4 A laparoscopic spatula (blue arrow) and two spatulated retractors for pancreatic enucleation. (Courtesy from Gumbs, AA and Inabnet, WB. Laparoscopic Pancreatic Enucleation/ Resection for Neuroendocrine Tumor)

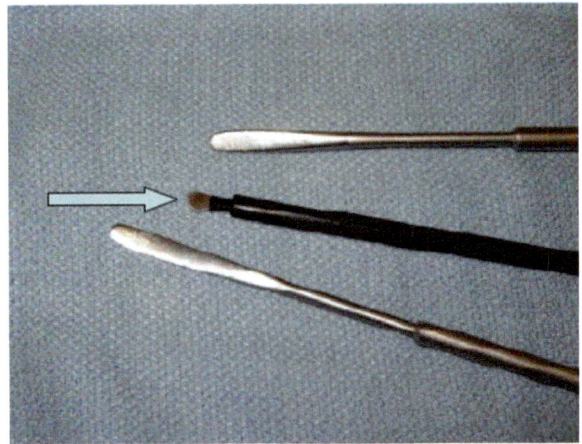

Fig. 27.5 Port placements for laparoscopic enucleation of pancreatic tumor. Working ports 15 mm, assistance and optic port 5 mm

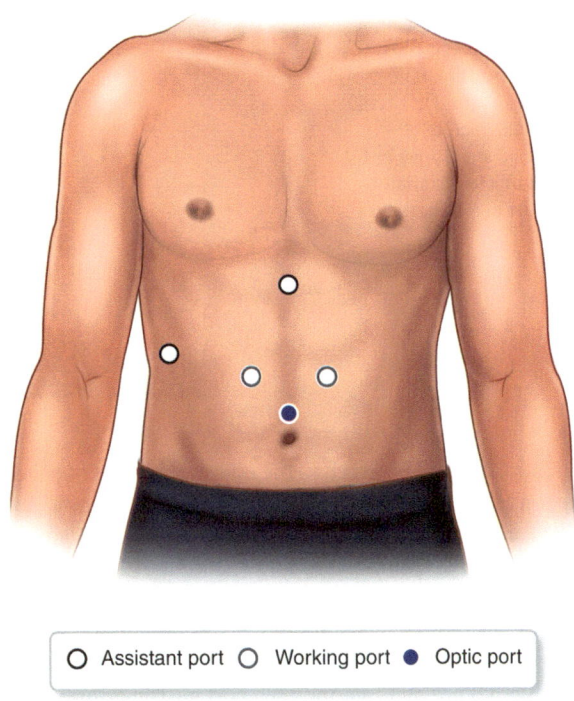

○ Assistant port ○ Working port ● Optic port

expose the entire pancreas. Lesions that locate at the head and the uncinate process may require takedown of the hepatic flexure to expose the third portion of the duodenum and thus allow full examination of the lesion using the ultrasound. Exposure of the superior mesenteric vein may be done to prevent iatrogenic injury during enucleation. If the lesions are benign, there will be a regular border "halo" sign that delineates that plane between normal pancreatic parenchyma and neoplasm. Extra

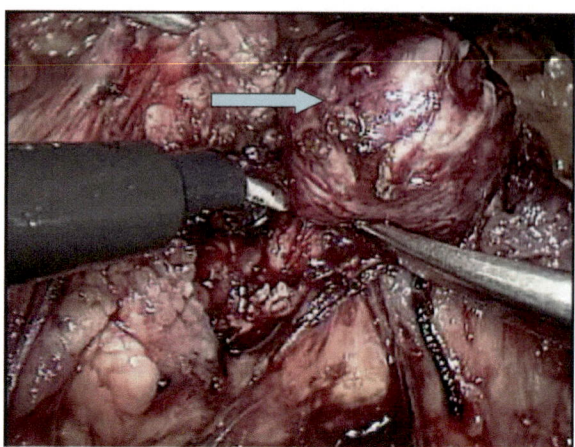

Fig. 27.6 Enucleation of a pancreatic lesion (an arrow) using a laparoscopic monopolar spatula on the left and a spatulated retractor on the right. (Courtesy from Gumbs, AA and Inabnet, WB. Laparoscopic Pancreatic Enucleation/ Resection for Neuroendocrine Tumor)

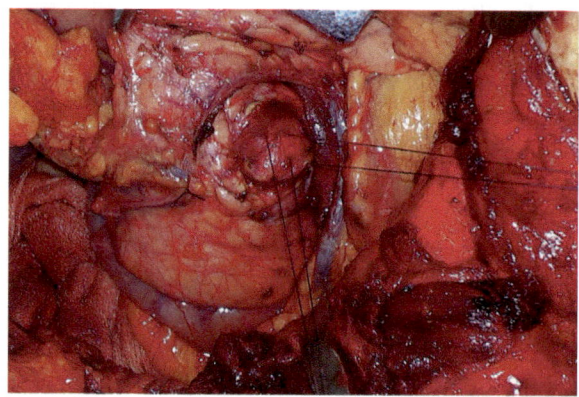

Fig. 27.7 A pancreatic lesion retracted by silk sutures for dissection. (Courtesy from Dr. Nicolo Pecorelli, Faculty of Medicine and Surgery of San Raffaele Scientific Institute in Milan, Italy)

attention should be given to the communication between the pancreatic duct and the lesion of interest. Using the monopolar laparoscopic spatula, a ring is scored around the lesion and hemostasis is controlled with the bipolar cautery forceps (Fig. 27.6). The use of a 2-0 silk suture for retraction of the lesion during the dissection reduces any iatrogenic injury to the pancreatic duct, as depicted in Fig. 27.7.

For lesions in the body/tail of the pancreas, the gastrocolic ligament may be required to be divided as far to the left and sometimes including taking down the splenic flexure and ligating the short gastric arteries to gain exposure to the pancreatic tail. Once the lesion is identified, the monopolar scissor should be used to score a desired distance from the lesion. If the lesion is isolated to the tail, sometimes, a distal pancreatectomy with or without splenectomy is recommended.

Robotic Enucleation

Patient Positioning

The use of the DaVinci Robotic System for laparoscopic procedures has increased over the past few years due to smaller incisions and a more precise dissection due to the greater degree of movement. It also reduces surgeon fatigue during long procedures when compared to conventional laparoscopic procedures. Similarly, the patient will be placed in a supine well-padded position with lower extremities abducted, 15–20% reverse Trendelenburg position with right side slightly up. Both arms of the patient should be tucked. Depending on the position of the boom, the robotic arms should be oriented cephalically, as depicted in Fig. 27.8.

Procedure

Preoperative preparation is similar to laparoscopic procedure. After gaining intra-abdominal access with a 5 mm port optical view trocar slightly 2 cm above and to the right of the umbilicus and then exchange with a 12 mm robotic port for robotic camera. Three additional 8 mm robotic trocars are placed at the same level on the robotic camera for pancreatic head lesions (Fig. 27.9a). One additional 5 mm port can be placed in the right anterior axillary line for liver retraction if needed. Then two assistant ports are placed halfway between each spino-umbilical line (SUL) for needles or ultrasound access.

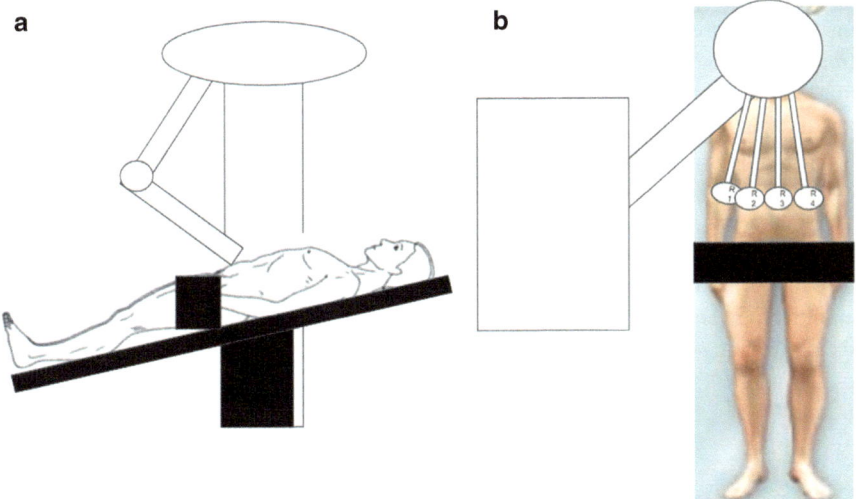

Fig. 27.8 Position of DaVinci Xi boom relative to patient. (**a**) Side view. (**b**) Top view

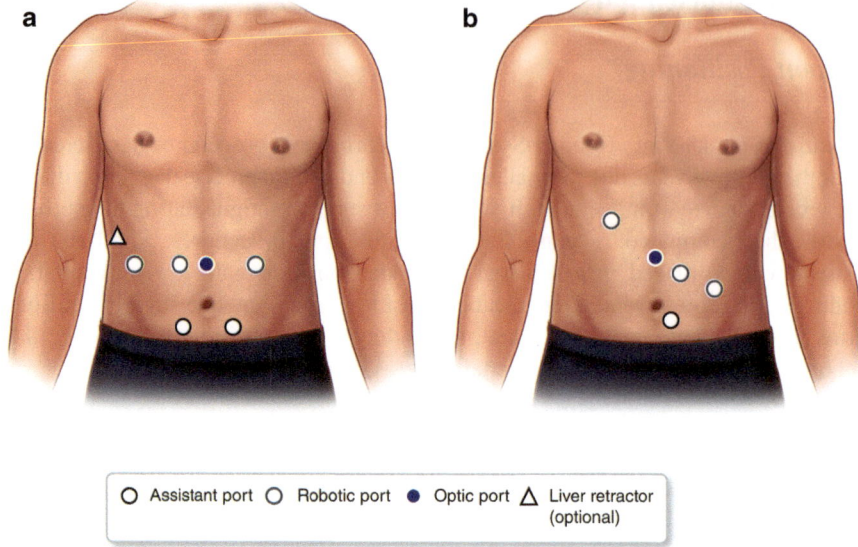

| ○ Assistant port | ○ Robotic port | ● Optic port | △ Liver retractor (optional) |

Fig. 27.9 Ports placement for DaVinci Xi robotic resection. (**a**) Pancreatic head lesion. (**b**) Pancreatic lesions located in the pancreatic body or tail. Robotic port 8 mm, Optic port 5 mm exchanged to robotic port after entry. Assistant port 5 mm

For pancreatic lesions located in the body or the tail, the optical view trocar is placed in a similar fashion as pancreatic head lesion. Three additional 8 mm robotic trocars are placed in a linear fashion from the right subcostal area to the left lower quadrant as depicted in Fig. 27.9b. One or two additional assistant ports can be placed approximately halfway along the SUL. Then the robot cart is docked. The instruments are monopolar hook (dissection and enucleation), bipolar forceps (retraction and hemostasis), fenestrated Prograsper forceps or tip-up grasper (retraction), ultrasonic scalpel (transection), and intraoperative ultrasound (through one of the assistant ports).

After the removal of the lesion and if there are any concerns for possible pancreatic duct injury/communications, intraoperative ultrasound can be used to inspect the deeper margin or the use of secretin intraoperatively can be administered and monitored for any sign of leak around the surgical area. If confirmed, the area can be oversewn with non-absorbable suture or formal resection may be needed using an ultrasonic shear. The use of fibrin glue is also popular among surgeons to use at the pancreatic stump. When in doubt, always leave a surgical drain for monitoring.

Pitfalls of Minimally Invasive Procedures

When compared to open procedures, the fistula rate is higher in laparoscopy. One possible explanation is the lack of tactile examination of pancreatic tissues increases the risk for potential pancreatic duct injuries and missed lesions and thus proper localization of lesion prior to surgery, accurate use of intraoperative ultrasound, and prior placement of a pancreatic duct stent are recommended for a successful procedure.

Open Enucleation

The indications for open enucleation include surgeon preference, patient's comorbidities, and prior abdominal surgeries. Intraoperatively, conversion to open may be required because of uncontrolled bleeding, major injuries to pancreatic or nearby structures that cannot be safely done laparoscopically, and the inability to tolerate pneumoperitoneum. Patients are placed in the same supine position with upper midline (pancreatic head) or left subcostal incision (pancreatic body/tail). The rest of the parenchymal resection is done in a similar fashion as a laparoscopic procedure utilizing the monopolar electrocautery (Fig. 27.10).

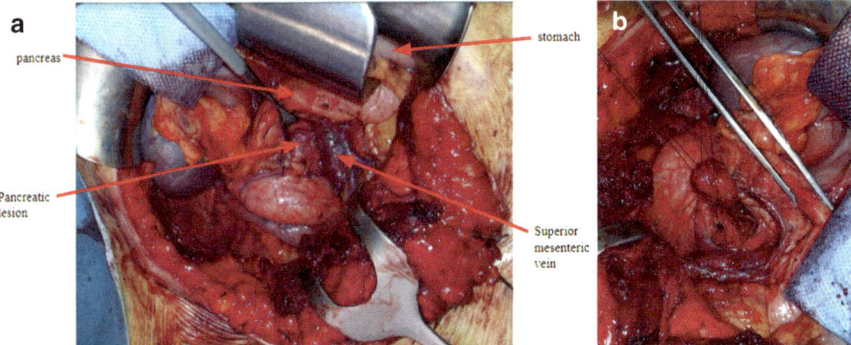

Fig. 27.10 Pancreatic lesion located in the uncinate process of the pancreas. (**a**) Uncinate process lesion located to the right of the superior mesenteric vein. (**b**) Silk sutures are used for retraction during dissection. (Courtesy from Dr. Nicolo Pecorelli, Faculty of Medicine and Surgery of San Raffaele Scientific Institute in Milan, Italy)

Postoperative Management

Postoperatively, an enhanced after surgery pathway is suggested. The nasogastric tube is removed at the end of surgery, while the Foley catheter is usually maintained. Patients can be managed on the floor unless there are pre-existing comorbidities that require intensive care monitoring. Patients are encouraged to mobilize out of bed as soon as possible and ambulate on postoperative day 1. Oral diet can be initiated early, and Foley can be removed once tolerating diet and fully resuscitated postoperatively. Daily chemistries and complete blood count are obtained and repleted as needed. Prophylactic low molecular weight heparin continues based on institutional protocols. Surgical drain fluid is sent for amylase analysis on POD #1, #3, and #5 to determine the occurrence of a pancreatic fistula and guide the timing of removal.

Postoperative Outcomes

Postoperatively, both enucleation and anatomical pancreatic resection have similar overall complication rates. For patients who underwent enucleation, the length of operation and hospital stay, blood loss, and both postoperative endocrine and exocrine insufficiency are reduced when compared to surgical resection group [1, 2, 6]. In some studies, it shows that enucleation has a higher postoperative pancreatic fistula (POPF) rate; however, this increase does not result in higher morbidity or mortality rate. Instead, if pancreatic enucleation is performed in a high volume center (which is defined as >20 cases and more than 4 cases per year), the overall POPF rate is similar among the two groups. Other measured outcomes include overall complications, reoperation rate and delayed gastric emptying are equivalent between the two groups [1, 2, 6].

When comparing both MIS enucleation and open approach, the MIS approach is proved to have reduced blood loss, better postoperative pain control, shorter hospital stay, and faster patient recovery. According to the same studies, MIS enucleation is preferred for small and benign pancreatic lesions, especially for pNET (pancreatic neuroendocrine tumors); however, if the size of the lesion is greater than 30–40 mm, a careful approach is recommended along with intraoperative frozen section. If lesion is malignant or non-pNET, an open enucleation or anatomical resection is encouraged. During MIS enucleation, the use of intraoperative US to delineate the distance between the lesion and main pancreatic duct can lower the risk of POPF. The risk increases with a distance that is less than 3 mm. Moreover, open enucleation or resection will provide better anatomy for lesions around the pancreatic head when compared to body or tail [6–8]. Currently, there are no randomized controlled studies comparing the exact safe distance between the pancreatic duct and lesion, advantages of MIS versus open procedure for pancreatic head lesions, or tumor recurrence rate for MIS vs open approach. Overall, multiple studies have shown that MIS enucleation can be considered a safe and comparable approach for small and benign pancreatic lesions, especially in high volume centers.

Acknowledgments Thank Dr. Pecorelli Nicolò (Faculty of Medicine and Surgery of San Raffaele Scientific Institute in Milan, Italy) for contributing intraoperative images for this article.

Financial Disclosures Drs. Mei Zhen Cao, Andrew Gumbs, Romulo Genato, and Luca Milone have no financial disclosures.

References

1. Chua TC, Yang TX, Gill AJ, Samra JS. Systematic review and meta-analysis of enucleation versus standardized resection for small pancreatic lesions. Ann Surg Oncol. 2016;23(2):592–9.
2. Hüttner FJ, et al. Meta-analysis of surgical outcome after enucleation versus standard resection for pancreatic neoplasms. Br J Surg. 2015;102(9):1026–36.
3. Kaiser J, Fritz S, Klauss M, Bergmann F, Hinz U, Strobel O, Schneider L, Büchler MW, Hackert T. Enucleation: a treatment alternative for branch duct intraductal papillary mucinous neoplasms. Surgery. 2017;161(3):602–10. Epub 2016 Nov 22.
4. Partelli S, Bartsch DK, Capdevila J, Chen J, Knigge U, Niederle B, Nieveen van Dijkum EJM, Pape UF, Pascher A, Ramage J, Reed N, Ruszniewski P, Scoazec JY, Toumpanakis C, Kianmanesh R, Falconi M, Antibes Consensus Conference Participants. ENETS consensus guidelines for standard of care in neuroendocrine tumours: surgery for small intestinal and pancreatic neuroendocrine tumours. Neuroendocrinology. 2017;105(3):255–65. Epub 2017 Feb 25.
5. Heeger K, Falconi M, Partelli S, et al. Increased rate of clinically relevant pancreatic fistula after deep enucleation of small pancreatic tumors. Langenbecks Arch Surg. 2014;399:315–21.
6. Shen X, Yang X. Comparison of outcomes of enucleation vs standard surgical resection for pancreatic neoplasms: a system review and meta-analysis. Front Surg. 2022;8:744316.
7. Dalla Valle R, Cremaschi E, Lamecchi L, Guerini F, Rosso E, Iaria M. Open and minimally invasive pancreatic neoplasms enucleation: a systematic review. Surg Endosc. 2019;33(10):3192–9.
8. Roesel R, et al. Minimally-invasive versus open pancreatic enucleation: systematic review and metanalysis of short-term outcomes. HPB (Oxford). 2023;25(6):603–13.

Chapter 28
Minimally Invasive Central Pancreatectomy

Vincent Butano, Iswanto Sucandy, Sharona Ross, and Alexander Rosemurgy

Introduction

A central pancreatectomy (CP) is a relatively uncommon operation in the United States, indicated for benign and low malignant potential pancreatic body tumors [1, 2]. CP either undertaken via "open" or minimally invasive method is proposed and utilized as an alternative surgical treatment to a distal pancreatectomy to preserve pancreatic parenchyma. The CP has declined in popularity due concerns of increased morbidity specifically related to postoperative pancreatic leak and fistula relative to non-parenchymal sparing techniques [3]. As imaging technology of computed tomography (CT) and magnetic resonance (MR) scans continue to improve, detection rate of small, mid-body pancreatic lesions increases and becomes a more relevant clinical question in daily clinical practice of pancreatic surgery. Additionally, nuclear medicine modality such as Dotatate scan has demonstrated the ability to improve detection of small pancreatic neuroendocrine tumors as well [4, 5]. It stands to reason that as detection of these lesions becomes more common, a central pancreatectomy may have a developing role in the management of these patients.

The advent and rapid adoption of robotic hepatopancreatobiliary surgery in the US changes the choice of surgical techniques in pancreatic surgery. The increased

V. Butano
Digestive Health Institute at AdventHealth, Tampa, FL, USA

I. Sucandy (✉)
Department of Surgery, University of Central Florida, Orlando, FL, USA
e-mail: iswanto.sucandy@adventhealth.com

S. Ross · A. Rosemurgy
Department of Surgery, University of Central Florida, Orlando, FL, USA

Department of Surgery, Nova Southeastern University, Fort Lauderdale, FL, USA

© The Author(s), under exclusive license to Springer Nature Switzerland AG 2025
E. P. Ceppa et al. (eds.), *The SAGES Manual of Evolving Techniques in Pancreatic Surgery*, https://doi.org/10.1007/978-3-031-78409-5_28

visualization, improved precision in delicate vascular dissection, and the ability to complete a fine pancreaticojejunostomy anastomosis allow a paradigm shift in the decision making between distal pancreatectomy versus central pancreatectomy for pancreatic body tumors. In this chapter, we describe indications, preoperative preparation, and surgical techniques of central pancreatectomy.

Indications

Careful patient selection is essential to maximize derived benefit. Risk and benefit must be carefully weighed for each individual patient since there are no absolute indications for central pancreatectomy for the appropriate biology. Historically, distal pancreatectomy had been the standard treatment for pancreatic body malignant tumors. Parenchymal-preserving central pancreatectomies then came as an alternative method for benign or low-risk malignant tumors (such as pancreatic neuroendocrine tumors, intraductal papillary mucinous neoplasms, mucinous cystic neoplasms, and solid pseudopapillary neoplasm) confined to the neck or proximal body of the pancreas [2]. The most classical indication for CP would be a central pancreatic mass of a tumor type which would typically be amenable to enucleation; however, due to its depth within the pancreatic parenchyma, or proximity to the main duct, enucleation would be impossible or carry a significant risk of pancreatic duct leak with its subsequent morbidities. The inherent benefit of pancreatic preservation and reduced risk of postoperative pancreatic insufficiency must justify the potential morbidity.

Preoperative Assessment

Patients diagnosed with suspicious lesions in the neck of the pancreas should undergo a thorough preoperative evaluation before any surgical intervention is offered. Many of these patients will be found to have metastatic disease or vascular involvement, precluding surgical resection. A multi-disciplinary approach to these central lesions is paramount to assess the patient's comorbidities, preoperative risk, the role of radiologic and endoscopic interventions, clinical staging, and potential role for neoadjuvant or adjuvant therapies.

Serologic Testing

- All patients should have standard preoperative labs including CBC, chemistry, hepatic panel, and PT/INR.
- Any patient with a suspicious pancreatic mass should have preoperative tumor markers (CA19-9, Chromogranin A, metanephrines, catecholamines).

Imaging and Additional Diagnostic Studies

- The initial imaging modality of choice is triphasic CT abdomen pelvis with 1 mm cuts. The CT is completed with intravenous contrast and timed for the arterial, venous, and portal venous phases. A non-contrast CT chest may be performed at the same time to rule out pulmonary lesions. This study is widely available and can be used both for diagnosis and staging. The ability of the CT scan to define the tumor location, size, extension, biliary and pancreatic obstruction, and vascular involvement make this study the most valuable in terms of information and efficiency.

- MRI/MRCP can be obtained to provide additional information on the status of biliary tree, proximity of lesion to the main pancreatic duct, and potential hepatic metastasis should there be any concerns on the initial CT. The MRI is not as useful in gleaning information regarding vascular involvement, and this study is not required prior to resection.

- Endoscopic ultrasound (EUS) has become routine in obtaining a tissue sample, assessing the lymph nodes near the mass, and vascular involvement. This modality is especially useful for ruling out non-surgical masses such as lymphoma as well as assessing the vasculature if the CT is equivocal. Should the tumor be found unresectable, a definitive tissue diagnosis can be obtained by the EUS to guide administration of systemic chemotherapy. This will allow the patient's therapy to be tailored to the specific tumor biology and potentially allow the patient to be downstaged for a potentially later resection.

- PET/CT may be indicated in the setting of a mass that has a high likelihood of metastasis; however, some tumors are not PET avid thus making this evaluation somewhat controversial. It is generally our practice to obtain a PET/CT for the majority of our preoperative patients, but this is not an absolute requirement. DOTATATE contrasted PET/CT has become the gold standard for suspected or confirmed pancreatic neuroendocrine tumors (pNET), and we recommend all patients with neuroendocrine tumors undergo this study as pNET have a high likelihood of regional and distant metastatic disease at presentation. Findings of extrapancreatic metastasis do not necessarily preclude resection; however, it helps identify other resectable lesions. DOTATATE also has an important role in detecting multifocal disease in patients at increased risk due to genetic syndrome (e.g., Multiple Endocrine Neoplasia type 1).

- Preoperative nutritional assessment is essential for all patients undergoing pancreatic resection. This is especially useful in those undergoing a central pancreatectomy as they are at higher risk for a pancreatic leak. A preoperative dietician consult and dietary modification with appropriate protein supplementation should be performed as indicated.

- In many patients with pancreatic masses, the preoperative glucose may be elevated requiring control. Improved glycemic control has been shown to decrease wound complications and other postoperative complications in many trials [3].

- Cardiology evaluation should be performed in patients with a history of cardiac disease. It is our practice to request a cardiology evaluation for all patients over the age of 50 to assess for any underlying cardiac abnormalities requiring intervention as well as preoperative risk stratification.

Surgical Management

In our institution, we undertake this operation using a robotic platform, which facilitates precise vascular dissection, stable platform, and increased manual dexterity for suturing of pancreaticojejunostomy anastomosis [6–9].

Patient Preparation

- Patients are positioned supine, arms outstretched, secured to the operating table.
- A single shot of intra-thecal morphine sulfate is injected prior to induction.
- Following endotracheal intubation, a Foley catheter and a nasogastric tube is inserted.
- Prophylactic antibiotics are given within 30 min of incision and sequential compression devices are applied to prevent deep vein thrombosis (DVT).

Diagnostic Laparoscopy

- Following an 8 mm robotic trocar insertion at the umbilicus as a camera port (arm #2), a diagnostic laparoscopy with the robotic laparoscope is performed to exclude peritoneal carcinomatosis, liver metastasis, or other indicators of non-operative disease.
- If the diagnostic laparoscopy shows localized disease without contraindications for resection, further trocars are inserted (Fig. 28.1):
  - Arm #1: 8 mm trocar lateral to the right midclavicular line at the level of the umbilicus
  - Arm #2: Robotic laparoscope
  - Arm #3: 12 mm at the left midclavicular line at the level of the umbilicus
  - Arm #4: 8 mm left anterior axillary line slightly cephalad to the level of the umbilicus
  - 5 mm AirSeal® Access Port (ConMed Inc., Utica, NY) in the right anterior axillary line in the subcostal region for liver and stomach retraction
  - An Advanced Access Gelport® (Applied Medical, Rancho Santa Margarita, CA) is inserted between arms #1 and #2 caudal to the umbilicus

Fig. 28.1 Port placement

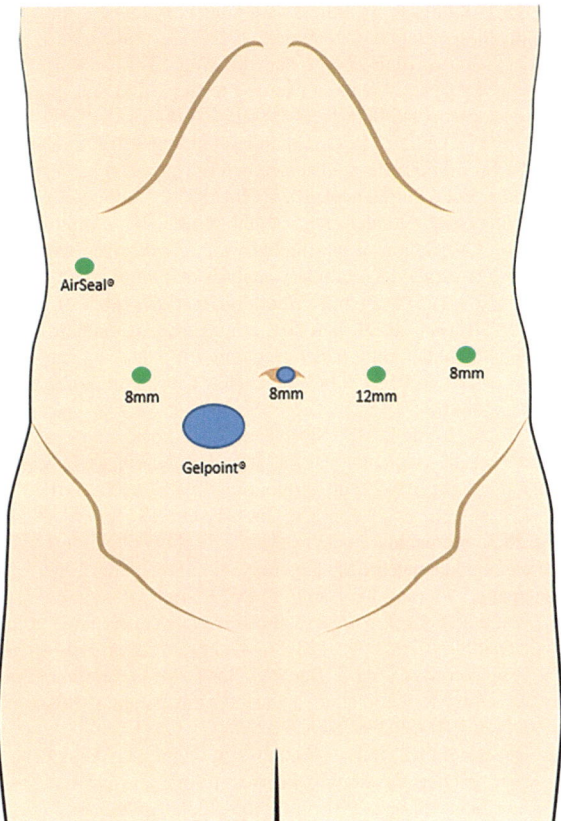

Surgical Steps

Step 1: Gastric Mobilization

- Arms setup:
  - Arm #1: Fenestrated bipolar
  - Arm #2: Camera
  - Arm #3: Monopolar scissors/hook cautery/vessel sealer
  - Arm #4: Small grasping retractor
  - Bedside assistant: Laparoscopic bowel grasper and suctioning device
- The lesser sac is entered by dividing the gastrocolic ligament using a combination of monopolar scissors, hook cautery, and the vessel sealer (Fig. 28.2).
- Once the lesser sac is entered, the dissection is carried laterally in order to mobilize the stomach cephalad. Caution should be taken during this mobilization in order to preserve the gastroepiploic vessels. The mobilization is complete once the stomach can sufficiently be retracted cephalad in order to view the neck and

Fig. 28.2 Stomach mobilization

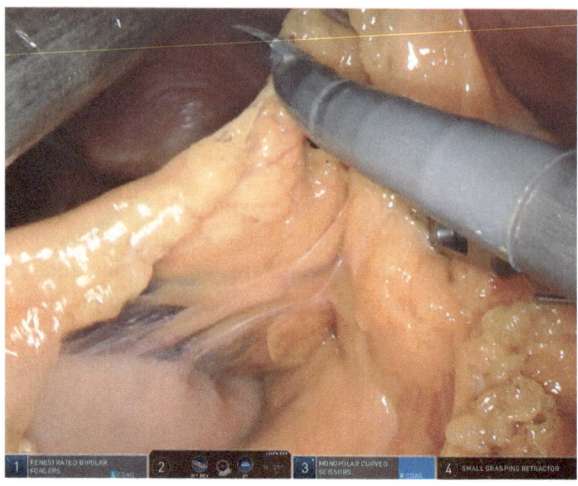

Fig. 28.3 Stomach retraction and exposure of pancreas

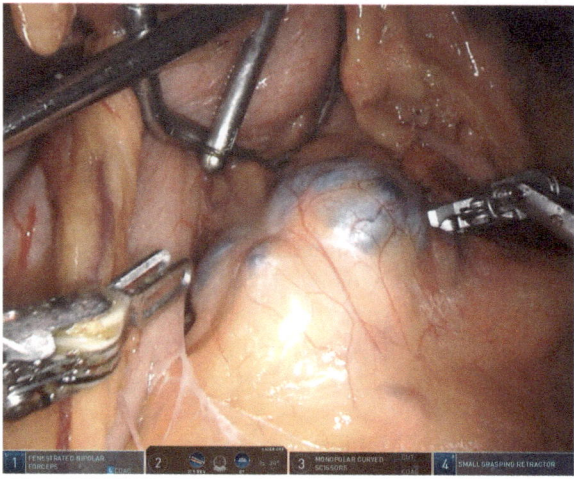

mid-body of the pancreas. This retraction can be obtained using a laparoscopic liver retractor via the 5 mm AirSeal® Port in the right upper quadrant subcostal region. Both the stomach and the left lateral sector (segment 2 and 3) of the liver can be both retracted together (Fig. 28.3).

Step 2: Pancreatic Resection

- Arms setup:
  - Arm #1: Fenestrated bipolar
  - Arm #2: Camera
  - Arm #3: Hook cautery/robotic stapling device

Fig. 28.4 Ultrasonographic examination of the pancreas

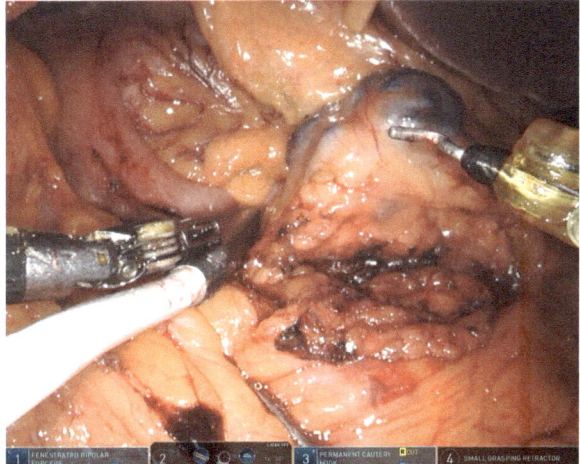

Fig. 28.5 Dissection of inferior border of pancreas

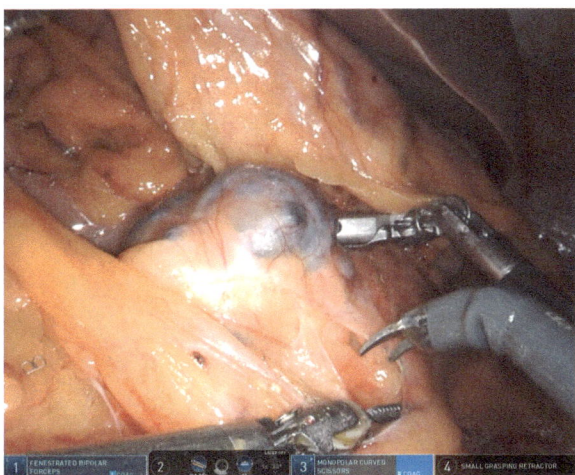

- Arm #4: Small grasping retractor
- Bedside assistant: Laparoscopic bowel grasper, suctioning device, intraoperative ultrasound probe

• The lesion is assessed with ultrasound and the corresponding location can be marked on the pancreatic parenchyma with the hook cautery (Fig. 28.4). After this, the resection lines can also be marked, and the dissection can begin.

• The dissection of the proximal pancreas is carried along the inferior edge of the pancreatic neck. The superior mesenteric vein (SMV) is identified, and the dissection is carried under the pancreatic neck over the SMV and portal vein (PV) (Fig. 28.5). The assistant may use the laparoscopic suction device through the Gelport® to retract and expose the SMV and PV to facilitate the dissection until the retropancreatic tunnel is developed (Fig. 28.6).

Fig. 28.6 Dissection of retropancreatic tunnel

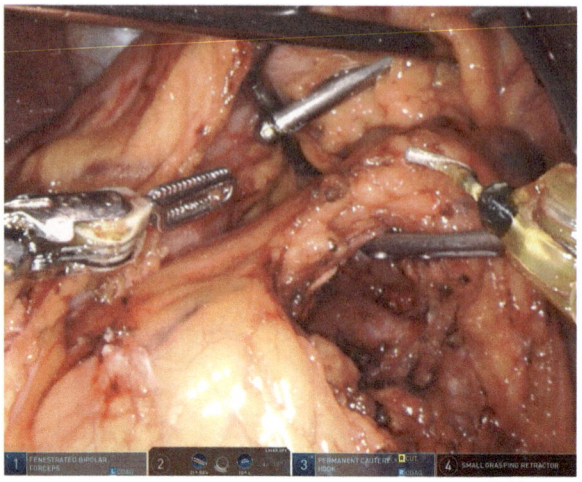

Fig. 28.7 Proximal pancreatic transection

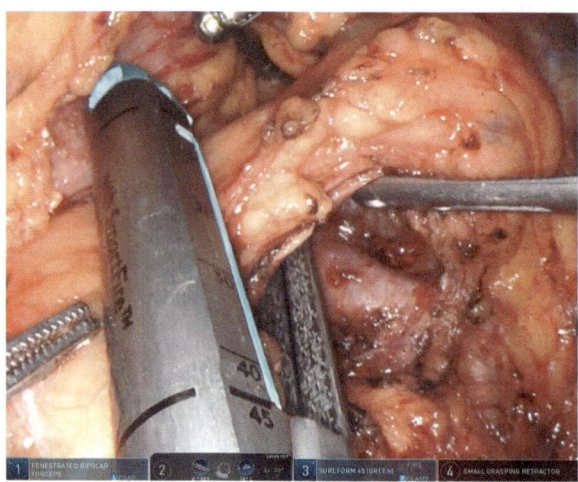

- The pancreatic neck may now be divided using a robotic stapling device. The pancreatic duct and the underlying vessels dorsal to the pancreas must be identified during pancreatic resection to prevent injury to the SMV or PV (Fig. 28.7).
- The pancreatic parenchyma should then be separated from the splenic artery and vein for a sufficient length to reach the previously marked transection point distal to the lesion (Fig. 28.8).
- The distal transection should be performed with the hook cautery in order identify the pancreatic duct for reconstruction (Fig. 28.9).
- At this point, the specimen should be placed into the EndoCatch™ (Medtronic, Minneapolis, MN) bag and sent to pathology to ensure that the resection margins are not involved by the disease before reconstruction can begin.

Fig. 28.8 Lateral
retropancreatic dissection

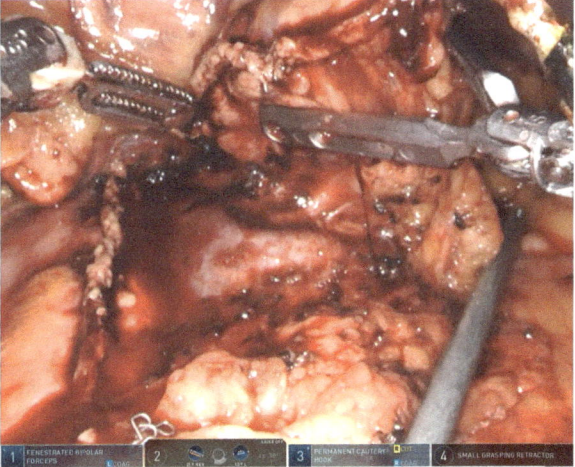

Fig. 28.9 Distal pancreatic
transection

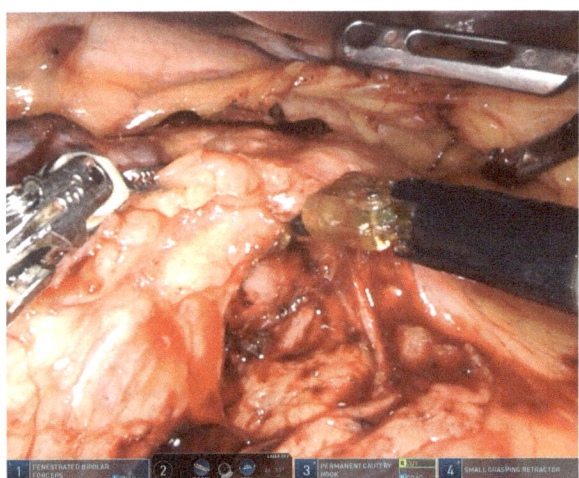

Step 3: Reconstruction

- Arms setup:
  - Arm #1: Needle driver
  - Arm #2: Camera
  - Arm #3: Needle driver/robotic stapling device/vessel sealer
  - Arm #4: Small grasping retractor
  - Bedside assistant: Laparoscopic bowel grasper and suctioning device
- Roughly 40 cm past the ligament of treitz the jejunum is transected with the robotic stapler and the mesentery divided using the vessel sealer.

Jejunojejunostomy

- First, the proximal jejunum is anastomosed to the distal jejunum to create a side-to-side stapled jejunojejunostomy. Using the scissors, an enterotomy is made in the proximal and distal jejunum. The enterotomies are enlarged to fit the two ends of the robotic 45 mm blue load stapler. The robotic stapler is then inserted into both ends and fired (Fig. 28.10).
- The staple line is checked for hemostasis and the common enterotomy is closed with 3-0 non-absorbable V-Loc™ sutures in a running fashion (Fig. 28.11).

Fig. 28.10 Side-to-side stapled jejunojejunostomy

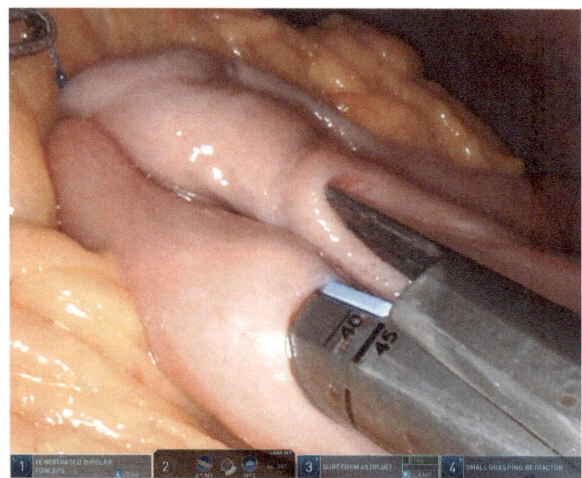

Fig. 28.11 Closure of common enterotomy

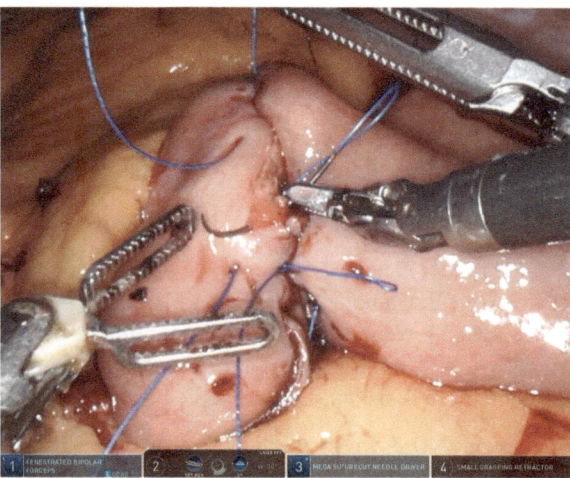

Pancreaticojejunostomy

- The distal jejunum is brought up to the distal pancreatic stump preferably in an antecolic fashion. Should there be tension, the jejunum may need to be brought to the distal pancreatic stump in a retrocolic fashion.
- The posterior-outer layer of the anastomosis is started with a running 3-0 non-absorbable V-Loc™ suture between the pancreatic capsule and substance to the seromuscular layer of the jejunum, with caution not to include or compress the pancreatic duct (Fig. 28.12).
- Using the scissors, a small enterotomy is made in the distal jejunal limb across from the pancreatic duct. The inner layer of the anastomosis is constructed with full-thickness, 3-0 or 4-0, interrupted absorbable V-Loc™ suture which are placed between the pancreatic duct and the enterotomy so that the duct is continuous with the bowel in a duct-to-mucosa fashion (Fig. 28.13).

Fig. 28.12 Outer layer of pancreaticojejunostomy

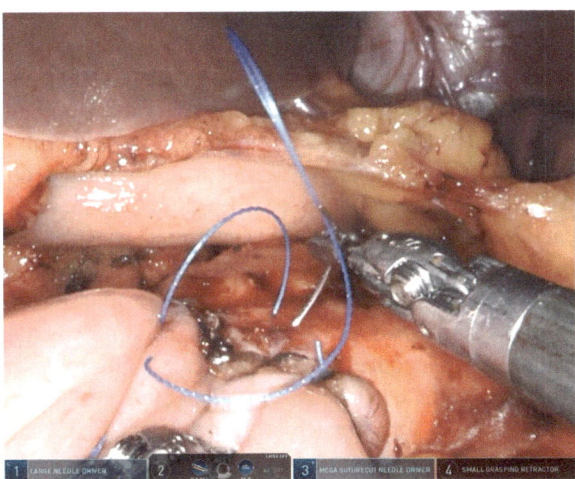

Fig. 28.13 Inner layer of pancreaticojejunostomy

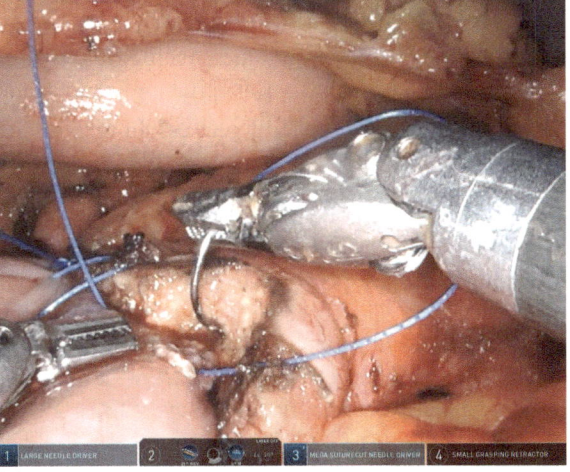

- We place four interrupted sutures between the pancreatic duct and the jejunot-omy, at four quadrants of the pancreatic duct in a 6-, 9-, 3-, and 12-o'clock order. The sutures are tied on the extra-luminal surface.
- A running 3-0 non-absorbable V-Loc™ suture is then used to form the anterior-outer layer between the pancreatic capsule and substance to the seromuscular layer of the jejunal limb, in a similar fashion as the posterior layer. The anterior and posterior outer-layer sutures are then tied together.
- A 10 Fr closed suction drain is placed near the proximal pancreatic stump and pancreaticojejunostomy. A final check for hemostasis is performed and the abdomen is desufflated. All port sites larger than 8 mm are closed and the opera-tion is complete.

Discussion

Central pancreatectomy brings several advantages when compared to other standard pancreatic resection techniques (pancreatoduodenectomy and distal pancreatec-tomy), mainly attributed to the preservation of pancreatic parenchyma. These include a reduced incidence of postoperative exocrine and endocrine insufficiency, as well as the avoidance of splenectomy-related complications [10–13], while enabling excision of pancreatic body tumors otherwise could not have been safely excised via enucleation. The first reported case of a laparoscopic CP was published by Baca and Bokan in 2003 for cystadenoma [14]. The first robotic CP was reported by Giulianotti et al. from Misericordia Hospital in Grosseto a year later [15]. Since then, there have been only few reports on minimally invasive CP surgical techniques and clinical outcomes. In this chapter, we aim to describe surgical steps of central pancreatectomy and discuss important clinical aspects of this operation.

Relative to distal pancreatectomy, central pancreatectomy has higher rates of overall and severe morbidity, overall and clinically relevant pancreatic fistula, hem-orrhage, and longer length of stay, which limits its widespread application and adoption [2, 16]. Other complications may include issues related to the reconstruc-tion such as enteric leak, bowel obstruction, or internal hernia. The technical demand of fine suturing skills during the creation of pancreaticojejunostomy anastomosis further deters surgeons from undertaking laparoscopic CP. The advent of robotic surgical systems facilitates fine suturing, which ameliorates this technical issue; however, the availability of the robotic platform is still not universal currently.

In 2018, Xio et al. conducted a systematic review which included 50 studies and 1305 patients undergoing CP. The outcomes of these patients were compared with those undergoing distal pancreatectomy and pancreaticoduodenectomy. The overall morbidity, mortality, postoperative pancreatic fistula, and reoperation rate was 51%, 0.5%, 35%, and 4%, respectively. Endocrine and exocrine insufficiency occurred in only 4% and 5% of patients, respectively [2]. Further subgroup meta-analysis of CP versus distal pancreatectomy favored CP with regard of blood loss and lower rate of postoperative endocrine insufficiency (OR = 0.13, $p < 0.001$) and exocrine insufficiency (OR = 0.38, $p < 0.001$); however, CP was associated with high pancreatic leak rate. In comparison to pancreatoduodenectomy, CP also had a lower risk of postoperative endocrine (OR = 0.14, $p < 0.001$) and exocrine insufficiency (OR = 0.14, $p < 0.001$), but higher pancreatic leak rate (OR = 1.6, $p = 0.015$). The authors concluded that CP maintains pancreatic endocrine and exocrine function better than distal pancreatectomy and pancreatoduodenectomy, but it is associated with a high pancreatic leak rate.

The most recent systematic review and meta-analysis published by Rompianesi et al. includes 13 series and 265 patients undergoing robotic central pancreatectomy. In all cases but one, robotic CP was undertaken to excise benign or low-grade tumors. Clinically relevant postoperative pancreatic fistula occurred in 42.3% of patients. The overall complications were 57.5%; however, only 9.4% were Clavien-Dindo ≥3 grades [17]. Despite the high rate of pancreatic fistula, the incidence of new-onset diabetes mellitus after the CP was only 0.3% with negligible mortality. This finding was consistent with long-term endocrinologic benefits of pancreatic parenchymal preservation offered by CP.

The conclusion is minimally invasive central pancreatectomy is safe and feasible as an alternative option to distal pancreatectomy and pancreatoduodenectomy for benign or low malignant potential pancreatic neck/body tumors. The ultimate benefit of CP is preservation of pancreatic endocrine and exocrine function, despite a higher incidence of postoperative pancreatic leak.

Acknowledgments Kaitlyn Crespo, BS; Cameron Syblis, BS; and Jacob Lambdin, MD for contributions of the images and preparation of the manuscript.

References

1. Dragomir MP, Sabo AA, Petrescu GED, Li Y, Dumitrascu T. Central pancreatectomy: a comprehensive, up-to-date meta-analysis. Langenbecks Arch Surg. 2019;404(8):945–58.
2. Xiao W, Zhu J, Peng L, Hong L, Sun G, Li Y. The role of central pancreatectomy in pancreatic surgery: a systematic review and meta-analysis. HPB (Oxford). 2018;20:896–904. https://doi.org/10.1016/j.hpb.2018.05.001.
3. Ambiru S, Kato A, Kimura F, Shimizu H, Yoshidome H, Otsuka M, et al. Poor postoperative blood glucose control increases surgical site infections after surgery for hepato-biliary-pancreatic cancer: a prospective study in a high-volume institute in Japan. J Hosp Infect. 2008;68(3):230–3.
4. Sadowski SM, Millo C, Cottle-Delisle C, Merkel R, Yang LA, Herscovitch P, et al. Results of (68)Gallium-DOTATATE PET/CT scanning in patients with multiple endocrine neoplasia type 1. J Am Coll Surg. 2015;221(2):509–17.
5. Werba G, Napolitano MA, Sparks AD, Lin PP, Johnson LB, Vaziri K. Impact of preoperative biliary drainage on 30 day outcomes of patients undergoing pancreaticoduodenectomy for malignancy. HPB (Oxford). 2022;24(4):478–88.
6. Ross S, Rayman S, Sucandy I, Syblis C, Rosemurgy A. Whipple's operation and distal pancreatectomy. In: Costello T, editor. Principles and practice of robotic surgery. Philadelphia: Elsevier; 2024.

7. Ross S, Rosemurgy A, Wecowski J, Bourdeau T, Sucandy I. Robotic pylorus-preserving pancreaticoduodenectomy and cholecystectomy. In: Atlas of robotic general surgery. Elsevier; 2021. p. 309–22.
8. Ross SB, Downs D, Sucandy I, Rosemurgy AS. Robotic pylorus-preserving pancreaticoduodenectomy. In: Fong Y, Woo Y, Hyung W, Lau C, Strong V, editors. The SAGES atlas of robotic surgery. Cham: Springer; 2018. p. 319–34.
9. Rosemurgy A, Ross S, Bourdeau T, Craigg D, Spence J, Alvior J, et al. Robotic pancreaticoduodenectomy is the future: here and now. J Am Coll Surg. 2019;228:613–24.
10. Crippa S, Bassi C, Warshaw AL, Falconi M, Partelli S, Thayer SP, Pederzoli P, Fernández-del Castillo C. Middle pancreatectomy: indications, short- and long-term operative outcomes. Ann Surg. 2007;246(1):69–76. https://doi.org/10.1097/01.sla.0000262790.51512.57.
11. Iacono C, Verlato G, Ruzzenente A, Campagnaro T, Bacchelli C, Valdegamberi A, Bortolasi L, Guglielmi A. Systematic review of central pancreatectomy and meta-analysis of central versus distal pancreatectomy. Br J Surg. 2013;100(7):873–85. https://doi.org/10.1002/bjs.9136.
12. Xu SB, Zhu YP, Zhou W, Xie K, Mou YP. Patients get more long-term benefit from central pancreatectomy than distal resection: a meta-analysis. Eur J Surg Oncol. 2013;39(6):567–74. https://doi.org/10.1016/j.ejso.2013.02.003. Epub 2013 Mar 7.
13. Santangelo M, Esposito A, Tammaro V, Calogero A, Criscitiello C, Roberti G, Candida M, Rupealta N, Pisani A, Carlomagno N. What indication, morbidity and mortality for central pancreatectomy in oncological surgery? A systematic review. Int J Surg. 2016;28(Suppl 1):S172–6. https://doi.org/10.1016/j.ijsu.2015.12.046. Epub 2015 Dec 18.
14. Baca I, Bokan I. Laparoskopische Pankreassegmentresektion bei Pankreaszystadenom [Laparoscopic segmental pancreas resection and pancreatic cystadenoma]. Chirurg. 2003;74(10):961–5. German. https://doi.org/10.1007/s00104-003-0690-y.
15. Giulianotti PC, Sbrana F, Bianco FM, Addeo P, Caravaglios G. Robot-assisted laparoscopic middle pancreatectomy. J Laparoendosc Adv Surg Tech A. 2010;20(2):135–9. https://doi.org/10.1089/lap.2009.0296.
16. Rompianesi G, Montalti R, Giglio MC, Caruso E, Ceresa CD, Troisi RI. Robotic central pancreatectomy: a systematic review and meta-analysis. HPB (Oxford). 2022;24(2):143–51. https://doi.org/10.1016/j.hpb.2021.09.014. Epub 2021 Sep 24.
17. Lv A, Qian HG, Qiu H, Wu JH, Hao CY. Is central pancreatectomy truly recommendable? A 9-year single-center experience. Dig Surg. 2018;35(6):532–8. https://doi.org/10.1159/000485806. Epub 2017 Dec 22.

Chapter 29
Palliation of Pancreatic Cancer

Imad Elkhatib and Marc Mesleh

Key Points
- Increasing number of patients with pancreatic cancer will require palliation of symptoms as more effective chemotherapeutic options became available.
- Endoscopically placed metal stents are the preferred method of palliating malignant biliary obstruction.
- Biliary metal stents have varying durations of patency and will require varying types of maintenance.
- Surgical gastrojejunostomy is an effective method of palliation.
- Palliation of duodenal obstruction via duodenal metal stent placement vs surgical bypass based on the expected prognosis.
- Cancer-related abdominal pain most often responds to narcotics, but may be palliated with EUS-guided celiac plexus neurolysis.

Introduction

Each year more than 62,000 patients in the United States develop cancer of the pancreas, and of these patients, only 11% are expected to survive 5 years from diagnosis [1]. Pancreatic cancer portends a poor prognosis regardless of stage, with an estimated 3–6-month survival for those patients presenting with metastatic disease and a 9–12-month survival for those with locally advanced, unresectable disease

I. Elkhatib
Advanced/Therapeutic Endoscopy, Advocate Christ Medical Center, Oak Lawn, IL, USA

M. Mesleh (✉)
Department of Surgery, University of Illinois Chicago (UIC), Chicago, IL, USA

Advocate Christ Medical Center, Oak Lawn, IL, USA
e-mail: marc.mesleh@aah.org

© The Author(s), under exclusive license to Springer Nature Switzerland AG 2025
E. P. Ceppa et al. (eds.), *The SAGES Manual of Evolving Techniques in Pancreatic Surgery*, https://doi.org/10.1007/978-3-031-78409-5_29

Table 29.1 Categories of cancer-related symptoms and endoscopic palliation options

Cancer-related problem	Symptoms	Role of endoscopic treatment	Role of surgical treatment
Biliary obstruction	– Jaundice – Pruritis – Cholangitis	– Biliary stenting – EUS-guided choledocoduodenostomy	– Hepaticojejunostomy
Duodenal obstruction	– Nausea/emesis – Anorexia – Esophagitis	– Endoluminal stenting – Venting PEG – EUS-guided gastrojejunostomy	– Gastrojejunostomy
Neural invasion	– Abdominal pain	– Celiac plexus neurolysis	– Celiac plexus block

[2]. Resection offers the only potential for cure, but even after pancreaticoduodenectomy for curative intent, the 5-year survival remains low at 27%. Therefore, the management of many patients with pancreatic cancer will involve palliation of cancer-related symptoms. Due to patients surviving longer with newer chemotherapy and radiation treatments, the prevalence of these symptoms continues to increase. The role of palliative therapy is becoming increasingly important to offer an acceptable quality of life.

The approach to palliating cancer-related symptoms in patients with pancreatic cancer is a multidisciplinary one and involves the combination of medical oncologists, radiation oncologists, surgical oncologists, interventional gastrointestinal endoscopists, interventional radiologists, pain management physicians, and medical palliative care teams. The focus of this chapter will be on the options for endoscopic and surgical techniques in palliation of cancer-related symptoms.

The most common cancer-related symptoms from pancreatic adenocarcinoma which requires intervention include biliary obstruction, duodenal obstruction, and pain from neural involvement of locally advanced disease (Table 29.1). Deciding on the best intervention for each patient depends on several factors and should be discussed in a multidisciplinary team.

Biliary Obstruction

Given the intra-pancreatic course of the common bile duct, biliary obstruction due to tumor invasion is the most common cancer-related complication of pancreatic cancer. In fact, given that 75–85% of new diagnoses of pancreatic cancer involve the head of the pancreas, up to 70% of patients will develop some degree of biliary obstruction, which is commonly symptomatic, causing jaundice and pruritus [3]. Severe biliary obstruction can lead to liver dysfunction and coagulopathy. This coagulopathy must be diagnosed and treated before invasive procedures can be safely performed.

While there are multiple pharmacologic options for the treatment of pruritis including hydroxyzine, diphenhydramine, benzodiazepines, cholestyramine, and ursodeoxycholic acid [4], these are seldom effective given the progressive obstructive nature of the jaundice. Therefore, it is reserved for patients who are not able to receive endoscopic or surgical interventions.

Endoscopic Interventions

Endoscopic biliary stenting provides an effective means of palliating jaundice and pruritis due to malignant biliary obstruction from pancreatic cancer. It is the most common therapy for this indication. Biliary stenting can be performed via endoscopic or percutaneous routes. There are mixed data regarding the benefits of the endoscopic route as compared to the percutaneous route [5–7]. An early randomized trial showed an 81% success rate of endoscopic decompression versus a rate of 61% via the percutaneous route, with a higher mortality in the percutaneous group which was mainly attributed to complications such as bile leaks and liver hematomas [5]. Another important consideration is that with percutaneous stenting the patient will require an external drain, at least initially, which in addition to inconvenience, pain, and leaking may also lead to infection, nutrient deficiencies, malnutrition, dehydration, and electrolyte imbalance.

Endoscopic biliary decompression is done via the placement of a biliary stent through the ampulla of Vater using a side viewing duodenoscope during Endoscopic Retrograde Cholangiopancreatography (ERCP). The procedure can be done with moderate sedation or general anesthesia and procedure time can vary, with a mean length of 30 min. Prior to biliary cannulation, the endoscopist must decide on whether to place a metal or plastic stent, a covered or uncovered stent as well as decide on the length of stent to be used.

Plastic Versus Metal Stents

Plastic stents are effective and inexpensive (<$20). They can be removed if needed and they are relatively easy to exchange. Plastic stents eventually develop occlusion by a combination of bacterial biofilm and sludge, with a resultant patency life of approximately 3 months [8]. This necessitates repeated ERCPs with stent exchange, which can impart a substantial financial and quality of life burden on the patient. The effect of stent diameter on time until occlusion was studied, and it appeared that 11.5 Fr stents were non-superior to 10 Fr stents in regard to rate of occlusion [9], and in practice 11.5 Fr stents are seldom used as they are technically challenging to place with no additional benefit.

Self-expanding metal stents (SEMS) are highly effective, expensive (>$1000) and come with an increased patency of approximately 6 months [8, 10]. Metal stents are composed of laser-cut nitinol and are available as uncovered, partially covered, or fully covered types (Figs. 29.1 and 29.2). The uncovered metal stents have an open mesh or cell configuration that embed in the biliary wall and are therefore not removable, whereas the fully covered stent is easily removable should the need arise. SEMS are available in diameter sizes of 6, 8, and 10 mm diameter (much larger than the plastic counterparts), with lengths ranging from 4 to 10 cm. They are deployed via through-the-scope (TTS) delivery systems.

The decision to use a plastic versus metal stent is made after consideration of the expected length of survival, anticipated treatment plan, costs, and physician expertise. That being said, the majority of endoscopists are now predominately using SEMS for palliation of malignant biliary obstructions. A systematic review and meta-analysis showed that metal stents had a lower risk of recurrent obstruction [10] although success rate and complication rate were not statistically different between SEMS use and plastic stents. As the majority of patients with pancreatic cancer at the time of bile duct obstruction are surviving longer than 2–6 months, metal stents are becoming a more desirable option (especially with hopes of decreased need to hold chemotherapy in event of biliary blockage resulting in cholangitis). Even if the therapeutic plan for the patient is still unclear at the time of ERCP, placement of a short length (4–6 cm long) SEMS will not interfere with future surgical resection. A Monte Carlo decision analysis compared multiple approaches to patients with obstructive jaundice from pancreatic cancer in whom the surgical plan was undetermined and results showed that placement of a short length SEMS is the preferred initial treatment for overall cost reduction [11]. In a high-volume center, there should be a standardized approach to pre-op stenting based on the endoscopist and surgeon preferences.

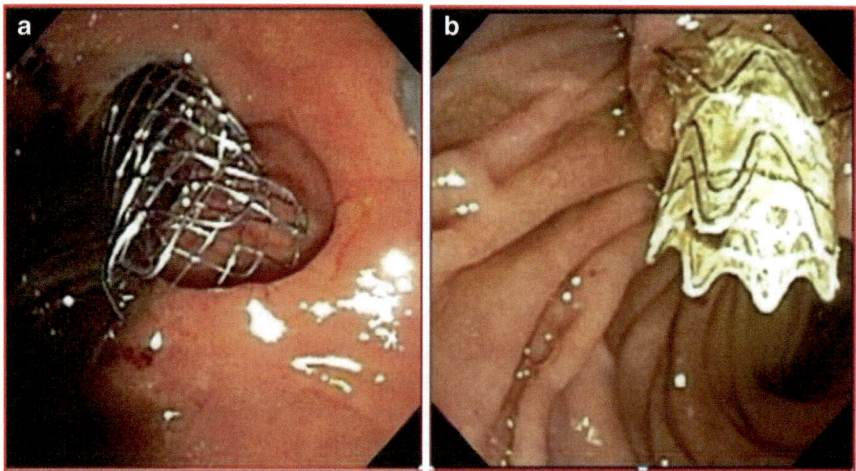

Fig. 29.1 Endoscopic appearance of an fully uncovered (**a**) and fully covered (**b**) self-expanding metal biliary stent

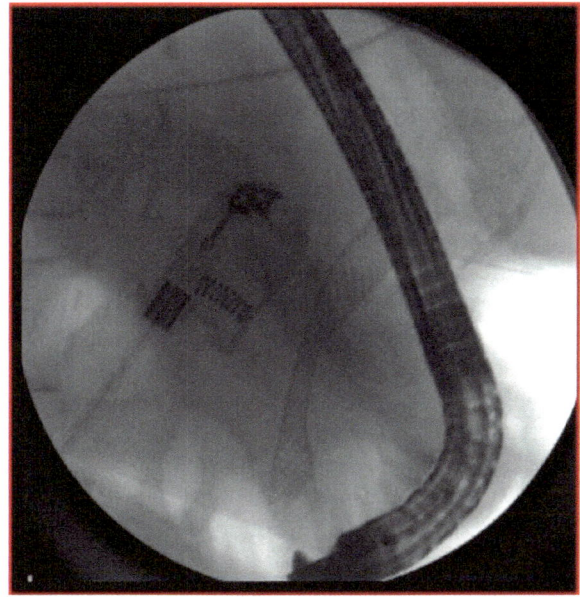

Fig. 29.2 Fluoroscopic image of a fully uncovered non-laser-cut self-expanding metal stent placed across a 3 cm long distal biliary stricture from pancreas head cancer. Note the appropriate "waist-sign" in the mid-line of the stent

Covered Versus Uncovered Metal Stents

Covered Self-Expanding Metal Stents (CSEMS) were developed with the goal of increasing patency duration over Uncovered Self-Expanding Metal Stents (USEMS). Tumor in-growth and overgrowth are examples of reasons SEMS can become occluded. There have been multiple randomized controlled trials comparing the two, yet these trials failed to show increased patency rates for CSEMS [12–14]. For example, in one of the trials evaluated 400 patients that had stent placement for malignant distal biliary obstruction; the authors found no difference between types in regard to stent patency or patient survival. Both CSEMS and USEMS had a near-identical stent failure rate (24% versus 23%) and no statistical difference between the time it took for 25% of the stents to occlude (145 days for CSEMs, versus 199 days for the USEMS). Furthermore, median survival time of the patients was similar (116 versus 174 days), but stent migration was more common in the patients with CSEMS (3% versus 0%) [15]. While a more recent meta-analysis in 2011 of five multicenter randomized trials comparing CSEMS and USEMS suggested a modest benefit to CSEMS over USEMS in regard to stent patency the increased risk of stent migration likely outweighs this marginal trend towards increased patency [16].

It has been suggested that patients with intact gallbladders should receive uncovered SEMS, with the intent of reducing the risk of cystic duct obstruction and resultant cholecystitis, although no strong data exists to support this. This may be of more concern when contrast is seen in the gallbladder during ERCP. There is a risk of acute cholecystitis due to cystic duct outflow obstruction. Surgery is typically not a first resort and may not be an option at all. A common option is placement of a cholecystostomy tube with interventional radiology. This drain will likely never come out and a newer option is EUS-guided cholecystostomy using an axios stent to decompress the gallbladder into the duodenum. This therefore is not an option if the duodenum is also obstructed.

Biliary stenting in the setting of malignant obstruction can be challenging due to tumor involvement of the duodenal wall or duodenal obstruction that prevents access to the ampulla. In these cases, interventional radiology with percutaneous biliary access has traditionally been used. However, recently a variety of EUS-guided techniques have been used to access the biliary system and place stents [17–19]. The endosonographic approach can be either a transgastric or transduodenal puncture of the biliary tree to pass a guide wire antegrade though the papilla for stent placement or creation of a choledocho-duodenostomy or hepatico-gastrostomy. Of note, the current complication rate of these approaches is about 20% and needs to be performed in a tertiary care center with extensive interventional endoscopic experience. Immediate interventional radiology and surgical back up should be available [20].

Stent Obstruction

As pancreatic cancer patients with biliary stents live longer due to improved oncologic treatment options, the concern for developing cholangitis or biliary obstruction has increased. This is due to either accumulation of biofilm and sludge or related to food impaction. Recent studies suggest that the chance of stent occlusion and cholangitis at 1 year is as high as 46% [21, 22]. If patients are actively receiving treatment with chemotherapy, the immunosuppression can increase the severity of their illness. Patients should be instructed that any shaking chills (rigors) or fevers likely represent biliary obstruction. Sometimes this is transient with relatively normal liver tests, and sometimes will be associated with jaundice and elevated liver tests. Patients with severe symptoms need to go to the emergency room for evaluation and probable hospitalization, while those with mild symptoms can sometimes be managed with outpatient oral antibiotics. Patients with suspected stent occlusion should be considered for repeat ERCP in order to sweep out any debris/food from the stent and/or place a new stent. Occasionally for long-term management or repeatedly occluding metal stents, the patient will be placed on oral ursodeoxycholic acid (to increase biliary secretion and flow) and/or prophylactic ERCP biliary stent cleaning with balloon sweep.

Future directions in palliative biliary stenting include potential endoscopic placement of drug-eluting stents to increase stent patency and deliver local therapy as well as radio frequency ablation of the tumor in-growth within the stents. Newer stents and instruments may allow quick and effective endoscopic choledocho-duodenostomy or hepatico-gastrostomy with expanding opportunity of endoscopic therapy for proximal biliary blockage from metastatic disease.

Surgical Options

Surgical options for biliary decompression include hepaticojejunostomy, choledo-chojejunostomy and cholecystojejunostomy. The choice of which type of surgical procedure to perform depends on the common bile duct diameter and surgeon's preference. The efficacy of surgical bypass in successfully decreasing hyperbilirubinemia has been estimated at up to 90% [23]. Even with this very effective technique, as the tumor progresses, the new anastomosis can become occluded as the malignancy progresses. For tumors in the head of the pancreas, a hepaticojejunostomy may be preferred because it will be anatomically more distant from the tumor.

Traditionally, a hepaticojejunostomy is created in an end-to-side or side-to-side anastomosis between the bile duct and Roux-en-Y loop of jejunum. An end-to-side anastomosis is easy to visualize and ensures a widely patent anastomosis but requires circumferential dissection around the bile duct. If this circumferential dissection is difficult due to tumor progression or lymphadenopathy, then a side-to-side anastomosis may be favorable. Knowledge of the vasculature to the bile duct is important during dissection to decrease ischemia, which may lead to leak or stenosis.

The Roux limb may be brought up to the hepatic hilum in an ante-colic or retro-colic fashion. Ideally, the roux limb should be distanced as much as possible from the primary tumor to decrease the future risk of roux limb occlusion if the tumor progresses. The anastomosis should be constructed with an absorbable suture to decrease the risk of stricture and stone formation. The choice of running vs interrupted suture will depend on the duct size and surgeon preference.

While this surgical bypass has been historically done in an open fashion, the increasing usage of minimally invasive surgery may decrease length of stay, wound infection rate and postoperative pain. The biliary anastomosis can be performed laparoscopic or robotically in high-volume centers with appropriate experience.

The risks of surgery include bleeding, biliary leak, and anastomotic stricture. In addition, the risks of general anesthesia are pertinent in patients who may have a poor performance status due to their advanced malignancy. These risks are critical for consideration when discussing options with the patient and treatment team.

Endoscopic Versus Surgical Intervention

Endoscopy is the more effective initial approach. Compared to surgical bypass, endoscopic biliary drainage has been shown to have a decreased length of stay, lower morbidity, lower mortality, and improved quality of life [24]. This can help initiate chemotherapy sooner since recovery from a major operation is not needed.

There are multiple factors which need to be considered when deciding on an optimal approach. The most obvious decision may be based on the technical feasibility of the technique. If there is a large bulky pancreatic malignancy that is extending into the hepatic hilum, a surgical bypass may not be technically possible due to the inability to safely access uninvolved hepatic ducts. Alternatively, if the patient has had previous gastric surgery, such as a Roux-en-Y gastric bypass, the ampulla and biliary system may not be approachable via traditional endoscopic approach. In this case, a surgical bypass may be the preferred approach.

Another technical consideration involves the extent of disease. In the setting of stage IV pancreatic adenocarcinoma with carcinomatosis and malignant ascites, a surgical approach to biliary bypass would be contraindicated due to the significant abdominal burden of disease.

Based on the invasive nature of surgery, this approach is associated with increased morbidity and mortality. However, compared to stenting, surgical bypass tends to last longer after the first intervention. As patients continue to live longer due to improved chemotherapy regimens, surgical bypass has the theoretical advantage of not requiring multiple re-interventions due to stent occlusion. But this has not been proven yet in randomized control trials.

Historically, patients who were brought to surgery for an oncologic resection but were found to be locally unresectable or with metastatic disease may have received a palliative biliary bypass. But this situation is becoming less frequent due to the increasing use of neoadjuvant chemotherapy, and often already having an endoscopically placed biliary stent already in place at the time of any surgery. When a patient already has an endoscopic drain in place, the benefits of performing a surgical bypass are unclear.

Duodenal Obstruction

The head, neck, and uncinate process of the pancreas are directly adjacent to all segments of the duodenum. For this reason, duodenal obstruction from either tumor invasion or extrinsic compression is common in locally advanced pancreatic cancer, leading to gastric outlet obstruction and symptoms of nausea, vomiting, dehydration, esophagitis, and oral intake intolerance. Despite not commonly being present on diagnosis, up to 20–40% of patients with pancreatic cancer will develop this cancer-related complication during their course [23].

Initial symptoms could be as mild as nausea, but progress to daily large volume vomiting. Imaging (plain films or CT) reveals a massively distended, fluid-filled stomach. Endoscopy plays an important role in management of this complication by helping establish diagnosis by visualization of retained food in the stomach and often the inability to pass the endoscope beyond the stomach or duodenum. It also offers different therapeutic options like placing enteric stents and/or a venting gastrostomy tube.

As was the case with biliary obstruction, medical management for advanced duodenal obstruction is ineffective, and complete NPO status may be mandatory for symptomatic control in this setting. However, gastric and salivary secretions continue, and even when patients have no oral intake, symptoms of obstruction will persist. Thus, concomitant upper intestinal decompression is often required, using a nasogastric tube to gravity or pump suction, or a venting (decompressive) gastrostomy tube (PEG).

In addition to being uncomfortable to the patient, a major disadvantage of nasogastric tube decompression is the unstable nature of the tube, which often is dislodged. For this reason, nasogastric tube gastric decompression is only used as a temporary solution or in patients in whom death is imminent.

Duodenal Stents

Over the past decade, duodenal stenting has evolved to become the most favored and most natural option for the management of duodenal obstruction in patients with unresectable pancreatic cancer. There have been many studies published evaluating the efficacy, feasibility, and safety of endoscopically deployed duodenal stents, all of which have shown a significant palliative benefit, a relatively low morbidity profile, decreased length of hospitalization, and significant overall cost reduction, especially when compared to surgical gastrojejunostomy [25–28]. In one study, the median survival time for patients with pancreatic cancer who underwent duodenal stent placement compared with those who underwent surgical gastrojejunostomy was 94 and 92 days, charges were $9921 and $28,173, and duration of hospitalization was 4 and 14 days, respectively (p value <0.005) [25]. The majority of the published experience with enteric stenting is derived from mostly small comparative studies and case series. A systematic review of 44 studies that looked at enteric stenting (1046 patients) versus gastrojejunostomy (297 patients) noted there were no significant differences between stent placement and gastrojejunostomy in regard to technical success (96% versus 100%, respectively), early complications (7% versus 6%) or late complications (18% versus 17%). Initial clinical success (i.e., symptomatic control) was higher after stent placement (89% versus 72%) although recurrent obstructive symptoms were more common after stent placement (18% versus 1%) [29].

After stent placement, the vast majority of patients will be able to tolerate soft solids or a full diet [30]. Despite initial rapid clinical success, anywhere from 15% to 40% of patients who receive enteric stenting for malignant obstruction will require re-intervention for recurrent symptoms of obstruction. In the only multicenter randomized controlled trial comparing enteral stenting to surgical gastrojejunostomy, the median duration of relief was 50 days for the stent group compared to 72 days for the surgical group [25]. The reasons for symptom recurrence included tumor in-growth into stent, stent migration, multifocal obstructions distal to duodenum, diffuse peritoneal carcinomatosis with bowel encasement, and functional gastroparesis due to tumor effect on regional neural networks (celiac axis). Thus, the endoscopic placement of self-expanding enteric stents for the palliation of gastric outlet obstruction in patients with unresectable pancreatic cancer is an effective intervention, with decreased length of hospitalization and overall costs as compared to surgery, although with a moderate re-intervention rate after 2 months. In-stent tumor growth can usually be managed by placement of additional stents through the original stent, and stent migration is a rare occurrence.

There are several FDA-approved dedicated duodenal stents commercially available in the United States, all of which are uncovered self-expandable metal stents (Figs. 29.3 and 29.4). The available diameters range from 20 to 22 mm, with length options including 6, 9, and 12 cm. The stents can be deployed through the accessory channel of a therapeutic endoscope or colonoscope and are deployed via a 10 Fr 160 cm or 225 cm long delivery system. Length of procedure varies highly, depending on the amount of difficulty the endoscopist encounters in trying to traverse the stricture, aspirate gastric contents, but an average of 1 h of endoscopy time should be allotted. Procedures should be done in rooms equipped with fluoroscopy and in the presence of skilled nurses trained in ERCP and advanced procedure skills. Stents can be deployed through the scope under direct visualization or via fluoroscopic guidance of catheter deployment over a guide wire.

In settings in which both biliary and enteric stenting is anticipated, biliary stent placement should be performed prior to enteral stenting, when possible, in order to increase the odds of technical success in biliary cannulation. Occasionally, duodenal stents may be placed prior to ERCP to facilitate passage of ERCP scope and biliary stent placement. In such a situation, biliary cannulation may be facilitated by EUS-guided antegrade passage of guide wire for cannulation.

Risks of enteral stenting for malignancy-induced gastroduodenal obstructions include bleeding, perforation, and distal stent migration, in addition to stent obstruction, which is mainly due to tumor infiltration. A systematic review of 606 patients in whom an enteral stent was placed revealed severe complications (bleeding and perforation) in 1.2% of cases and stent migration in 5%. Stent obstruction occurred

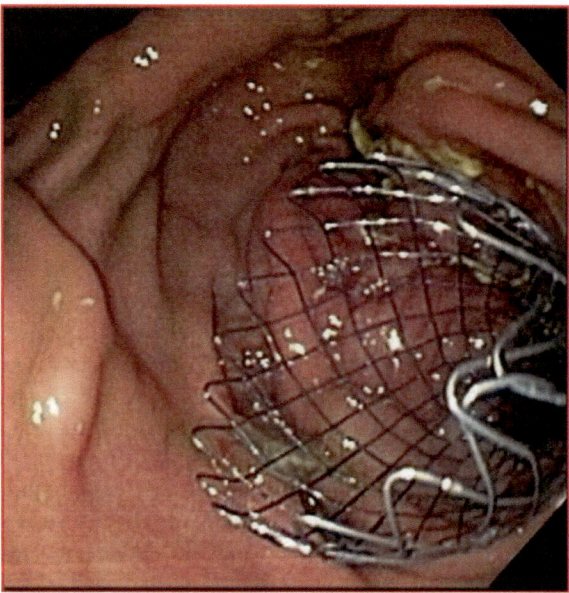

Fig. 29.3 Endoscopic view of a fully deployed fully uncovered metal duodenal stent

Fig. 29.4 Fluoroscopic image of a metal duodenal stent with central wasting in region of tumor

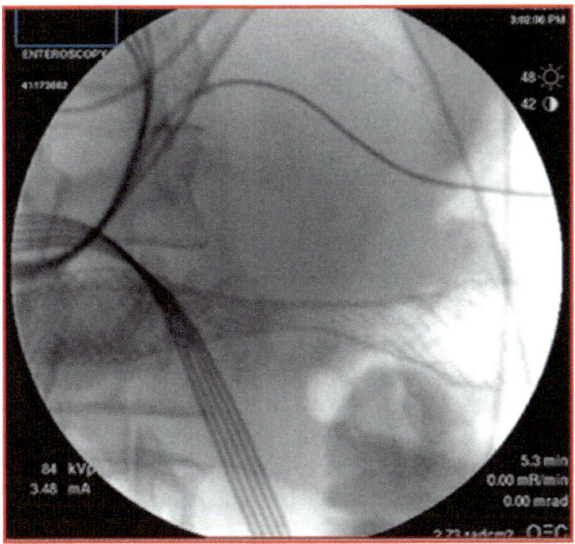

in 18% of cases. There was 0% case-related mortality. Mean survival period was 12.1 weeks [31]. With improved devices and equipment, these complications are likely to be even fewer in number.

A newer option has emerged with endoscopic ultrasonography-guided gastroenterostomy. Not all centers have the equipment or expertise, but this endoscopic gastrojejunostomy is gaining traction. An international multicenter randomized controlled trial (NCT03823690) from 2023 showed in patients with malignant gastric outlet obstruction, endoscopic ultrasonography-guided gastroenterostomy can reduce the frequency of re-intervention, improve stent patency, and result in better patient-reported eating habits compared with duodenal stenting, and the procedure should be used preferentially over duodenal stenting when expertise and required devices are available [32].

Venting Percutaneous Gastrostomy Tubes (PEG)

Decompressive PEG tubes can be placed endoscopically, percutaneously via fluoroscopy or surgically, and allow for a more stable access route to the stomach [33]. The access port can then be used for intermittent decompression throughout the day, usually to gravity, and can remain clamped when asymptomatic. Decompressive PEG tubes have been used with good efficacy and relatively low complication rate for malignant gastric outlet obstructions although the majority of the published studies are from gynecologic malignancies [34]. One study that did look at the effect of venting PEG tubes for decompression of outlet obstruction from gastrointestinal malignancies, including pancreatic cancer, showed a technical and clinical success rate of 89% (41 of 46 patients) and tube utilization duration on average of 60 ± 91 days. In addition, 88% of patients were able to remain on a liquid and soft food diet [35]. The authors use a special fenestrated 24 Fr tube to maximize drainage, which is not currently commercially available.

If the degree of outlet obstruction permits, a gastrojejunal tube (GJ tube or PEG-J tube) can be placed via the PEG site, in which there is jejunal access for feeding, and a separate intragastric portion which can be used for decompression.

Thus, a combination of medical management with anti-nausea and anti-secretory therapies combined with a decompressive PEG tube is a management option for patients needing palliation for pancreatic cancer-related gastric outlet obstruction, despite a lack of published literature on the matter. This approach results in an externally positioned tube over the patient's abdomen, and severely limits the patient's ability to tolerate a normal diet. There are also risks involved in PEG placement such as bleeding, infection, perforation, and is not always technically possible. In patients with carcinomatosis with malignant ascites, this is a relative contraindication to PEG placement.

Surgical Gastrojejunostomy (Duodenal Bypass)

Patients may have symptomatic duodenal obstruction at presentation or may develop an obstruction while on treatment due to tumor progression from an advanced pancreatic malignancy. For these patients, surgical bypass with a gastrojejunostomy should be considered. Most experts advocate for a loop side-to-side gastrojejunostomy. The anastomosis can be done either hand-sewn or stapled anastomosis, with neither showing any clear superiority. Care must be taken to not cause angulation of the outflow limb of the jejunum or narrowing the anastomosis during the construction.

Even after surgical bypass, there can be significant delayed gastric emptying. Therefore, we recommend an isoperistaltic, retro-colic, and retrogastric anastomosis to decrease this risk [36]. Typically, a loop of jejunum approximately 30–40 cm distal to the ligament of Treitz is brought up through a defect in the transverse mesocolon. The posterior wall of the stomach is exposed, and an anastomosis is created to the posterior wall, near the greater curve. This can be done in an open, laparoscopic or robotic fashion (Fig. 29.5). The benefits of minimally invasive surgery include decreased length of stay and postoperative pain.

In patients who do not have a symptomatic duodenal obstruction, there is controversy around prophylactic surgical bypass. Prophylactic gastrojejunostomy is sometimes done during an attempted oncologic surgery if the patient is found to have unresectable disease, in order to prevent impending (or treat) duodenal obstruction [23]. A meta-analysis of several prospective studies evaluated the benefit of prophylactic surgical gastrojejunostomy plus biliodigestive anastomosis versus no bypass or biliary anastomosis alone. In the prophylactic gastrojejunostomy group, the risk of developing gastric outlet obstruction during follow-up was significantly

Fig. 29.5 Laparoscopic gastrojejunostomy. Retro-colic and retrogastric anastomosis

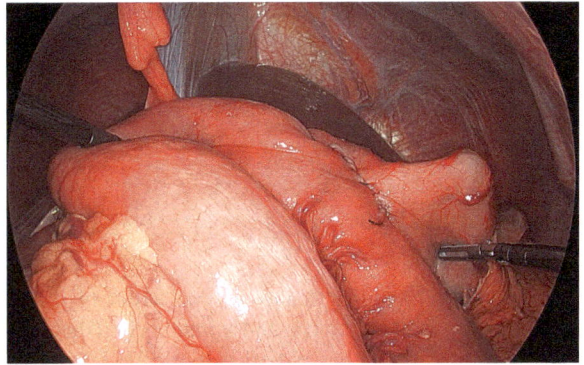

lower than the group without surgical bypass (odds ratio [OR] 0.06, 95% confidence interval 0.02–0.21; $p < 0.001$) and mortality rates were similar for both groups [37]. For this reason, many surgeons advocate prophylactic gastrojejunostomy for prevention of gastric outlet obstruction in patients in whom exploratory laparotomy reveals unresectable disease.

There are critics to this approach, who question the true benefit of prophylactic surgery in these patients, citing the high rate of delayed gastric emptying postoperatively (up to 50% of patients in one study) [38], the increased length of hospitalization [31], as well as the fact that a large portion of patients with pancreatic cancer will not develop outlet obstruction until the terminal weeks of their disease [39]. A single-center study examined a group of 155 consecutive patients who underwent laparoscopic staging for pancreatic adenocarcinoma, and the presence of subsequent surgical bypass was documented after a mean follow-up length of 5.9 months. During this follow-up period, 81% of patients died from their disease (125 patients). Only three patients (2%) required a subsequent gastrojejunostomy for outlet obstruction [40]. The authors of that study advocated against the use of prophylactic gastrojejunostomy as a routine practice, but rather, to be used in the setting of documented obstruction.

Endoscopic Versus Surgical Intervention

The decision regarding ideal intervention for patients with advanced malignancy causing duodenal obstruction must be personalized for each patient. A multidisciplinary discussion, including the patient's wishes, is critical. Some patients may want to avoid surgery and associated morbidity at all costs.

There may be technical aspects that are contraindications for surgery. For example, significant carcinomatosis or malignant ascites increase the morbidity of surgical bypass. Specifically, there is an increased risk of anastomotic failure leading to life-threatening gastric leak. Additionally, the anastomosis may not be technically possible because of tumor involvement on the surface of the stomach or bowel.

Conversely, because of the higher long-term patency rates, for patients in whom survival is expected to extend beyond 6–9 months, surgical bypass may be a more appropriate consideration. This would prevent repeat endoscopic interventions associated with duodenal stenting.

Abdominal Pain

Abdominal pain can be a significant feature of patients with unresectable locally advanced pancreatic cancer and a major contributor to decreased quality of life in these patients. The celiac plexus is located below and anterior to the diaphragm and surrounds the origin of the celiac trunk and is responsible for transmitting the sensation of pain for the pancreas. Pain in pancreatic cancer comes from nociceptive stimulation of the nerves that supply the pancreas, which in turn transmit this pain signal to the celiac plexus and from there travel to the thalamus and cortex of the brain, ending in the perception of pain [41].

Management of malignancy-related pain in pancreatic cancer can be achieved via tumor therapy with chemotherapy and radiation therapy, with medical therapy (narcotic pain medications), or with nerve blocks (i.e., celiac plexus neurolysis (CPN), celiac ganglia blocks). CPN may be achieved via percutaneous, surgical, or endoscopic means [42]. It is important to note that medical management of pancreatic cancer-induced pain using narcotics is highly effective. Non-opioid analgesics, on the other hand, are rarely capable of controlling patients' symptoms [43]. The use of narcotics is sometimes associated with several side-effects, such as constipation and nausea, which in turn require symptomatic control with additional medications. Co-management of terminal pancreatic cancer patients with a Pain Management specialist or Palliative Service specialist, where opioid analgesics are given in an effective and satisfactory manner and potential side-effects are managed appropriately. This approach tends to increase the yield of noninvasive management of cancer-related pain even further.

Celiac Plexus Neurolysis

CPN involves the direct injection of ethanol into the area of the celiac plexus and can be done via Endoscopic Ultrasound (EUS) or via percutaneous injection, often with image guidance, such as Computer Tomography (CT). EUS has the theoretical advantage of augmenting needle localization and spread of the ethanol injectate. There have been no large trials that have directly compared EUS-guided CPN to percutaneous CPN in order to reliably compare differences in efficacy and safety profile. However, in the setting of palliation of pancreatic cancer pain, it does appear that EUS-guided CPN is a safe and effective option, although infrequently needed with current oncologic management.

There have been multiple small trials evaluating the efficacy of EUS-guided CPN in patients with pancreatic cancer. Two meta-analyses noted the percentage of patients with pain relief between 73% and 80% [44, 45]. There were no randomized placebo-controlled trials among the studies evaluated, and pain relief was often objectively quantified using visual pain analogs and amount of narcotic use. One study looked at patients' pain scores at 2, 4, 8, and 12 weeks after EUS CPN compared to baseline, and noted that at each follow-up time point, 82–91% of patients required the same or less pain medication and 79–88% of patients had persistent improvement in their pain score [46]. Another prospective study followed patients for up to 6 months after EUS CPN and noted a sustained effect of decreased pain scores for up to a median of 24 weeks [47]. In all studies, no patients reported complete resolution of pain, and no patients were able to completely discontinue systemic narcotics.

Early use of CPN has been associated with an improved response rate, with the theory that as cancer progresses, the etiology of the pain becomes more multifactorial and less responsive to loco-regional therapies, such as CPN [48]. In a randomized double-blind controlled trial comparing early EUS-guided CPN (done at the time of staging EUS) to standard narcotic therapy in 96 patients (48 per study arm), pain relief scores were greater at 3 months in the CPN arm, whereas Quality of Life, survival, and morphine consumption were not statistical significant between the two groups. Other factors that may predict a poor response to EUS-guided CPN include direct invasion of cancer into the celiac plexus and unilateral injection of ethanol [49].

In the future, as more advances are made in the understanding of pain pathophysiology and newer management tools (narcotics, spinal stimulators), endoscopy might not play a significant role.

Serious complications with EUS-guided CPN are rare and include asymptomatic hypotension, severe self-limited post-procedural pain, and retroperitoneal abscess. The incidence of these complications is low, with one series of 230 EUS-guided CPN or CPB showing an overall complication rate of 1.8% (1 patient developed retroperitoneal abscess, 1 patient developed hypotension, and 2 patients developed pain) [50].

Transient diarrhea, lasting usually up to 7 days, is common after EUS CPN, occurring in up to 44% of patients, and reflects the sympathetic blockade that can occur after injection [50]. This same sympathetic blockade is responsible for the transient orthostatic hypotension that can occur. There does not seem to be any reports of cardiac arrhythmias after CPN.

Surgical Celiac Plexus Block

In patients who are already in the operating room for surgical palliation of biliary or duodenal obstruction, the option of a surgical celiac plexus block is also available. The technique can be performed in a minimally invasive or open surgery. In laparoscopic or robotic surgery, the use of an ultrasound probe can assist in finding the origin of the celiac axis along the aorta. Then using this imaging guidance, the celiac plexus can be injected with 50% ethanol. Typically, bilateral injections along the aorta, near the celiac origin are needed. Access to this area can be achieved by opening the gastrohepatic ligament and following the left gastric artery down to the celiac axis.

In open surgery, palpation of the aorta and celiac origin are useful to guide the injection. The surgeon uses their non-dominant hand to palpate the aorta and holds it stable while injecting. Typically, neurolysis is similarly performed with injection of 50% ethanol. This can be injected into the retroperitoneum to the right and left sides of the aorta. While the risks are low, they do include bleeding, paraplegia, and anterior spinal syndrome [51].

With the increasing expertise of interventional gastroenterology, EUS-guided celiac neurolysis has replaced surgical block in most institutions.

Summary

As patients with pancreatic cancer live longer with improved oncologic therapy, there are increasing numbers of patients with unresectable disease who develop complications of biliary obstruction, duodenal obstruction and pain. Palliative procedures for pancreatic cancer are continuing to develop and the options for endoscopic and surgical palliation are improving. There are several safe, effective, and beneficial options for patients. A multidisciplinary discussion with surgeons, interventional gastroenterology, interventional radiology, medical oncology, radiation oncology, and the patient are critical to deciding which intervention will provide the best palliation for these patients.

References

1. Howlader N, Noone A, Krapcho M, Neyman N, Aminou R, Waldron W, et al. SEER cancer statistics review, 1975–2008. Bethesda, MD: National Cancer Institute; 2010.
2. Schmidt CM, Powell ES, Yiannoutsos CT, Howard TJ, Wiebke EA, Wiesenauer CA, et al. Pancreaticoduodenectomy: a 20-year experience in 516 patients. Arch Surg. 2004;139(7):718–25; discussion 725–7.
3. Sarr MG, Cameron JL. Surgical palliation of unresectable carcinoma of the pancreas. World J Surg. 1984;8(6):906–18.
4. Bergasa NV. Medical palliation of the jaundiced patient with pruritus. Gastroenterol Clin N Am. 2006;35(1):113–23.
5. Speer AG, Cotton PB, Russell RC, Mason RR, Hatfield AR, Leung JW, et al. Randomised trial of endoscopic versus percutaneous stent insertion in malignant obstructive jaundice. Lancet. 1987;2(8550):57–62.

6. Saluja SS, Gulati M, Garg PK, Pal H, Pal S, Sahni P, et al. Endoscopic or percutaneous biliary drainage for gallbladder cancer: a randomized trial and quality of life assessment. Clin Gastroenterol Hepatol. 2008;6(8):944–950.e3.
7. Pinol V, Castells A, Bordas JM, Real MI, Llach J, Montana X, et al. Percutaneous self-expanding metal stents versus endoscopic polyethylene endoprostheses for treating malignant biliary obstruction: randomized clinical trial. Radiology. 2002;225(1):27–34.
8. Levy MJ, Baron TH, Gostout CJ, Petersen BT, Farnell MB. Palliation of malignant extra-hepatic biliary obstruction with plastic versus expandable metal stents: an evidence-based approach. Clin Gastroenterol Hepatol. 2004;2(4):273–85.
9. Kadakia SC, Starnes E. Comparison of 10 French gauge stent with 11.5 French gauge stent in patients with biliary tract diseases. Gastrointest Endosc. 1992;38(4):454–9.
10. Moss AC, Morris E, Leyden J, MacMathuna P. Malignant distal biliary obstruction: a systematic review and meta-analysis of endoscopic and surgical bypass results. Cancer Treat Rev. 2007;33(2):213–21.
11. Chen VK, Arguedas MR, Baron TH. Expandable metal biliary stents before pancreaticoduodenectomy for pancreatic cancer: a Monte-Carlo decision analysis. Clin Gastroenterol Hepatol. 2005;3(12):1229–37.
12. Yoon WJ, Lee JK, Lee KH, Lee WJ, Ryu JK, Kim YT, et al. A comparison of covered and uncovered Wallstents for the management of distal malignant biliary obstruction. Gastrointest Endosc. 2006;63(7):996–1000.
13. do Park H, Kim MH, Choi JS, Lee SS, Seo DW, Kim JH, et al. Covered versus uncovered wallstent for malignant extrahepatic biliary obstruction: a cohort comparative analysis. Clin Gastroenterol Hepatol. 2006;4(6):790–6.
14. Telford JJ, Carr-Locke DL, Baron TH, Poneros JM, Bounds BC, Kelsey PB, et al. A randomized trial comparing uncovered and partially covered self-expandable metal stents in the palliation of distal malignant biliary obstruction. Gastrointest Endosc. 2010;72(5):907–14.
15. Kullman E, Frozanpor F, Soderlund C, Linder S, Sandstrom P, Lindhoff-Larsson A, et al. Covered versus uncovered self-expandable nitinol stents in the palliative treatment of malignant distal biliary obstruction: results from a randomized, multicenter study. Gastrointest Endosc. 2010;72(5):915–23.
16. Saleem A, Leggett CL, Murad MH, Baron TH. Meta-analysis of randomized trials comparing the patency of covered and uncovered self-expandable metal stents for palliation of distal malignant bile duct obstruction. Gastrointest Endosc. 2011;74(2):321–327.e1–3.
17. Shami VM, Kahaleh M. Endoscopic ultrasound-guided cholangiopancreatography and rendezvous techniques. Dig Liver Dis. 2010;42(6):419–24.
18. Maranki J, Hernandez AJ, Arslan B, Jaffan AA, Angle JF, Shami VM, et al. Interventional endoscopic ultrasound-guided cholangiography: long-term experience of an emerging alternative to percutaneous transhepatic cholangiography. Endoscopy. 2009;41(6):532–8.
19. Shah JN, Marson F, Weilert F, Bhat YM, Nguyen-Tang T, Shaw RE, et al. Single-operator, single-session EUS-guided anterograde cholangiopancreatography in failed ERCP or inaccessible papilla. Gastrointest Endosc. 2012;75(1):56–64.
20. Gupta K, Mallery S, Hunter D, Freeman ML. Endoscopic ultrasound and percutaneous access for endoscopic biliary and pancreatic drainage after initially failed ERCP. Rev Gastroenterol Disord. 2007;7(1):22–37.
21. Buxbaum JL, Biggins SW, Bagatelos KC, Inadomi JM, Ostroff JW. Inoperable pancreatic cancer patients who have prolonged survival exhibit an increased risk of cholangitis. JOP. 2011;12(4):377–83.
22. Pola S, Muralimohan R, Cohen B, Fehmi S, Savides T. Cholangitis is common in cancer survivors with metal biliary stents. Gastrointest Endosc. 2011;73(4 Suppl):AB360.
23. Singh SM, Longmire WP Jr, Reber HA. Surgical palliation for pancreatic cancer. The UCLA experience. Ann Surg. 1990;212(2):132–9.
24. Smith AC, Dowsett JP, Rusell RC, et al. Randomized trial of endoscopic stenting versus surgical bypass in malignant low bile duct obstruction. Lancet. 1994;344:1655–60.

25. Yim HB, Jacobson BC, Saltzman JR, Johannes RS, Bounds BC, Lee JH, et al. Clinical outcome of the use of enteral stents for palliation of patients with malignant upper GI obstruction. Gastrointest Endosc. 2001;53(3):329–32.
26. Holt AP, Patel M, Ahmed MM. Palliation of patients with malignant gastroduodenal obstruction with self-expanding metallic stents: the treatment of choice? Gastrointest Endosc. 2004;60(6):1010–7.
27. Mosler P, Mergener KD, Brandabur JJ, Schembre DB, Kozarek RA. Palliation of gastric outlet obstruction and proximal small bowel obstruction with self-expandable metal stents: a single center series. J Clin Gastroenterol. 2005;39(2):124–8.
28. Adler DG, Baron TH. Endoscopic palliation of malignant gastric outlet obstruction using self-expanding metal stents: experience in 36 patients. Am J Gastroenterol. 2002;97(1):72–8.
29. Jeurnink SM, van Eijck CH, Steyerberg EW, Kuipers EJ, Siersema PD. Stent versus gastrojejunostomy for the palliation of gastric outlet obstruction: a systematic review. BMC Gastroenterol. 2007;7:18.
30. Dormann A, Meisner S, Verin N, Wenk Lang A. Self-expanding metal stents for gastroduodenal malignancies: systematic review of their clinical effectiveness. Endoscopy. 2004;36(6):543–50.
31. de Rooij PD, Rogatko A, Brennan MF. Evaluation of palliative surgical procedures in unresectable pancreatic cancer. Br J Surg. 1991;78(9):1053–8.
32. Teoh AYB, Lakhtakia S, Tarantino I, Perez-Miranda M, Kunda R, Maluf-Filho F, Dhir V, Basha J, Chan SM, Ligresti D, Ma MTW, de la Serna-Higuera C, Yip HC, Ng EKW, Chiu PWY, Itoi T. Endoscopic ultrasonography-guided gastroenterostomy versus uncovered duodenal metal stenting for unresectable malignant gastric outlet obstruction (DRA-GOO): a multicentre randomised controlled trial. Lancet Gastroenterol Hepatol. 2023. pii: S2468-1253(23)00242-X; https://doi.org/10.1016/S2468-1253(23)00242-X.
33. Itkin M, DeLegge MH, Fang JC, McClave SA, Kundu S, d'Othee BJ, et al. Multidisciplinary practical guidelines for gastrointestinal access for enteral nutrition and decompression from the Society of Interventional Radiology and American Gastroenterological Association (AGA) Institute, with endorsement by Canadian Interventional Radiological Association (CIRA) and Cardiovascular and Interventional Radiological Society of Europe (CIRSE). Gastroenterology. 2011;141(2):742–65.
34. Marks WH, Perkal MF, Schwartz PE. Percutaneous endoscopic gastrostomy for gastric decompression in metastatic gynecologic malignancies. Surg Gynecol Obstet. 1993;177(6):573–6.
35. Herman LL, Hoskins WJ, Shike M. Percutaneous endoscopic gastrostomy for decompression of the stomach and small bowel. Gastrointest Endosc. 1992;38(3):314–8.
36. Sohn TA, Lillemoe KD, Cameron JL, et al. Surgical palliation of unresectable periampullary adenocarcinoma in the 1990s. J Am Coll Surg. 1999;188:658–66.
37. Huser N, Michalski CW, Schuster T, Friess H, Kleeff J. Systematic review and meta-analysis of prophylactic gastroenterostomy for unresectable advanced pancreatic cancer. Br J Surg. 2009;96(7):711–9.
38. Doberneck RC, Berndt GA. Delayed gastric emptying after palliative gastrojejunostomy for carcinoma of the pancreas. Arch Surg. 1987;122(7):827–9.
39. Weaver DW, Wiencek RG, Bouwman DL, Walt AJ. Gastrojejunostomy: is it helpful for patients with pancreatic cancer? Surgery. 1987;102(4):608–13.
40. Espat NJ, Brennan MF, Conlon KC. Patients with laparoscopically staged unresectable pancreatic adenocarcinoma do not require subsequent surgical biliary or gastric bypass. J Am Coll Surg. 1999;188(6):649–55; discussion 655–7.
41. Nagakawa T, Mori K, Nakano T, Kadoya M, Kobayashi H, Akiyama T, et al. Perineural invasion of carcinoma of the pancreas and biliary tract. Br J Surg. 1993;80(5):619–21.
42. Wang PJ, Shang MY, Qian Z, Shao CW, Wang JH, Zhao XH. CT-guided percutaneous neurolytic celiac plexus block technique. Abdom Imaging. 2006;31(6):710–8.
43. Nabal M, Librada S, Redondo MJ, Pigni A, Brunelli C, Caraceni A. The role of paracetamol and nonsteroidal anti-inflammatory drugs in addition to WHO Step III opioids in the control of pain in advanced cancer. A systematic review of the literature. Palliat Med. 2011;26:305.

44. Kaufman M, Singh G, Das S, Concha-Parra R, Erber J, Micames C, et al. Efficacy of endo-scopic ultrasound-guided celiac plexus block and celiac plexus neurolysis for managing abdominal pain associated with chronic pancreatitis and pancreatic cancer. J Clin Gastroenterol. 2010;44(2):127–34.

45. Puli SR, Reddy JB, Bechtold ML, Antillon MR, Brugge WR. EUS-guided celiac plexus neu-rolysis for pain due to chronic pancreatitis or pancreatic cancer pain: a meta-analysis and systematic review. Dig Dis Sci. 2009;54(11):2330–7.

46. Harada N, Wiersema MJ, Wiersema LM. Endosonography-guided celiac plexus neurolysis. Gastrointest Endosc Clin N Am. 1997;7(2):237–45.

47. Gunaratnam NT, Sarma AV, Norton ID, Wiersema MJ. A prospective study of EUS-guided celiac plexus neurolysis for pancreatic cancer pain. Gastrointest Endosc. 2001;54(3):316–24.

48. Wyse JM, Carone M, Paquin SC, Usatii M, Sahai AV. Randomized, double-blind, controlled trial of early endoscopic ultrasound-guided celiac plexus neurolysis to prevent pain progres-sion in patients with newly diagnosed, painful, inoperable pancreatic cancer. J Clin Oncol. 2011;29(26):3541–6.

49. Iwata K, Yasuda I, Enya M, Mukai T, Nakashima M, Doi S, et al. Predictive factors for pain relief after endoscopic ultrasound-guided celiac plexus neurolysis. Dig Endosc. 2011;23(2):140–5.

50. Eisenberg E, Carr DB, Chalmers TC. Neurolytic celiac plexus block for treatment of cancer pain: a meta-analysis. Anesth Analg. 1995;80(2):290–5.

51. Davies DD. Incidence of major complications of neurolytic coeliac plexus block. J R Soc Med. 1993;86:264–6.

Part VII
Perioperative Considerations—
Perioperative Management

Chapter 30
Preoperative Risk Stratification to Prehabilitation

Maximiliano Servin-Rojas and Motaz Qadan

An Introduction to Prehabilitation in Pancreatic Cancer

Prehabilitation refers to the optimization of patients' functional capacity before surgery [1]. A study published in 1946 in the *British Medical Journal* appears to be the first in the medical literature to adopt this term [2]. In this study, the British Army reported encouraging results after providing young military recruits with a better diet, hygiene, recreational activities, and physical training to prepare them for war. While the program was initially directed at improved physical fitness, the results of the intervention transcended beyond physical conditioning to include cognitive benefits. In the same way, prehabilitation in medicine intends to prepare patients to endure an assault with a physiological stressor, such as a major operation. It was not until the early 2000s that prehabilitation was formally introduced as an intervention to improve outcomes in surgical patients [3]. Current evidence suggests that prehabilitation is associated with decreased length of stay, postoperative pain, and postoperative complications. The benefit of prehabilitation is thought to be predominantly related to cardiorespiratory fitness, which has been identified as an independent predictor of surgical complications [4, 5]. Cardiorespiratory aerobic training leads to increased cardiac output, increased arteriovenous oxygen difference, and ultimately, increased maximal oxygen consumption [1]. The increased functional capacity is believed to facilitate the adaptation toward increased energy and oxygen expenditure during the postoperative period.

M. Servin-Rojas
Department of Surgery, Massachusetts General Hospital, Boston, MA, USA

M. Qadan (✉)
Division of Surgical Oncology, Department of Surgery, Massachusetts General Hospital, Boston, MA, USA
e-mail: mqadan@mgh.harvard.edu

The management of pancreatic cancer has become increasingly complex over the last decades. To achieve prolonged survival rates, patients must undergo multimodal treatment, composed of a combination of systemic therapy, provided as neoadjuvant, adjuvant, or perioperative therapy, radiation therapy, and surgical resection [6]. Furthermore, complete aggressive therapy requires patients to have an adequate functional capacity, which is often complicated given that nearly half of the patients with pancreatic cancer have cachexia, loss of appetite, fatigue, and deconditioning as a result of their disease at the time of presentation [7]. The chemotherapeutic regimens and surgery can further deteriorate patient's functional and physical capacity, further jeopardizing their opportunities to complete multimodal treatment, undergo operative intervention, and recover from any treatment toxicities and complications, thereby compromising quality of life, oncologic outcomes, and, ultimately, survival [8, 9]. Given the recent increase in the utilization of neoadjuvant therapy, including total neoadjuvant therapy, in the management of borderline resectable and locally advanced pancreatic cancer, in addition to upfront resectable disease, it is these authors' view that a unique window of opportunity exists during neoadjuvant therapy to improve patients' physical and mental fitness through prehabilitation prior to arrival to surgery. In this chapter, we will review existing tools for risk stratification and different prehabilitation strategies that multidisciplinary teams can employ to manage patients with pancreatic cancer.

Patient Risk Stratification

The first step in managing pancreatic cancer patients includes a thorough history and physical examination. During the initial visit, patients should be screened for risk factors that could place them at higher risk of postoperative complications, such as cardiorespiratory fitness and exercise tolerance, nutritional status, alcohol and illicit substance consumption, cigarette smoking, and psychological status. After the initial screening, an objective evaluation is necessary to best determine baseline functional status. These steps are crucial to tailor interventions according to patients' individual risk status. Table 30.1 summarizes the available screening and assessment tools.

Risk Screening and Assessment Tools

Before carrying out a more in-depth objective assessment, utilizing a surgical risk calculator is a reasonable first step in screening patients who might require a more detailed evaluation and preoperative attention. These tools are readily available and easy to utilize. Many multidisciplinary prehabilitation teams employ the American College of Surgeons National Surgical Quality Improvement Program (ACS

Table 30.1 Preoperative risk factors and screening/assessment tools

	Cardiorespiratory	Nutrition	Smoking	Alcohol	Psychological
Screening	Weekly physical activity: • 150 minutes of moderate intensity, aerobic physical activity • 75 minutes of vigorous intensity, aerobic physical activity • Two muscle-strengthening exercises per week	Preoperative Nutrition Score (PONS)	Inquire about current smoking habits	Inquire about weekly alcohol consumption. Over 14 units[a] per week is considered hazardous	Screening for illness behavior questionnaire (SIBQ)[b] Perceived stress scale
Assessment	Suspected low cardiorespiratory function: Cardiopulmonary exercise testing (CPET) Low-risk patients or CPET not available: Non-exercise prediction models (e.g., Jackson equation [21]), 6-min walking test	Subjective Global Assessment (SGA) or patient-generated SGA[c]	Fagerström test for nicotine dependence	Alcohol use disorders identification test (AUDIT)	Computerized adaptive test-mental health (CAT-MH)[b]

[a] One unit is equivalent to 10 mL or 8 g of pure alcohol
[b] Has not been validated for surgical patients
[c] Training required for application and interpretation

NSQIP) risk calculator as part of the initial consultation. The ACS NSQIP risk calculator is a web-based tool that estimates the risk of postoperative complications based on patient demographics, comorbidities, and surgery-specific factors [10]. Studies have shown that this calculator reliably predicts short-term postoperative complications after hepatopancreatobiliary surgery [11, 12].

Poor cardiorespiratory fitness is an adverse predictor of postoperative complications and all-cause mortality [13]. Habitual physical activity can be considered a surrogate marker for cardiorespiratory fitness [14]. Thus, a reasonable screening approach is to inquire about weekly physical activity. Adult patients are recommended to perform at least 150 min of moderate or 75 min of weekly vigorous intensity, aerobic physical activity and at least two muscle-strengthening exercises per week [15]. Patients who fail to fulfill these criteria should be strongly encouraged to increase their weekly physical activity. Cardiopulmonary exercise with ventilatory expired gas analysis is the most accurate way of assessing cardiorespiratory fitness. However, it is complex, resource-intensive, and not widely available [16]. Cardiorespiratory fitness can be estimated from clinical variables using non-exercise-based equations [17]. Other less resource-intensive ways to measure cardiorespiratory fitness include the 400-m 6-min walking test. Studies have demonstrated an association between increased postoperative complications and inability to complete the 6-min walk distance test [18, 19]. Patients suspected of having low baseline cardiorespiratory fitness levels should be strongly considered for cardiorespiratory exercise testing, as calculations tend to overestimate cardiorespiratory fitness in these patients [16].

Malnutrition is common among patients with pancreatic cancer due to the metabolic dysregulations caused by inflammatory cytokine production, exocrine dysfunction, biliary obstruction, and mass effect on the stomach resulting in early satiety [20]. Weight loss is a near universal symptom among these patients [21]. Several studies have demonstrated the association between malnutrition and increased postoperative morbidity and mortality [7, 20, 22, 23]. Early recognition of malnutrition is critical to optimize outcomes and improve quality of life. Out of the several screening tools that have been described and validated [24–28], only the Preoperative Nutrition Score (PONS) was specifically developed for surgical patients [28]. Patients can be further assessed with the subjective global assessment (SGA) or the patient-generated SGA [29, 30]. Assessment by a nutritionist as part of the initial multidisciplinary consultation is preferred, as these tools can be challenging to utilize and interpret. Body composition measurements derived from CT scans can be utilized as other surrogate markers of nutritional status [31, 32]. Studies have shown that both muscle mass and quality have been associated with improved outcomes in patients with pancreatic cancer. On the other hand, obesity and sarcopenia have been associated with worse prognosis [31]. Therefore, imaging can play a significant role in identifying patients who may benefit from nutritional or exercise interventions to improve postoperative outcomes.

Alcohol consumption and tobacco smoking have been consistently associated with an increased risk of postoperative wound infection, pneumonia, readmission, and death [33–36]. In particular, smoking has been associated with a higher incidence of postoperative pancreatic fistula [37]. Patients should be interviewed about their smoking and drinking habits during the initial consultation. At least 4 weeks of cessation are typically recommended and required prior to surgery to decrease postoperative complications associated with smoking [38, 39]. With respect to alcohol, patients who consume greater than 14 units per week should undergo further assessment using the alcohol use disorders identification test (AUDIT) [40, 41]. Nicotine dependence can be objectively assessed using the Fagerström Test for Nicotine Dependence [42].

While highly heterogeneous, evidence linking postoperative outcomes to patients' psychological status is emerging [43]. To date, no validated screening or assessment tools have been developed specifically for surgical patients. The perceived stress scale (PSS) can be utilized to identify patients who might be good candidates for mindfulness practices [44]. The screening for illness behavior questionnaire (SIBQ) was recently evaluated in a study evaluating postoperative complications in general surgery patients [45]. The authors found a significant correlation between screening scores and persistent postoperative pain. An assessment tool is currently being developed for surgical patients. While results from the pilot study are promising, the tool requires further testing prior to incorporation into clinical practice [46].

Frailty Assessment

Frailty is a clinical syndrome in which patients are at increased risk of developing adverse outcomes, dependence, and mortality [47, 48]. More than half of the patients with pancreatic cancer are diagnosed after age 60, putting them at some risk for frailty [49]. In fact, it is estimated that this clinical syndrome afflicts nearly 40% of patients with hepatobiliary and pancreatic malignancies [50]. Studies reported an increased risk of postoperative complications and death in frail patients undergoing pancreatoduodenectomy [51, 52]. In addition, frailty is an independent predictor of cancer-specific mortality in PDAC [53]. The deleterious effects of frailty along with advancing age render patients with pancreatic malignancies who are ideal candidates for prehabilitation. Interim results from a non-randomized clinical trial suggest that prehabilitation may improve the frail phenotype and protect patients from chemotherapy-associated physiologic deterioration [54]. Thus, early recognition of frailty is paramount to counter its deleterious effects through mitigation measures, such as prehabilitation.

Most frailty assessment tools are based on two major concepts [55]. The first concept is biologic, what has been described as the frail phenotype by Fried and colleagues [56]. The phenotype is distinguished by weight loss, sarcopenia, weakness, slowness, and reduced physical activity. Rookwood and colleagues defined the second concept as an accumulation of deficits in the functional, cognitive, social, and physical spheres [57]. Out of the wide variety of frailty assessment tools utilized in the surgical literature, the risk analysis index (RAI-C) has been validated in the hepatobiliary and pancreatic field [11, 58]. Besides predicting short-term postoperative outcomes, RAI-C was also designed to identify patients who might benefit from prehabilitation [11]. While RAI-C does not measure physical status, and there is criticism about inclusion of physical status in accurately determining frailty, recent evidence suggests that physical status strongly correlates with frailty scores [59]. Furthermore, it is neither resource-intensive nor cost-intensive, making it easy to implement [55]. Some of the most commonly utilized frailty assessment tools are summarized in Table 30.2.

Table 30.2 Frailty assessment tools

Assessment tool	Items	Scoring
Rockwood's Brief Frailty Instrument [57]	Dependency on mobility and daily activities Continence Cognition	Four levels (0–3); increasing frailty with higher scores
Fried's Physical Frailty Phenotype [56]	Weight loss/sarcopenia Weakness Exhaustion Slowness Low activity	One or two criteria: pre-frail Three or more criteria: frail
Risk Analysis Index (RAI-C)	Items divided into four compartments: A. Age, sex, and cancer B. Medical comorbidities C. Cognition, residence, and activities of daily living D. Activities of daily living and cognitive decline	Score from 0 to 81. Increasing frailty with higher scores

Indications for Prehabilitation

Under ideal circumstances, prehabilitation should be offered to any patient whose definitive treatment includes surgical resection, although even this criterion can, and likely will be, expanded. The intensity of the intervention depends on the initial risk screening as highlighted above combined with formal evaluation results. Some patients might require interventions in multiple domains, while others may require only counseling. The Royal College of Anaesthetists has proposed a tiered approach (Fig. 30.1) [60].

Prehabilitation offers potential benefits to patients where upfront resection or neoadjuvant therapy is the primary treatment strategy. In patients undergoing upfront resection, it is estimated that almost half of the patients who are taken into the operating room develop postoperative complications that render them unable to receive adjuvant therapy [61]. Despite the limited time available between diagnosis and surgery, prehabilitation can be implemented during this period; most prehabilitation programs for cancer patients usually last 4–6 weeks [60, 62]. While this time period might seem unreasonable because of the concerns of pancreatic cancer's rapid progression [63], surgical waiting times of 30 or more days are not uncommon and are not necessarily associated with worse oncologic outcomes, particularly if optimization of patient health occurs during that time frame [64, 65]. Current evidence suggests that patients with higher risk profiles for postoperative complications can safely proceed to prehabilitation, without compromising their oncologic outcomes.

On the other hand, neoadjuvant therapy is becoming increasingly popular because of the associated survival benefits, increased R0 resection rates, increased nodal downstaging rates, and increased completion of systemic therapies [66–68].

Fig. 30.1 Tiered approach to prehabilitation intervention. The arrow direction represents the direction of the intervention depending on the number and severity of risk factors. Universal interventions are directed to any patient with pancreatic cancer; targeted are directed to patients acute chronic, long-term conditions, or treatment adverse effects; specialist care is warranted for patients with complex needs or severe impairments

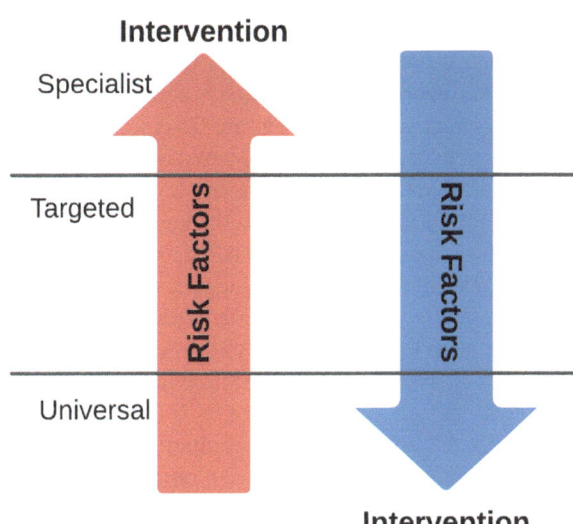

Naturally, surgery is delayed until completion of neoadjuvant treatment, after which time resectability is evaluated [6]. While there are numerous merits to neoadjuvant strategies in the management of solid gastrointestinal tumors, patients receiving neoadjuvant therapy may suffer from chemotherapy-associated deconditioning, thereby reducing their suitability for surgery and increasing their chances of postoperative complications [69]. Early evidence suggests that prehabilitation could protect patients from chemotherapy-associated deconditioning [54]. In addition, the hiatus between diagnosis to surgery provides a unique opportunity for prehabilitation, both to mitigate the deleterious effects of chemotherapy and optimize patients for surgery independent of receipt of systemic therapy.

Prehabilitation Programs

Prehabilitation programs can be classified according to the multitude of interventions. Single-intervention programs are classified as unimodal, while those with more than one intervention are multimodal. Multimodal interventions are usually preferred over unimodal programs because, as previously discussed, patients with PDAC are usually frail and harbor numerous comorbidities, in addition to the deleterious effects of the disease process itself [70]. Thus, unimodal interventions should be reserved for fit patients with a low-risk profile, as the evidence supporting these interventions in frail patients is limited [71]. Programs can be further classified as supervised or unsupervised. To our knowledge, supervised and unsupervised interventions have not been compared in the hepatobiliary and pancreatic populations. Evidence from other surgical populations suggests that supervised interventions are associated with improvements in physical function, symptom severity, pain, and physical activity compared to unsupervised programs [72–74]. However, direct supervision might not always be feasible or easy to implement; when this is the case, unsupervised intervention is a reasonable alternative. In our prehabilitation program, exercise interventions are designed in tiers of increasing intensity (beginner, intermediate, and advanced) based on the initial physical assessment. The exercise regimens include a warmup, cardiovascular, and resistance training. Similarly, we conduct nutritional interventions based on each individual patient's nutritional needs. Our main goal is to provide a nutritious diet, optimize glycemic control, and increase protein intake through supplementation with whey or vegetable-based protein [70]. While we do not include immunonutrition in our program, available evidence suggests that it could lead to fewer postoperative infections and reduce length of stay [75]. Nutritional interventions are supervised by physicians and licensed dietitians.

The optimal duration of prehabilitation programs for pancreatic cancer is yet to be determined. Programs have been reported to be as short as 5 days or as long as 6 months in duration [62]. Shorter duration might be more appropriate for patients whose primary treatment strategy is upfront resection followed by adjuvant therapy. On the other hand, patients treated with neoadjuvant therapy are better candidates for lengthier interventions. While some form of prehabilitation standardization is required, it is important to note that, like many other principles in medicine, a "one-size-fits-all" approach is unlikely to be successful in prehabilitation. Thus, the number of interventions, type of supervision, and program duration should be customized according to the patient's risk profile, clinical judgment, and, most importantly, patient preference, providing tiers for interventions based on need, as well as available resources.

Reassessment

As mentioned in the section "Patient Risk Stratification," surgical risk should be assessed during the initial visit. However, surgical risk is dynamic and varies along the course of therapy. The overarching objective of a prehabilitation program is to improve a patient's global status across the different surgical risk spheres (Table 30.1). If the intervention is successful, it is reasonable to assume that some patients will possess a lower risk during the time leading to their operation. On the other hand, despite best efforts, some patients might suffer from refractory deconditioning because of treatment-associated toxicity, underlying disease, or even disease progression. While patients should be continuously followed during the program, reassessment is typically carried out after finishing the intervention or before undergoing definitive surgical treatment at the very least. In our prehabilitation phase II program, we conduct sequential reassessments at critical time points during treatment that coincide with treatment intervals to minimize the burden on patients and caregivers alike. Following the initial evaluation that occurs during the initial visit, we reassess patients halfway through neoadjuvant systemic therapy

(8 weeks), followed by a second reassessment after finishing the eighth and final cycle (16 weeks). Given that we routinely include radiation therapy at our institution, another assessment is carried out at the end of radiation therapy. Finally, patients are reevaluated for the last time 1 month following surgical resection [8, 9]. Such frequent assessments allow us to tightly monitor patient progress along with clinical results. The program thus effectively supports patients through all aspects of aggressive therapy regimen with rigorous oversight.

Integrating a Prehabilitation Program into Clinical Practice

Establishing a prehabilitation program is a challenging process. Bundred and colleagues accurately highlighted the paucity of funds available for these programs [76]. In the same study, the authors demonstrated that physicians involved in the care of patients with cancer are frequently unaware of the availability of these services. In addition, many surveyed surgeons were reluctant to integrate prehabilitation into their practices [76]. This is problematic, as participation and adherence improve among patients with improved surgeon buy-in and uptake [77]. It is our strict belief that prehabilitation programs should be seamlessly integrated into institutions' any pre-existing clinical workflow. Otherwise, an increased workload and workflow disruption may lead to reluctance to participate among clinical staff. Implementation requires strong support from patients, surgical staff, and clinical leaders within institutions. Reduction in costly postoperative complications alone provides a hugely compelling argument to provide funding for these programs, including from hospital and insurance company sources.

In this section, we will provide two examples of prehabilitation programs that we carry out in our institution. The first is an in-person prehabilitation program implemented as part of a registered, ongoing, phase II clinical trial (NCT0386587), aiming to assess the feasibility and benefits of prehabilitation during neoadjuvant treatment. The second is a home-based program that was developed in response to the COVID-19 coronavirus pandemic. These examples might serve as a guide for surgeons interested in developing or modifying a prehabilitation program at their respective institutions. Both programs are multimodal interventions and consist of combinations of a standardized fitness program, nutrition supplementation program, smoking (and alcohol and other substances) cessation program, and mindfulness practices program. The main difference between both programs is that patients in the in-person program undergo supervised interventions. While there are reports of better results among supervised programs, these might, understandably, not be feasible to implement in resource-constrained setting [72, 74]. Our multidisciplinary team consists of physicians specializing in oncologic disciplines, physical medicine and rehabilitation, physical therapists, and cancer nutritionists. An example timeline that both programs follow is summarized in Fig. 30.2.

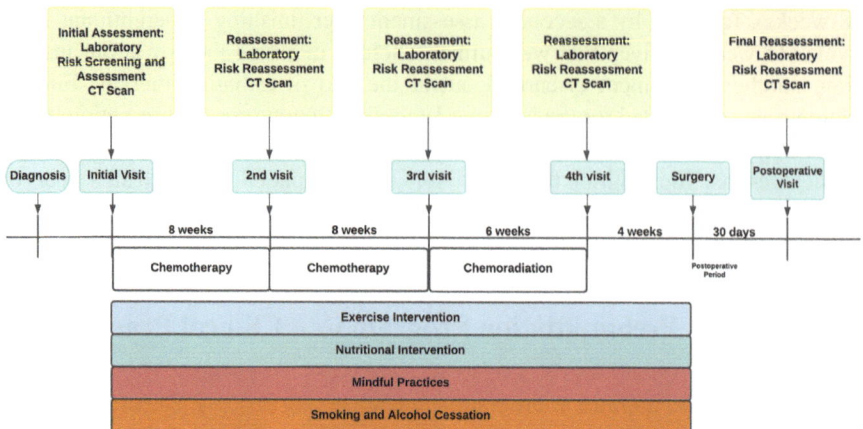

Fig. 30.2 Timeline of a multimodal prehabilitation program in patients undergoing neoadjuvant chemotherapy

Outcomes of Prehabilitation Trials

To date, there are 17 registered clinical trials, including our own, evaluating prehabilitation in patients with pancreatic adenocarcinoma. While current data appear to be promising, most studies suffer from small sample sizes and heterogeneous interventions. Mikami and colleagues evaluated postoperative complications among 26 patients with pancreatic cancer scheduled for surgery [78]. Patients exhibited an increase in peak oxygen consumption and 6-min walk distances, and none developed wound infection, respiratory complications, or deep venous thrombosis. Ausania and colleagues conducted a randomized controlled trial among 40 patients undergoing pancreatoduodenectomy [79]. Twenty-two patients were randomized into the prehabilitation group followed by surgery and 18 were treated with the standard of care. The authors did not find any differences in the risk of developing a pancreatic leak. However, the risk for delayed gastric emptying was significantly smaller in the prehabilitation group (5.6% vs. 40.9%, $p = 0.01$). Gade and colleagues evaluated the effect of a unimodal nutritional intervention in patients with pancreatic cancer [80]. Patients were supplemented with 1.5 g protein/kg of bodyweight. No differences were found between groups. However, only 40% of the patients were deemed to be at nutritional risk. Lastly, Baimas-George and colleagues reported interim results of a multimodal prehabilitation program in patients with hepatobiliary and pancreatic malignancies [54]. They found that multimodal prehabilitation significantly improved frailty and concluded that prehabilitation can protect patients from the physiologic deterioration associated with chemotherapy administration. While the results from some of these studies are promising, further evidence is required to determine which patients will truly benefit from prehabilitation and to allow prehabilitation to become a widespread, universal, and reimbursable mainstay treatment in pancreatic cancer and other solid tumors.

In conclusion, prehabilitation serves to enhance and optimize patients' functional capacity prior to major operative intervention with the intent of mitigating the risk of postoperative complications. Risk screening and assessment are needed to tailor the intervention accordingly. While prehabilitation should be offered to everyone, patients undergoing neoadjuvant chemotherapy are ideal candidates because of the treatment-associated toxicities and the unique opportunity present between diagnosis and surgical treatment. Finally, implementing a prehabilitation program can be a challenge but efforts to integrate these programs with clinical workflow and buy-in from healthcare providers will be critical.

References

1. Banugo P, Amoako D. Prehabilitation. BJA Educ. 2017;17(12):401–5. https://doi.org/10.1093/bjaed/mkx032.
2. Prehabilitation, rehabilitation, and revocation in the army. Br Med J. 1946;1:192–7.
3. Ditmyer MM, Topp R, Pifer M. Prehabilitation in preparation for orthopaedic surgery. Orthop Nurs. 2002;21(5):43–51; quiz 52. https://doi.org/10.1097/00006416-200209000-00008.
4. Moran J, Wilson F, Guinan E, McCormick P, Hussey J, Moriarty J. Role of cardiopulmonary exercise testing as a risk-assessment method in patients undergoing intra-abdominal surgery: a systematic review. Br J Anaesth. 2016;116(2):177–91. https://doi.org/10.1093/bja/aev454.
5. Mans CM, Reeve JC, Elkins MR. Postoperative outcomes following preoperative inspiratory muscle training in patients undergoing cardiothoracic or upper abdominal surgery: a systematic review and meta analysis. Clin Rehabil. 2015;29(5):426–38. https://doi.org/10.1177/0269215514545350.
6. Tempero MA, Malafa MP, Al-Hawary M, et al. Pancreatic adenocarcinoma, version 2.2021. J Natl Compr Cancer Netw. 2021;19(4):439–57. https://doi.org/10.6004/jnccn.2021.0017.
7. Bachmann J, Heiligensetzer M, Krakowski-Roosen H, Büchler MW, Friess H, Martignoni ME. Cachexia worsens prognosis in patients with resectable pancreatic cancer. J Gastrointest Surg. 2008;12(7):1193–201. https://doi.org/10.1007/s11605-008-0505-z.
8. Lawrence VA, Hazuda HP, Cornell JE, et al. Functional independence after major abdominal surgery in the elderly. J Am Coll Surg. 2004;199(5):762–72. https://doi.org/10.1016/j.jamcollsurg.2004.05.280.
9. Couwenberg AM, de Beer FSA, Intven MPW, et al. The impact of postoperative complications on health-related quality of life in older patients with rectal cancer; a prospective cohort study. J Geriatr Oncol. 2018;9(2):102–9. https://doi.org/10.1016/j.jgo.2017.09.005.
10. Bilimoria KY, Liu Y, Paruch JL, et al. Surgical risk calculator: a decision aide and informed consent tool for patients and surgeons. J Am Coll Surg. 2013;217(5):833–842.e3. https://doi.org/10.1016/j.jamcollsurg.2013.07.385.
11. van der Windt DJ, Bou-Samra P, Dadashzadeh ER, Chen X, Varley PR, Tsung A. Preoperative risk analysis index for frailty predicts short-term outcomes after hepatopancreatobiliary surgery. HPB. 2018;20(12):1181–8. https://doi.org/10.1016/j.hpb.2018.05.016.
12. Choi M, Kang CM, Chong JU, Hwang HK, Yoon DS, Lee WJ. Rates of serious complications estimated by the ACS-NSQIP surgical risk calculator in predicting oncologic outcomes of patients treated with pancreaticoduodenectomy for pancreatic head cancer. J Gastrointest Surg. 2019;23(6):1180–7. https://doi.org/10.1007/s11605-018-4041-1.
13. DeFina LF, Haskell WL, Willis BL, et al. Physical activity versus cardiorespiratory fitness: two (partly) distinct components of cardiovascular health? Prog Cardiovasc Dis. 2015;57(4):324–9. https://doi.org/10.1016/j.pcad.2014.09.008.

14. Haskell WL, Lee IM, Pate RR, et al. Physical activity and public health: updated recommendation for adults from the American College of Sports Medicine and the American Heart Association. Med Sci Sports Exerc. 2007;39(8):1423–34. https://doi.org/10.1249/mss.0b013e3180616b27.

15. Physical activity guidelines for Americans. Okla Nurse. 2008;53(4):25. https://doi.org/10.1249/fit.0000000000000472.

16. Ross R, Blair SN, Arena R, et al. Importance of assessing cardiorespiratory fitness in clinical practice: a case for fitness as a clinical vital sign: a scientific statement from the American Heart Association. Circulation. 2016;134. https://doi.org/10.1161/CIR.0000000000000461.

17. Jackson AS, Blair SN, Mahar MT, Wier LT, Ross RM, Stuteville JE. Prediction of functional aerobic capacity without exercise testing. Med Sci Sports Exerc. 1990;22(6):863–70. https://doi.org/10.1249/00005768-199012000-00021.

18. Gillis C, Fenton TR, Gramlich L, et al. Older frail prehabilitated patients who cannot attain a 400 m 6-min walking distance before colorectal surgery suffer more postoperative complications. Eur J Surg Oncol. 2021;47(4):874–81. https://doi.org/10.1016/j.ejso.2020.09.041.

19. Ramos RJ, Ladha KS, Cuthbertson BH, Shulman MA, Myles PS, Wijeysundera DN. Association of six-minute walk test distance with postoperative complications in non-cardiac surgery: a secondary analysis of a multicentre prospective cohort study. Can J Anesth. 2021;68(4):514–29. https://doi.org/10.1007/s12630-020-01909-9.

20. Lee DU, Hastie DJ, Fan GH, et al. Effect of malnutrition on the postoperative outcomes of patients undergoing pancreatectomy for pancreatic cancer: propensity score–matched analysis of 2011–2017 US hospitals. Nutr Clin Pract. 2022;37(1):117–29. https://doi.org/10.1002/ncp.10816.

21. Bye A, Jordhøy MS, Skjegstad G, Ledsaak O, Iversen PO, Hjermstad MJ. Symptoms in advanced pancreatic cancer are of importance for energy intake. Support Care Cancer. 2013;21(1):219–27. https://doi.org/10.1007/s00520-012-1514-8.

22. Lee B, Han HS, Yoon YS, Cho JY, Lee JS. Impact of preoperative malnutrition, based on albumin level and body mass index, on operative outcomes in patients with pancreatic head cancer. J Hepatobiliary Pancreat Sci. 2021;28(12):1069–75. https://doi.org/10.1002/jhbp.858.

23. Zhang YX, Yang YF, Han P, Ye PC, Kong H. Protein-energy malnutrition worsens hospitalization outcomes of patients with pancreatic cancer undergoing open pancreaticoduodenectomy. Updat Surg. 2022;74:0123456789. https://doi.org/10.1007/s13304-022-01293-7.

24. Ferguson M, Capra S, Bauer J, Banks M. Development of a valid and reliable malnutrition screening tool for adult acute hospital patients. Nutrition. 1999;15(6):458–64. https://doi.org/10.1016/S0899-9007(99)00084-2.

25. Rubenstein LZ, Harker JO, Salvà A, Guigoz Y, Vellas B. Screening for undernutrition in geriatric practice: developing the short-form mini-nutritional assessment (MNA-SF). J Gerontol A Biol Sci Med Sci. 2001;56(6):366–72. https://doi.org/10.1093/gerona/56.6.M366.

26. Malnutrition Advisory Group (MAG). MAG. The "MUST" explanatory booklet; 2011.

27. Kondrup J, Ramussen HH, Hamberg O, et al. Nutritional risk screening (NRS 2002): a new method based on an analysis of controlled clinical trials. Clin Nutr. 2003;22(3):321–36. https://doi.org/10.1016/S0261-5614(02)00214-5.

28. Wischmeyer PE, Carli F, Evans DC, et al. American Society for Enhanced recovery and perioperative quality initiative joint consensus statement on nutrition screening and therapy within a surgical enhanced recovery pathway. Anesth Analg. 2018;126(6):1883–95. https://doi.org/10.1213/ANE.0000000000002743.

29. Detsky AS, Mclaughlin J, Baker JP, et al. What is subjective global assessment of nutritional status? J Parenter Enter Nutr. 1987;11(1):8–13. https://doi.org/10.1177/014860718701100108.

30. Abbott J, Teleni L, McKavanagh D, Watson J, McCarthy AL, Isenring E. Patient-Generated Subjective Global Assessment Short Form (PG-SGA SF) is a valid screening tool in chemotherapy outpatients. Support Care Cancer. 2016;24(9):3883–7. https://doi.org/10.1007/s00520-016-3196-0.

31. Bettinelli A, Campisi A, Guarneri G, et al. Prognostic value of preoperative CT scan derived body composition measures in resected pancreatic cancer. Eur J Surg Oncol. 2024;50:106848. https://doi.org/10.1016/j.ejso.2023.02.005.

32. Salinas-Miranda E, Deniffel D, Dong X, et al. Prognostic value of early changes in CT-measured body composition in patients receiving chemotherapy for unresectable pancreatic cancer. Eur Radiol. 2021;31:8662–70.

33. Henriksen NA, Bisgaard T, Helgstrand F. Smoking and obesity are associated with increased readmission after elective repair of small primary ventral hernias: a nationwide database study. Surgery (United States). 2020;168(3):527–31. https://doi.org/10.1016/j.surg.2020.04.012.

34. Hawn MT, Houston TK, Campagna EJ, et al. The attributable risk of smoking on surgical complications. Ann Surg. 2011;254(6):914–20. https://doi.org/10.1097/SLA.0b013e31822d7f81.

35. DeLancey JO, Blay E, Hewitt DB, et al. The effect of smoking on 30-day outcomes in elective hernia repair. Am J Surg. 2018;216(3):471–4. https://doi.org/10.1016/j.amjsurg.2018.03.004.

36. Eliasen M, Grønkjær M, Skov-Ettrup LS, et al. Preoperative alcohol consumption and postoperative complications: a systematic review and meta-analysis. Ann Surg. 2013;258(6):930–42. https://doi.org/10.1097/SLA.0b013e3182988d59.

37. Rozich NS, Landmann A, Butler CS, et al. Tobacco smoking associated with increased anastomotic disruption following pancreaticoduodenectomy. J Surg Res. 2019;233:199–206. https://doi.org/10.1016/J.JSS.2018.07.047.

38. Lindström D, Azodi OS, Wladis A, et al. Effects of a perioperative smoking cessation intervention on postoperative complications: a randomized trial. Ann Surg. 2008;248(5):739–45. https://doi.org/10.1097/SLA.0b013e3181889d0d.

39. Møller AM, Villebro N, Pedersen T, Tønnesen H. Effect of preoperative smoking intervention on postoperative complications: a randomised clinical trial. Lancet. 2002;359(9301):114–7. https://doi.org/10.1016/S0140-6736(02)07369-5.

40. Durrand J, Singh SJ, Danjoux G. Prehabilitation. Clin Med (Northfield IL). 2017;17(6):458–64.

41. Babor TF, Higgins-Biddle JC, Saunders JB, Monteiro MG. The alcohol use disorders identification test guidelines for use in primary care. Published online 2001.

42. Heatherton TF, Kozlowski LT, Frecker RC, Fagerstrom K-O. The Fagerström test for nicotine dependence: a revision of the Fagerstrom tolerance questionnaire. Br J Addict. 1991;86(9):1119–27. https://doi.org/10.1111/j.1360-0443.1991.tb01879.x.

43. Mavros MN, Athanasiou S, Gkegkes ID, Polyzos KA, Peppas G, Falagas ME. Do psychological variables affect early surgical recovery? PLoS One. 2011;6(5):e20306. https://doi.org/10.1371/journal.pone.0020306.

44. Chan SF, La Greca AM. Perceived stress scale (PSS). In: Encyclopedia of behavioral medicine. Published online 2020. p. 1646–8. https://doi.org/10.1007/978-3-030-39903-0_773.

45. Aspari AR, Lakshman K. Effects of pre-operative psychological status on post-operative recovery: a prospective study. World J Surg. 2018;42(1):12–8. https://doi.org/10.1007/s00268-017-4169-2.

46. Bass V, Brown F, Beiser DG, Peterson T, Gibbons RD, Nagele P. Preoperative assessment of anxiety and depression using computerized adaptive screening tools: a pilot prospective cohort study. Anesth Analg. 2022;134(4):853–7. https://doi.org/10.1213/ANE.0000000000005844.

47. Ghignone F, Hernandez P, Mahmoud NN, Ugolini G. Functional recovery in senior adults undergoing surgery for colorectal cancer: assessment tools and strategies to preserve functional status. Eur J Surg Oncol. 2020;46(3):387–93. https://doi.org/10.1016/j.ejso.2020.01.003.

48. Walston J, Buta B, Xue QL. Frailty screening and interventions. Clin Geriatr Med. 2018;34(1):25–38. https://doi.org/10.1016/j.cger.2017.09.004.

49. Wang H, Liu J, Xia G, Lei S, Huang X, Huang X. Survival of pancreatic cancer patients is negatively correlated with age at diagnosis: a population-based retrospective study. Sci Rep. 2020;10(1):1–9. https://doi.org/10.1038/s41598-020-64068-3.

50. Komici K, Cappuccio M, Scacchi A, et al. The prevalence and the impact of frailty in Hepatobiliary pancreatic cancers: a systematic review and meta-analysis. J Clin Med. 2022;11(4). https://doi.org/10.3390/jcm11041116.

51. Augustin T, Burstein MD, Schneider EB, et al. Frailty predicts risk of life-threatening complications and mortality after pancreatic resections. Surgery (United States). 2016;160(4):987–96. https://doi.org/10.1016/j.surg.2016.07.010.
52. Nakano Y, Hirata Y, Shimogawara T, et al. Frailty is a useful predictive marker of postoperative complications after pancreaticoduodenectomy. World J Surg Oncol. 2020;18(1):1–10. https://doi.org/10.1186/s12957-020-01969-7.
53. Yamada S, Shimada M, Morine Y, et al. Significance of frailty in prognosis after surgery in patients with pancreatic ductal adenocarcinoma. World J Surg Oncol. 2021;19(1):1–8. https://doi.org/10.1186/s12957-021-02205-6.
54. Baimas-George M, Watson M, Thompson K, et al. Prehabilitation for hepatopancreatobiliary surgical patients: interim analysis demonstrates a protective effect from neoadjuvant chemotherapy and improvement in the frailty phenotype. Am Surg. 2021;87(5):714–24. https://doi.org/10.1177/0003134820952378.
55. Nidadavolu LS, Ehrlich AL, Sieber FE, Oh ES. Preoperative evaluation of the frail patient. Anesth Analg. 2020;130(6):1493–503. https://doi.org/10.1213/ANE.0000000000004735.
56. Fried LP, Tangen CM, Walston J, et al. Frailty in older adults: evidence for a phenotype. J Gerontol A Biol Sci Med Sci. 2001;56(3):146–57. https://doi.org/10.1093/gerona/56.3.m146.
57. Mitnitski AB, Mogilner AJ, Rockwood K. Accumulation of deficits as a proxy measure of aging. ScientificWorldJournal. 2001;1:323–36. https://doi.org/10.1100/tsw.2001.58.
58. Hall DE, Arya S, Schmid KK, et al. Development and initial validation of the risk analysis index for measuring frailty in surgical populations. JAMA Surg. 2017;152(2):175–82. https://doi.org/10.1001/jamasurg.2016.4202.
59. Perlmutter BC, Ali J, Cengiz TB, et al. Correlation between physical status measures and frailty score in patients undergoing pancreatic resection. Surgery (United States). 2022;171(3):711–7. https://doi.org/10.1016/j.surg.2021.10.030.
60. Macmillan, Royal College of Anaesthetists, National Institute for Health Research Cancer and Nutrition Collaboration. Principles and guidance for prehabilitation within the management and support of people with cancer. Published online 2019. p. 1–84.
61. Wu W, He J, Cameron JL, et al. The impact of postoperative complications on the administration of adjuvant therapy following pancreaticoduodenectomy for adenocarcinoma. Ann Surg Oncol. 2014;21(9):2873–81. https://doi.org/10.1245/s10434-014-3722-6.
62. Bundred JR, Kamarajah SK, Hammond JS, Wilson CH, Prentis J, Pandanaboyana S. Prehabilitation prior to surgery for pancreatic cancer: a systematic review. Pancreatology. 2020;20(6):1243–50. https://doi.org/10.1016/j.pan.2020.07.411.
63. Yu J, Blackford AL, Dal Molin M, Wolfgang CL, Goggins M. Time to progression of pancreatic ductal adenocarcinoma from low-to-high tumour stages. Gut. 2015;64(11):1783–9. https://doi.org/10.1136/gutjnl-2014-308653.
64. Kirkegård J, Mortensen FV, Hansen CP, Mortensen MB, Sall M, Fristrup C. Waiting time to surgery and pancreatic cancer survival: a nationwide population-based cohort study. Eur J Surg Oncol. 2019;45(10):1901–5. https://doi.org/10.1016/j.ejso.2019.05.029.
65. Marchegiani G, Andrianello S, Perri G, et al. Does the surgical waiting list affect pathological and survival outcome in resectable pancreatic ductal adenocarcinoma? HPB. 2018;20(5):411–7. https://doi.org/10.1016/j.hpb.2017.10.017.
66. Versteijne E, Van Dam JL, Suker M, et al. Neoadjuvant chemoradiotherapy versus upfront surgery for resectable and borderline resectable pancreatic cancer: long-term results of the Dutch randomized PREOPANC trial. J Clin Oncol. 2022;40(11):1220–30. https://doi.org/10.1200/JCO.21.02233.
67. van Dam JL, Janssen QP, Besselink MG, et al. Neoadjuvant therapy or upfront surgery for resectable and borderline resectable pancreatic cancer: a meta-analysis of randomised controlled trials. Eur J Cancer. 2022;160:140–9. https://doi.org/10.1016/j.ejca.2021.10.023.
68. Aquina CT, Ejaz A, Tsung A, Pawlik TM, Cloyd JM. National trends in the use of neoadjuvant therapy before cancer surgery in the US from 2004 to 2016. JAMA Netw Open. 2021;4(3):e211031. https://doi.org/10.1001/JAMANETWORKOPEN.2021.1031.

69. Stonko DP, He J, Zheng L, Blair AB. A contemporary evidence basis for neoadjuvant chemotherapy in upfront resectable pancreatic adenocarcinoma: a systematic review of the literature. J Pancreatol. 2020;3(1):12–20. https://doi.org/10.1097/JP9.0000000000000037.
70. Sell NM, Silver JK, Rando S, Draviam AC, Mina DS, Qadan M. Prehabilitation telemedicine in neoadjuvant surgical oncology patients during the novel COVID-19 coronavirus pandemic. Ann Surg. 2020;272(2):e81–3. https://doi.org/10.1097/SLA.0000000000004002.
71. Norris CM, Close JCT. Prehabilitation for the frailty syndrome: improving outcomes for our Most vulnerable patients. Anesth Analg. 2020;130(6):1524–33. https://doi.org/10.1213/ANE.0000000000004785.
72. Minetama M, Kawakami M, Teraguchi M, et al. Supervised physical therapy vs. home exercise for patients with lumbar spinal stenosis: a randomized controlled trial. Spine J. 2019;19(8):1310–8. https://doi.org/10.1016/j.spinee.2019.04.009.
73. Awasthi R, Minnella EM, Ferreira V, Ramanakumar AV, Scheede-Bergdahl C, Carli F. Supervised exercise training with multimodal pre-habilitation leads to earlier functional recovery following colorectal cancer resection. Acta Anaesthesiol Scand. 2019;63(4):461–7. https://doi.org/10.1111/aas.13292.
74. Lacroix A, Hortobágyi T, Beurskens R, Granacher U. Effects of supervised vs. unsupervised training programs on balance and muscle strength in older adults: a systematic review and meta-analysis. Sport Med. 2017;47(11):2341–61. https://doi.org/10.1007/s40279-017-0747-6.
75. De Luca R, Gianotti L, Pedrazzoli P, et al. Immunonutrition and prehabilitation in pancreatic cancer surgery: a new concept in the era of ERAS® and neoadjuvant treatment. Eur J Surg Oncol. 2023:49. https://doi.org/10.1016/j.ejso.2022.12.006.
76. Provan D, McLean G, Moug SJ, Phillips I, Anderson AS. Prehabilitation services for people diagnosed with cancer in Scotland—current practice, barriers and challenges to implementation. Surgeon. 2021;20:284. https://doi.org/10.1016/j.surge.2021.08.005.
77. Shaughness G, Howard R, Englesbe M. Patient-centered surgical prehabilitation. Am J Surg. 2018;216(3):636–8. https://doi.org/10.1016/j.amjsurg.2017.04.005.
78. Mikami Y, Kouda K, Kawasaki S, et al. Preoperative in-hospital rehabilitation improves physical function in patients with pancreatic cancer scheduled for surgery. Tohoku J Exp Med. 2020;251(4):279–85. https://doi.org/10.1620/tjem.251.279.
79. Ausania F, Senra P, Meléndez R, Caballeiro R, Ouviña R, Casal-Núñez E. Prehabilitation in patients undergoing pancreaticoduodenectomy: a randomized controlled trial. Rev Esp Enfermedades Dig. 2019;111(8):603–8. https://doi.org/10.17235/REED.2019.6182/2019.
80. Gade J, Levring T, Hillingsø J, Hansen CP, Andersen JR. The effect of preoperative oral immunonutrition on complications and length of hospital stay after elective surgery for pancreatic cancer—a randomized controlled trial. Nutr Cancer. 2016;68(2):225–33. https://doi.org/10.1080/01635581.2016.1142586.

Chapter 31
Enhanced Recovery Pathways: What's the Evidence?

Didier Roulin ⓘ, David Martin ⓘ, and Nicolas Demartines ⓘ

Introduction

Enhanced Recovery After Surgery (ERAS) is a standardized pathway guiding multidisciplinary and multimodal perioperative care after surgery. The main objective is to offer patients all required support to reduce the major stress induced by surgery with reduced complications and fasten functional recovery [1]. The implementation and application of ERAS principles are challenging processes with specific evidence-based recommendations covering the entire perioperative pathway, from the first contact of the patient with the hospital prior to surgery until full postoperative recovery.

Over 20 years ago, Kehlet described a multimodal approach [2], called "fast-track surgery," allowing to discharge patients within 2 days after open colectomy [3]. However, readmission rate was about 20% leading to the concept of enhancement rather than speed. With this purpose, Ljungqvist and Fearon gathered several academic surgeons from Northern Europe and formed the ERAS® Study group [4]. They noticed a big knowledge-to-practice gap [5] and published the first evidence-based ERAS recommendation for colon surgery in 2005 [6]. As implementation of ERAS pathway led to significant improvement of postoperative outcome [7], the group grew over time with the creation in 2010 of the International ERAS Society. Further guidelines in other surgical specialties were developed and in-turn 2022, 28 up-to-date guidelines covering many areas of abdominal (colorectal, hepatobiliary and pancreatic, upper gastrointestinal, and emergency laparotomy), urology, gynecology, cardiac and thoracic surgery, as well as anesthesia and neonatal surgery have been implemented. All guidelines were elaborated by worldwide experts and

D. Roulin · D. Martin · N. Demartines (✉)
Department of Visceral Surgery, Lausanne University Hospital CHUV, University of Lausanne, Lausanne, Switzerland
e-mail: didier.roulin@chuv.ch; david.martin@chuv.ch; demartines@unil.ch

© The Author(s), under exclusive license to Springer Nature Switzerland AG 2025
E. P. Ceppa et al. (eds.), *The SAGES Manual of Evolving Techniques in Pancreatic Surgery*, https://doi.org/10.1007/978-3-031-78409-5_31

are freely available on the website of the ERAS® Society (https://erassociety.org/guidelines/). The main objective of an enhanced recovery pathway is to gather all healthcare providers involved in the patient's journey to provide the best evidence and comprehensive patient-centered care, especially anesthetist, surgeons, and nursing staff.

The present chapter will go through the current state of ERAS recommendations for pancreatic surgery and will focus on the main ERAS items, the benefits, and challenges of ERAS in pancreatic surgery, as well as the existing controversies and will explore future directions.

Current State of Guidelines and Recommendations for Enhanced Recovery After Pancreatic Surgery

In pancreatic surgery, especially pancreatoduodenectomy (PD) is an extensive and highly complex procedure. Despite low in-hospital mortality (less than 2%) after PD in high-volume centers, the morbidity remains high (more than 70%) according to a multicenter benchmark study for pancreatic surgery [8]. Moreover, pancreatic surgery is associated with specific complications such as postoperative pancreatic fistula (POPF), delayed gastric emptying (DGE), and post-pancreatectomy hemorrhage (PPH). In pancreatic surgery, the potential effect of implementing optimized perioperative care such as ERAS pathway could lead to significant improvement.

While the very first ERAS guidelines for colorectal surgery were published in 2005 [6], and updated in 2009 [9], the potential of ERAS in pancreatic surgery was identified early, and specific recommendations for ERAS in PD were first published in 2012 [10] as third guideline endorsed by the ERAS Society. However, at that time, most evidence for ERAS in pancreatic surgery was extrapolated from previous observations coming from colorectal surgery. Those guidelines were more based on expert consensus than on scientific evidence. Nevertheless, this allowed the development of standardized perioperative care after PD paving the road to many further studies, including an international multicenter cohort [11] evaluating the compliance to the enhanced recovery pathway in over 400 pancreatic surgeries. With data emergence, the guidelines were updated in 2019 [12] with 27 evidence-based elements supporting ERAS perioperative management for PD.

Perioperative Elements

The ERAS pathway currently contains 27 perioperative items [12] that cover the pre-, intra-, and postoperative phases (Table 31.1). To apply enhanced recovery principles to pancreatic surgery, several main issues differ from other surgical specialties like preoperative biliary drainage, minimally invasive surgery, prophylactic

Table 31.1 Enhanced Recovery After Surgery (ERAS) items for pancreas surgery

	Pancreas
Preoperative items	
Counseling	Dedicated (multimedia) preoperative counseling
Prehabilitation	Prehabilitation program 3–6 weeks before surgery (extrapolation from other types of abdominal surgery)
Biliary drainage	Avoidance of preoperative drainage unless decompression is needed (bilirubin >250 µmol/L, preoperative cholangitis, neoadjuvant treatment)
Smoking and alcohol consumption	Smoking and alcohol consumption, abstention at least 4 weeks before surgery
Nutrition	Nutritional status assessment based on BMI and weight loss. Preoperative nutritional intervention if severe weight loss (>15% weight loss or BMI <18.5 kg/m^2)
Immunonutrition	Not recommended
Fasting and carbohydrate drinks	Clear fluids until 2 h, solids 6 h before surgery. Carbohydrate loading on evening and 2 h before surgery
Preanesthetic medication	No anxiolytics. Opioid-sparing multimodal medication (acetaminophen and single dose gabapentinoid)
Anti-thrombotic prophylaxis	Low molecular weight heparin (LMWH) or unfragmented heparin (UFH) 2–12 h before surgery and until hospital discharge. Mechanical measures are advised in addition. Four weeks thromboprophylaxis is advised in case of cancer
Intraoperative items	
Antimicrobial prophylaxis and skin preparation	Single dose intravenous antibiotic less than 60 min before skin incision, and repeated intraoperative doses depending on the duration of the procedure. Intraoperative bile culture if preoperative biliary stenting. Therapeutic postoperative antibiotics if positive bile culture. Use of alcohol-based preparations and wound protectors
Epidural	Thoracic epidural analgesia for open surgery
Wound catheter	Preperitoneal wound catheter as alternative to epidural for open surgery
Minimally invasive surgery	Laparoscopic surgery only in highly experienced high-volume center. No recommendation for robotic-assisted surgery
Hypothermia prevention	Active warming (cutaneous and perfusions warming) to maintain body temperature ≥36 °C
Nasogastric intubation	Not recommended
Postoperative items	
Analgesia	Multimodal opioid-sparing analgesia
Postoperative nausea and vomiting (PONV) prophylaxis	Multimodal PONV prophylaxis adapted to risk factors (female, non-smoking status, history of PONV or motion sickness, and postoperative opioid use) patients with ≥2 risk factors should receive a combination of two antiemetics
Glycemic control	Glucose levels should be maintained as close to normal as possible with treatments that reduce insulin resistance without causing hypoglycemia

(continued)

Table 31.1 (continued)

	Pancreas
Fluid balance	A goal-directed fluid therapy algorithm using intra- and postoperative noninvasive monitoring is recommended to avoid fluid overload
Abdominal drains	Routine intraoperative placement. Drain removal at 72 h in low-risk patients (amylase content <5000 U/L postoperative day 1)
Somatostatin analogs	Systematic use not recommended
Urinary catheter	Early urinary catheter removal
Delayed gastric emptying (DGE)	No acknowledged prophylactic strategy. Early diagnosis and treatment of intra-abdominal complications. Artificial nutrition in case of prolonged DGE
Stimulation of bowel movement	Use of chewing gum, alvimopan, or mosapride
Diet	Normal diet after surgery without restrictions according to tolerance. Artificial nutrition should be considered as an individual approach, and the enteral route should be preferred
Mobilization	Early and active mobilization from operative day
Audit	Regular audit and feedback based on an electronic database (EIAS: ERAS Interactive Audit System)

abdominal drainage, systematic nasogastric decompression, somatostatin analogs, fluid management, and delayed gastric emptying (DGE) management. The present subchapter does not go through all evidence behind every item of the ERAS protocol but focuses on the evidence supporting the specific items related to pancreatic surgery, while the others are discussed in summary form or in other chapters.

Preoperative Elements

Counseling, Prehabilitation, Smoking and Alcohol Consumption, Nutrition, Immunonutrition, Fasting and Carbohydrate Drinks, Preanesthetic Medication, Anti-thrombotic Prophylaxis

Preoperatively, counseling and initiation of a 3–6-week prehabilitation program with physical exercise and nutritional supplements should be offered whenever possible. Modalities of prehabilitation and nutritional supports are described in Chaps. 30 and 32, respectively. Patients should quit smoking and heavy alcohol consumption at least 4 weeks before surgery. Immunonutrition is no longer recommended, and preoperative fasting allows solids until 6 h and clear fluids until 2 h before surgery. Carbohydrate loads are given the previous evening and 2 h before surgery. Premedication (anxiolytics) is avoided, but an opioid-sparing multimodal medication in the form of acetaminophen and a single dose of gabapentin may be delivered. Low molecular weight heparin or unfragmented heparin anti-thrombotic prophylaxis is to be started 2–12 h before surgery and continued 4 weeks after surgery in case of cancer. Additionally, mechanical measures are advised during hospital stay.

However, the evidence is limited in pancreatic surgery, especially in terms of prophylaxis timing. A randomized study (PREPOSTEROUS Trial: Pre- vs. Postoperative Thromboprophylaxis in Pancreatic Surgery, NCT05245877) is currently underway and may soon provide data.

Biliary Drainage

The question of the biliary drain arises at the time of biliary obstruction and pathological diagnosis (ampullary adenoma, neoplasia, and chronic inflammatory remodeling). An increased number of patients with pancreatic ductal carcinoma require neoadjuvant chemotherapy (borderline tumor), and in those patients, biliary drainage is mandatory and not an option [12]. In other cases, preoperative drainage is associated with increased postoperative complications. A systematic review already performed a decade ago included four randomized controlled trials (RCTs) focusing on percutaneous transhepatic biliary drainage and two RCTs on endoscopic sphincterotomy and stenting [13]. There was no difference in postoperative mortality, but morbidity rates were higher in the preoperative biliary drainage group. In another more recent meta-analysis, percutaneous biliary drainage was inferior to endoscopic drainage without advantage of postoperative complications while causing significant discomfort to patients [14]. In addition, there was no difference between plastic and metallic stent. According to a RCT, resection should be performed without prior endoscopic stenting for asymptomatic patients with bilirubin level below 250 µmol/L [15].

Intraoperative Elements

Antimicrobial Prophylaxis and Skin Preparation, Epidural, Wound Catheter, Hypothermia Prevention

Antimicrobial intravenous prophylaxis is administered less than 60 min before skin incision and repeated depending on the duration of the procedure. Alcohol-based preparations and wound protectors are recommended. Intraoperative bile culture should be sent for microbiological analysis in case of preoperative biliary stenting. If positive, therapeutic antibiotics should be given postoperatively. Analgesia uses thoracic epidural for open pancreatic surgery or preperitoneal wound catheters in case of contraindication. To prevent hypothermia, active warming (cutaneous and perfusion warming) is used to maintain body temperature above 36 °C.

Minimally Invasive Surgery

The continuous growth and interest in a minimally invasive approach for pancreatic surgery led to extensive studies about its feasibility and safety, which have been gathered in two guidelines: the International Miami [16] and the European Brescia [17] consensus. The DIPLOMA randomized trial [18] showed non-inferiority of a minimally invasive distal pancreatectomy (DP), with comparable postoperative outcomes, radical resection rate, and overall outcome. For robotic pancreatoduodenectomy (PD), the consensus concluded that robotic PD had similar perioperative mortality, complication rates, and oncological outcomes, with reduced length of stay, less blood loss, and prolonged operative time when compared to open. These minimally invasive approaches are discussed in several chapters.

Nasogastric Intubation

There is high-level evidence that prophylactic nasogastric intubation increases the risk of pulmonary atelectasis and pneumonia and alters return of bowel function in abdominal surgery [19]. Specifically, in PD, one recent randomized clinical trial including 111 patients displayed no difference in postoperative complication occurrence until 90 days after surgery, suggesting that avoiding systematic nasogastric decompression was safe and should be the standard of care [20]. Concerning distal pancreatectomy, there is a lack of high-level evidence, but keeping with the previous data, nasogastric tubes placed during the surgery should be removed before the end of the anesthesia. There is still debate concerning the insertion of feeding tubes intraoperatively, through the gastrojejunal anastomosis, to initiate early postoperative enteral nutrition. An ongoing randomized controlled trial should provide data in the coming years [21].

Postoperative Elements

Analgesia, Postoperative Nausea and Vomiting (PONV) Prophylaxis, Glycemic Control, Diet, Stimulation of Bowel Movement, Urinary Catheter, Mobilization

Postoperative multimodal opioid-sparing analgesia is recommended, associated with PONV prophylaxis adapted to risk factors. Glucose levels should be maintained as close to normal with treatments that reduce insulin resistance without causing hypoglycemia. A normal diet is recommended after surgery without restrictions, according to tolerance. Artificial nutrition should be considered as an individual approach and the enteral route preferred. Modalities of perioperative nutrition management are further described in Chap. 32. Chewing gum and pharmacological agents (alvimopan and mosapride) may accelerate bowel function. The urinary catheter should be removed early after surgery, and active mobilization started from the operative day.

Fluid Balance

It has been suggested that fluid overload may cause interstitial fluid shift with consequent bowel wall edema that triggers inflammatory response with decreased anastomotic stability [22]. Several observational studies reported an increased rate of pancreatic fistula in case of perioperative fluid overload [23–25]. However, different definitions of restrictive protocol were used, and some of the protocols were only applied during the intra- or postoperative phase. In a retrospective study within an ERAS pathway, more than 4400 mL of intravenous fluid during the first 24 h following PD was an independent predictor of overall postoperative complications [26]. A recent RCT on fluid therapy for PD in ERAS patients compared fluid therapy with or without a cardiac output goal-directed therapy [27]. Length of stay and number of complications were decreased in the restrictive fluid therapy group. More studies on the definition of fluid balance and overload are required for pancreatic surgery within ERAS, but currently, perioperative hemodynamic optimization that preserves cardiac output and organ perfusion pressure by goal-directed fluid therapy and rational use of vasoactive drugs and inotropic drugs is recommended.

Abdominal Drains

The use of prophylactic drains placed close to the biliary and pancreatic anastomoses is still considered mandatory by many surgeons. More than two decades ago, a first randomized trial compared prophylactic drainage versus no drainage after pancreatic resection for pancreatic cancer [28]. This study showed the absence of significant difference in mortality or morbidity with or without intraperitoneal drainage. Another randomized trial comparing PD with or without routine drainage was interrupted because of increased mortality in the patients without drainage [29]. A recent meta-analysis showed that for patients undergoing PD, the drain group had lower mortality but higher rate of International Study Group of Pancreatic Surgery (ISGPS) grades B/C clinically relevant pancreatic fistula than the no-drain group [30]. For patients undergoing distal pancreatectomy, the drain group had higher rates of clinically relevant fistula, wound infection, and readmission. There were no significant differences in bile leak, hemorrhage, and DGE for both types of surgery, PD and DP. A recurring limitation is that most trials did not mention the proportion of these fistulas that were clinically significant, meaning grades B and C according to the ISGPS [31].

The Fistula Risk Score (FRS) is a ten-point score predicting the risk of developing ISGPF grades B/C clinically relevant pancreatic fistulas following PD and is based on gland texture, pathology, pancreatic duct diameter, and intraoperative blood loss [32]. A selective drain management approach has been suggested, with no-drain management in negligible/low-risk patients (FRS 0–2), a drain-dependent regimen for medium-/high-risk patients (FRS 3–10) with early drain removal on day 3 in case of low amylase levels (<5000 U/L at day 1) or later at surgeons' discretion (amylase >5000 at day 1) [33]. Further trials based on FRS and ISGPS definitions are required to establish adequate drainage management. Meanwhile, a conservative approach with systematic use of drainage catheters and early removal in patients at low risk of fistula is recommended.

Somatostatin Analogs

Somatostatin analogs reduce splanchnic blood flow and pancreatic secretion. A Cochrane review from 2013 included 21 trials with 2348 patients and showed no significant difference in perioperative mortality in patients who did receive somatostatin analogs even if the incidence of pancreatic fistula was lower [34]. Subgroup analyses for the variability in the texture and duct size of the pancreas were not available in most studies. More recently, pasireotide, a somatostatin analog with longer half-life than octreotide, was assessed in a randomized trial including 300 patients [35]. The rate of clinically significant pancreatic fistulas, leaks, or abscess was significantly lower in the pasireotide group. However, these results have not been validated yet, and similarly to intraperitoneal drainage management, further trials with FRS subgroup analyses are necessary to assess the role of systematic somatostatin analogs in the prevention of pancreatic fistula.

Delayed Gastric Emptying (DGE)

The definition of DGE described by the ISGPS is based on the duration of the need for nasogastric tube and is related to postoperative complications like pancreatic fistulas and intra-abdominal infections [36–38]. A relation between DGE and several surgical techniques has not been observed. There are no differences of DGE incidence based on gastrojejunostomy reconstruction type (antecolic versus retrocolic), pancreaticojejunostomy versus pancreaticogastrostomy, or pylorus-preserving resection versus classical Whipple's procedure [39–41]. Similarly, minimally invasive PD does not influence the occurrence of DGE compared with open surgery [42]. There are no known strategies to prevent DGE. Once diagnosed, treatment of intra-abdominal complications reduces the duration of DGE, and administration of supplemental nutrition improves outcomes [43]. If possible, enteral feeding beyond the gastrojejunostomy is to be preferred over parenteral nutrition. A RCT is currently assessing if early postoperative enteral nutrition can decrease complications after PD compared to oral nutrition within an ERAS program [21].

Monitoring and Audit

A proper and structured data monitoring with audit system is essential, including prospective database maintenance, and regular internal and external audits, to provide feedback and adherence to the ERAS recommendations. The existence of an evidence-based protocol is not enough to change practice and old dogmas, and reporting of adherence to the protocol (compliance) should be standard practice [44].

Outcomes of Enhanced Recovery in Pancreatic Surgery: Who Benefits and How?

The impact of ERAS pathway can be assessed by various outcomes. Initially, the main outcomes were length of stay (LOS) and readmission rate. However, these metrics present a high variability, as individual factors like local habits and logistics can highly influence the length of stay. The occurrence of perioperative morbidity, with complications graded according to Clavien classification [45] or Comprehensive Complication Index [46], provides a very useful evaluation of the impact of an ERAS pathway on clinical outcomes. In addition, functional metrics such as "ready-to-discharge" or "functional recovery" based on predefined criteria are accurately reflecting the patient's recovery. The report and usage of functional outcomes are encouraged. In addition, economic analysis can give insight into the cost-effectiveness of ERAS, which is the basis to convince healthcare administrators to implement ERAS. The effect of ERAS on clinical outcome, cost-effectiveness, and long-term functional and oncological benefits will be discussed.

Clinical Outcome

To the best of our knowledge, there are now at least seven available meta-analyses [47–52] assessing the impact of ERAS on clinical outcomes and the last published [49] included 26 observational case-control studies and five randomized controlled trials, with more than 5000 patients. As summarized in Table 31.2, all these meta-analyses systematically reported that enhanced recovery pathway in pancreatic surgery was associated with a reduction of overall morbidity and length of stay, with similar readmission rate, mortality, and reoperation rate. Looking at which type of complications was reduced by ERAS, two meta-analyses [50, 53] identified mild complications (Clavien grade I–II), but not major complications (Clavien grade III–V). Cao et al. observed that ERAS reduced incisional and pulmonary infections, but not abdominal infections [48]. Regarding pancreatic surgery, specific complications like DGE and POPF, most meta-analyses reported a decreased rate of DGE and similar rate of POPF with enhanced recovery [49–53]. Only one meta-analysis reported a reduced rate of POPF and a non-different rate of DGE in the enhanced recovery group [48]. Different inclusion criteria could explain this as this meta-analysis also included patients after distal pancreatectomy (DP). Interestingly, the latest meta-analysis focused on functional recovery and the ERAS pathway was

Table 31.2 Summary of enhanced recovery meta-analysis for pancreatic surgery

First author	Studies (N)	Patients (N)	Surgery	LOS, MD (95% CI)	Morbidity (95% CI)	DGE (95% CI)	POPF (95% CI)
Coolsen (2013)	4	996	PD, DP, TP	–	RD −0.083[a] (−0.15, −0.02)	–	–
Xiong (2016)	14	2719	PD	−4.17[a] (−5.72, −2.61)	OR 0.63[a] (0.54, 0.74)	OR 0.56[a] (0.44, 0.71)	OR 0.90 (0.74, 1.10)
Ji (2018)	20	3694	PD and DP	−4.45[a] (−5.99, −2.91)	OR 0.57[a] (0.45, 0.72)	OR 0.58[a] (0.48, 0.72)	OR 0.87 (0.74, 1.03)
Cao (2019)	19	3387	PD and DP	−3.89[a] (−4.98, −2.81)	–	OR 0.65 (0.40, 1.06)	OR 0.79[a] (0.67, 0.95)
Sun (2020)	20	3613	PD	−4.27[a] (−4.81, −3.73)	OR 0.62[a] (0.53, 0.74)	OR 0.51[a] (0.42- 0.63)	OR 0.86 (0.69, −1.06)
Wang (2020)	22	4147	PD	−5.07[a] (−6.71, −3.43)	RR 0.80[a] (0.72, 0.88)	RR 0.69[a] (0.55, 0.88)	RR 0.86 (0.73, 1.01)
Kuemmerli (2022)	31	5854	PD	−2.33[a] (−2.98, −1.69)	RD -0.04[a] (−0.08, −0.01)	RD 0.11[a] (0.22, 0.01)	RD 0.01 (−0.03, 0.02)

[a] Indicates statistically significance

LOS length of stay, *MD* median days, *OR* odds ratio, *CI* confidence interval, *DGE* delayed gastric emptying, *POPF* postoperative pancreatic fistula, *PD* pancreatoduodenectomy, *DP* distal pancreatectomy, *TP* total pancreatectomy, *RR* risk ratio, *RD* risk difference

found to be associated with shorter time to liquid and solid intake and earlier bowel recovery [49]. This meta-analysis also reported a reduced rate of complications (but not minor or major complications individually), as well as a decreased occurrence of incisional and intra-abdominal infections with ERAS. Moreover, fewer pulmonary complications occurred in the subgroup of patients with classic PD.

Despite the growing body of evidence, there are some limitations in the available evidence of ERAS in pancreatic surgery. First, the inclusion criteria of the studies on ERAS in pancreatic surgery differed widely, with some including distal pancreatectomy (DP) together with PD. Another limitation is the wide variation of the number of enhanced recovery elements used and reported by each study, which varied from 4 to 15 [54] out of the 27 evidence-based elements. Moreover, in a recent international survey, only around 60% of the surgeons used ERAS pathway for PD [55]. Thus, significant effort is still required to extend the dissemination of ERAS practice in pancreatic resection.

Economical Outcome

The implementation of ERAS pathway is a time and financial investment. Time needed to establish a pathway, train and build a dedicated team, and to allow continuous improvement of the process based on a database audit. However, the in-hospital cost reduction induced not only by the reduction of length of stay but also by the decrease of complications [56] allows an early return on investment. In addition, liberating hospital beds earlier with a shorter length of stay, allowing further admission of patients, creates a substantial cost opportunity. In pancreatic surgery, a dedicated systematic review [57] including five retrospective studies identified a net cost savings of 7020 USD per patient using enhanced recovery. Among included studies, Kagedan et al. [58] performed a detailed cost-minimization analysis and identified a significant decrease in cost of laboratory tests, medical imaging investigations, pharmaceuticals, and patient food. A recent meta-analysis assessed the cost-effectiveness of enhanced recovery for PD [59] with a mean cost saving of 4280 USD per patient based on nine studies in Europe, Asia, and America. Based on our own hospital's data [57], the extrapolated net saving was around 4 million USD over 8 years since the implementation of ERAS in pancreatic surgery. In conclusion, the implementation of enhanced recovery pathways represents a dominant cost-effective intervention, with decreased cost and improved patient outcomes. This strong positive economic impact was reproduced throughout various countries and healthcare systems.

Long-Term and Oncological Outcome

The positive impact of ERAS on short-term outcomes after pancreatic surgery is well established. The potential long-term advantage of improved recovery on the functional and oncological outcome would be of utmost interest, as most pancreatic surgery is performed in patients with cancer. The surgical resection of malignant cells has the potential risk of dissemination of circulating tumor cells, but also the induction of a temporary immunosuppression window, exposing the patients to higher risk of local and systemic tumor recurrence [60]. In pancreatic cancer surgery, a decrease in total lymphocyte count and an increase in neutrophil-to-lymphocyte ratio were observed in the early postoperative period [61]. It recovered within 4 days. As ERAS pathways were elaborated to mitigate surgical stress [62], a positive effect on cancer progression could be hypothesized. This was first suggested by a cohort study of over 900 colorectal patients in which compliance to ERAS ≥70% was related to improved oncological 5-year survival [63]. Similar evidence for pancreatic surgery is scarce. For example, an observational study could not observe any difference in oncological survival following ERAS implementation in PD [64]. However, faster recovery can also allow earlier beginning of postoperative chemotherapy. A recent observational study reported that ERAS led to faster time to recovery and earlier time to chemotherapy beginning after PD [65]. Another retrospective study described that ERAS compliance ≥67% tended to be associated with a reduction in the delay to adjuvant chemotherapy in young patients with hepatobiliary and pancreatic malignancies [66]. However, the translation of earlier return to chemotherapy into survival advantage for pancreatic cancer surgery still needs further assessment. The concept of improved long-term and oncological outcomes with ERAS seems appealing, but further data on large multicenter cohorts are needed to evaluate its pertinence.

Does One Pathway for Pancreatic Surgery Suit All?

Most available literature on enhanced recovery in pancreatic surgery is mainly focusing on classical or pylorus-preserving PD. For example, distal pancreatectomy (DP) is a completely different intervention without an anastomosis and an increased application of minimally invasive approach. A case-control study assessed that adding ERAS pathway in laparoscopic DP could be impactful. Patients after laparoscopic DP within enhanced recovery had shorter LOS (3 vs 6 days) with faster functional recovery and reduced overall complication rate compared to those with traditional care [67]. A retrospective study by Pecorelli et al. [68] reported a shorter functional recovery without difference in complications and length of stay in patients undergoing DP within an enhanced recovery pathway. The compliance to ERAS elements was reported, and the most challenging ones were intraoperative balanced fluid (defined as <6 mL/kg/h), mobilization out of bed on postoperative day 1 (>2 h) and urinary catheter removal (postoperative day 2) with a compliance of 15%, 33%, and 37%, respectively. The benefit of ERAS after DP seems appealing, but further studies are needed to address the specific needs for DP dedicated enhanced recovery pathway as opposed to PD.

For more seldom pancreatic resections like duodenum-preserving pancreatic head resection, segmental/central pancreatectomy, or total pancreatectomy (TP), only few available observational studies on enhanced recovery included these procedures (Porter et al. [69]: 12 TP; Berberat et al. [70]: 25 duodenum sparing, 9 segmental, 15 TP; di Sebastiano et al. [71]: 4 duodenum preserving, 3 central pancreatectomy, 10 TP; Agarwal et al. [72]: 3 central, 2 TP). However, their outcome was integrated in an overall group with PD ± DP, and the feasibility and impact of ERAS on these specific pancreatic resections could not be detailed. Further studies detailing specific outcomes for ERAS in duodenum-preserving pancreatic head resection, segmental/central pancreatectomy, or total pancreatectomy (TP) are needed.

Hot Topics, Controversies, and Future Advances

Compliance

ERAS programs may be heterogeneous in terms of number and definition of outcomes and items included. Furthermore, data like time to functional recovery and adherence to the perioperative elements are frequently omitted in the literature. The statement "we do ERAS" without measuring adherence or presenting an audit is often debated during discussions at international congresses. In pancreatic surgery, only few studies reported the compliance to ERAS program. It seems that compliance to pre- and intraoperative ERAS items is high (70–100%), but the postoperative items are more difficult to implement with success (38–66%), and the level of compliance is correlated with postoperative outcomes [73–75]. A multicenter study including 404 patients showed that a level of adherence of more than 70% was associated with significantly shorter length of stay and significantly fewer overall and major complications [11]. Only postoperative items were independent predictors of complications. These results highlight the interest in measuring compliance to improve outcomes but challenging and should be assessed in the near future.

Outcomes

Identification of the facilitators and barriers to ERAS implementation is a key element. It has been suggested in two qualitative studies that key points associated with a successful implementation with sustained adherence were the patient-related factors (demographics, comorbidities) and expectations; the staff-related factors (education, change of habits); the practice-related issues (communication, standardized protocol); and the health system resources [76, 77]. Future qualitative studies specifically evaluating this aspect in pancreatic surgery are required, without forgetting patient-reported outcomes measures (PROMs). PROMs go beyond the traditional clinical and oncological endpoints and ascertain perceptions of the patient's health status, perceived impairment, disability, and quality of life [78]. In 2019, a multicenter Delphi study including both patients and healthcare providers identified eight PROMs: general quality of life, general health, physical ability, ability to work/do usual activities, fear of recurrence, satisfaction with services/care organization, abdominal complaints, and relationship with partner/family [79]. These findings should facilitate the design of future pancreatic cancer trials and outcomes research. ERAS could also be assessed through patient-reported experience measures (PREMs), which gather information on patients' views of their care, using satisfaction scales, whereas PROMs provide reports from patients about their own health.

Future studies on ERAS should adhere to the RECOvER (Reporting on ERAS Compliance, Outcome, and Elements Research) checklist with the report of the clinical pathway and adherence auditing [80]. However, difficulties in conducting randomized trials on ERAS are to be emphasized, as the program applies the best-evidence care to all patients without exclusion criteria. In consequence, the control group would receive more traditional and conservative treatment. This raises an ethical issue, to be addressed and discussed and in the future, depending on the economic resources and politics of different health systems and countries.

Mobile Health

To facilitate and follow patient's perceptions (PROMs and PREMs), mobile health technology allowing recording in real time will be an important add. In a recent systematic review of 40 studies focusing on adult patients with pancreatic cancer, telemedicine has been proposed in multiple clinical settings, demonstrating high levels of patient and health professional satisfaction [81]. Successful applications were tele-rehabilitation and nutritional assessment, remote symptom control, tele-discharge after pancreatic surgery, tele-education and medical mentoring regarding pancreatic disease, as well as tele-pathology. Based on these suggestions, new data will provide more insight from the patient's perspective. In this direction, the Perioperative Quality Initiative (POQI) workgroup from North America and Europe detailed the incorporation of patient-centered outcomes within ERAS [82].

Elderly and Frailty

Most of the patients operated for pancreatic disease are elderly. A retrospective study showed that the application of ERAS was feasible in elderly patients undergoing pancreatic resection, even if older than 80 years [75]. However, perioperative management of elderly patients presents specific challenges related to their associated comorbidities [83]. Due to the heterogeneity of this population, decisions regarding surgical treatment cannot rely solely on treatment guidelines but must consider patient frailty, geriatric impairments, and resilience [84]. Frailty is defined as a clinically recognizable state of increased vulnerability, resulting from aging-associated decline in reserve and function across multiple physiologic systems [85]. Fried and colleagues suggested frailty as a condition meeting three of the five criteria: low grip strength, low energy, slowed walking speed, low physical activity, and unintentional weight loss [86]. Although scarcely investigated, frailty seems to be associated with negative short- and long-term treatment outcomes in older patients undergoing pancreatic surgery [84]. Frailty is currently not a routine part of the clinical preoperative assessment. Future studies should include frailty investigation, to determine the type and way of necessary assessment tool, specifically within an ERAS program.

Conclusion

The implementation of ERAS requires a multidisciplinary team and a structured implementation strategy with regular monitoring and audits. This program in pancreatic surgery is feasible and leads to significant reduction in postoperative complications and length of stay, both for pancreatoduodenectomy and distal pancreatectomy. Initially, many of the principles of the ERAS pathway were extrapolated from colorectal surgery. However, there are important differences in pancreatic surgery, like the role of systematic nasogastric or abdominal drainage, fluid balance, minimally invasive surgery, and nutrition management. After the first official ERAS pancreas guidelines published in 2012 and updated in 2019, the protocol could be studied and validated in various forms, including clinical and oncological outcomes. The current evidence reports improved postoperative outcomes with shorter length of stay, lower incidence of delayed gastric emptying, and overall complications without increasing readmission rates or mortality in ERAS patients. Its impact on postoperative pancreatic fistulas is not established, but it is associated with significant cost savings and represents an interesting argument for health care management. The extension of ERAS benefits to oncological outcomes as well as patient-reported outcomes remains to be investigated.

References

1. Ljungqvist O, Scott M, Fearon KC. Enhanced recovery after surgery a review. JAMA Surg. 2017;152(3):292–8.
2. Kehlet H. Multimodal approach to control postoperative pathophysiology and rehabilitation. Br J Anaesth. 1997;78(5):606–17.
3. Kehlet H, Mogensen T. Hospital stay of 2 days after open sigmoidectomy with a multimodal rehabilitation programme. Br J Surg. 1999;86(2):227–30.
4. Ljungqvist O, Young-Fadok T, Demartines N. The history of enhanced recovery after surgery and the ERAS society. J Laparoendosc Adv Surg Tech. 2017;27(9):860–2.
5. Lassen K, Hannemann P, Ljungqvist O, Fearon K, Dejong CH, von Meyenfeldt MF, et al. Patterns in current perioperative practice: survey of colorectal surgeons in five northern European countries. BMJ. 2005;330(7505):1420–1.
6. Fearon KC, Ljungqvist O, Von Meyenfeldt M, Revhaug A, Dejong CH, Lassen K, et al. Enhanced recovery after surgery: a consensus review of clinical care for patients undergoing colonic resection. Clin Nutr. 2005;24(3):466–77.
7. Hendry PO, Hausel J, Nygren J, Lassen K, Dejong CH, Ljungqvist O, et al. Determinants of outcome after colorectal resection within an enhanced recovery programme. Br J Surg. 2009;96(2):197–205.
8. Sanchez-Velazquez P, Muller X, Malleo G, Park JS, Hwang HK, Napoli N, et al. Benchmarks in pancreatic surgery: a novel tool for unbiased outcome comparisons. Ann Surg. 2019;270(2):211–8.
9. Lassen K, Soop M, Nygren J, Cox PB, Hendry PO, Spies C, et al. Consensus review of optimal perioperative care in colorectal surgery: Enhanced Recovery After Surgery (ERAS) Group recommendations. Arch Surg. 2009;144(10):961–9.

10. Lassen K, Coolsen MM, Slim K, Carli F, de Aguilar-Nascimento JE, Schafer M, et al. Guidelines for perioperative care for pancreaticoduodenectomy: Enhanced Recovery After Surgery (ERAS(R)) Society recommendations. World J Surg. 2013;37(2):240–58.
11. Roulin D, Melloul E, Wellg BE, Izbicki J, Vrochides D, Adham M, et al. Feasibility of an enhanced recovery protocol for elective pancreatoduodenectomy: a multicenter international cohort study. World J Surg. 2020;44(8):2761–9.
12. Melloul E, Lassen K, Roulin D, Grass F, Perinel J, Adham M, et al. Guidelines for perioperative care for pancreatoduodenectomy: enhanced recovery after surgery (ERAS) recommendations 2019. World J Surg. 2020;44:2056–84.
13. Fang Y, Gurusamy KS, Wang Q, Davidson BR, Lin H, Xie X, et al. Pre-operative biliary drainage for obstructive jaundice. Cochrane Database Syst Rev. 2012;9(9):CD005444.
14. Lee PJ, Podugu A, Wu D, Lee AC, Stevens T, Windsor JA. Preoperative biliary drainage in resectable pancreatic cancer: a systematic review and network meta-analysis. HPB (Oxford). 2018;20(6):477–86.
15. van der Gaag NA, Rauws EA, van Eijck CH, Bruno MJ, van der Harst E, Kubben FJ, et al. Preoperative biliary drainage for cancer of the head of the pancreas. N Engl J Med. 2010;362(2):129–37.
16. Asbun HJ, Moekotte AL, Vissers FL, Kunzler F, Cipriani F, Alseidi A, et al. The Miami international evidence-based guidelines on minimally invasive pancreas resection. Ann Surg. 2020;271(1):1–14.
17. Abu Hilal M, van Ramshorst TME, Boggi U, Dokmak S, Edwin B, Keck T, et al. The Brescia internationally validated European guidelines on minimally invasive pancreatic surgery (EGUMIPS). Ann Surg. 2024;279(1):45–57.
18. Korrel M, Jones LR, van Hilst J, Balzano G, Björnsson B, Boggi U, et al. Minimally invasive versus open distal pancreatectomy for resectable pancreatic cancer (DIPLOMA): an international randomised non-inferiority trial. Lancet Reg Health Eur. 2023;6(31):100673.
19. Nelson R, Edwards S, Tse B. Prophylactic nasogastric decompression after abdominal surgery. Cochrane Database Syst Rev. 2007;2007(3):CD004929.
20. Bergeat D, Merdrignac A, Robin F, Gaignard E, Rayar M, Meunier B, et al. Nasogastric decompression vs no decompression after pancreaticoduodenectomy: the randomized clinical IPOD trial. JAMA Surg. 2020;155(9):e202291.
21. Joliat GR, Martin D, Labgaa I, Melloul E, Uldry E, Halkic N, et al. Early enteral vs. oral nutrition after Whipple procedure: study protocol for a multicentric randomized controlled trial (NUTRIWHI trial). Front Oncol. 2022;12:855784.
22. Kulemann B, Fritz M, Glatz T, Marjanovic G, Sick O, Hopt UT, et al. Complications after pancreaticoduodenectomy are associated with higher amounts of intra- and postoperative fluid therapy: a single center retrospective cohort study. Ann Med Surg (Lond). 2017;16:23–9.
23. Bruns H, Kortendieck V, Raab HR, Antolovic D. Intraoperative fluid excess is a risk factor for pancreatic fistula after partial pancreaticoduodenectomy. HPB Surg. 2016;2016:1601340.
24. Winer LK, Dhar VK, Wima K, Lee TC, Morris MC, Shah SA, et al. Perioperative net fluid balance predicts pancreatic fistula after pancreaticoduodenectomy. J Gastrointest Surg. 2018;22(10):1743–51.
25. Han IW, Kim H, Heo J, Oh MG, Choi YS, Lee SE, et al. Excess intraoperative fluid volume administration is associated with pancreatic fistula after pancreaticoduodenectomy: a retrospective multicenter study. Medicine (Baltimore). 2017;96(22):e6893.
26. Gilgien J, Hübner M, Halkic N, Demartines N, Roulin D. Perioperative fluids and complications after pancreatoduodenectomy within an enhanced recovery pathway. Sci Rep. 2020;10(1):17898.
27. Weinberg L, Ianno D, Churilov L, Chao I, Scurrah N, Rachbuch C, et al. Restrictive intraoperative fluid optimisation algorithm improves outcomes in patients undergoing pancreaticoduodenectomy: a prospective multicentre randomized controlled trial. PLoS One. 2017;12(9):e0183313.

28. Conlon KC, Labow D, Leung D, Smith A, Jarnagin W, Coit DG, et al. Prospective randomized clinical trial of the value of intraperitoneal drainage after pancreatic resection. Ann Surg. 2001;234(4):487–93; discussion 93–4.
29. Van Buren G 2nd, Bloomston M, Hughes SJ, Winter J, Behrman SW, Zyromski NJ, et al. A randomized prospective multicenter trial of pancreaticoduodenectomy with and without routine intraperitoneal drainage. Ann Surg. 2014;259(4):605–12.
30. Liu X, Chen K, Chu X, Liu G, Yang Y, Tian X. Prophylactic intra-peritoneal drainage after pancreatic resection: an updated meta-analysis. Front Oncol. 2021;11:658829.
31. Pulvirenti A, Ramera M, Bassi C. Modifications in the International Study Group for Pancreatic Surgery (ISGPS) definition of postoperative pancreatic fistula. Transl Gastroenterol Hepatol. 2017;2:107.
32. Callery MP, Pratt WB, Kent TS, Chaikof EL, Vollmer CM Jr. A prospectively validated clinical risk score accurately predicts pancreatic fistula after pancreatoduodenectomy. J Am Coll Surg. 2013;216(1):1–14.
33. McMillan MT, Malleo G, Bassi C, Allegrini V, Casetti L, Drebin JA, et al. Multicenter, prospective trial of selective drain management for pancreatoduodenectomy using risk stratification. Ann Surg. 2017;265(6):1209–18.
34. Gurusamy KS, Koti R, Fusai G, Davidson BR. Somatostatin analogues for pancreatic surgery. Cochrane Database Syst Rev. 2013;2013(4):CD008370.
35. Allen PJ, Gönen M, Brennan MF, Bucknor AA, Robinson LM, Pappas MM, et al. Pasireotide for postoperative pancreatic fistula. N Engl J Med. 2014;370(21):2014–22.
36. Wente MN, Veit JA, Bassi C, Dervenis C, Fingerhut A, Gouma DJ, et al. Postpancreatectomy hemorrhage (PPH): an International Study Group of Pancreatic Surgery (ISGPS) definition. Surgery. 2007;142(1):20–5.
37. Parmar AD, Sheffield KM, Vargas GM, Pitt HA, Kilbane EM, Hall BL, et al. Factors associated with delayed gastric emptying after pancreaticoduodenectomy. HPB (Oxford). 2013;15(10):763–72.
38. Qu H, Sun GR, Zhou SQ, He QS. Clinical risk factors of delayed gastric emptying in patients after pancreaticoduodenectomy: a systematic review and meta-analysis. Eur J Surg Oncol. 2013;39(3):213–23.
39. Hüttner FJ, Klotz R, Ulrich A, Büchler MW, Diener MK. Antecolic versus retrocolic reconstruction after partial pancreaticoduodenectomy. Cochrane Database Syst Rev. 2016;9(9):CD011862.
40. Lei P, Fang J, Huang Y, Zheng Z, Wei B, Wei H. Pancreaticogastrostomy or pancreaticojejunostomy? Methods of digestive continuity reconstruction after pancreaticoduodenectomy: a meta-analysis of randomized controlled trials. Int J Surg. 2014;12(12):1444–9.
41. Hackert T, Probst P, Knebel P, Doerr-Harim C, Bruckner T, Klaiber U, et al. Pylorus resection does not reduce delayed gastric emptying after partial pancreatoduodenectomy: a blinded randomized controlled trial (PROPP Study, DRKS00004191). Ann Surg. 2018;267(6):1021–7.
42. Lei P, Wei B, Guo W, Wei H. Minimally invasive surgical approach compared with open pancreaticoduodenectomy: a systematic review and meta-analysis on the feasibility and safety. Surg Laparosc Endosc Percutan Tech. 2014;24(4):296–305.
43. Beane JD, House MG, Miller A, Nakeeb A, Schmidt CM, Zyromski NJ, et al. Optimal management of delayed gastric emptying after pancreatectomy: an analysis of 1,089 patients. Surgery. 2014;156(4):939–46.
44. Martin D, Roulin D, Addor V, Blanc C, Demartines N, Hübner M. Enhanced recovery implementation in colorectal surgery-temporary or persistent improvement? Langenbecks Arch Surg. 2016;401(8):1163–9.
45. Clavien PA, Barkun J, de Oliveira ML, Vauthey JN, Dindo D, Schulick RD, et al. The Clavien-Dindo classification of surgical complications: five-year experience. Ann Surg. 2009;250(2):187–96.
46. Slankamenac K, Graf R, Barkun J, Puhan MA, Clavien PA. The comprehensive complication index: a novel continuous scale to measure surgical morbidity. Ann Surg. 2013;258(1):1–7.

47. Coolsen MM, van Dam RM, van der Wilt AA, Slim K, Lassen K, Dejong CH. Systematic review and meta-analysis of enhanced recovery after pancreatic surgery with particular emphasis on pancreaticoduodenectomies. World J Surg. 2013;37(8):1909–18.
48. Cao Y, Gu HY, Huang ZD, Wu YP, Zhang Q, Luo J, et al. Impact of enhanced recovery after surgery on postoperative recovery for pancreaticoduodenectomy: pooled analysis of observational study. Front Oncol. 2019;9:687.
49. Kuemmerli C, Tschuor C, Kasai M, Alseidi AA, Balzano G, Bouwense S, et al. Impact of enhanced recovery protocols after pancreatoduodenectomy: meta-analysis. Br J Surg. 2022;109(3):256–66.
50. Sun Y-M, Wang Y, Mao Y-X, Wang W. The safety and feasibility of enhanced recovery after surgery in patients undergoing pancreaticoduodenectomy: an updated meta-analysis. Biomed Res Int. 2020;2020:1–15.
51. Wang XY, Cai JP, Huang CS, Huang XT, Yin XY. Impact of enhanced recovery after surgery protocol on pancreaticoduodenectomy: a meta-analysis of non-randomized and randomized controlled trials. HPB. 2020;22:1373–83.
52. Xiong J, Szatmary P, Huang W, de la Iglesia-Garcia D, Nunes QM, Xia Q, et al. Enhanced recovery after surgery program in patients undergoing pancreaticoduodenectomy: a PRISMA-compliant systematic review and meta-analysis. Medicine (Baltimore). 2016;95(18):e3497.
53. Ji HB, Zhu WT, Wei Q, Wang XX, Wang HB, Chen QP. Impact of enhanced recovery after surgery programs on pancreatic surgery: a meta-analysis. World J Gastroenterol. 2018;24(15):1666–78.
54. Pecorelli N, Nobile S, Partelli S, Cardinali L, Crippa S, Balzano G, et al. Enhanced recovery pathways in pancreatic surgery: state of the art. World J Gastroenterol. 2016;22(28):6456–68.
55. Groen JV, Henrar RB, Hanna Sawires RG, AlEassa E, Martini CH, Bonsing BA, et al. Pain management, fluid therapy and thromboprophylaxis after pancreatoduodenectomy: a worldwide survey among surgeons. HPB (Oxford). 2022;24(4):558–67.
56. Roulin D, Donadini A, Gander S, Griesser AC, Blanc C, Hübner M, et al. Cost-effectiveness of the implementation of an enhanced recovery protocol for colorectal surgery. Br J Surg. 2013;100(8):1108–14.
57. Joliat GR, Labgaa I, Petermann D, Hübner M, Griesser AC, Demartines N, et al. Cost-benefit analysis of an enhanced recovery protocol for pancreaticoduodenectomy. Br J Surg. 2015;102(13):1676–83.
58. Kagedan DJ, Devitt KS, Tremblay St-Germain A, Ramjaun A, Cleary SP, Wei AC. The economics of recovery after pancreatic surgery: detailed cost minimization analysis of an enhanced recovery program. HPB. 2017;19(11):1026–33.
59. Karunakaran M, Jonnada PK, Chandrashekhar SH, Vinayachandran G, Kaambwa B, Barreto SG. Enhancing the cost-effectiveness of surgical care in pancreatic cancer: a systematic review and cost meta-analysis with trial sequential analysis. HPB (Oxford). 2022;24(3):309–21.
60. Coffey JC, Wang JH, Smith MJ, Bouchier-Hayes D, Cotter TG, Redmond HP. Excisional surgery for cancer cure: therapy at a cost. Lancet Oncol. 2003;4(12):760–8.
61. Kim EY, Hong TH. Changes in total lymphocyte count and neutrophil-to-lymphocyte ratio after curative pancreatectomy in patients with pancreas adenocarcinoma and their prognostic role. J Surg Oncol. 2019;120(7):1102–11.
62. Ljungqvist O. Insulin resistance and outcomes in surgery. J Clin Endocrinol Metab. 2010;95(9):4217–9.
63. Gustafsson UO, Oppelstrup H, Thorell A, Nygren J, Ljungqvist O. Adherence to the ERAS protocol is associated with 5-year survival after colorectal cancer surgery: a retrospective cohort study. World J Surg. 2016;40(7):1741–7.
64. Passeri M, Lyman WB, Murphy K, Iannitti D, Martinie J, Baker E, et al. Implementing an ERAS protocol for pancreaticoduodenectomy does not affect oncologic outcomes when compared with traditional recovery. Am Surg. 2019;86:E81–3.

65. Li M, Wang X, Shen R, Wang S, Zhu D. Advancing the time to the initiation of adjuvant chemotherapy and improving postoperative outcome: enhanced recovery after surgery in pancreaticoduodenectomy. Am Surg. 2020;86(4):293–9.
66. St-Amour P, St-Amour P, Joliat GR, Eckert A, Labgaa I, Roulin D, et al. Impact of ERAS compliance on the delay between surgery and adjuvant chemotherapy in hepatobiliary and pancreatic malignancies. Langenbecks Arch Surg. 2020;405(7):959–66.
67. Richardson J, Di Fabio F, Clarke H, Bajalan M, Davids J, Abu HM. Implementation of enhanced recovery programme for laparoscopic distal pancreatectomy: feasibility, safety and cost analysis. Pancreatology. 2015;15(2):185–90.
68. Pecorelli N, Capretti G, Balzano G, Castoldi R, Maspero M, Beretta L, et al. Enhanced recovery pathway in patients undergoing distal pancreatectomy: a case-matched study. HPB. 2017;19(3):270–8.
69. Porter GA, Pisters PW, Mansyur C, Bisanz A, Reyna K, Stanford P, et al. Cost and utilization impact of a clinical pathway for patients undergoing pancreaticoduodenectomy. Ann Surg Oncol. 2000;7(7):484–9.
70. Berberat PO, Ingold H, Gulbinas A, Kleeff J, Muller MW, Gutt C, et al. Fast track—different implications in pancreatic surgery. J Gastrointest Surg. 2007;11(7):880–7.
71. di Sebastiano P, Festa L, De Bonis A, Ciuffreda A, Valvano MR, Andriulli A, et al. A modified fast-track program for pancreatic surgery: a prospective single-center experience. Langenbecks Arch Surg. 2011;396(3):345–51.
72. Agarwal V, Thomas MJ, Joshi R, Chaudhari V, Bhandare M, Mitra A, et al. Improved outcomes in 394 pancreatic cancer resections: the impact of enhanced recovery pathway. J Gastrointest Surg. 2018;22(10):1732–42.
73. Braga M, Pecorelli N, Ariotti R, Capretti G, Greco M, Balzano G, et al. Enhanced recovery after surgery pathway in patients undergoing pancreaticoduodenectomy. World J Surg. 2014;38(11):2960–6.
74. Bai X, Zhang X, Lu F, Li G, Gao S, Lou J, et al. The implementation of an enhanced recovery after surgery (ERAS) program following pancreatic surgery in an academic medical center of China. Pancreatology. 2016;16(4):665–70.
75. Scarsi S, Martin D, Halkic N, Demartines N, Roulin D. Enhanced recovery in elderly patients undergoing pancreatic resection: a retrospective monocentric study. Medicine (Baltimore). 2022;101(23):e29494.
76. Lyon A, Solomon MJ, Harrison JD. A qualitative study assessing the barriers to implementation of enhanced recovery after surgery. World J Surg. 2014;38(6):1374–80.
77. Martin D, Roulin D, Grass F, Addor V, Ljungqvist O, Demartines N, et al. A multicentre qualitative study assessing implementation of an enhanced recovery after surgery program. Clin Nutr. 2018;37(6 Pt A):2172–7.
78. Martin D, Demartines N, Hübner M. Patient perspectives in cancer surgery. J Clin Med. 2022;11(3):789.
79. van Rijssen LB, Gerritsen A, Henselmans I, Sprangers MA, Jacobs M, Bassi C, et al. Core set of patient-reported outcomes in pancreatic cancer (COPRAC): an international Delphi study among patients and health care providers. Ann Surg. 2019;270(1):158–64.
80. Elias KM, Stone AB, McGinigle K, Tankou JI, Scott MJ, Fawcett WJ, et al. The reporting on ERAS compliance, outcomes, and elements research (RECOvER) checklist: a joint statement by the ERAS(®) and ERAS(®) USA societies. World J Surg. 2019;43(1):1–8.
81. Tripepi M, Pizzocaro E, Giardino A, Frigerio I, Guglielmi A, Butturini G. Telemedicine and pancreatic cancer: a systematic review. Telemed J E Health. 2022;29:352.
82. Abola RE, Bennett-Guerrero E, Kent ML, Feldman LS, Fiore JF Jr, Shaw AD, et al. American Society for Enhanced Recovery and Perioperative Quality Initiative Joint Consensus Statement on patient-reported outcomes in an enhanced recovery pathway. Anesth Analg. 2018;126(6):1874–82.

83. Robinson TN, Eiseman B, Wallace JI, Church SD, McFann KK, Pfister SM, et al. Redefining geriatric preoperative assessment using frailty, disability and co-morbidity. Ann Surg. 2009;250(3):449–55.
84. Rostoft S, van Leeuwen B. Frailty assessment tools and geriatric assessment in older patients with hepatobiliary and pancreatic malignancies. Eur J Surg Oncol. 2021;47(3 Pt A):514–8.
85. Xue QL. The frailty syndrome: definition and natural history. Clin Geriatr Med. 2011;27(1):1–15.
86. Pedone C, Costanzo L, Cesari M, Bandinelli S, Ferrucci L, Incalzi RA. Are performance measures necessary to predict loss of Independence in elderly people? J Gerontol A Biol Sci Med Sci. 2016;71(1):84–9.

Chapter 32
Perioperative Nutrition in Pancreatic Surgery

Alessia Vallorani, Martina Abati, Chiara Limongi, and Nicolò Pecorelli

Introduction

Pancreatic resection is a major operation, thus a major trauma for the patients due to the extent of surgical dissection, resection, and the duration of surgery leading to a significant alteration of patient homeostasis. The neuroendocrine stress response and the inflammatory cascade elicited by tissue damage induce insulin resistance and a catabolic state with protein loss, ultimately leading to muscle depletion and loss of function that may persist until adequate nutritional substrates are introduced. Therefore, the nutritional status represents an important factor in all perioperative phases for any patient undergoing pancreatic surgery.

Pancreatic cancer patients are often older with preexisting comorbidities such as diabetes, obesity, and subclinical organ dysfunction and may have experienced a long course of chemotherapy, which all decrease physiological reserves further contributing to poor postoperative recovery. In addition, patients presenting with

A. Vallorani · C. Limongi
Vita-Salute San Raffaele University, Milan, Italy

M. Abati
Division of Pancreatic Surgery, Pancreas Translational and Clinical Research Center, San Raffaele Scientific Institute, Milan, Italy

Nutrition Service, San Raffaele Scientific Institute, Milan, Italy

N. Pecorelli (✉)
Vita-Salute San Raffaele University, Milan, Italy

Division of Pancreatic Surgery, Pancreas Translational and Clinical Research Center, San Raffaele Scientific Institute, Milan, Italy

Pancreas Translational & Clinical Research Center, San Raffaele Scientific Institute, Vita-Salute San Raffaele University, Milan, Italy
e-mail: pecorelli.nicolo@hsr.it

E. P. Ceppa et al. (eds.), *The SAGES Manual of Evolving Techniques in Pancreatic Surgery*, https://doi.org/10.1007/978-3-031-78409-5_32

malnutrition before surgery have very limited reserve resulting in poor healing, altered immune function, and delayed functional recovery after surgery. Therefore, the preoperative nutritional status represents an important preoperative optimization target to improve postoperative outcomes.

In the present chapter, we will mainly focus on two phases in the surgical patient continuum of care: (a) the preoperative phase including the use of screening tools to identify patients at risk for malnutrition and the nutritional interventions to optimize patient conditions and reduce postoperative morbidity risks; (b) the postoperative phase encompassing nutritional prescription in uneventful or complicated postoperative course, considering also intraoperative strategies to favor postoperative tolerance of oral intake or initiate artificial nutrition if necessary.

Preoperative Nutritional Evaluation and Intervention

Nutritional care before surgery should operate ensuring a safe and effective intervention, following a well-defined method. There are four phases of work that characterize the nutritional care process: nutritional screening, nutritional evaluation (assessment), nutritional treatment, monitoring, and evaluation of the results (follow-up). Each of these phases assumes the previous one has been completed, although the process is not linear as it is advisable to review, re-evaluate, and modify one of the previous phases of the ongoing process, according to the needs of the patients. Figure 32.1 shows the different phases of nutritional evaluation and intervention that will be covered in this section of the chapter.

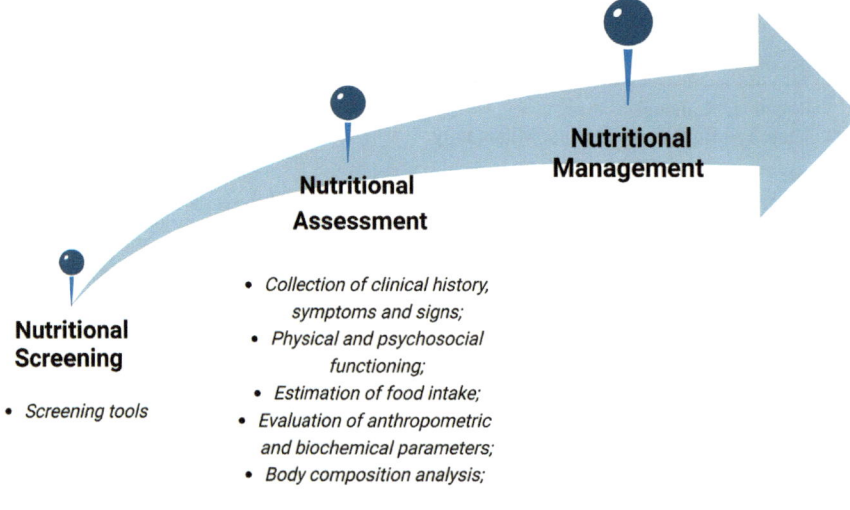

Fig. 32.1 From nutritional screening to intervention

Nutritional Screening

The first step in assessing malnutrition is nutritional screening [1]. Through proper nutritional screening, patients at immediate risk for malnutrition can be easily identified. Selected patients should then be referred for a comprehensive assessment of their nutritional status [2]. Nutritional screening uses relatively simple and quick tools such as questionnaires that can be filled out with patients or family members. Nutritional status screening must be performed in all patients at the time of cancer diagnosis and repeated at different timepoints. Screening can be done by the attending physician, the surgery or oncology clinic nurses, or any trained healthcare professional according to the clinical setting. After screening, patients found to be at malnutrition risk should be evaluated by the nutritionist through a formal nutritional assessment. Even if alterations in nutritional status are not present at disease onset, patients' conditions can change due to the secondary effects of cancer treatment and/or disease progression; therefore, screening should be performed periodically. Many validated nutritional status screening tools are available in the literature: Mini Nutritional Assessment (MNA) [3], Nutritional Risk Screening 2002 (NRS-2002) [4], Patient Generated-Subjective Global Assessment (PG-SGA) [5], Preoperative Nutrition Screen (PONS), and the Malnutrition Universal Screening Tool (MUST) [1, 6]. They have been developed to identify malnourished patients or those at risk of malnutrition using simple questions. Screening tools should be both sensitive and specific and if possible useful to monitor changes after nutritional interventions. The Mini Nutritional Assessment (MNA) provides a rapid assessment of nutritional status and has been recommended especially for elderly patients. The MNA test is composed of brief questions including only six items that can be completed in few minutes. In addition to a dietary and body weight assessment, MNA-SF also includes a questionnaire on physical and mental aspects that might affect the nutritional status. The sum of the MNA score stratifies different levels of malnutrition risk: adequate nutritional status (MNA $\geq$12), at risk of malnutrition (MNA between 8 and 11), and protein-calorie malnutrition (MNA $\leq$7). Some studies suggest that the MNA scoring could possibly predict mortality and hospital cost [3, 7].

The Nutritional Risk Screening 2002 (NRS 2002) is a screening tool recommended by the European Society for Clinical Nutrition and Metabolism (ESPEN) to identify surgical patients who may benefit from nutritional support [4]. Its validity in detecting undernutrition at the time of hospitalization, or the risk of developing in-hospital malnutrition, was supported by more than 100 randomized controlled trials. The first part of the questionnaire represents a pre-screening test which includes four questions. If even one question has an affirmative answer, a complete screening, comprehensive of surrogate measures of nutritional status, which consider static and dynamic parameters and the severity of the disease, must be performed. Each part scores from 0 to 3 points, and an age $\geq$70 years is considered as a further risk factor, raising the final score of one point. The NRS-2002 score ranges from 0 to 7, and a score $\geq$3 points identifies patients at risk of malnutrition or malnourished. According to ESPEN society guidelines, a score greater than 5 points suggests a severe malnutrition status.

The Patient-Generated Subjective Global Assessment Short Form (PG-SGA SF) [5], a component of the full PG-SGA, has recently been receiving attention as a valid screening tool for nutritional risk. The PG-SGA SF consists of four boxes: box 1, questions regarding body weight (scored 0–5); box 2, food intake (score 0–4); box 3, symptoms affecting oral food intake (scored 0–23); and box 4, regarding activities and function. The PG-SGA classifies patients into three categories: (A) well-nourished; (B) moderately malnourished; or (C) severely malnourished.

A targeted perioperative nutrition screening tool, the Perioperative Nutrition Score (PONS), which is a modified version of the Malnutrition Universal Screening Tool (MUST), has recently been proposed by an international consortium, the American Society for Enhanced Recovery (ASER) and Perioperative Quality Initiative (PQI) and has demonstrated predictive validity for postoperative outcomes [6]. PONS evaluates the presence of nutrition risk based on four different parameters: patient's body mass index (BMI), recent body weight changes, decrease in dietary intake, and preoperative serum albumin level. The PONS tool suggests a formal nutritional evaluation if the patient has any of the following risk factors: BMI lower than 18.5 (or lower than 20 if the patient is 65 or older), unplanned weight loss exceeding 10% body weight over the previous 6 months, dietary intake was less than 50% in the previous week, and albumin levels are below 3.0 g/dL. Serum albumin has been consistently reported in literature as a valid predictor of postoperative complications. However, recent studies showed controversial results, as albumin levels are influenced by a series of factors outside of its plain synthesis and degradation. Most of all, inflammation, which induces a shift in protein synthesis toward acute phase proteins that increase vascular permeability and extravascular leakage.

Nutritional Assessment

Nutritional assessment should be performed by a trained nutritionist. It should include collecting information about patient nutritional habits (dietary history, food and nutrient intake methods), overall health (anthropometric measurements and biochemical data, physical and clinical conditions, physiological and pathological state), and functional and behavioral status (social and cognitive function, psychological and emotional factors, quality of life, and willingness to change). Food intake is measured during the first interview through retrospective methods (24-h recall interview) or longitudinal methods (3-day food diary).

Evaluation of patient body composition is also suggested relying on validated tools such as multi-frequency bioelectrical impedance analysis (BIA) or preoperative cross-sectional imaging with quantification of body compartment areas using specific segmentation software [8–10]. Measurement of body composition gives important additional information compared to simple anthropometric parameters for both prognosis and nutritional intervention and follow-up.

BIA is a simple, easy-to-perform, non-invasive, and reproducible method that analyzes body composition and hydration status [11]. The BIA is based on the principle that body compartments offer different electrical conductivity to the passage of electrical current expressed by tissue resistance (R, Ohm) and reactance (X_c, Ohm). Lean tissues with high content of water and electrolytes provide low resistance (R), whereas fat, bone, and skin have low conductivity [12]. The R component is associated with hydration status, whereas the X_c component is related to the electrical capacitance (i.e., cell membrane integrity). Figure 32.2 shows the BIA nomogram for identifying the main features of patient body composition.

BIA is performed by placing two distal current or signal-introducing electrodes on the dorsal surfaces of the hand and foot close to the metacarpal-phalangeal and metatarsal-phalangeal joints, respectively. It is conventionally performed on the right side of the body. Some factors may interfere with BIA parameters such as position of the body and limbs, moderate to intense level of physical activity/exercise before BIA measurements (last exercise activity should be performed at least 12 h previously), medical conditions and medication that have an impact on the fluid and electrolyte balance; infection and cutaneous disease that may alter the

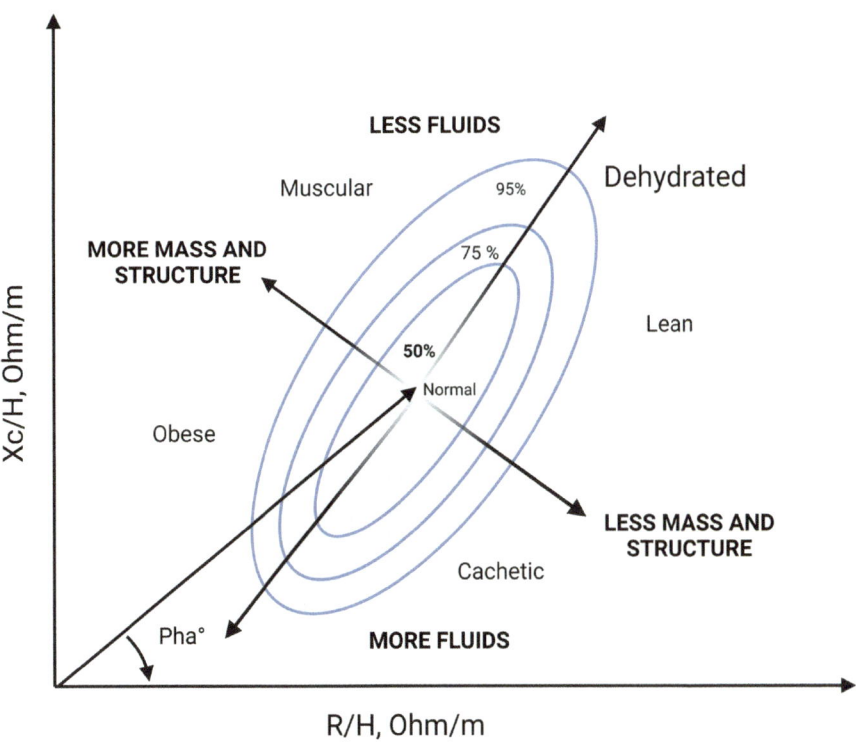

BIA nomogram

Fig. 32.2 The bioelectrical impedance analysis nomogram

electrical transmission between electrode and skin. Multiple BIA parameters are estimated from the impedance value via software algorithm including body cell mass (BCM), extracellular mass (ECM), fat-free mass (FFM), fat mass (FM), phase angle (PhA), skeletal muscle mass (SMM), and total body water (TBW).

BCM is the metabolically active component of fat-free mass, which represents the cell mass involved in O_2 consumption, CO_2 production, and energy expenditure [13]. Since it is closely related to energy expenditure, BCM could also represent a good reference value for the calculation of nutrient requirements. ECM includes bone, cartilage, ligaments, and non-metabolically active tissues, along with extracellular water. FFM represents about 75–80% of the total body weight and is mainly composed by water, minerals, muscles, organs, and bones [13]. FM indicates the amount of fat present in the body. Under normal conditions, this amount should not exceed 25% of the total weight. FM is indirectly estimated as the difference between body weight and FFM. PhA reflects the relative contributions of fluid (resistance) and cellular membranes (capacitance) of the human body. The phase angle is positively associated with capacitance and negatively associated with resistance. Lower PhA suggests cell death or decreased cell integrity, whereas higher PhA suggests large quantities of intact cell membranes. Phase angle has been found to be a prognostic marker in several clinical conditions, such as HIV infection, liver cirrhosis, chronic obstructive pulmonary disease, hemodialysis, sepsis, and lung cancer and is also correlated with markers for inflammation and oxidative stress. Research suggests that PhA is correlated with muscle area and muscle composition. Standardized phase angle (SPA) refers to PhA adjusted for sex and age and some studies suggest that it could be an independent prognostic indicator in cancer patients receiving chemotherapy treatment, even after adjustment for other prognostic variables. There is an increasing interest in estimating SMM, as it may reflect nutritional status, body protein reserves and function in disease-related malnutrition, cachexia, and sarcopenia better than FFM [14]. SMM accounts for 30–40% of total BW and correlates with physical functions and health status. Approximately 75% of SMM is located in the appendicular areas, defined as Appendicular Muscle Mass (ASMM) [14]. A reduction of ASMM leads to negative health consequences such as weakness, disability, impaired QoL, and mortality resulting in increased health care burden [15]. TBW represents the overall percentage of body fluids relative to the total body water of the subject. Physiological values are considered between 60% and 70% (during childhood the value reaches 77% and progressively decreases with age), while lower percentages are due to conditions of dehydration, loss of lean mass, or increase in FM (since most of the TBW is contained in lean body mass). Intracellular and extracellular water (ICW and ECW), expressed as a percentage of the TBW, allow to evaluate the distribution ratio of body fluids between the intra- and extracellular compartments. The values are in physiological range when the ICW is equal to 60% and the ECW is 40% [8].

In patients undergoing pancreatic resection, BIA has been mainly investigated as a predictive tool for postoperative complications. In a multicenter Italian study, preoperative SPA was significantly lower in patients who experienced severe postoperative morbidity than who did not [16]. In a further study by the same research group, preoperative FM measured at BIA was significantly higher in patients who developed clinically relevant postoperative pancreatic fistula as compared to patients who did not develop a fistula [17].

The recently published nutritional support and therapy in pancreatic surgery position paper by the International Study Group on Pancreatic Surgery also recommends measurement of body composition and the ratio of the different body compartments using quantitative abdominal CT scan along with weight loss and BMI estimation, as sarcopenia and sarcopenic obesity are strong predictors of short-term and long-term outcomes [18]. Evaluation of body composition through preoperative cancer staging abdominal CT scan provides an accurate quantitative measure of muscle mass and visceral fat. The prevalence of imaging low muscle mass (i.e., sarcopenia) in pancreatic cancer patients undergoing surgery can be as high as 65% [19]. Multiple studies have shown a consistent association between CT measured sarcopenic obesity and poor outcomes after pancreatoduodenectomy, with increased risk of pancreatic fistula, severe complications, and prolonged postoperative recovery [10]. In fact, visceral obesity is associated with a systemic inflammatory status and an increased risk of pancreatic anastomosis failure, while sarcopenia is part of the frailty syndrome delineating a patient with limited physiological reserves and ability to cope with stressful events.

Preoperative Nutritional Intervention

Pancreatic resection significantly affects pancreatic function and patients' nutritional status. Unlike starvation in absence of inflammation, in which body fat is mobilized in response to prolonged negative energy balance, surgery triggers a catabolic state inducing an inflammatory response. Therefore, skeletal muscle is broken down and hepatic uptake of amino acids supports gluconeogenesis and synthesis of acute-phase proteins. The inflammatory response to surgery is amplified by poor protein and energy intake, particularly in elderly patients or patients with preexisting malnutrition or low muscle mass [13].

Preoperative nutrition status influences a patient's surgical stress tolerance, wound healing, postoperative physical recovery, and the risk of postoperative complications [20, 21]. Poor nutrition status can also adversely affect humoral and cell-mediated immune responses, which, in turn, impair normal functioning of neutrophils and the ability of inflammatory cells to respond to infection. These immune processes are sensitive to changes in nutritional status and even a short period of protein-energy malnutrition induces negative immunological changes in the surgical patient in a prolonged fasting or malnourished state [22]. Preoperative nutritional interventions to enhance patient nutritional status aim at meeting an adequate protein target by improving diet or adding high-protein oral nutritional supplements, since proteins are most used in surgical stress situations [16, 20]. After assessing the nutrition and functional status, attention needs to be focused on implementing strategies and interventions to prepare patients to face the surgical stress and favor their recovery process. Preoperative conditioning, also known as prehabilitation, is defined as the process of enhancing physical fitness and well-being via a multimodal intervention including exercise training, diet, and psychological support. A full chapter dedicated to prehabilitation is available in this Manual, therefore we will only focus on preoperative nutritional interventions.

First, preoperatively patients should reach both an adequate caloric intake and protein target. For this purpose, the best solution is enriching daily diet with high-quality proteins (e.g., whey proteins and casein) that favor anabolism and muscle synthesis. The aim is to reach an intake of at least 1.5–2.0 g of protein/kg/day that is approximately 25–35 g of proteins for each meal [16, 22]. However, if the goal is not met with oral diet alone, high-protein content Oral Nutritional Supplements (ONS) should be prescribed. These products are available in many different energy and protein concentration formulas. Additionally, it is still debated if there is a role for preoperative immunonutrition [23]. Immunonutrition is an oral supplementation of specific nutrients such as arginine, nucleotides, and omega-3 fatty acids. Arginine is a conditional amino acid, as they represent more than 70% of the amino acids mobilized during the stress response. Their biological functions include stimulation of the immune system and promotion of wound healing. They also serve as nitric oxide precursors whose action is to improve microvascular perfusion through vasodilation. Omega-3 fatty acids comprising docosahexaenoic acid (DHA) and eicosapentaenoic acid (EPA) are known to be positive modulators of the inflammatory response. Combined immunonutrition formulas have a positive influence on the immune and inflammatory response as well as encouraging protein synthesis, suggesting a synergic effect. A recent meta-analysis on preoperative immunonutrition in gastrointestinal cancer only has demonstrated a significant reduction in postoperative infectious complications [24]. However, there is conflicting evidence regarding the actual benefit of immunonutrition in a modern perioperative care setting such as ERAS (Enhanced Recovery After Surgery) programs [25]. For this reason, the European Society for Clinical Nutrition and Metabolism (ESPEN) [26] guidelines suggest that peri- or at least postoperative administration of immunonutrition should be given in malnourished patients undergoing major cancer surgery. Although further research is needed to determine the benefit and optimal duration of immunonutrition, current data suggests that administration should be initiated at least 5–7 days before surgery, and a minimum treatment of 14 days in patients with severe malnutrition [23].

When supplementation is not possible via the oral route, a preoperative nutritional intervention can be administered via enteral route following the placement of a feeding tube for a period of at least 7 days. The enteral route is always preferable to the parenteral one, when feasible, due to the many benefits in terms of intestinal barrier permeability and preservation of the gut immune system and microbiota. If neither oral nutrition supplementation via ONS nor enteral nutrition (EN) is possible, or when protein or calories requirement cannot be adequately reached by the discussed strategies, parenteral nutrition should be administrated for a period of 7–14 days [23, 27].

Widespread integration of Enhanced Recovery After Surgery (ERAS) guidelines has increased awareness of the importance of preoperative nutrition optimization [25, 28]. ERAS programs are standardized, multimodal, multidisciplinary coordinated, and planned care approaches that integrate various evidence-based interventions in the perioperative period. Among ERAS nutritional interventions, limited preoperative fasting to 6 h for solids and 2 h for clear liquids before induction of anesthesia can attenuate insulin resistance compared to prolonged fasting. Carbohydrate loading administered a few hours before surgery has also been proposed as a measure to increase glycogen storage and decrease insulin resistance. The PROCY RCT compared carbohydrate loading and placebo in 800 non-diabetic patients undergoing major abdominal surgery. They found no difference in postoperative morbidity and infection rate; however, the control group required significantly more insulin postoperatively confirming the role of this intervention in blunting perioperative insulin resistance and maintaining euglycemia [29].

Postoperative Nutrition

Following the introduction of ERAS protocols in most surgical specialties, early and sustained oral feeding after pancreatic surgery has also become common [6]. Several nutritional interventions have been embedded in care pathways to facilitate postoperative recovery [30], including avoidance of nasogastric tube (NGT) decompression, postoperative nausea and vomiting (PONV) prophylaxis to facilitate oral food "at will" from the early postoperative days, stimulation of bowel movements, and use of artificial nutrition in selected patients [31].

Early Oral Feeding

The latest ESPEN guidelines on clinical nutrition in surgery recommend that oral intake shall be initiated within hours after surgery in most patients (grade of recommendation A) [32]. This statement is supported by data from recent meta-analyses showing significant benefits concerning the risk of nausea and vomit, return of bowel function, infections, and morbidity rate, without negative effects on anastomotic dehiscence. Focusing on pancreatic resection, early resumption of oral intake is both feasible and safe, as demonstrated by multiple studies and systematic reviews [33–35]. However, it is challenging to establish whether early oral feeding alone is associated with improved outcomes, as the data derived from studies where multiple ERAS interventions are implemented. According to most care pathways, patients can resume eating solid food from the first or second day after surgery, presuming nasogastric decompression is omitted. In an open-label, randomized clinical trial, the IPOD study (Impact of the Absence of Nasogastric Decompression After Pancreaticoduodenectomy), no difference was found in postoperative complications between systematic nasogastric decompression and no nasogastric decompression after pancreaticoduodenectomy. In the no-NGT group, patients had a significantly lower time to tolerance of oral liquids and solid food [36].

Despite the safety of avoiding nasogastric decompression and starting oral feeding as soon as tolerated, most patients fail to reach adequate energy (25 kcal/kg of body weight per day) and protein (1.5 g/kg of body weight per day) intakes during the first postoperative week. In a prospective study of 50 patients who underwent major abdominal surgery, protein and energy consumption were recorded in the first week postoperatively showing that caloric (82%) and protein intakes (90%) were largely inadequate. In addition, more Clavien-Dindo III complications were observed in the patients who did not achieve the protein target [37].

Optimal functional recovery after surgery requires an adequate amount of lean body mass, which can only be achieved with a sufficient protein intake. Thus, the addition of high-protein oral nutritional supplements has been suggested by multiple studies on postoperative nutrition. A recent trial in colorectal surgery demonstrated that adding high-protein ONS postoperatively was associated with a significant reduction in length of hospital stay [6]. However, few data on ONS supplementation are available for pancreatic surgery patients, where adherence to resuming oral feeding in the first few days after pancreatoduodenectomy is reported as low as 53%, but compliance decreases even more in patients with complications [38]. In fact, adherence to ONS may be difficult in patients not tolerating oral intake such as those experiencing delayed gastric emptying (DGE) on top of common postoperative symptoms including loss of appetite and taste, belching, gas and diarrhea [20].

Artificial Nutritional Support

The available evidence suggests that nutritional intake using only early oral feeding within an ERAS protocol after pancreatic surgery may be only partially adequate. Therefore, according to international guidelines [32], artificial nutritional support should be implemented early postoperatively in malnourished patients or those patients at high risk of developing malnutrition, in those who develop early severe postoperative complications, and in well-nourished patients who do not tolerate at least 50% of their caloric and protein requirement by postoperative day 7 for any reason.

When the need for postoperative nutritional support is determined, enteral nutrition is the preferred route. The delivery of nutritional substrates in the gastrointestinal tract stimulates the release of metabolic and regulatory gastrointestinal hormones, which can maintain gut contractility and blood flow, preserve the gut mucosal barrier function, and prevent bacterial translocation. There is not sufficient evidence suggesting that the composition of enteral formulas can affect outcome after pancreatic resection. Some clinicians suggest using peptide-based formulas compared to standard polymeric enteral formulas. Peptide-based or semi-elemental formulas contain proteins that have been enzymatically hydrolyzed to dipeptides and tripeptides. These hydrolyzed proteins are combined with higher medium-chain triglyceride content to generate an enteral formula that is essentially easier to absorb and utilize, especially in patients with pancreatic exocrine insufficiency. A recent meta-analysis on immunonutrition after major abdominal surgery suggests that this approach may decrease postoperative morbidity, infection rate, and duration of hospitalization in malnourished patients who underwent hepatobiliary and pancreatic operations. This topic, however, needs more investigation to robustly support the use of these more expensive feeds [39].

EN is not always well tolerated as bloating and diarrhea may occur preventing achievement of energy and protein goals. It is recommended to start enteral nutrition with a low flow rate (e.g., 10–20 mL/h) and progressively increase based on intestinal tolerance. The time to reach the target intake can be very different and may take up to 5 days. When nutrition goals are not met with oral and enteral intake alone, a combination of enteral and parenteral nutrition is recommended. Parenteral nutrition shall be administered as soon as possible if nutrition therapy is indicated and there is a contraindication for enteral nutrition (e.g., ileus or bowel obstruction or absence of a feeding tube) or enteral nutrition is not tolerated. Parenteral nutrition provides an excellent and complete nutritional formula, but is associated with many potential complications (hyperglycemia, metabolic acidosis, fluid overload, and vascular catheter-related infections) [18]. The beneficial effects of enteral compared with parenteral nutrition are well documented in numerous RCTs [40], with the most consistent being a reduction in infectious morbidity, a faster recovery of gastrointestinal function, and decreased hospital costs. Recent studies are now challenging the superiority of enteral to parenteral nutrition in the postoperative period. Gao et al. randomized 230 patients at increased nutritional risk or with poor tolerance to enteral nutrition after abdominal surgery to early (postoperative day 3) or late (postoperative day 8) supplemental parenteral nutrition. Patients who received early parenteral nutrition were at significantly lower risk of hospital-acquired infection (risk difference: 9.7%; 95% CI: 0.9–18.5; $p = 0.04$) although no difference was observed for secondary outcomes including infectious complications, length of hospital stay, and cost of admission [41]. Although early parenteral nutrition showed some benefits is this group of surgical patients, further studies are needed clarify these findings. In pancreatoduodenectomy patients, results from two multicenter randomized trials are expected: the first is evaluating the impact of early administration of parenteral nutrition versus usual care (oral intake alone) on postoperative morbidity in patients treated within an ERAS pathway [42] and the second is comparing early enteral with oral nutrition alone [43].

Techniques for Placement of an Enteral Feeding Tube After Pancreatic Surgery

The easiest way of delivering enteral nutrition is the placement of a nasogastric tube. However, as previously discussed, patients requiring artificial feeding after pancreatic resection are those not tolerating oral intake and experiencing complications such as DGE. In these patients, enteral nutrition cannot be delivered in the stomach as it would not be tolerated and increase the risk of aspiration. Thus, post-pyloric, jejunal feeding is necessary.

Post-pyloric enteral access can be achieved through the insertion of a nasoenteric feeding tube or more invasive methods including operative, laparoscopic, percutaneous, or endoscopic techniques. Examples include the operative insertion of a feeding jejunostomy during pancreatic surgery or a percutaneous or endoscopic gastrostomy with a jejunal extension. Each technique comes with its own set of complications influencing decision-making. Studies comparing different techniques favor nasojejunal (NJ) tubes considering severity of complications and recovery of digestive function [18]. However, after pancreatoduodenectomy, anatomy is altered and placement of NJ feeding tubes usually requires endoscopic or fluoroscopic guidance based on local expertise. In addition, failure of NJ feeding is reported in up to 34% of the cases within the first week mostly due to dislodgement or blockage [18]. Nonetheless, performing more invasive procedures such as endoscopic gastrostomy with a jejunal extension or surgical placement of a feeding tube jejunostomy can have more severe morbidity such as bowel perforation or obstruction from internal hernias or gut torsion.

In the authors' experience, postoperative artificial nutritional support after pancreatoduodenectomy is required in 15–20% patients. Most of these patients are experiencing prolonged DGE secondary to other intra-abdominal complication such as pancreatic fistula and peripancreatic fluid collections. In patients not tolerating oral feeding after the first five postoperative days, our management includes first to start parenteral nutrition from a peripheral IV line to satisfy patient daily energy and protein requirements. Second, a NJ tube is placed endoscopically and enteral nutrition is started at a low flow rate, with daily increases to reach nutritional targets based on patient tolerance and symptoms. Parenteral nutrition is then progressively withdrawn, usually within 3–5 days from the start of NJ feeding if enteral nutrition is tolerated.

Considering that pancreatic cancer is linked to significant metabolic disturbances known as cancer anorexia-cachexia syndrome, and the prolonged impairment of the patient's ability to consume food orally when experiencing severe postoperative complication, some authors suggest intraoperative placement of a feeding tube at the time of resection in selected patients [18]. Certainly, patients who are malnourished at the time of operation will benefit from receiving artificial nutrition support from the start, as supported by evidence. For patients at high risk of developing postoperative complications, the benefit of intraoperative placement of a feeding tube such as a NJ tube or a needle catheter jejunostomy is still uncertain. Surgeons can effectively assess risk factors that influence the likelihood of developing pancreas-specific complications during surgery and stratify patient into different risk categories (e.g., using the Fistula Risk Score). In patients with a very high risk of fistula identified by a Fistula Risk Score of 7 or higher, the authors support intraoperative placement of a feeding tube, but prospective data are needed to evaluate the actual benefit of this strategy.

Nutritional Management During Postoperative Complications and Post-discharge Support

As discussed in the previous sections, preoperative nutritional screening and prehabilitation together with early perioperative nutritional support majorly contribute to the optimization of the recovery process. Nonetheless, there are some important strategies that can be applied when postoperative complications occur and in late postoperative and post-discharge phases, that shall be acknowledged.

Even though in some settings it has been demonstrated that early oral nutrition and enteral feeding can contribute to the prevention of morbidity [44], the question is still debated in the presence of a clinically relevant POPF (CR-POPF), given that, intuitively, oral intake increases the production of pancreatic enzymes, that can exacerbate this condition. Despite that, a recent multicenter RCT comparing a group of 30 patients who were treated with oral dietary intake versus another group of 29 patients on total parenteral nutrition after occurrence of POPF found no significant differences in terms of nutritional indices up to 3 weeks after surgery, progression to a more CR-POPF, or development of intra-abdominal bleeding. As expected, a difference in the drain output was observed, with a higher volume in the oral intake group [45]. Moreover, recent evidence suggests that infections with certain microorganisms, such as Enterococcus, Pseudomonas, and Candida, can increase the development and severity of a POPF [46, 47]. In this setting, enteral fasting results in the growth and increased risk of translocation of these species, and consequently in a greater chance of infection.

There is currently no evidence of whether oral intake should be avoided in patients experiencing CR-POPF after proximal or distal pancreatectomy, and no specific criteria were identified to determine when oral diet can be considered both safe and helpful. Generally, it is accepted that in stable patients with a grade A or B POPF oral diet should always be attempted. Unstable or more severe CR-POPFs should accordingly be managed on a case-by-case basis [18].

Perhaps, one of the most intricate complications related to nutrition is delayed gastric emptying, with an incidence of 19–44% after pancreatic surgery [48]. Although primary DGE pathophysiology has not been clarified yet, it is often a coexisting condition with POPF and intra-abdominal infections [49–51]. Traditionally, early oral intake was considered a risk factor for its development, but currently the concept has largely been overcome, as demonstrated by a recent high-quality analysis [52]. In the presence of prolonged DGE, recommendations suggest starting artificial nutrition within 10 days, preferably via enteral routes beyond the gastro-jejunostomy over parenteral routes [53, 54].

Post-pancreatectomy hemorrhage (PPH), that can occur in up to 8% of cases [55], can be considered the most dreadful complication after pancreatic resections and is strictly related to the presence of a CR-POPF. In this context, interesting evidence emerged in literature regarding nutritional aspects. Despite the small retrospective series, Rayar et al. reported lower rates of PPH in patients treated with EN [56].

Recovery to baseline functional status after pancreatic surgery is a lengthy process, that is significantly affected by complications. In fact, post-pancreatectomy morbidity negatively influences patients' overall performance, mental and nutritional status. POPF and DGE may also persist beyond hospital stay, resulting in a subset of patients that no longer require hospitalization but may benefit from the continuation of home enteral and parenteral nutritional support. When adequate healthcare support is present, patients can be educated on home management of a feeding NJ tube or jejunostomy to continue with nutritional treatment.

As previously stated, patients undergoing pancreatic resections mostly for malignant diseases are characterized by a pathologic catabolic and inflammation state, that contributes to the depletion of nutritional substrates. This is exacerbated by surgical stress and coexisting oncological treatments. In this setting, it is likely that even uncomplicated patients that were able to resume normal oral diet, may not reach an adequate calory target and lose considerable weight after discharge. ESPEN recommends "regular reassessment of nutritional status during hospital stay and, if necessary, a continuation of nutritional support therapy including qualified dietary counseling after discharge, in patients who have received nutritional support therapy perioperatively and still do not cover appropriately their energy requirements via the oral route" [32]. In fact, to meet the nutritional needs of the challenging recovery process, high-protein ONS prescriptions must be part of any postoperative discharge care plan [57, 58]. For patients who underwent major surgery, it is suggested to continue postoperative high-protein ONS for 4–8 weeks minimum, and as long as 3–6 months postoperatively in more severely malnourished patients or those with prolonged hospital stays. In all these cases, a nutritional follow-up is always advocated to monitor the trajectory of recovery and eventually to introduce tailored support strategies.

Conclusion

This chapter has analyzed the importance and potential impact of perioperative nutrition in patients undergoing pancreatic surgery. Although many factors unrelated to patient nutritional status influence a patient perioperative course and the benefit of nutritional interventions may not be straightforward, marginal gains achieved from nutrition care should not be discounted. When considered cumulatively, small gains are likely to surmount to clinically meaningful outcomes, especially when nutrition is optimized throughout the pre-, peri-, postoperative, and post-discharge phases.

References

1. Prado CM, Ford KL, Gonzalez MC, Murnane LC, Gillis C, Wischmeyer PE, Morrison CA, Lobo DN. Nascent to novel methods to evaluate malnutrition and frailty in the surgical patient. JPEN J Parenter Enteral Nutr. 2023;47(Suppl 1):S54–68. https://doi.org/10.1002/jpen.2420.
2. Cederholm T, Jensen GL, Correia MITD, Gonzalez MC, Fukushima R, Higashiguchi T, Baptista G, Barazzoni R, Blaauw R, Coats A, Crivelli A, Evans DC, Gramlich L, Fuchs-Tarlovsky V, Keller H, Llido L, Malone A, Mogensen KM, Morley JE, Muscaritoli M, Nyulasi I, Pirlich M, Pisprasert V, de van der Schueren MAE, Siltharm S, Singer P, Tappenden K, Velasco N, Waitzberg D, Yamwong P, Yu J, Van Gossum A, Compher C. GLIM criteria for the diagnosis of malnutrition—a consensus report from the global clinical nutrition community. Clin Nutr. 2019;38:1–9. https://doi.org/10.1016/j.clnu.2018.08.002.
3. Vellas B, Guigoz Y, Garry PJ, Nourhashemi F, Bennahum D, Lauque S, Albarede JL. The Mini Nutritional Assessment (MNA) and its use in grading the nutritional state of elderly patients. Nutrition. 1999;15:116–22. https://doi.org/10.1016/s0899-9007(98)00171-3.
4. Reber E, Gomes F, Vasiloglou MF, Schuetz P, Stanga Z. Nutritional risk screening and assessment. J Clin Med. 2019;8. https://doi.org/10.3390/jcm8071065.
5. Zhang Q, Li X-R, Zhang X, Ding J-S, Liu T, Qian L, Song M-M, Song C-H, Barazzoni R, Tang M, Wang K-H, Xu H-X, Shi H-P. PG-SGA SF in nutrition assessment and survival prediction for elderly patients with cancer. BMC Geriatr. 2021;21:687. https://doi.org/10.1186/s12877-021-02662-4.
6. Wischmeyer PE, Carli F, Evans DC, Guilbert S, Kozar R, Pryor A, Thiele RH, Everett S, Grocott M, Gan TJ, Shaw AD, Thacker JKM, Miller TE, Hedrick TL, McEvoy MD, Mythen MG, Bergamaschi R, Gupta R, Holubar SD, Senagore AJ, Abola RE, Bennett-Guerrero E, Kent ML, Feldman LS, Fiore JFJ. American Society for Enhanced Recovery and Perioperative Quality Initiative Joint Consensus Statement on nutrition screening and therapy within a surgical enhanced recovery pathway. Anesth Analg. 2018;126:1883–95. https://doi.org/10.1213/ANE.0000000000002743.
7. Hung C-Y, Hsueh S-W, Lu C-H, Chang P-H, Chen P-T, Yeh K-Y, Wang H-M, Tsang N-M, Huang P-W, Hung Y-S, Chen S-C, Chou W-C. A prospective nutritional assessment using mini nutritional assessment-short form among patients with head and neck cancer receiving concurrent chemoradiotherapy. Support Care Cancer. 2021;29:1509–18. https://doi.org/10.1007/s00520-020-05634-3.
8. Di Somma S, Lukaski HC, Codognotto M, Peacock WF, Fiorini F, Aspromonte N, Ronco C, Santarelli S, Lalle I, Autunno A, Piccoli A. Consensus paper on the use of BIVA (Bioeletrical Impendance Vector Analysis) in medicine for the management of body hydration. Emerg Care J. 2011;7:6. https://doi.org/10.4081/ecj.2011.4.6.
9. Walter-Kroker A, Kroker A, Mattiucci-Guehlke M, Glaab T. A practical guide to bioelectrical impedance analysis using the example of chronic obstructive pulmonary disease. Nutr J. 2011;10:35. https://doi.org/10.1186/1475-2891-10-35.
10. Guarneri G, Pecorelli N, Bettinelli A, Campisi A, Palumbo D, Genova L, Gasparini G, Provinciali L, Della Corte A, Abati M, Aleotti F, Crippa S, De Cobelli F, Falconi M. Prognostic value of preoperative CT scan derived body composition measures in resected pancreatic cancer. Eur J Surg Oncol. 2024;50:106848. https://doi.org/10.1016/j.ejso.2023.02.005.
11. de Medeiros GOC, de Sousa IM, Chaves GV, Gonzalez MC, Prado CM, Fayh APT. Comparative assessment of abdominal and thigh muscle characteristics using CT-derived images. Nutrition. 2022;99–100:111654. https://doi.org/10.1016/j.nut.2022.111654.
12. Bundred J, Kamarajah SK, Roberts KJ. Body composition assessment and sarcopenia in patients with pancreatic cancer: a systematic review and meta-analysis. HPB (Oxford). 2019;21:1603–12. https://doi.org/10.1016/j.hpb.2019.05.018.
13. Prado CM, Landi F, Chew STH, Atherton PJ, Molinger J, Ruck T, Gonzalez MC. Advances in muscle health and nutrition: a toolkit for healthcare professionals. Clin Nutr. 2022;41:2244–63. https://doi.org/10.1016/j.clnu.2022.07.041.

14. Cruz-Jentoft AJ, Gonzalez MC, Prado CM. Sarcopenia ≠ low muscle mass. Eur Geriatr Med. 2023;14:225–8.
15. Bahat G, Tufan A, Tufan F, Kilic C, Akpinar TS, Kose M, Erten N, Karan MA, Cruz-Jentoft AJ. Cut-off points to identify sarcopenia according to European Working Group on Sarcopenia in Older People (EWGSOP) definition. Clin Nutr. 2016;35:1557–63. https://doi.org/10.1016/j.clnu.2016.02.002.
16. Sandini M, Paiella S, Cereda M, Angrisani M, Capretti G, Casciani F, Famularo S, Giani A, Roccamatisi L, Viviani E, Caccialanza R, Montorsi M, Zerbi A, Bassi C, Gianotti L. Perioperative interstitial fluid expansion predicts major morbidity following pancreatic surgery: appraisal by bioimpedance vector analysis. Ann Surg. 2019;270:923–9. https://doi.org/10.1097/SLA.0000000000003536.
17. Angrisani M, Sandini M, Cereda M, Paiella S, Capretti G, Nappo G, Roccamatisi L, Casciani F, Caccialanza R, Bassi C, Zerbi A, Gianotti L. Preoperative adiposity at bioimpedance vector analysis improves the ability of Fistula Risk Score (FRS) in predicting pancreatic fistula after pancreatoduodenectomy. Pancreatology. 2020;20:545–50. https://doi.org/10.1016/j.pan.2020.01.008.
18. Gianotti L, Besselink MG, Sandini M, Hackert T, Conlon K, Gerritsen A, Griffin O, Fingerhut A, Probst P, Abu Hilal M, Marchegiani G, Nappo G, Zerbi A, Amodio A, Perinel J, Adham M, Raimondo M, Asbun HJ, Sato A, Takaori K, Shrikhande SV, Del Chiaro M, Bockhorn M, Izbicki JR, Dervenis C, Charnley RM, Martignoni ME, Friess H, de Pretis N, Radenkovic D, Montorsi M, Sarr MG, Vollmer CM, Frulloni L, Büchler MW, Bassi C. Nutritional support and therapy in pancreatic surgery: a position paper of the International Study Group on Pancreatic Surgery (ISGPS). Surgery. 2018;164:1035–48. https://doi.org/10.1016/j.surg.2018.05.040.
19. Carrara G, Pecorelli N, De Cobelli F, Cristel G, Damascelli A, Beretta L, Braga M. Preoperative sarcopenia determinants in pancreatic cancer patients. Clin Nutr. 2017;36:1649–53. https://doi.org/10.1016/j.clnu.2016.10.014.
20. Ford KL, Prado CM, Weimann A, Schuetz P, Lobo DN. Unresolved issues in perioperative nutrition: a narrative review. Clin Nutr. 2022;41:1578–90. https://doi.org/10.1016/j.clnu.2022.05.015.
21. Capurso G, Pecorelli N, Burini A, Orsi G, Palumbo D, Macchini M, Mele R, de Cobelli F, Falconi M, Arcidiacono PG, Reni M. The impact of nutritional status on pancreatic cancer therapy. Expert Rev Anticancer Ther. 2022;22:155–67. https://doi.org/10.1080/14737140.2022.2026771.
22. Caccialanza R, Laviano A, Bosetti C, Nardi M, Casalone V, Titta L, Mele R, De Pergola G, De Lorenzo F, Pedrazzoli P. Clinical and economic value of oral nutrition supplements in patients with cancer: a position paper from the Survivorship Care and Nutritional Support Working Group of Alliance Against Cancer. Support Care Cancer. 2022;30:9667–79. https://doi.org/10.1007/s00520-022-07269-y.
23. De Luca R, Gianotti L, Pedrazzoli P, Brunetti O, Rizzo A, Sandini M, Paiella S, Pecorelli N, Pugliese L, Pietrabissa A, Zerbi A, Salvia R, Boggi U, Casirati A, Falconi M, Caccialanza R. Immunonutrition and prehabilitation in pancreatic cancer surgery: a new concept in the era of ERAS® and neoadjuvant treatment. Eur J Surg Oncol. 2023;49:542–9. https://doi.org/10.1016/j.ejso.2022.12.006.
24. Stannard D. Early enteral nutrition within 24 hours of lower gastrointestinal surgery versus later commencement for length of hospital stay and postoperative complications. J Perianesth Nurs. 2020;35:541–2. https://doi.org/10.1016/j.jopan.2020.07.003.
25. Bozzetti F, Mariani L. Perioperative nutritional support of patients undergoing pancreatic surgery in the age of ERAS. Nutrition. 2014;30:1267–71. https://doi.org/10.1016/j.nut.2014.03.002.
26. Weimann A, Braga M, Carli F, Higashiguchi T, Hübner M, Klek S, Laviano A, Ljungqvist O, Lobo DN, Martindale RG, Waitzberg D, Bischoff SC, Singer P, Zanetti M, Gianotti L, Martindale R, Waitzberg DL. Linea guida pratica ESPEN: nutrizione clinica in chirurgia Basata su (ESPEN guideline: clinical nutrition in surgery). Clin Nutr. 2017;36:623–50.

27. Paiella S, Azzolina D, Trestini I, Malleo G, Nappo G, Ricci C, Ingaldi C, Vacca PG, De Pastena M, Secchettin E, Zamboni G, Maggino L, Corciulo MA, Sandini M, Cereda M, Capretti G, Casadei R, Bassi C, Mansueto G, Gregori D, Milella M, Zerbi A, Gianotti L, Salvia R. Body composition parameters, immunonutritional indexes, and surgical outcome of pancreatic cancer patients resected after neoadjuvant therapy: a retrospective, multicenter analysis. Front Nutr. 2023;10:1065294. https://doi.org/10.3389/fnut.2023.1065294.
28. Gianotti L, Sandini M, Romagnoli S, Carli F, Ljungqvist O. Enhanced recovery programs in gastrointestinal surgery: actions to promote optimal perioperative nutritional and metabolic care. Clin Nutr. 2020;39:2014–24. https://doi.org/10.1016/j.clnu.2019.10.023.
29. Gianotti L, Biffi R, Sandini M, Marrelli D, Vignali A, Caccialanza R, Viganò J, Sabbatini A, Di Mare G, Alessiani M, Antomarchi F, Valsecchi MG, Bernasconi DP. Preoperative oral carbohydrate load versus placebo in major elective abdominal surgery (PROCY): a randomized, placebo-controlled, multicenter, phase III trial. Ann Surg. 2018;267:623–30. https://doi.org/10.1097/SLA.0000000000002325.
30. Pecorelli N, Nobile S, Partelli S, Cardinali L, Crippa S, Balzano G, Beretta L, Falconi M. Enhanced recovery pathways in pancreatic surgery: state of the art. World J Gastroenterol. 2016;22:6456–68. https://doi.org/10.3748/wjg.v22.i28.6456.
31. Melloul E, Lassen K, Roulin D, Grass F, Perinel J, Adham M, Wellge EB, Kunzler F, Besselink MG, Asbun H, Scott MJ, Dejong CHC, Vrochides D, Aloia T, Izbicki JR, Demartines N. Guidelines for perioperative care for pancreatoduodenectomy: enhanced recovery after surgery (ERAS) recommendations 2019. World J Surg. 2020;44:2056.
32. Weimann A, Braga M, Carli F, Higashiguchi T, Hübner M, Klek S, Laviano A, Ljungqvist O, Lobo DN, Martindale RG, Waitzberg D, Bischoff SC, Singer P. ESPEN practical guideline: clinical nutrition in surgery. Clin Nutr. 2021;40:4745–61. https://doi.org/10.1016/j.clnu.2021.03.031.
33. Halle-Smith JM, Pande R, Powell-Brett S, Pathak S, Pandanaboyana S, Smith AM, Roberts KJ. Early oral feeding after pancreatoduodenectomy: a systematic review and meta-analysis. HPB (Oxford). 2022;24:1615.
34. Gerritsen A, Besselink MGH, Gouma DJ, Steenhagen E, Borel Rinkes IHM, Molenaar IQ. Systematic review of five feeding routes after pancreatoduodenectomy. Br J Surg. 2013;100:589.
35. Lassen K, Kjæve J, Fetveit T, Tranø G, Sigurdsson HK, Horn A, Revhaug A. Allowing normal food at will after major upper gastrointestinal surgery does not increase morbidity: a randomized multicenter trial. Ann Surg. 2008;247:721–9. https://doi.org/10.1097/SLA.0b013e31815cca68.
36. Bergeat D, Merdrignac A, Robin F, Gaignard E, Rayar M, Meunier B, Beloeil H, Boudjema K, Laviolle B, Sulpice L. Nasogastric decompression vs no decompression after pancreaticoduodenectomy: the randomized clinical IPOD trial. JAMA Surg. 2020;155:e202291. https://doi.org/10.1001/jamasurg.2020.2291.
37. Constansia RDN, Hentzen JEKR, Hogenbirk RNM, van der Plas WY, Campmans-Kuijpers MJE, Buis CI, Kruijff S, Klaase JM. Actual postoperative protein and calorie intake in patients undergoing major open abdominal cancer surgery: a prospective, observational cohort study. Nutr Clin Pract. 2022;37:183–91. https://doi.org/10.1002/ncp.10678.
38. Braga M, Pecorelli N, Ariotti R, Capretti G, Greco M, Balzano G, Castoldi R, Beretta L. Enhanced recovery after surgery pathway in patients undergoing pancreaticoduodenectomy. World J Surg. 2014;38:2960–6. https://doi.org/10.1007/s00268-014-2653-5.
39. Probst P, Ohmann S, Klaiber U, Hüttner FJ, Billeter AT, Ulrich A, Büchler MW, Diener MK. Meta-analysis of immunonutrition in major abdominal surgery. Br J Surg. 2017;104:1594–608. https://doi.org/10.1002/bjs.10659.
40. For personal use. Only reproduce with permission from The Lancet Publishing Group. Enteral nutrition parenteral nutrition.
41. Gao X, Liu Y, Zhang L, Zhou D, Tian F, Gao T, Tian H, Hu H, Gong F, Guo D, Zhou J, Gu Y, Lian B, Xue Z, Jia Z, Chen Z, Wang Y, Jin G, Wang K, Zhou Y, Chi Q, Yang H, Li M, Yu J, Qin

H, Tang Y, Wu X, Li G, Li N, Li J, Pichard C, Wang X. Effect of early vs late supplemental parenteral nutrition in patients undergoing abdominal surgery: a randomized clinical trial. JAMA Surg. 2022;157:384–93. https://doi.org/10.1001/jamasurg.2022.0269.

42. Gianotti L, Paiella S, Frigerio I, Pecorelli N, Capretti G, Sandini M, Bernasconi DP. ERAS with or without supplemental artificial nutrition in open pancreatoduodenectomy for cancer. A multicenter, randomized, open labeled trial (RASTA study protocol). Front Nutr. 2023;10. https://doi.org/10.3389/fnut.2023.1113723.

43. Joliat GR, Martin D, Labgaa I, Melloul E, Uldry E, Halkic N, Fotsing G, Cristaudi A, Majno-Hurst P, Vrochides D, Demartines N, Schäfer M. Early enteral vs. oral nutrition after Whipple procedure: study protocol for a multicentric randomized controlled trial (NUTRIWHI trial). Front Oncol. 2022;12. https://doi.org/10.3389/fonc.2022.855784.

44. Kehlet H. Fast-track colorectal surgery. Lancet. 2008;371:791–3. https://doi.org/10.1016/S0140-6736(08)60357-8.

45. Fujii T, Nakao A, Murotani K, Okamura Y, Ishigure K, Hatsuno T, Sakai M, Yamada S, Kanda M, Sugimoto H, Nomoto S, Takeda S, Morita S, Kodera Y. Influence of food intake on the healing process of postoperative pancreatic fistula after pancreatoduodenectomy: a multi-institutional randomized controlled trial. Ann Surg Oncol. 2015;22:3905–12. https://doi.org/10.1245/s10434-015-4496-1.

46. Sato A, Masui T, Nakano K, Sankoda N, Anazawa T, Takaori K, Kawaguchi Y, Uemoto S. Abdominal contamination with Candida albicans after pancreaticoduodenectomy is related to hemorrhage associated with pancreatic fistulas. Pancreatology. 2017;17:484–9. https://doi.org/10.1016/j.pan.2017.03.007.

47. Yamashita K, Sasaki T, Itoh R, Kato D, Hatano N, Soejima T, Ishii K, Takenawa T, Hiromatsu K, Yamashita Y. Pancreatic fistulae secondary to trypsinogen activation by Pseudomonas aeruginosa infection after pancreatoduodenectomy. J Hepatobiliary Pancreat Sci. 2015;22:454–62. https://doi.org/10.1002/jhbp.223.

48. Qu H, Sun GR, Zhou SQ, He QS. Clinical risk factors of delayed gastric emptying in patients after pancreaticoduodenectomy: a systematic review and meta-analysis. Eur J Surg Oncol. 2013;39:213–23. https://doi.org/10.1016/j.ejso.2012.12.010.

49. Liu Q-Y, Li L, Xia H-T, Zhang W-Z, Cai S-W, Lu S-C. Risk factors of delayed gastric emptying following pancreaticoduodenectomy. ANZ J Surg. 2016;86:69–73. https://doi.org/10.1111/ans.12850.

50. Riediger H, Makowiec F, Schareck WD, Hopt UT, Adam U. Delayed gastric emptying after pylorus-preserving pancreatoduodenectomy is strongly related to other postoperative complications. J Gastrointest Surg. 2003;7:758–65. https://doi.org/10.1016/s1091-255x(03)00109-4.

51. Park Y-C, Kim S-W, Jang J-Y, Ahn YJ, Park Y-H. Factors influencing delayed gastric emptying after pylorus-preserving pancreatoduodenectomy. J Am Coll Surg. 2003;196:859–65. https://doi.org/10.1016/S1072-7515(03)00127-3.

52. Shen Y, Jin W. Early enteral nutrition after pancreatoduodenectomy: a meta-analysis of randomized controlled trials. Langenbecks Arch Surg. 2013;398:817–23. https://doi.org/10.1007/s00423-013-1089-y.

53. Liu C, Du Z, Lou C, Wu C, Yuan Q, Wang J, Shu G, Wang Y. Enteral nutrition is superior to total parenteral nutrition for pancreatic cancer patients who underwent pancreaticoduodenectomy. Asia Pac J Clin Nutr. 2011;20:154–60.

54. Beane JD, House MG, Miller A, Nakeeb A, Schmidt CM, Zyromski NJ, Ceppa E, Feliciano DV, Pitt HA. Optimal management of delayed gastric emptying after pancreatectomy: an analysis of 1,089 patients. Surgery. 2014;156:939–46. https://doi.org/10.1016/j.surg.2014.06.024.

55. Wente MN, Veit JA, Bassi C, Dervenis C, Fingerhut A, Gouma DJ, Izbicki JR, Neoptolemos JP, Padbury RT, Sarr MG, Yeo CJ, Büchler MW. Postpancreatectomy hemorrhage (PPH): an International Study Group of Pancreatic Surgery (ISGPS) definition. Surgery. 2007;142:20–5. https://doi.org/10.1016/j.surg.2007.02.001.

56. Rayar M, Sulpice L, Meunier B, Boudjema K. Enteral nutrition reduces delayed gastric emptying after standard pancreaticoduodenectomy with child reconstruction. J Gastrointest Surg. 2012;16:1004–11. https://doi.org/10.1007/s11605-012-1821-x.
57. Cawood AL, Elia M, Stratton RJ. Systematic review and meta-analysis of the effects of high protein oral nutritional supplements. Ageing Res Rev. 2012;11:278–96. https://doi.org/10.1016/j.arr.2011.12.008.
58. Stratton RJ, Hébuterne X, Elia M. A systematic review and meta-analysis of the impact of oral nutritional supplements on hospital readmissions. Ageing Res Rev. 2013;12:884–97. https://doi.org/10.1016/j.arr.2013.07.002.

Part VIII
Postoperative Complications

Chapter 33
Short-Term Morbidity After Pancreatectomy

Heather E. Matheny and Amir H. Fathi

Introduction

Pancreatic surgery, specifically pancreatoduodenectomy, has been considered a formidable surgical endeavor for many years [1]. The introduction of minimally invasive techniques and recent gradual adoption of the robotic approach in pancreatic surgery have added to its complexity.

Early publications from the 1960s have reported postoperative morbidity rates of 60% and mortality rates up to 25% [2]. However, sustained refinements of the surgical approach and improvement of patient modifiable risk factors have resulted in continued decline of these numbers. Crist et al. (1987) observed that, over a 17-year period, there was a gradual reduction of mortality from 11% to 2% as well as complications from 41% to 36%, respectively [3]. More recent series have corroborated these numbers and are confirmatory of continued downward trends in high-volume centers for pancreatic surgery [4].

Although the majority of perioperative complications are not life-threatening, they can result in prolonged hospitalizations and healthcare expenditures, and delays in adjuvant therapy for cancer patients, which have been proven imperative.

In this chapter, we seek to address the short-term complications associated with pancreatic surgery that are not addressed by the International Study Group of Pancreatic Surgery. These include surgical site infections, biliary fistulas, chyle leaks, and gastrointestinal anastomotic leaks after pancreatic resection.

H. E. Matheny
Vascular Surgery, University of Washington, Seattle, WA, USA
e-mail: HMatheny@uw.edus

A. H. Fathi (✉)
University of California San Francisco, Fresno MEP, Fresno, CA, USA
e-mail: Amir.Fathi@ucsf.edu

© The Author(s), under exclusive license to Springer Nature Switzerland AG 2025
E. P. Ceppa et al. (eds.), *The SAGES Manual of Evolving Techniques in Pancreatic Surgery*, https://doi.org/10.1007/978-3-031-78409-5_33

Surgical Site Infection After Pancreatectomy

Definition

Infectious complications associated with pancreatic surgery, such as superficial wound infections or deep incisional or organ/space infections, can result in decreased quality of life and other adverse effects including, but not limited to, increased healthcare costs, prolonged hospital stay, and in rare cases, increased mortality [4, 5].

The incidence of wound infection after pancreatoduodenectomy has been reported to be 6–17%, and intra-abdominal infection has been reported to occur in 2.5–23.3% of patients [1–7]. Anecdotally, these wide ranges in the infectious complication rates were attributed to the lack of uniform criteria to define infection after pancreatectomy [5].

In 1992, the Centers for Disease Control and Prevention (CDC) and National Nosocomial Infections Surveillance (NNIS) system modified the definition of surgical wound infection and changed the nomenclature to surgical site infection (SSI) [8]. Subsequently, in 1999, the Guidelines for Prevention of SSI were revised by the CDC. These guidelines define SSI as an infection occurring within 30- or 90-days following surgery where an implant is involved. This infection could involve the skin or subcutaneous tissue of the incisional region, deep soft tissues (e.g., fascial and muscle layers), or any part of the cavity, such as organ or spaces other than the incision, that was created or intervened during the operation [4, 9]. Therefore, SSIs are classified into three categories: superficial (i.e., skin or subcutaneous tissues), deep incisional (i.e., deep tissues of an incision), or organ/space (i.e., intra-abdominal) infections. Table 33.1 summarizes the CDC classification, definition, and criteria for diagnosis of these infections. To date, a plethora of publications have addressed the SSI in the general or gastrointestinal surgery field. However, few reports have evaluated the incidence and risk factors associated with SSI following pancreatic surgery according to the CDC's definitions and guidelines. In this section, we aim to outline the important findings of available publications.

Risk Factors

Among major pancreatic resections, pancreatoduodenectomy has been studied most frequently to determine the risk factors associated with SSIs. Nevertheless, the other types of pancreatic surgery share the majority of these findings. Table 33.2 summarizes the recent published studies that outline this association and risk factors. These risks factors include male sex, age over 70 years, malnutrition, perioperative biliary stents and drainage, pancreatic fistula, body mass index (BMI) indicating overweight or obesity, prior abdominal surgery, prolonged operative time (>480 min, >7 h), blood transfusion, and neoadjuvant systemic therapy [4, 5, 10–18]. It is worth

Table 33.1   Centers for Disease Control and Prevention (CDC) and Surgical Site Infection (SSI) classification, diagnostic criteria, and treatment suggestions

	Timeline	Location	Diagnostic criteria	Treatment
Superficial incisional SSI	Within 30 days after operation	Skin and subcutaneous tissue of the incision	Patient has at least **one** of the following: (a) Purulent drainage from the superficial incision (b) Organism(s) identified by a culture or non-culture-based microbiologic testing (c) Superficial incision that is deliberately opened by a provider and culture or non-culture-based testing of the incision is not performed **AND** patient has at least one of the following signs or symptoms: Localized pain or tenderness; localized swelling; erythema; or heat (d) Diagnosis of a superficial incisional SSI by a provider	Wound exploration, drainage of abscess/collection, obtaining cultures, debridement, and wash out Possible antibiotic therapy
Deep SSI	Within 30 or days after operation	Deep soft tissues of the incision (e.g., fascial and muscle layers)	Patient has at least one of the following: (a) Purulent drainage from the deep incision (b) A deep incision that spontaneously dehisces, or is deliberately opened or aspirated by a provider **AND** organism(s) identified from the deep soft tissues of the incision by a culture or non-culture-based microbiologic testing. **AND** patient has at least one of the following signs or symptoms: Fever (>38 °C); localized pain or tenderness (c) An abscess or other evidence of infection involving the deep incision that is detected on gross anatomical or histopathologic exam, or imaging test	Wound exploration in the operating room, drainage, debridement, and wash out Possible percutaneous drainage Possible exploratory laparotomy for source control Antibiotic therapy

(continued)

Table 33.1 (continued)

	Timeline	Location	Diagnostic criteria	Treatment
Organ/space SSI	Within 30 or days after operation	Any part of the body deeper than the fascial/muscle layers that are opened or manipulated during the operative procedure	Patient has at least one of the following: (a) PURULENT drainage from a drain that is placed into the organ/space (e.g., closed suction drainage system, open drain, T-tube drain, CT-guided drainage) (b) Organism(s) identified from fluid or tissue in the organ/space by a culture or non-culture-based microbiologic testing (c) An abscess or other evidence of infection involving the organ/space that is detected on gross anatomical or histopathologic exam, or imaging test evidence suggestive of infection **AND** meets at least one criterion for a specific organ/space infection site such as intra-abdominal infection	Possible percutaneous drainage High suspicion for leaks Possible exploratory laparotomy for source control Antibiotic therapy

mentioning that all the studies outlined in Table 33.2 are retrospective in nature. Differences in practice patterns such as type and frequency of prophylactic antibiotic dosing and redosing, quantity and frequency of abdominal irrigation throughout the case or before the closure, and the number of studied patients could impact the published association of risk factors with SSI in this table. Additionally, the relationship between blood transfusions and SSI is debatable since the data in the literature are contradictory.

Recently, neoadjuvant systemic therapy has been gaining popularity in the treatment of pancreatic cancer. Neoadjuvant chemotherapy has been identified as a risk factor for SSI in surgical treatment of rectal and breast cancer [16]. However, it has not previously been associated with SSI after pancreatic surgery [6, 16]. Based on their institutional data, Poruk et al. (2016) developed an innovative and internally validated risk stratification score for accurate prediction of the risk of SSI after pancreatoduodenectomy. The risk stratification score is established on neoadjuvant chemotherapy and biliary stent/drain placement. Based on their study utilizing this risk stratification score, a patient who received neoadjuvant chemotherapy and a preoperative biliary stent or drain had an estimated SSI risk of 64% [16]. The presence of one or both risk factors may account for the high rates of SSI after pancreatoduodenectomy and emphasizes the need for improved perioperative management [16].

Table 33.2 Risk factors associated with surgical site infection in recent publications

Author (year)	# of patients	Incidence of SSI (%)	Risk factor for SSI
Burkhart (2017) [10]	394	19.8	Preoperative biliary drainage, neoadjuvant therapy, prior abdominal surgery
Suragul (2020) [6]	280	32	Preoperative biliary drainage, pancreatic fistula, and preoperative cholangitis
Barreto (2015) [11]	277	35	Preoperative biliary stent, non-diabetic endocrine co-morbidity
Sugiura (2012) [5]	408	51	Long operative time, high BMI, pancreatic fistula, semi-close suction drain, main pancreatic duct <3 mm, abdominal wall fat thickness >10 mm
Zhang (2016) [12]	212	29	Pancreatic fistula, blood transfusion
Shinkawa (2018) [13]	106	14.2	Malnutrition, pancreatic fistula
Okano (2015) [14]	4147	27.1	Male sex, age 70 years or more, body mass index at least 25 kg/m^2, other previous malignancy, liver disease, bile contamination, duration of surgery 7 h or longer, intraoperative blood transfusion, soft pancreas
Gavazzi (2016) [15]	180	52.3	Preoperative biliary stent, cardiac disease, high BMI
Poluk (2016) [16]	679	17.2	Preoperative biliary drainage, neoadjuvant chemotherapy, neoadjuvant radiation, operative time >7 h, and blood transfusion, concomitant vascular resection, and absence of a superficial wound vacuum dressing

SSI Preventive Strategies

General Recommendations

The Surgical Care Improvement Project (SCIP) was implemented in 2006 with the goal of reducing surgical complications by 25% by the year 2010. However, multiple studies have suggested that implementation of the SCIP infection prevention measures did not yield measurable improvement in SSI at the patient or hospital levels [19]. Since then, there has been significant gravitation toward utilizing evidence-based measures such as care bundles (i.e., set of evidence-informed practices performed collectively and reliably to improve the quality of care) to improve surgical outcomes and decrease SSI. To date, unlike colorectal or cardiac surgery, no care bundles have been established for pancreatic surgery in order to reduce the incidence of SSI.

In 2017, the CDC updated their guidelines for the prevention of surgical site infections [20]. These guidelines are intended to provide new and updated evidence-based recommendations for the prevention of SSI. The pertinent recommendations to pancreatic surgery are briefly addressed below:

Antibiotic Prophylaxis

- The CDC recommends preoperative administration of parenteral antimicrobial prophylaxis in accordance with evidence-based standards.
- Evidence suggests uncertain trade-offs between the benefits and harms regarding intraoperative antimicrobial irrigation (e.g., intra-abdominal, deep, or subcutaneous tissues) for the prevention of SSI.
- The CDC recommends against application of antimicrobial agents (e.g., ointments, solutions, or powders) to the surgical incision for the prevention of SSI.

Glycemic Control

- The CDC recommends implementation of perioperative glycemic control and use of blood glucose target levels less than 200 mg/dL in patients with and without diabetes.

Normothermia

- The CDC recommends maintenance of perioperative normothermia. However, CDC does not identify randomized controlled trials that have evaluated strategies to achieve and maintain normothermia, the lower limit of normothermia, or the optimal timing and duration of normothermia for the prevention of SSI.

Oxygenation

- The CDC recommends administration of increased FiO_2 during surgery and after extubation in the immediate postoperative period for patients with normal pulmonary function undergoing general anesthesia with endotracheal intubation. The goal is to optimize tissue oxygen delivery.

Antiseptic Prophylaxis

- The CDC advises patients to shower or bathe (i.e., full body) with soap (e.g., antimicrobial or non-antimicrobial) or an antiseptic agent at least the night before the operation.

Pancreatectomy-Specific Recommendations

Modifiable Risk Factors

The extensive list of risk factors associated with SSI after pancreatic surgery under-lines the necessity of enhanced SSI risk stratification for these patients. Preoperative identification of the higher risk patients and implementation of optimization and preventative strategies are imperative to decrease SSI in the postoperative period. Special attention should be given to identification and optimization of patients' modifiable risk factors such as smoking, hypertension, diabetes, physical inactivity, and malnutrition prior to pancreatic surgery.

Preoperative Biliary Drainage and Antibiotic Prophylaxis

Bile provides an optimal substrate for many bacteria and fungi, particularly when the biliary tract has been instrumented. Preoperative diagnostic and therapeutic bili-ary system procedures such as biliary stenting and drainage have been associated with a significantly increased risk for various postoperative complications, includ-ing wound infections and intra-abdominal abscesses [15, 18]. Standard preoperative antibiotic prophylaxis for pancreatic surgery includes a first- or second-generation cephalosporin such as cefazolin or cefoxitin. However, recent studies have chal-lenged this standard approach in these patients. Our literature review suggests that piperacillin-tazobactam is an appropriate perioperative antibiotic for pancreatic operations [18]. Furthermore, a randomized control trial demonstrated that piperacillin-tazobactam significantly reduces SSIs compared to cefoxitin in patients undergoing open pancreatoduodenectomy. The trial also demonstrated lower SSI rates, reduced postoperative pancreatic fistula, and fewer complications such as *C. difficile* colitis and sepsis with piperacillin-tazobactam, supporting its use as standard care for these patients [21].

A study by Donald et al. (2013) has shown that the most common isolates from SSI after pancreatoduodenectomy are *Enterococcus* and *Enterobacter* species, which are not covered by SCIP-approved cephalosporins [22]. In support, a study by Ellis et al. (2023) has shown that reductions in SSI and clinically relevant post-operative pancreatic fistula in patients receiving piperacillin-tazobactam may be due to its effectiveness against cefoxitin-resistant biliary pathogens, particularly Enterobacter spp. and Enterococcus spp. [23]. This highlights the importance of selecting appropriate antibiotic prophylaxis based on pathogen resistance profiles to improve outcomes in pancreatoduodenectomy patients.

Furthermore, contrary to SCIP recommendation regarding discontinuation of prophylactic antibiotics within 24 h after the surgery end time, some studies suggest prolonged duration of antibiotic therapy up to 72 h postoperatively, especially in patients who have undergone preoperative biliary instrumentation. Japanese surgeons who use 72 h of perioperative antibiotics believe that surgical stress might weaken the host immune system, thereby increasing the risk of postoperative complications, including surgical site infections [18, 24].

The Role of Wound Protectors in Pancreatoduodenectomy

In pancreatoduodenectomy surgeries, the use of dual-ring wound protectors has been investigated as a method to reduce surgical site infections (SSIs), especially in patients with intrabiliary stents. Randomized clinical trials and systematic reviews have provided evidence supporting their efficacy [25–27]. These studies have demonstrated that intraoperative wound protectors can significantly lower the risk of SSIs by creating a physical barrier that minimizes direct contact between the surgical incision and potential infectious agents. This intervention has been highlighted as a simple yet effective strategy to enhance postoperative outcomes by reducing infection rates in such complex abdominal surgeries.

Prophylactic Negative Pressure Wound Therapy (NPWT)

In patients who are at high risk for wound complications, NPWT for closed abdominal fascial incisions may reduce SSI compared with conventional closure. In a meta-analysis of 31 trials, prophylactic NPWT reduced SSI compared with standard dressings [28]. Poruk et al. (2016) also determined that the use of a superficial vacuum-assisted closure device as NPWT markedly decreased the SSI rate in patients undergoing pancreatoduodenectomy. However, other studies have challenged the benefits associated with this type of prophylactic therapy and show no difference [29].

Diagnosis and Treatment

When SSI is suspected in a postoperative wound, the affected area should be examined meticulously by visual and tactile inspection. In a post-pancreatectomy patient, depending upon severity of signs and symptoms, the risk of other potential complications such as leaks or fistulas (e.g., pancreatic, biliary, and chyle) and anastomotic disruptions should be highly considered and ruled-out. Therefore, in the presence of clinical signs of a systemic infection, a low threshold is needed for ordering cross-sectional imaging.

The treatment options for SSIs are better delineated based on the type and extent of the involved tissue. Table 33.1 summarizes the potential treatment options based on the SSI classification.

The role of percutaneous and endoscopic drainage in managing fluid collections and treating organ and space SSIs following pancreatoduodenectomy is increasingly recognized [30]. These minimally invasive techniques offer an effective alternative to surgical intervention, reducing the patient's recovery time and improving outcomes. Recent publications have emphasized their importance in the postoperative management of pancreatic surgery complications, underscoring the advantages of these approaches in terms of both safety and efficacy in draining postoperative collections and mitigating the risk of infection.

Given the complexity of pancreatic surgeries and the high risk of SSIs, incorporating percutaneous and endoscopic drainage into the treatment algorithm can significantly impact patient care. By offering a less invasive means to address postoperative complications, these methods align with the broader goals of enhancing patient recovery, minimizing hospital stays, and reducing the overall burden of complications associated with pancreatoduodenectomy. Recent studies and systematic reviews have further validated these techniques, highlighting their role in improving surgical outcomes and patient quality of life post-surgery.

In summary, SSI can be classified into three categories: superficial (e.g., skin or subcutaneous tissues), deep (e.g., deep tissues of an incision), or organ/space (e.g., intra-abdominal) infections according to CDC criteria [31]. However, this is not specific for pancreatic surgery. Neoadjuvant chemotherapy and biliary stent/drain placement place patients at high risk for developing a SSI. In regard to pancreatic surgery, perioperative antibiotic prophylaxis should have broad coverage to include gram-negative isolates commonly identified within the biliary tract and may need to be continued up to 72 h after pancreatic surgery, unlike other intra-abdominal surgeries. Minimally invasive techniques, including percutaneous and endoscopic drainage, are frequently used to mitigate postoperative fluid collections. Lastly, SSI in any post-pancreatectomy patient should be evaluated for a concomitant complication.

Biliary Fistula

Definition

Biliary fistulas (synonymous with biliary leak and hepaticojejunostomy anastomotic leak) have been underreported and under-investigated in pancreatic surgery literature. This complication is rare when compared to the three most common complications (i.e., pancreatic fistula, delayed gastric emptying, and post-pancreatectomy hemorrhage) after pancreatectomy, leading to a paucity of data in the literature. Biliary fistula after pancreatectomy is reported with an incidence of 3–8% [32–34]. Similar to postoperative pancreatic fistulas and other pancreatectomy-specific complications, biliary fistulas range in severity from benign and of little clinical significance to severe and life-threatening. These usually pursue a benign course, but rarely may represent a life-threatening event, such as intra-abdominal sepsis, especially when associated with a second complication [35, 36].

Experience from high-volume centers has identified that patients with a biliary fistula were more likely to have a concomitant complication. Specific complications associated with biliary fistulas include pancreatic fistula, wound infection, delayed gastric emptying, and sepsis [32, 36]. Additionally, clinically insignificant, transient biliary fistulas following pancreatoduodenectomy can elevate the risk of developing biliary anastomotic stricture [34]. This association underlines the importance of closely monitoring and managing biliary fistulas post-surgery to mitigate the potential for long-term complications such as strictures, which can significantly impact patient outcomes and quality of life after this complex abdominal surgery. Even more pertinent, an accompanying complication must be ruled-out, as misdiagnosis of the actual location of the leak and possibility of increased morbidity might occur. For example, postoperative pancreatic fistula may present as bilious drainage from the intra-abdominal drains as bile leaks through a defect in the pancreaticojejunostomy. In this situation, obtaining a fistulogram through the abdominal drain can aid in the correct diagnosis and demonstrate the location of the leak [35, 37]. Taking into consideration the serious complications that may result from a biliary fistula, care must be taken to recognize the complication early and identify ways to reduce the occurrence and mitigate further sequelae with aggressive treatment.

Diagnosis

While there is no consensus, the International Study Group for Liver Surgery (ISGLS) has proposed that the diagnosis of a biliary fistula may be established using clinical and laboratory analysis, being defined as "a bilirubin concentration in the drain fluid at least three times the serum bilirubin concentration on or after postoperative day 3, or as the need for radiologic or operative intervention resulting from biliary collections or bile peritonitis" [38]. In the majority of patients in one case series, the diagnosis was suggested with bilious drainage noted in a surgically placed drain [36]. Compared to duodenojejunal leaks, which typically present more than a week after surgery, biliary leaks present much sooner. On average, a biliary leak can be identified by postoperative day 5 (range: postoperative day 1–17) [39]. In most patients, placement of an intra-abdominal drain at the time of surgery not only allowed for the detection of an early biliary fistula, but these patients were less ill during the postoperative course. This was likely due to the early drainage of the biliary fistula. Furthermore, by having a drain already in place, there was a decreased need for additional interventions [36]. The routine placement of abdominal drains for this purpose is still a topic that requires further elucidation.

Biliary fistulas can also be identified with various imaging modalities when the diagnosis cannot be made by bilious drainage. A computed tomography (CT) scan may show a fluid collection near the hepaticojejunostomy anastomosis. However, given its adjacency to the pancreatic anastomosis, it can be difficult to delineate between a biliary fistula and pancreatic fistula based on CT scan findings alone. Fistulogram is another useful imaging technique whereby passage of a contrast medium through the biliary anastomosis from the surgical drainage can demonstrate the passage of contrast medium into the jejunal limb and the biliary tract through the biliary anastomosis, identifying the leak and supporting the diagnosis [39]. Magnetic resonance imaging is another option, which can demonstrate the presence of a fluid collection and, in combination with the use of liver-specific contrast agents (e.g., gadobenate dimeglumine and gadoxetate disodium), also support the diagnosis of a biliary fistula [37].

Classification

The utility of classification systems permits for proper evaluation and risk stratification and offers proposed management for various disease processes and complications. Unfortunately, there is no currently standardized classification or grading of biliary fistula after pancreatectomy. There are, however, three different classifications reported in the literature (Table 33.3). These include a system proposed by the ISGLS (2011), the classification by Burkhart et al. (2013), which is modeled after the International Study Group on Pancreatic Surgery (ISGPS) for postoperative pancreatic fistula, and the Modified Accordion Classification, proposed by Miller et al. (2013), which applies to all fistulas different from postoperative pancreatic fistula following pancreatoduodenectomy [40]. The modified accordion assigns each patient from grade 1 to 6 based on the severity of the complication profile. Each of these classifications has been validated by an independent research group and noted to be reliable and accurate, albeit with some overlap observed between the classification groups [32].

Comparison of biliary fistula classification systems Table 33.3.

The ISGLS proposed classification will be discussed further in this chapter as it relates to diagnosis and management. This classification system grades biliary fistulas, grade A to C, after biliary and pancreatic surgery based on the significance this complication has on a patients' clinical management.

Grade A bile leaks can be mild or be of little significance to the overall health of the patient. These leaks tend to be low volume, with the amount decreasing over time. Radiologic imaging (CT scans, fistulograms) is not needed in most cases. If CT imaging is performed, normal postoperative findings may be seen (e.g., perihepatic fluid collection, acute anastomotic edema, and peripancreatic fat stranding), which are usually not associated with clinical findings [37]. Fistulograms may be better able to facilitate a diagnosis as they are better able to define anatomy. Management generally requires continued abdominal drainage and may require drain repositioning or upsizing. Moreover, if a drain is found to be in contact with the leak, the drain may need to be withdrawn from the leak to allow for closure of the fistula. Antibiotics are generally not necessary. Persistent drainage via an

Table 33.3 Comparison of current biliary fistula classifications

ISGLS classification	Burkhart et al. classification	Modified accordion classification
A. Bile leak requiring no or little change in patients' clinical management	A. Bilious drainage, no infection Diagnosed with fistulogram Continue drainage via surgical drains	0. Evidence of leak, but no intervention
		1. Discharge with original surgical drain or treatment of fistula by NPO alone
B. Bile leak requiring a change in patients' management (additional diagnostic or interventional procedure) but without re-laparotomy or bile leak that lasts more than 1 week	B. Bile leak requiring a change in patients' management (additional diagnostic or interventional procedure) but without re-laparotomy or bile leak that lasts more than 1 week	2. Use of therapeutic octreotide, antibiotic, artificial nutrition
		3. Percutaneous drain placement, interventional procedures, any short general anesthesia needed for leak management (e.g., complex wound management)
C. Bile leak that requires re-laparotomy	C. Severe infection, increased level of care in ICU, output >250 mL/day for three or more days, patient death. Diagnosed with CT scan and fistulogram	4. Reoperation or single organ failure secondary to the leak
		5. Reoperation with single organ failure secondary to the leak Multi-system (2 or more) organ failure secondary to the leak
		6. Death attributable to the leak

intra-abdominal drain after the seventh postoperative day should be classified as a Grade B bile leak.

Grade B bile leaks are defined as a complication requiring an alteration in the patients' clinical management that does not require re-laparotomy. The illness severity of the patient is moderately increased as a result of an uncontrolled leak. These patients may present with signs of mild infection, such as fever and/or abdominal discomfort. Radiologic imaging can be performed and may demonstrate perianastomotic fluid. Surgically placed drains are commonly left in place, yet, they may not be adequately controlling the leak. Thus, additional procedures such as percutaneous transhepatic biliary drainage, endoscopic retrograde cholangiography with intrahepatic stent placement, or percutaneous intra-abdominal drainage of fluid collections may be warranted. Antibiotics may be needed to control infection if present. These patients also have extended hospital stays and may need to be discharged with a drain in place and close outpatient follow-up.

Grade C bile leaks are the most severe and require re-laparotomy to control the leak. Patients often have signs of sepsis, severe abdominal pain, or biliary peritonitis. It may be associated with multisystem organ failure and can be life-threatening. These patients should be closely monitored in an intensive care unit. Radiographic imaging should be obtained, and findings would be similar to those seen in Grade B leaks. Attempts at surgical control might include suture reinforcement of leakage sites, washout of intra-abdominal fluid collections, and reconstruction of the anastomosis if needed. Continued abdominal drainage is essential. Similar to Grade B bile leaks, percutaneous and/or endoscopic interventions may be beneficial in management. Nutritional support is also essential after a re-laparotomy, and patients may benefit from a needle catheter jejunostomy of nasojejunal feeding tube placed at the time of surgical revision. Finally, these patients also have prolonged hospital courses given the severity of disease and the resultant complications that follow.

Risk Factors

Biliary fistulas appear to have a multifactorial etiology, with several studies reporting different risk factors [32, 36, 39]. Patient factors such as male gender, older age, low preoperative albumin (i.e., marker of nutrition status), high BMI, and combined liver resection have been associated with the risk of developing a biliary fistula [36, 39, 41]. Technical factors during the operation also appear to contribute to the success or failure of a hepaticojejunostomy. Smaller size of the common bile duct (≤5 mm) is consistently reported as a risk factor for biliary leak, while the level of duct transection and condition of remaining blood supply have also been traditionally reported as an important variable. Theoretically, anastomoses created well below the hilum (e.g., choledochojejunostomy) have a higher risk of leak compared to hepaticojejunostomy, but the supporting literature is very limited [42]. Excessive dissection and skeletonization of the common bile duct, as well as ligation of the hepatic arteries can lead to ischemic cholangiopathy. To achieve adequate vascularization, the bile duct should be resected at the level of the hepatic duct, above the cystic duct but below the confluence. The common hepatic duct blood supply comes from the hepatic arteries, in contrast to the right and left hepatic ducts, which are supplied by hilar plate vessels. Furthermore, the inferior portion of the common bile duct is vascularized by the gastroduodenal artery, which is ligated during a pancreatoduodenectomy, thus increasing the risk of ischemic cholangiopathy and consequently increasing the risk of biliary fistula in the early postoperative course and stricture later on [39]. Careful handling of tissues and meticulous attention to suture placement and knot tying have also been reported to decrease rates of biliary fistula [36].

Mitigating Factors and Treatment Options

When a biliary fistula occurs, a technical error must always be considered. These may include suture line disruption, failure to include adequate bile duct within the anastomosis, and ischemia of the bile duct as previously mentioned. Meticulous suture technique with duct-to-mucosa anastomosis prevents a large proportion of fistulas. In addition, secondary causes, such as adjacent abscess formation and tissue ischemia, either from the duct or bowel, can contribute to suture line disruption. Again, it is imperative to determine whether the fistula is exclusively biliary, or whether a concomitant pancreatic leak is present. Hepaticojejunostomy and combined leaks following pancreatoduodenectomy, though less common than pancreatojejunostomy leaks, significantly elevate the risk of major morbidity and mortality [43]. These complications necessitate prompt recognition and management to mitigate adverse outcomes and ensure patient recovery. Their rarity does not diminish the critical nature of their impact, underscoring the need for meticulous surgical technique and vigilant postoperative care.

Reconstruction techniques such as running suture versus interrupted suture, size of suture (i.e., 5–0 versus 6–0), temporary placement of a biliary stent during suture placement, percutaneous biliary drainage, and intraoperative T-tube placement are among many attempted protective measures with minimal effect [35, 39]. However, to date there is no data from randomized trials comparing interrupted versus continuous suture technique in hepaticojejunostomy, thus most surgeons prefer to fashion the anastomosis with a continuous running suture for dilated bile ducts and interrupted for non-dilated ($\leq$5 mm). It is worth mentioning that a group in Japan evaluated intraoperative hepaticojejunostomy leak testing using indwelling transhepatic biliary drainage catheters [44]. When a leak test was performed and was normal, these authors did not observe a bile leak suggesting that this step may decrease its incidence, although further validation is needed.

In summary, biliary fistulas are rare. They can be minor and associated with no additional morbidity to the patient, or they can be severe and life-threatening. The presence of bile in the postsurgical intra-abdominal drain is an important finding to suggest this complication. Biliary fistulas rarely occur alone and may be associated with a second complication, and thus it is important to consider the differential diagnosis when a biliary fistula is suspected. Meticulous surgical technique with consideration of specific risk factors can help reduce the incidence of biliary fistula after pancreatectomy. There is a notable correlation between transient biliary fistula and an elevated risk of biliary anastomotic stricture among patients undergoing pancreatoduodenectomy. This association underscores the potential of transient biliary fistula as a significant predictor of postoperative complications, emphasizing the importance of early detection and management of transient biliary fistula to mitigate the risk of biliary anastomotic stricture development and improve patient outcomes following pancreatoduodenectomy. While there is no consensus on classification, several models exist that can aid in diagnosis and treatment. Treatment decisions should reflect the degree of leak and clinical status of the patient. For instance, mild leaks do not necessarily require percutaneous interventions, while critically ill patients require prompt and aggressive care, potentially with repeat laparotomy.

Chyle Leak

Definition

Chyle leaks are an important clinical complication after pancreatic surgery. However, chyle leaks are not limited to pancreatic surgery and can be a complication seen in many operations including thoracic (e.g., aortic and esophageal) and abdominal operations that involve retroperitoneal dissection or extensive lymph node dissections. The incidence of chyle leak after pancreatectomy varies widely in the literature from 1% to 11% [45–48]. This may be due to lack of standardized definition at the time of publications, surgical case volume, differences in surgical techniques, extent of lymph node dissection, differences in postoperative management, and time to enteral intake. Post-pancreatectomy chyle leaks may be attributable to the close vicinity of the cisterna chyli and its tributaries [49, 50].

Chyle consists of intestinal lymphatic fluid that is high in fat-soluble vitamins and long-chain triglycerides carried by chylomicrons. Its milky appearance is attributable to its high fat component. Therefore, with the loss of chyle, patients are susceptible to malnutrition. Lymphatic fluid also contains lymphocytes and immunoglobulins, which is also relevant because loss of chyle by way of a leak results in lymphocytopenia, predisposing these patients to infection-related complications [51]. Therefore, early diagnosis and appropriate treatment are imperative.

Diagnosis

Using the ISGPS definition of chyle leak, the diagnosis is generally simple to make and can often be established by the character of the drain output in the correct clinical context. When the definition is used (i.e., triglyceride level at least 110 mg/dL), a large percentage of chyle leaks also demonstrate a milky or white appearance of the drainage outflow [53]. The typical manifestation of a chyle leak is the new onset of milky, white drainage from a drain that was once transparent peritoneal fluid. It is important to note that this can occur around the same time that a postoperative pancreatic fistula is typically diagnosed: postoperative day 5–7, when a patient has usually returned to oral feeding with solid food [52]. Generally, characterization of the drain output is all that is needed to distinguish between these two leaks (i.e., clear to cloudy tan pancreatic fluid versus milky white chylous fluid). To further support the diagnosis of a chyle leak, a sample of fluid from the drain can be sent to the laboratory and analyzed for triglyceride level, where a value of 110 mg/dL is needed to confirm the diagnosis. Likewise, drain fluid should be analyzed for amylase as a concomitant postoperative pancreatic fistula may be present.

After a chyle leak is diagnosed, it is important to determine if the leak is contained or free-flowing ascites, again, because the treatments are often different. A detailed history and physical examination can aid in differentiating between the two. Chylous ascites can present with painless and worsening abdominal distention in the postoperative period. Studies have reported that the most common complaint is abdominal distension followed by pain or peritonitis [45]. If the diagnosis is still not clear, a CT scan can be obtained showing peritoneal ascites [50].

Classification

At the same time the ISGPS derived a definition for chyle leak, they also defined a classification system, Grade A to C, based on severity and management of this complication (Table 33.4) [52]. Grade A leak is defined as one that can be managed conservatively by dietary restrictions. These leaks have little clinical implication and no increase in length of hospital stay. Grade B leak requires one of the following criteria: nasoenteral nutrition with dietary restriction and/or total parenteral nutrition (TPN), maintenance of the surgical drains or placement of new percutaneous catheter drainage by interventional radiology, or pharmacotherapy (e.g., octreotide) to control the chyle leak. These patients also have prolonged hospitalizations. Furthermore, patients may be discharged with an intra-abdominal drain. Grade C leaks require additional treatment which may include an interventional radiology procedure such as lymphatic embolization (also known as sclerosis) and/or reoperation. Patients who are initially classified as Grade B but later require additional invasive treatment should be reclassified as Grade C. These patients can be critically ill, necessitating admission to an intensive care unit, and have prolonged hospital courses. While this classification system has clinical relevance to isolated chyle leaks, it remains cognizant that patients may be harboring concomitant complications. In situations where more than one complication exists (e.g., postoperative pancreatic fistula with high drain amylase and chyle leak with high drain triglycerides), simultaneous use of grading systems should be utilized.

Table 33.4 ISGPS consensus grading system for isolated chyle leak after pancreatic resection

	Grade A	Grade B	Grade C
Therapeutic consequence	None or oral dietary restrictions[a]	Nasoenteral nutrition with dietary restriction[a] and /or TPN, percutaneous drainage by IR, maintenance of surgical drains, or drug (e.g., octreotide) treatment	Other invasive in-hospital treatment[b], admission to ICU and/or mortality[c]
Discharge with (surgical) drain or readmission[c]	No	Possibly	Possibly
Prolonged hospital stay[c]	No	Yes	Yes

TPN total parenteral Nutrition, IR interventional radiology, ICU intensive care unit [H]
[a] No-fat diet with/without medium-chain-triglyceride
[b] Interventional radiology (excluding percutaneous drainage) or reoperation
[c] Related directly to the chyle leak

ISGPS consensus grading system for isolated chyle leak after pancreatic resection. TPN, total parenteral nutrition; IR, interventional radiology, ICU intensive care unit [52] Table 33.4.

Risk Factors

Review of literature regarding the risk for development of chyle leak reveals insight into several factors. First, patient demographics, such as age, sex, American Society of Anesthesiologists grade III–IV, and higher BMI, have inconsistent conclusions [52, 54–56]. The significance of neoadjuvant therapy on chyle leak largely remains unknown [56]. Open versus minimally invasive technique, vascular resection, and splenectomy versus spleen-preservation, did affect the reported leak rate in a recent systematic review [47]. Pathology-related risk factors predicting increased risk include lymph node dissection (i.e., dissection of paraaortic nodes, increased number of positive nodes, and total number of lymph nodes harvested), dissection within root of superior mesenteric artery, malignant diseases, lymphovascular invasion, and chronic pancreatitis [46, 52, 53, 56].

A more thorough discussion on operative risk factors is warranted as direct operative trauma to the main chyle duct, its branches, or lymph node basins is believed to be a major cause of chyle leak [52]. As briefly mentioned above, the risk increases with extended resections and has been demonstrated to positively correlate with the number of lymph nodes harvested [45, 46, 48]. The cisterna chyli, or origin of the thoracic duct, is located deep to the head of the pancreas; therefore, it is vulnerable during pancreatic surgery and lymph node dissection [42, 52]. Dissection around the pancreas can lead to disruption of the mesenteric lymphatic plexus. However, there are conflicting studies regarding this as a potential etiology despite the anatomic reasoning. Assumpcao et al. (2008) reported that extensive lymph node harvesting during pancreatic surgery increased the relative risk of chyle leak, while in contrast, [57] reported similar numbers of harvested lymph nodes between the chyle leak and non-chyle-leak groups. Thus, more investigation is warranted.

Mitigating Factors and Treatment Options

There is currently no consensus on the treatment of chyle leaks. Management of chyle leaks can often be achieved with conservative measures and dietary modifications. The treatment is intended to control drain output until the leak closes. Enteric lymphatics absorb long-chain triglycerides, so by initiating a low-fat diet or TPN, the lymph flow will decrease, thereby facilitating closure of the low volume leak [45, 58]. Medium-chain triglycerides are an acceptable source of calories because they are absorbed across enterocytes into the mesenteric venous circulation and not enteral lymphatics. Moreover, from a pathophysiologic standpoint, TPN is another practical treatment option as fat is delivered parenterally, thereby bypassing the enteral lymphatics. However, TPN is expensive and fraught with its own complications (e.g., peripherally inserted central catheter infections, liver toxicity, and electrolyte imbalances). The administration of somatostatin or octreotide (long-acting somatostatin) has also been reported to be beneficial since these hormones reduce intestinal fat absorption and decrease lymph excretion [45, 50]. The implementation of these as single modality treatments results in low success rates, but case reports have suggested that a combination of these treatments is more successful [45, 59]. Further guidance toward treatment can be made with the assessment of drain output as being low (i.e., <200 mL/day) or high (i.e., >200 mL/day). This determination will be helpful in guiding the route of nutrition (i.e., enteral versus TPN) and the need for somatostatin as patients with lower drain output can be treated with a low-fat diet or medium-chain triglycerides, compared to patients with higher drain output who are more likely to need TPN and/or somatostatin. High-volume output also necessitates more vigilant nutritional and electrolyte support since more fluid is lost.

The ISGPS has suggested a step-up approach beginning with dietary restrictions (e.g., restricted long-chain triglycerides, low-fat diet with medium-chain triglycerides). If no decrease in the drain output is seen over time, TPN can be considered. A small percentage of chyle leaks will be refractory to the conservative measures discussed above and may require more direct and invasive treatment strategies. These may include lymphatic embolization, a peritoneovenous shunt to decompress chyle from the peritoneum into the systemic circulation, and the use of lymphangiography to define the site of chyle leak for operative intervention [52]. Research is limited, and the reported results are poor [46, 58, 59]. Success from open surgical ligation of chyle leaks after pancreatectomy is very limited and is considered a last resort as it carries a high morbidity rate [46, 58].

Patients who are diagnosed with chylous ascites present a different problem as mentioned previously. The management of chylous ascites includes restricting oral intake, TPN, and octreotide [45, 47, 50]. The goal is to decrease the triglyceride content while also limiting caloric losses. Due to large volume losses, close attention should be placed on fluid and nutrient balance with appropriate adjustments made in TPN. The actual change in quantity of drain output will be more variable. The time to closure can take up to several months, so these patients should be prepared for prolonged treatment courses.

There are currently no evidence-based recommendations on the timing of drain removal. On the other hand, there are also no reported deleterious effects of early drain removal [60, 61]. Members of the ISGPS noted that drain removal can be attempted after negative cultures in combination with closure of past drain sites [52].

In summary, chyle leaks are a rare but potentially morbid complication associated with pancreatectomy. Early recognition is imperative to minimize effects of the associated malnutrition and immunosuppression due to loss of fats, lymphocytes, and immunoglobulins. The diagnosis can be made by observing milky drain output and/or by analyzing the triglyceride content in the drain fluid. It is important to further differentiate between a contained chyle leak and chylous ascites as the management and prognosis are different. The majority of chyle leaks will resolve on their own within a few weeks with conservative management (e.g., low-fat diet, TPN ± somatostatin, and drain management). For patients who are maintained on an enteral diet, long-chain triglycerides should be removed from the diet by either a nonfat diet or low-fat medium-chain triglyceride diet to decrease lymphatic flow. Refractory chyle leaks are most often associated with chylous ascites and may require additional interventions such as sclerotic embolization or open surgical ligation, which should be reserved as a last resort due to the high morbidity.

Gastrojejunal or Duodenojejunal Anastomotic Leak

Definition

A pancreatoduodenectomy is a complex and laborious operation because at least three anastomoses are performed after the disease has been resected. In a classic pancreatoduodenectomy according to Whipple, three anastomoses are made between the pancreas, biliary tract, and alimentary tract: pancreaticojejunal, hepaticojejunal, and gastrojejunal, respectively. Alternatively, in the pylorus-preserving operation, a duodenojejunal anastomosis is created instead of a gastrojejunal anastomosis. Failure of gastrojejunal or duodenojejunal anastomosis has a very low occurrence rate, reported in less than 1–2% of patients after a pancreatoduodenectomy [62–65], but reoperation is usually required leading to longer hospitalization and sequelae. To date, there are very few publications that have focused on this complication.

Although there is no consensus definition for enteric anastomotic leakage, several terms such as anastomotic failure, defect, or dehiscence have been used interchangeably to describe this complication. Gastrojejunal or duodenojejunal anastomotic failure in some studies has been defined as leakage confirmed during re-laparotomy or the radiological presence of perianastomotic air, fluid, or extravasation of contrast material [62, 64].

Diagnosis

Anastomotic leaks at the gastrojejunal or duodenojejunal location typically occur 7–10 days after the initial operation [62, 64]. The diagnosis or clinical suspicion of an anastomotic leak is generally based on clinical presentation alone. Cross-sectional imaging may be useful if the diagnosis remains uncertain. Clinical presentation may include non-specific signs such as tachycardia, fever, abdominal pain, purulent or increased drain output, oliguria, and nausea and/or vomiting [64]. Other possible, but less common signs are peritonitis or an enterocutaneous fistula through the surgical wound [62, 64]. In one published series of patients, leukocytosis was also a common finding, with nearly half of the patients demonstrating a white blood cell count greater than 30,000 cells/mm^2 [64].

Radiographic evidence for an anastomotic leak is usually present when imaging is obtained. Common findings include free air on plain film or CT scan, the presence of a fluid collection adjacent to the level of anastomosis or extravasation of contrast on a fistulogram or upper gastrointestinal series if oral contrast is used [37, 38, 66, 67]. Intra-abdominal abscesses may develop secondary to leakage from gastrojejunostomy or duodenojejunostomy anastomoses [64], but also from the pancreatic anastomosis lying posteriorly. It is also useful to understand normal postoperative CT scan findings obtained within the early postoperative period as they can appear similar to a pathologic process. Common benign CT findings include mild fluid, anastomotic edema, free air, and fluid collections [37, 67]. These early findings should not be misinterpreted as an anastomotic leak unless they are found in the correct clinical context.

Classification

There is currently no universal, objective classification or grading system for anastomotic leaks pertaining to gastrojejunal or duodenojejunal anastomosis after pancreatic surgery. Winter et al. (2008) and Eshius et al. (2014) assessed these complications according to the Clavien Dindo criteria (2004) and found that all patients were considered "severe," Grade III or greater. This contrasts with more frequently occurring complications such as pancreatic fistulas, in which only 25–40% of patients were classified as "severe" [63, 64]. Thus, given the high morbidity, pancreatic surgeons should be cognizant of this complication.

Risk Factors

The etiology of an anastomotic leak is multifactorial, but it has not yet been fully elucidated. There are several possible factors that have been identified. Preoperative risk factors include BUN-to-creatinine ratio >20, neoadjuvant radiotherapy, and low serum hemoglobin [62, 64], although results are not consistent across studies [63]. Intraoperative risk factors include intraoperative blood loss greater than 1000 mL, blood transfusion, longer operative time, total pancreatectomy, and additional surgical resections in addition to the pancreatectomy [62–64]. Taken as a whole, the majority of these risk factors are potential surrogates for impairment of anastomotic blood supply (e.g., preoperative hypovolemia, large volume blood loss, and perioperative hypotension) or gastric venous congestion (i.e., total pancreatectomy with splenectomy with ligation of splenic vein, short gastric vessels, and both right and left gastric veins). Furthermore, patients who are diagnosed with an anastomotic leak also have an increased incidence of concomitant leak from the pancreatic anastomosis which may also support the importance of maintaining an adequate blood supply. However, this may also be due to the erosive effect of the pancreatic enzymes on the nearby healing anastomoses; however, additional evidence is lacking, and anastomotic leaks still occur after total pancreatectomies [62, 63].

Mitigating Factors and Treatment Options

The ideal gastrojejunostomy or duodenojejunostomy technique for pancreatic surgery has not yet been identified. The literature comparing surgical techniques is limited, and no randomized control trials have been conducted to evaluate its impact on postoperative anastomotic leak. However, a few factors have been reported based on retrospective findings. Much of the field of surgery relies on surgeon experience, and meticulous adherence to operative techniques has been shown to serve an important role in decreasing complications. A large retrospective study on gastrojejunostomy leaks demonstrated an approximately 40% reduction in leaks as the surgeons gained more experience [68]. It is imperative to adhere to basic principles of surgical technique as all anastomoses need to have an adequate blood supply, be free from tension, and be properly oriented without twists or kinks.

There are also various techniques that can be used to create a gastroenteric or enteroenteric anastomosis. Depending on surgeon preference, either a stapled or two-layer hand-sewn anastomosis may be chosen without affecting the postoperative morbidity or mortality [69, 70]. Additionally, in the literature, there has been no significant difference reported between the pylorus-preserving pancreatoduodenectomy compared to the classic Whipple procedure in terms of anastomotic leakage rates [65, 71]. Nevertheless, given the sparse evidence that currently exists, which is principally retrospective studies, it is difficult to gather conclusive recommendations on the superiority of one anastomotic technique over the other.

When a leak is suspected, early surgical management is the mainstay of treatment to confirm and repair the leak, remove extraluminal enteric contents, and place closed-suction drains [62, 64]. At re-laparotomy, a distal gastrectomy with gastrojejunostomy is performed in most patients, with a minority of patients undergoing revision or repair of the failure site [62–64]. Repair of the anastomosis may be difficult due to friability of the acutely inflamed tissues. In such cases, placement of drains may be the safest option. It is also recommended to place a nasogastric tube to decompress the stomach during the first days after surgical revision and to fashion a needle catheter jejunostomy to provide adequate energy and protein intake via enteral nutrition, which represents a key aspect for postoperative tissue healing. Winter et al. (2008) reported one patient who was treated with multiple percutaneous drains alone to control intra-abdominal collection, yet this patient had a longer postoperative course compared to patients treated with re-laparotomy. There is additional limited literature discussing conservative management with improved outcomes, which may be due to advancements in radiological interventions and technology [63].

In summary, duodenojejunal and gastrojejunal leaks following major pancreatic resection have been poorly investigated compared to other more frequently occurring complications such as postoperative pancreatic fistula and post-pancreatectomy hemorrhage. There is no consensus definition, classification, or grading system. The diagnosis is based upon clinical signs and symptoms, and radiographic imaging. A high index of suspicion is necessary to make an early diagnosis of an anastomotic leak as they are associated with high morbidity and mortality. The majority of cases with this complication type require surgical reoperation.

References

1. Yeo CJ, Cameron JL, Sohn TA, Lillemoe KD, Pitt HA, Talamini MA, et al. Six hundred fifty consecutive pancreaticoduodenectomies in the 1990s: pathology, complications, and outcomes. Ann Surg. 1997;226(3):248–57; discussion 257–260
2. Stojadinovic A, Brooks A, Hoos A, Jaques DP, Conlon KC, Brennan MF. An evidence-based approach to the surgical management of resectable pancreatic adenocarcinoma. J Am Coll Surg. 2003;196(6):954–64.
3. Crist DW, Sitzmann JV, Cameron JL. Improved hospital morbidity, mortality, and survival after the Whipple procedure. Ann Surg. 1987;206(3):358–65.
4. Suragul W, Rungsakulkij N, Vassanasiri W, Tangtawee P, Muangkaew P, Mingphruedhi S, et al. Predictors of surgical site infection after pancreaticoduodenectomy. BMC Gastroenterol. 2020;20(1):201.
5. Sugiura T, Uesaka K, Ohmagari N, Kanemoto H, Mizuno T. Risk factor of surgical site infection after pancreaticoduodenectomy. World J Surg. 2012;36(12):2888–94.
6. Ho CK, Kleeff J, Friess H, Büchler MW. Complications of pancreatic surgery. HPB (Oxford). 2005;7(2):99–108.
7. Adam U, Makowiec F, Riediger H, Schareck WD, Benz S, Hopt UT. Risk factors for complications after pancreatic head resection. Am J Surg. 2004;187(2):201–8.
8. Horan TC, Gaynes RP, Martone WJ, Jarvis WR, Emori TG. CDC definitions of nosocomial surgical site infections, 1992: a modification of CDC definitions of surgical wound infections. Infect Control Hosp Epidemiol. 1992;13(10):606–8.
9. Mangram AJ, Horan TC, Pearson ML, Silver LC, Jarvis WR. Guideline for prevention of surgical site infection, 1999. Centers for disease control and prevention (CDC) hospital infection control practices advisory committee. Am J Infect Control. 1999;27(2):97–132. quiz 133–4; discussion 96
10. Burkhart RA, Javed AA, Ronnekleiv-Kelly S, Wright MJ, Poruk KE, Eckhauser F, et al. The use of negative pressure wound therapy to prevent post-operative surgical site infections following pancreaticoduodenectomy. HPB (Oxford). 2017;19(9):825–31.
11. Barreto SG, Singh MK, Sharma S, Chaudhary A. Determinants of surgical site infections following pancreatoduodenectomy. World J Surg. 2015;39(10):2557–63.
12. Zhang L, Liao Q, Zhang T, Dai M, Zhao Y. Blood transfusion is an independent risk factor for postoperative serious infectious complications after pancreaticoduodenectomy. World J Surg. 2016;40(10):2507–12.
13. Shinkawa H, Takemura S, Uenishi T, Sakae M, Ohata K, Urata Y, et al. Nutritional risk index as an independent predictive factor for the development of surgical site infection after pancreaticoduodenectomy. Surg Today. 2013;43(3):276–83.
14. Okano K, Hirao T, Unno M, Fujii T, Yoshitomi H, Suzuki S, et al. Postoperative infectious complications after pancreatic resection. Br J Surg. 2015;102(12):1551–60.

15. Gavazzi F, Ridolfi C, Capretti G, Angiolini MR, Morelli P, Casari E, et al. Role of preoperative biliary stents, bile contamination and antibiotic prophylaxis in surgical site infections after pancreaticoduodenectomy. BMC Gastroenterol. 2016;16:43.
16. Poruk KE, Lin JA, Cooper MA, He J, Makary MA, Hirose K, et al. A novel, validated risk score to predict surgical site infection after pancreaticoduodenectomy. HPB (Oxford). 2016;18(11):893–9.
17. Sutton JM, Kooby DA, Wilson GC, Squires MH, Hanseman DJ, Maithel SK, et al. Perioperative blood transfusion is associated with decreased survival in patients undergoing pancreatico-duodenectomy for pancreatic adenocarcinoma: a multi-institutional study. J Gastrointest Surg. 2014;18(9):1575–87.
18. Fathi AH, Jackson T, Siegel K, Siegel C. Incidence of postoperative infectious complications in complex hepatopancreatobiliary surgery utilizing preoperative broad spectrum antibiotic and antifungal coverage in conjunction with intraoperative cultures. HBP Surg. 2016;2016:3031749.
19. Hawn MT, Vick CC, Richman J, Holman W, Deierhoi RJ, Graham LA, et al. Surgical site infection prevention: time to move beyond the surgical care improvement program. Ann Surg. 2011;254(3):494–9; discussion 499–501
20. Berríos-Torres SI, Umscheid CA, Bratzler DW, Leas B, Stone EC, Kelz RR, et al. Centers for disease control and prevention guideline for the prevention of surgical site infection, 2017. JAMA Surg. 2017;152(8):784–91.
21. D'Angelica MI, Ellis RJ, Liu JB, Brajcich BC, Gönen M, Thompson VM, Cohen ME, Seo SK, Zabor EC, Babicky ML, Bentrem DJ, Behrman SW, Bertens KA, Celinski SA, Chan CHF, Dillhoff M, Dixon MEB, Fernandez-Del Castillo C, Gholami S, House MG, Karanicolas PJ, Lavu H, Maithel SK, McAuliffe JC, Ott MJ, Reames BN, Sanford DE, Sarpel U, Scaife CL, Serrano PE, Smith T, Snyder RA, Talamonti MS, Weber SM, Yopp AC, Pitt HA, Ko CY. Piperacillin-tazobactam compared with cefoxitin as antimicrobial prophylaxis for pancre-atoduodenectomy: a randomized clinical trial. JAMA. 2023;329(18):1579–88.
22. Donald GW, Sunjaya D, Lu X, Chen F, Clerkin B, Eibl G, et al. Perioperative antibiotics for surgical site infection in pancreaticoduodenectomy: does the SCIP-approved regimen provide adequate coverage? Surgery. 2013;154(2):190–6.
23. Ellis RJ, Brajcich BC, Bertens KA, Chan CHF, Castillo CF, Karanicolas PJ, Maithel SK, Reames BN, Weber SM, Vidri RJ, Pitt HA, Thompson VM, Gonen M, Seo SK, Yopp AC, Ko CY, D'Angelica MI. Association between biliary pathogens, surgical site infection, and pancreatic fistula: results of a randomized trial of perioperative antibiotic prophylaxis in patients undergoing pancreatoduodenectomy. Ann Surg. 2023;278(3):310–9.
24. Haga N, Ishida H, Ishiguro T, Kumamoto K, Ishibashi K, Tsuji Y, et al. A prospective randomized study to assess the optimal duration of intravenous antimicrobial prophylaxis in elective gastric cancer surgery. Int Surg. 2012;97(2):169–76.
25. Bressan AK, Aubin JM, Martel G, Dixon E, Bathe OF, Sutherland FR, Balaa F, Mimeault R, Edwards JP, Grondin SC, Isherwood S, Lillemoe KD, Saeed S, Ball CG. Efficacy of a dual-ring wound protector for prevention of surgical site infections after pancreaticoduodenectomy in patients with Intrabiliary stents: a randomized clinical trial. Ann Surg. 2018;268(1):35–40.
26. De Pastena M, Marchegiani G, Paiella S, Fontana M, Esposito A, Casetti L, Secchettin E, Manzini G, Bassi C, Salvia R. Use of an intraoperative wound protector to prevent surgical-site infection after pancreatoduodenectomy: randomized clinical trial. Br J Surg. 2020;107(9):1107–13.
27. Hassan K, Baloch S, Tan EJZ, Chamberlain J, Ashfaq A, Shah J, Hajibandeh S, Hajibandeh S. The effect of intraoperative wound protector use on the risk of surgical site infections in patients undergoing pancreatoduodenectomy: a systematic review and meta-analysis. Langenbeck's Arch Surg. 2022;407(2):459–68.
28. Norman G, Goh EL, Dumville JC, Shi C, Liu Z, Chiverton L, et al. Negative pressure wound therapy for surgical wounds healing by primary closure. Cochrane Database Syst Rev. 2020;2020(6):CD009261.

29. DeLeon G, Rao V, Duggan BS, Becker T, Pei K. American College of Surgeons National Surgical Quality Improvement Program (ACS-NSQIP) analysis of negative pressure wound therapy following pancreatectomy for pancreatic diagnoses. J Am Coll Surg. 2023;236(5):S37.

30. Al Efishat M, Attiyeh MA, Eaton AA, Gönen M, Covey AM, D'Angelica MI, DeMatteo RP, Kingham TP, Balachandran V, Jarnagin WR, Gerdes H, Allen PJ, Schattner MA. Endoscopic versus percutaneous drainage of post-operative peripancreatic fluid collections following pancreatic resection. HPB (Oxford). 2019;21(4):434–43.

31. Center for Disease Control and National Healthcare Safety Network, Surgical Site Infection Event. CDC.gov; 2022. https://www.cdc.gov/nhsn/pdfs/pscmanual/9pscssicurrent.pdf. Accessed 3 Aug 2022.

32. Andrianello S, Marchegiani G, Malleo G, Pollini T, Bonamini D, Salvia R, et al. Biliary fistula after pancreaticoduodenectomy: data from 1618 consecutive pancreaticoduodenectomies. HPB (Oxford). 2017;19(3):264–9.

33. Antolovic D, Koch M, Galindo L, Wolff S, Music E, Kienle P, et al. Hepaticojejunostomy—analysis of risk factors for postoperative bile leaks and surgical complications. J Gastrointest Surg. 2007;11(5):555–61.

34. Maatman TK, Loncharich AJ, Flick KF, Simpson RE, Ceppa EP, Nakeeb A, Nguyen TK, Schmidt CM, Zyromski NJ, House MG. Transient biliary fistula after pancreatoduodenectomy increases risk of biliary anastomotic stricture. J Gastrointest Surg. 2021;25(1):169–77.

35. El Nakeeb A, El Sorogy M, Hamed H, Said R, Elrefai M, Ezzat H, et al. Biliary leakage following pancreaticoduodenectomy: prevalence, risk factors and management. Hepatobiliary Pancreat Dis Int. 2019;18(1):67–72.

36. Burkhart RA, Relles D, Pineda DM, Gabale S, Sauter PK, Rosato EL, et al. Defining treatment and outcomes of hepaticojejunostomy failure following pancreaticoduodenectomy. J Gastrointest Surg. 2013;17(3):451–60.

37. Chincarini M, Zamboni GA, Pozzi MR. Major pancreatic resections: normal postoperative findings and complications. Insights Imaging. 2018;9(2):173–87.

38. Koch M, Garden OJ, Padbury R, Rahbari NN, Adam R, Capussotti L, et al. Bile leakage after hepatobiliary and pancreatic surgery: a definition and grading of severity by the international study group of liver surgery. Surgery. 2011;149(5):680–8.

39. Farooqui W, Penninga L, Burgdorf SK, Storkholm JH, Hansen CP. Biliary leakage following pancreatoduodenectomy: experience from a high-volume center. J Pancreat Cancer. 2021;7(1):80–5.

40. Miller BC, Christein JD, Behrman SW, Callery MP, Drebin JA, Kent TS, et al. Assessing the impact of a fistula after a pancreaticoduodenectomy using the post-operative morbidity index. HPB (Oxford). 2013;15(10):781–8.

41. Malgras B, Duron S, Gaujoux S, Dokmak S, Aussilhou B, Rebours V, et al. Early biliary complications following pancreaticoduodenectomy: prevalence and risk factors. HPB (Oxford). 2016;18(4):367–74.

42. Jarnagin WR. Blumgart's surgery of the liver, biliary tract, and pancreas. 6th ed. Philadelphia, PA: Elsevier; 2017.

43. Jester AL, Chung CW, Becerra DC, et al. The impact of hepaticojejunostomy leaks after pancreatoduodenectomy: a devastating source of morbidity and mortality. J Gastrointest Surg. 2017;21(6):1017–24.

44. Suzuki Y, Fujino Y, Tanioka Y, Ajiki T, Hiraoka K, Takada M, et al. Factors influencing hepaticojejunostomy leak following pancreaticoduodenal resection; importance of anastomotic leak test. Hepato-Gastroenterology. 2003;50(49):254–7.

45. van der Gaag NA, Verhaar AC, Haverkort EB, Busch ORC, van Gulik TM, Gouma DJ. Chylous ascites after pancreaticoduodenectomy: introduction of a grading system. J Am Coll Surg. 2008;207(5):751–7.

46. Assumpcao L, Cameron JL, Wolfgang CL, Edil B, Choti MA, Herman JM, et al. Incidence and management of chyle leaks following pancreatic resection: a high volume single-center institutional experience. J Gastrointest Surg. 2008;12(11):1915–23.

47. Weniger M, D'Haese JG, Angele MK, Kleespies A, Werner J, Hartwig W. Treatment options for chylous ascites after major abdominal surgery: a systematic review. Am J Surg. 2016;211(1):206–13.
48. Strobel O, Brangs S, Hinz U, Tausch T, Hüttner FJ, Diener MK, et al. Chyle leak after pancreatic surgery: incidence, risk factors, clinical relevance, and therapeutic implications. Pancreatology. 2016;16(3, Supplement 1):S74.
49. Loukas M, Wartmann CT, Louis RG, Tubbs RS, Salter EG, Gupta AA, et al. Cisterna chyli: a detailed anatomic investigation. Clin Anat. 2007;20(6):683–8.
50. Kuboki S, Shimizu H, Yoshidome H, Ohtsuka M, Kato A, Yoshitomi H, et al. Chylous ascites after hepatopancreatobiliary surgery. Br J Surg. 2013;100(4):522–7.
51. Aalami OO, Allen DB, Organ CH. Chylous ascites: a collective review. Surgery. 2000;128(5):761–78.
52. Besselink MG, van Rijssen LB, Bassi C, Dervenis C, Montorsi M, Adham M, et al. Definition and classification of chyle leak after pancreatic operation: a consensus statement by the international study group on pancreatic surgery. Surgery. 2017;161(2):365–72.
53. Strobel O, Brangs S, Hinz U, Pausch T, Hüttner FJ, Diener MK, et al. Incidence, risk factors and clinical implications of chyle leak after pancreatic surgery. Br J Surg. 2017;104(1):108–17.
54. Abu Hilal M, Layfield DM, Di Fabio F, Arregui-Fresneda I, Panagiotopoulou IG, Armstrong TH, et al. Postoperative chyle leak after major pancreatic resections in patients who receive enteral feed: risk factors and management options. World J Surg. 2013;37(12):2918–26.
55. Pan W, Yang C, Cai SY, Chen ZM, Cheng NS, Li FY, et al. Incidence and risk factors of chylous ascites after pancreatic resection. Int J Clin Exp Med. 2015;8(3):4494–500.
56. Varghese C, Wells CI, Lee S, Pathak S, Siriwardena AK, Pandanaboyana S. Systematic review of the incidence and risk factors for chyle leak after pancreatic surgery. Surgery. 2022;171(2):490–7.
57. Van der Gaag NA, Verhaar AC, Haverkort EB, Busch OR, van Gulik TM, et al. Chylous ascites after pancreaticoduodenectomy: introduction of a grading system. J Am Coll Surg; 2008;207:751–7.
58. Leibovitch I, Mor Y, Golomb J, Ramon J. The diagnosis and management of postoperative chylous ascites. J Urol. 2002;167(2 Pt 1):449–57.
59. Malik HZ, Crozier J, Murray L, Carter R. Chyle leakage and early enteral feeding following pancreatico-duodenectomy: management options. Dig Surg. 2007;24(6):418–22.
60. Bassi C, Molinari E, Malleo G, Crippa S, Butturini G, Salvia R, et al. Early versus late drain removal after standard pancreatic resections: results of a prospective randomized trial. Ann Surg. 2010;252(2):207–14.
61. He S, Xia J, Zhang W, Lai M, Cheng N, Liu Z, et al. Prophylactic abdominal drainage for pancreatic surgery. Cochrane Database Syst Rev. 2021;(12):CD010583. https://doi.org/10.1002/14651858.CD010583.pub5/full.
62. Mazza M, Crippa S, Pecorelli N, Tamburino D, Partelli S, Castoldi R, et al. Duodeno-jejunal or gastro-enteric leakage after pancreatic resection: a case-control study. Updat Surg. 2019;71(2):295–303.
63. Eshuis WJ, Tol JAMG, Nio CY, Busch ORC, van Gulik TM, Gouma DJ. Leakage of the gastro-enteric anastomosis after pancreatoduodenectomy. Surgery. 2014;156(1):75–82.
64. Winter JM, Cameron JL, Yeo CJ, Lillemoe KD, Campbell KA, Schulick RD. Duodenojejunostomy leaks after pancreaticoduodenectomy. J Gastrointest Surg. 2008;12(2):263–9.
65. Tran KTC, Smeenk HG, van Eijck CHJ, Kazemier G, Hop WC, Greve JWG, et al. Pylorus preserving pancreaticoduodenectomy versus standard Whipple procedure: a prospective, randomized, multicenter analysis of 170 patients with pancreatic and periampullary tumors. Ann Surg. 2004;240(5):738–45.
66. Gervais DA, Fernandez-del Castillo C, O'Neill MJ, Hahn PF, Mueller PR. Complications after pancreatoduodenectomy: imaging and imaging-guided interventional procedures. Radiographics. 2001;21(3):673–90.

67. Raman SP, Horton KM, Cameron JL, Fishman EK. CT after pancreaticoduodenectomy: spectrum of normal findings and complications. Am J Roentgenol. 2013;201(1):2–13.
68. Welsh LK, Murayama KM. Surgical management: Roux-en-Y reconstruction. In: Grams J, Perry KA, Tavakkoli A, editors. The SAGES manual of foregut surgery. Cham: Springer International Publishing; 2019. p. 695–707. https://doi.org/10.1007/978-3-319-96122-4_60.
69. Lee SH, Lee YH, Hur YH, Kim HJ, Choi BG. A comparative study of postoperative outcomes after stapled versus handsewn gastrojejunal anastomosis for pylorus-resecting pancreaticoduodenectomy. Ann Hepatobiliary Pancreat Surg. 2021;25(1):84–9.
70. Hajibandeh S, Hajibandeh S, Khan RMA, Malik S, Mansour M, Kausar A, et al. Stapled anastomosis versus hand-sewn anastomosis of gastro/duodenojejunostomy in pancreaticoduodenectomy: a systematic review and meta-analysis. Int J Surg. 2017;48:1–8.
71. Cameron JL, Pitt HA, Yeo CJ, Lillemoe KD, Kaufman HS, Coleman J. One hundred and forty-five consecutive pancreaticoduodenectomies without mortality. Ann Surg. 1993;217(5):430–5; discussion 435–438

Chapter 34
Prevention, Prediction, and Mitigation of Pancreatic Fistula

Fabio Casciani, Maxwell T. Trudeau, and Charles M. Vollmer

Definition and General Perspective

From a pathophysiological standpoint, pancreatic fistula is defind as an abnormal communication between the pancreatic ductal system and another epithelial surface, containing pancreas-derived, enzyme-rich fluid. Such a broad definition not only describes a complication occurring after a pancreatectomy, but also applies to any circumstance in which the integrity of the pancreatic ductal system is violated, for instance, in the case of pancreatic trauma, necrotizing pancreatitis or iatrogenic injuries occurring during non-surgical interventions. When a pancreatico-enteric anastomosis is constructed (namely, in the case of a Whipple procedure or central pancreatectomy), POPF is the consequence of a partial or complete dehiscence of the anastomosis, resulting in pancreatic and enteric juice spilling into the abdominal cavity. Conversely, in the case of distal pancreatectomy (DP), pancreatic enucleation, or ablative procedures, POPF represents the spillage of pancreatic fluid from the parenchymal cut-edge. Therefore, as opposed to the former, in this scenario there is no direct contamination of peripancreatic collections by the intestinal microbial flora, resulting in a usually sterile collection of enzyme-rich fluid.

F. Casciani
University of Verona, Verona, Italy

University of Pennsylvania Perelman School of Medicine, Philadelphia, PA, USA
e-mail: fabio.casciani@univr.it

M. T. Trudeau
University of Pennsylvania Perelman School of Medicine, Philadelphia, PA, USA

University of Connecticut School of Medicine, Farmington, CT, USA

C. M. Vollmer (✉)
University of Pennsylvania Perelman School of Medicine, Philadelphia, PA, USA
e-mail: Charles.Vollmer@pennmedicine.upenn.edu

E. P. Ceppa et al. (eds.), *The SAGES Manual of Evolving Techniques in Pancreatic Surgery*, https://doi.org/10.1007/978-3-031-78409-5_34

Moving from such a biological basis to a clinical definition, the International Study Group of Pancreatic Fistula (ISGPS) has recently updated practical, universally recognized diagnostic and grading criteria for POPF [1]. Diagnosis of POPF relies on the analysis of drain fluid to ascertain the presence of pancreas-derived enzymes on or after postoperative day 3. In fact, any volume of drain fluid with amylase level >3 times higher than the upper limit of normal (according to the local, institutional thresholds) defines a POPF. This implies that at least one intra-abdominal drain (placed either intraoperatively or postoperatively) must be in situ for fluid collection, or, alternatively, a certain volume of fluid discharging spontaneously from a skin incision to be analyzed.

The notion that a pancreatic fistula needs to be considered clinically "relevant" (CR) has been cemented in the latest 2016 ISGPS statement (Fig. 34.1). In fact, the clinical scenario where the presence of amylase-rich drain fluid is not associated with any deviation from the normal clinical course (which represented a grade A POPF in the previous ISGPS classification) has been renamed as "biochemical leak" and is no longer considered a meaningful fistula. Conversely, CR-POPF is now graded as B when medical treatment or minimally invasive procedures such as percutaneous drain placement are employed, whereas grade C events include reoperation, intensive care transfer for multiorgan failure or death directly attributable to the fistula. Notably, CR-POPF is graded only retrospectively based on the specific intervention enacted by the surgeon; such an approach enables the surgeon to express qualitatively the clinical severity of pancreatic fistulas, while also providing a standardized, common language for comparative studies. When applying the revised ISGPS criteria, incidence of CR-POPF following Whipple procedure is

Fig. 34.1 The 2016 International Study Group criteria for the diagnosis and grading of pancreatic fistula. (Adapted from Bassi C, Marchegiani G, Dervenis C, Sarr M, Abu Hilal M, Adham M, et al. The 2016 update of the International Study Group (ISGPS) definition and grading of postoperative pancreatic fistula: 11 Years After. Surgery. 2017;161 (3):584–91)

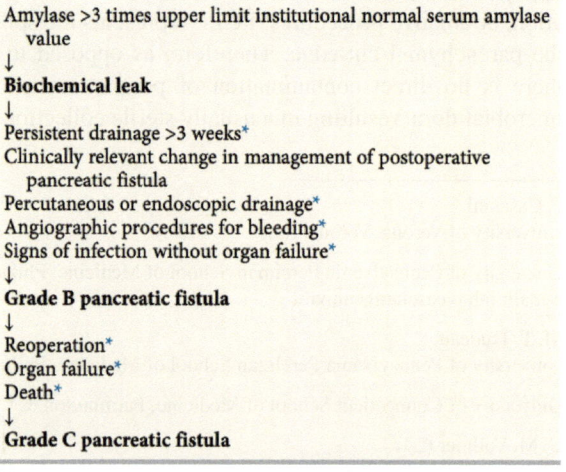

Amylase >3 times upper limit institutional normal serum amylase value
↓
Biochemical leak
↓
Persistent drainage >3 weeks*
Clinically relevant change in management of postoperative pancreatic fistula
Percutaneous or endoscopic drainage*
Angiographic procedures for bleeding*
Signs of infection without organ failure*
↓
Grade B pancreatic fistula
↓
Reoperation*
Organ failure*
Death*
↓
Grade C pancreatic fistula

*Treatment/event postoperative pancreatic fistula related.
Modified from Bassi, C, Marchegiani G, Dervenis C, et al. The 2016 update of the International Study Group (ISGPS) definition and grading of postoperative pancreatic fistula: 11 years after. *Surgery.* 2017;161:584–591.

established around 15% according to contemporary standards, while a higher 18–25% rate is considered reasonable in the case of DP.

A sequential, conceptual framework to address the issue of pancreatic fistula should be embraced by HPB surgeons. Practically, three consecutive phases of decision-making can be identified to reduce the burden of POPF, namely patient risk assessment and stratification, employment of risk-based techniques and mitigation strategies at time of anastomosis creation, and a modern, "step-up" approach for fistula management [2].

Risk Assessment and Stratification

Several risk factors for pancreatico-enteric anastomosis dehiscence have been documented. The most important, ubiquitously recognized predictor of CR-POPF development after a Whipple procedure is pancreatic parenchymal texture. Of note, this is an intrinsic, non-modifiable characteristic to deal with. A so-called *soft* parenchyma (namely, a friable pancreatic stump rich in active secretory glands and/or high adipose cellularity) is by far the most dangerous scenario for sewing an anastomosis when compared to a *hard*, fibrous, atrophic organ. In the former situation, passing the needle through the pancreas when constructing the anastomosis can easily cut the parenchyma, leading to laceration, bleeding, hematomas, and trauma of the anastomotic edge. From this comes the common expression that pancreatico-enteric anastomotic construction is somewhat like "sewing a stick of butter."

A soft pancreas is often associated with a non-dilated pancreatic duct, which also carries an increased risk of POPF. An inverse relationship exists between duct size and CR-POPF risk; a recent position paper by the ISGPS proposed a duct smaller than 3 mm as measured by the surgeon intraoperatively as critical factor for anastomotic failure, with a 23% observed CR-POPF rate when such a small duct and soft gland texture coexist [3]. In fact, a diminutive, 1 mm duct holds the largest risk odds for a leak occurring.

Other contributors to pancreatic fistula development include obesity (BMI ≥ 30) and/or visceral adiposity, as well as disease pathology different from pancreatic cancer and chronic pancreatitis, which are usually associated with a soft pancreatic parenchyma. Uncertainty exists regarding the contribution of diabetes and preoperative chemo-radiation therapy, which might positively impact anastomotic healing given a putative association with gland atrophy and firmness. Interestingly, even though the biological mechanisms whereby intraoperative blood loss could affect anastomotic healing are uncertain, high blood loss correlates with stepwise escalation in CR-POPF rates, as well as overall morbidity and mortality. Therefore, in contrast to the patient-specific characteristics, minimizing blood loss appears as an effective target for fistula prevention and performance improvement for the pancreatic surgeon. Furthermore, following the impact of some recent, innovative hypothesis-generating studies—as well as the established evidence regarding colorectal anastomoses—one of the most curious areas for future investigation is the relationship between intestinal microbiota and anastomotic failure.

Moving from initial, rudimentary attempts to identify risk factors for POPF development in isolation, several predictive scores have been generated to quantify the patient-specific, cumulative risk of POPF more usefully. Among them, only the fistula risk score (FRS) [4] has been employed thus far to design risk-stratified observational and randomized clinical studies and represents the most commonly employed predictive tool by experts in the field [2]. Proposed in 2013 and subsequently validated internationally, the FRS provides a ten-point scale which can be easily calculated by the operating surgeon at the time of anastomosis creation (Fig. 34.2). In detail, such a score is derived by summing the weighted contribution of gland texture (0 points for hard texture and 2 points for soft texture), duct diameter (acquired from direct measurement of the pancreatic duct in the pancreatic stump; 0–4 points—in an inverse manner), baseline pathology (0 points for pancreatic cancer/pancreatitis, and 1 point for any other diseases), and blood loss (estimated by the surgeon after consultation with the attending anesthesiologist; 0–3 points). Of note, besides correlating with a progressively higher risk of CR-POPF across the 0 to 10 point scale (namely from 0.7% to 41.7%), the FRS both allows the identification of eighty distinct scenarios to apply the customization of medical decisions tailored for the individual patient [5] and segregates four distinct risk zones which can be employed for the generation of comparative studies (FRS 0: negligible risk zone; FRS 1–2: low risk zone; FRS 3–6: intermediate risk score; FRS 7–10: high risk zone). In fact, given its substantial predictive capacity, the FRS has often been employed to evaluate fistula mitigation strategies and surgeon/institutional outcomes in methodologically sound risk-adjusted analyses. Some of the

Fig. 34.2 The fistula risk score for prediction of clinically relevant pancreatic fistula following pancreaticoduodenectomy. (Adapted from Callery MP, Pratt WB, Kent TS, Chaikof EL, Vollmer CM, Jr. A prospectively validated clinical risk score accurately predicts pancreatic fistula after pancreatoduodenectomy. J Am Coll Surg. 2013;216 (1):1–14)

Risk Factor	Parameter	Points
Gland Texture	Firm	0
	Soft	2
Disease Pathology	Pancreatic carcinoma/ pancreatitis	0
	Other	1
Pancreatic duct diameter (mm)	≥5	0
	4	1
	3	2
	2	3
	≤1	4
Estimated Blood Loss (mL)	≤400	0
	401–700	1
	701–1000	2
	≥1001	3

salient insights obtained thus far include the validation of a selective drain placement protocol and early removal in the case of negligible/low risk scenarios (FRS 0–2) [6], the ineffectiveness of internal stent placement [7], the definition of an optimal mitigation strategy bundle for high-risk patients [8], as well as the design of a randomized controlled trial investigating the optimal anastomotic reconstruction in high-risk scenarios (FRS 7–10—see below) [9]. More recently, risk-stratified outcome analyses employing the FRS have been conducted to compare proficiency and competency among pancreatic surgeons worldwide [10, 11].

It should be emphasized that only the implementation of an *intraoperative* predictive tool such as the FRS allows the surgeon to adapt their practice according to the predicted risk (namely employing optimal techniques and adjuncts for fistula mitigation), especially for patients residing in the high-risk cohort. Practically speaking, compared to other predictive scores available which require specific calculators, the FRS has the advantage of being easily computed on the fingertips or, alternatively, using a "cheat sheet" located in the operating room. To further facilitate fruition of the FRS in the daily practice, along with the opportunity to create a personal repository of data and a contemporary bibliography regarding pancreatic fistula, a dedicated website can be consulted (https://fistulariskscore.com), along with a free app recently made available for mobile devices (FRS App).

Furthermore, the Alternative FRS has been recently endorsed by the Dutch Pancreatic Cancer group on behalf of a multi-institutional collaborative, and subsequently updated (ua-FRS) in order to fit the increasing popularity of minimally invasive approaches for the Whipple procedures worldwide [12]. Such a tool encompasses the weighted contribution of BMI, gland texture, and duct diameter, providing a net probability (i.e., percentage) of CR-POPF development using an online platform (pancreascalculator.com). Despite having a predictive capacity comparable to that of the original FRS, there are no prospective studies available thus far encompassing the ua-FRS as a tool for fistula risk stratification and quality assessment. Therefore, whether the implementation of that score will be valuable in broader clinical practice, or will provide actual benefit for fistula mitigation, is yet to be determined.

Regarding DP, several factors have been associated with increased incidence of POPF, among which younger age, obesity, hypoalbuminemia, neuroendocrine or non-malignant pathology, concomitant splenectomy, and vascular resection [13]. Of note, no intraoperative technique (such as distinct transection methods either with, or without, suture ligation of the pancreatic duct, use of tissue sealants or autologous tissue patch) has yet resulted in a significant reduction of POPF incidence. A recent meta-analysis including 43 studies concluded that only non-diabetic patients and smokers have an increased likelihood of developing CR-POPF, whereas neither high BMI nor soft pancreatic texture did add a statistically significant risk [14]. As a matter of fact, only two risk scores have been generated and externally validated thus far to assess the risk of pancreatic fistula development following DP: the Distal Fistula Risk Score (D-FRS) [15] and the DISPAIR Score [16]. Interestingly, both tools are based on the evaluation of the parenchymal thickness, given a putative correlation between the gland antero-posterior diameter at the transection site and risk of developing POPF. Since they have been both just published in 2022, whether such scores will be employed for value in the clinical practice is yet to be ascertained.

Intraoperative Decision-Making for POPF Prevention and Mitigation Following Pancreatoduodenectomy

Most long-time pancreatic surgeons are used to saying that "when a pancreatic fistula has to occur, it will." With such a statement of resignation, they admit that, unfortunately, most efforts dedicated to preventing anastomotic dehiscence are eventually unsuccessful—at least, in the presence of high-stake, daunting scenarios. In fact, the only approach to *avoid* pancreatic fistula from the outset is committing to total pancreatectomy, thus accepting the consequences of a brittle diabetes and long-life pancreatic exocrine insufficiency. Traditionally, total pancreatectomy has been discouraged given its long-time sequelae due to the complete, prompt suppression of pancreatic function. Recently, the debate regarding the appropriateness and safety of total pancreatectomy for patients at high risk for CR-POPF (i.e., FRS 7–10) has been re-ignited, following the publication of studies reporting improved short- and long-term outcomes at high-volume institutions and the availability of long-acting insulin and modern pancreatic enzyme preparations [17]. Therefore, some authors now suggest performing a total pancreatectomy instead of constructing a high risk pancreatico-enteric anastomosis in highly selected, obese, older patients who may fail to thrive in the case of CR-POPF development, as well as those with pre-existing diabetes [17]. In order to provide a high quality, evidence-based ground to support the difficult decision to commit to total pancreatectomy in selected circumstances, in the PAN-IT trial [18], non-diabetic patients at high-risk for CR-POPF development (i.e., soft gland with a ≤3 mm duct) were randomized to receive either PD with pancreato-jejunostomy reconstruction or total pancreatectomy with islet auto-transplantation. Despite some design limitations, the PAN-IT study indicated a significant superiority for total pancreatectomy in reducing morbidity (60 vs. 90%) with no difference in disease-free and overall survival in the case of malignancy. The question as to whether total pancreatectomy reduces the burden associated with traditional pancreatico-enteric anastomosis reconstruction in high risk for pancreatic fistula cases is actually under scrutiny in other randomized controlled trials (NCT05212350, NCT05116072).

Apart from such an unconventional approach, it is important to stress the notion that the surgeon's mindset should generally revolve around the mitigation of pancreatic fistula *once it occurred*—rather than solely trying to prevent it. Multiple mitigation strategies have been scrutinized thus far to lower the burden of POPF following pancreatoduodenectomy.

The employment of an intraoperative, objective risk assessment tool such as the FRS allows the surgeon to implement distinct anastomotic techniques and adjuncts according to the patient-specific risk profile—rather than a dogmatic "one-size-fits-all" approach. For instance, in the case of high-risk scenarios (FRS 7–10), an optimal bundle of strategies available to reduce CR-POPF morbidity entails the construction of a pancreatico-jejunostomy (rather than a pancreatico-gastrostomy), the application of an externalized trans-anastomotic stent (compared to internal stents or stent omission), the use of peripancreatic drains, as well as omission of prophylactic somatostatin-analogues such as octreotide [8]. Notably, a recent, risk-adjusted randomized controlled trial reported higher fistula-related complication burden and major complication rates for patients receiving pancre-atico-gastrostomy compared to those assigned to the pancreatico-jejunostomy arm [9]. These conclusions are in line with previous RCTs that were unable to demonstrate the superiority of PG vs. PJ, suggesting to abandon such technique. Moreover, it should be acknowledged that, despite the lack of supporting evidence, most specialized pancreatic surgeons favor a selective use of trans-anastomotic stents in the case of challenging anastomoses, to divert pancreatic secretion in the case of overt anastomotic dehiscence. In the authors' experience [19], employment of specifically designed external stents with several holes on the sides and a proximal bulge to prevent displacement within the jejunal loop (Fig. 34.3) has displayed improved

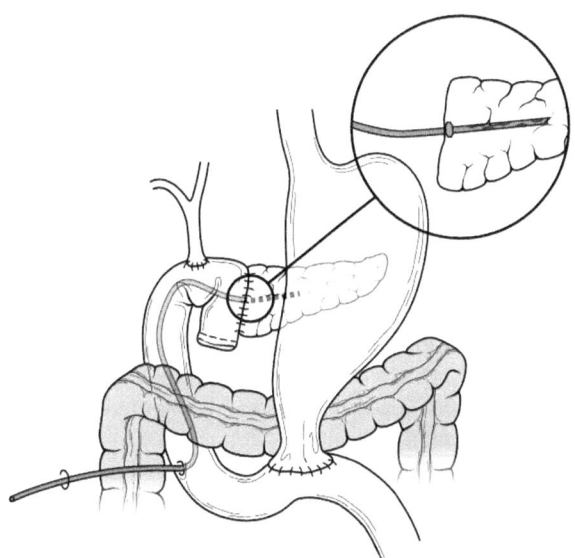

Fig. 34.3 Illustration displaying the surgical field after PD with pancreatico-jejunal anastomosis and trans-anastomotic externalized stent. It should be noted that the stent is characterized by the presence of several holes on the sides to facilitate pancreatic fluid drainage, and a proximal bulge to be placed within the pancreatic duct right before the pancreatic-enteric interface to prevent displacement (se detail in the upper right circle). (Adapted from Andrianello S, Marchegiani G, Malleo G, Masini G, Balduzzi A, Paiella S, et al. Pancreaticojejunostomy With Externalized Stent vs. Pancreaticogastrostomy With Externalized Stent for Patients With High-Risk Pancreatic Anastomosis: A Single-Center, Phase 3, Randomized Clinical Trial. JAMA Surg. 2020;155 (4):313–21)

performance in fistula management compared to less refined devices used in the past. Therefore, we suggest employing such stents routinely in high-risk scenarios (i.e. FRS 7–10) and selectively in the case of intermediate risk circumstances (FRS 3–6) when soft gland and/or diminutive duct are present.

Concerning the choice of anastomotic technique, most expert pancreatic surgeons recommend an end-to-side, double layer, duct-to-mucosa pancreatico-jejunostomy as the preferred approach, although the so-called Blumgart's duct-to-mucosa reconstruction technique has lately gained popularity. Importantly, the latter approach aims to reduce the risk of parenchymal laceration when tying trans-pancreatic sutures through the application of trans-parenchymal mattress sutures. Such a variant might be particularly useful in the case of a "flat," soft pancreas with an eccentrically situated duct and represents a feasible approach both for open and minimally invasive PD. Whether the Blumgart technique provides significant improvement in terms of CR-POPF rate/severity in high-risk scenarios, when compared to the standard duct-to-mucosa anastomosis, still needs to be ascertained by properly designed RCTs.

Furthermore, several options have been proposed over time to prevent and/or mitigate the impact of POPF, such as pancreatic duct occlusion throughout direct sutures or polymer injection, the use of Teres ligament and/or omental pedicled flaps, biological sealants, as well as the construction of an isolated pancreatico-enteric anastomosis on a Roux-en-Y jejunal loop to divert pancreatic and biliary secretions. In a randomized, controlled, German multicenter trial, 445 patients were randomly allocated in a 1:1 ratio to receive PD with pancreato-jejunostomy reconstruction with (intervention) or without (control) a falciform ligament wrap around the hepatic artery. The rate of clinically relevant post-pancreatectomy hemorrhage (PPH) from the hepatic artery or gastroduodenal artery stump in the per-protocol analysis was significantly lower in the intervention group (2 vs. 7.2%; odds ratio 0.26 [95% confidence interval 0.09–0.80]; $P = 0.017$), suggesting that a falciform ligament wrap may reduce PPH from the hepatic artery or gastroduodenal artery stump and should be considered during pancreatoduodenectomy to mitigate the sequelae of POPF [20]. However, the choice of employing this and other technical expedients is likely to be predicated by personal background, training, and comfort level, rather than sound scientific evidence.

A long-time debate is still open regarding drain placement following pancreatectomy. Of note, drainage of the perianastomotic space likely does not interfere with anastomotic healing (namely, it does not prevent fistula development), but rather mitigates its impact by evacuating purulent, enzyme- or bile-rich fluid which might be responsible for sepsis and peripancreatic vessel erosion. Therefore, a selective use of drains following pancreatoduodenectomy is now gaining popularity and is recommended by most expert surgeons in contrast to "all or nothing" policies. In fact, the omission of prophylactic drainage for patients with an intraoperatively calculated FRS ≤2—over a quarter of all patients—has demonstrated benefit in a prospective multicenter study, with no CR-POPF observed in such a cohort [6].

As opposed to a traditional, prolonged drainage, an early drain removal protocol based on drain fluid amylase (DFA) measurement and daily assessment of drain fluid characteristics has been implemented at the authors' institutions as an effective approach to improve outcomes [21]. Such an algorithm encompasses an FRS-based selective drain placement as explained above, followed by POD1 DFA assessment. Drain removal is suggested within POD3, if POD1 DFA is ≤5000 UI/mL. Deviation from such a protocol, consisting of prolonged drainage with further DFA assessment on POD3 and POD5, is at the operating surgeon's discretion, especially in the case of "sinister" drain fluid appearance suspicious for pancreatic and/or biliary fistulas, as well as a so-called sentinel bleed (see Fig. 34.4). The aforementioned perioperative dynamic drain management protocol provides a model for an optimized and individualized patient care after pancreatoduodenectomy.

Finally, a *caveat* should be made regarding the perioperative administration of somatostatin analogues as a prophylactic intervention to reduce POPF. Although this is still advocated as a theoretically reasonable approach by some HPB surgeons given the inhibition of pancreatic exocrine secretion exerted by octreotide and its derivatives, most evidence from contemporary research indicates a significant, detrimental effect of such in terms of fistula occurrence and associated morbidity [8]. Therefore, despite the biological mechanisms underlying such an effect being unknown, we currently discourage prophylactic use of somatostatin analogues, while, on the other hand, it might be taken in consideration in the case of overt, clinically manifest pancreatic anastomosis dehiscence with no signs of infection/sepsis, in order to reduce drain volume.

Bringing it all together, a conceptual playbook of mitigation approaches for fistula can be composed—applying a personalized medicine approach to pancreatic

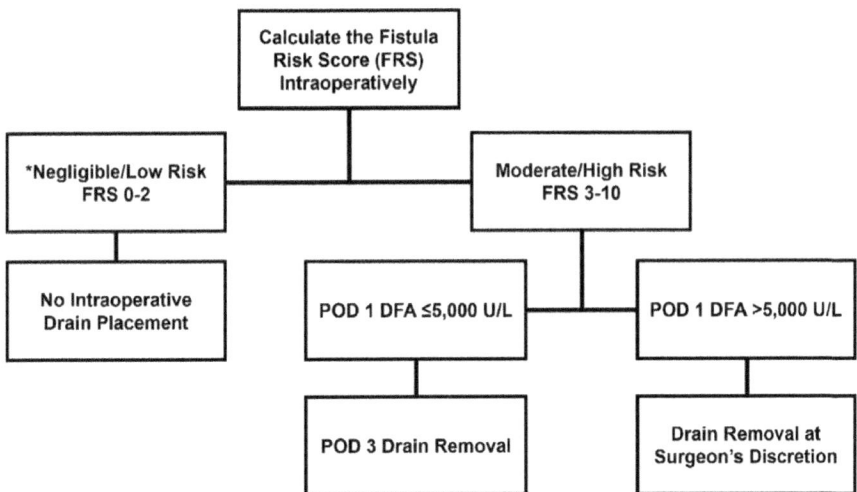

Fig. 34.4 Proposed algorithm for drain management following pancreatoduodenectomy, based on intraoperative fistula risk score (FRS) calculation and postoperative day one (POD1) drain fluid amylase level (DFA) measurement. (Adapted from McMillan MT, Malleo G, Bassi C, Allegrini V, Casetti L, Drebin J, et al. Multicenter, prospective trial of selective drain management for pancreatoduodenectomy using risk stratification. Ann Surg 2017;265 (6):1209–1218)

surgery. First, quantitatively assessing the likelihood of CR-POPF occurrence at the time of pancreatic anastomosis creation is paramount allowing the surgeon to implement risk-based, patient-specific approaches. Accounting for the cumulative contribution of four predictors, the fistula risk score can be easily computed to provide a 0–10 score. Interestingly, intraoperative blood loss is the single contributor under the surgeon's control; therefore, efforts for minimizing blood loss during the entire operation are influential. Moreover, a user-friendly tool such as the FRS App/website is now available to provide the highest level of granularity in risk stratification, as well as real-time, evidence-based support for decision-making.

Patients residing in the negligible (FRS 0—notably, the most frequent scenario, a surgeon can encounter on a given day) and low-risk zone (FRS 1–2) are unlikely to develop CR-POPF (0.7 and 5%, respectively). Technical adjuncts for anastomotic reconstruction and mitigation strategies are unlikely to provide value in the context of an overall protective biological situation. Patients can also benefit from omitting drains, unless other reasons for drain placement exist such as higher risk of biliary leak or bleeding, or the need for evacuating infected fluid. On the other hand, for those residing in the high-risk zone (FRS 7–10; predicted CR-POPF rate >30%), a mitigation strategy bundle including pancreatico-jejunostomy reconstruction with an externalized stent, intra-abdominal drain placement and octreotide omission represents the most effective approach to attenuate fistula occurrence and severity. The intermediate risk zone (FRS 3–6) is composed of a heterogeneous cohort of clinical scenarios, with observed CR-POPF rates escalating from 4% to 30%. Especially in the case of vulnerable circumstances when soft parenchyma and/or a small duct diameter are encountered, patients will benefit from the combination of pancreatico-jejunostomy, drain placement, and omission of prophylactic octreotide. Furthermore, an early drain removal algorithm can be safely implemented after assessing drain fluid amylase on POD1, with intraoperatively placed drains being removed in POD3 when POD1 DFA is below 5000 UI/L.

Intraoperative Decision-Making for POPF Prevention and Mitigation Following Distal Pancreatectomy

Given the unique physio-pathological characteristics of POPF development after a DP—which is not associated with any anastomotic dehiscence, but rather the spillage of pancreatic juice from the pancreatic stump cut-surface–prevention/mitigation approaches differ from those discussed above.

First, multiple techniques for pancreatic transection have been scrutinized over time. The dissemination of minimally invasive approaches for DP has substantially contributed to the abandonment of hand-closure techniques, demonstrating that the use of staplers is an easy, fast, and effective choice—also in open surgery. However, despite being the most frequently employed approach, superiority of staplers with respect to scalpel transection followed by hand-sewn closure of the pancreatic duct has not been demonstrated in randomized trials [22]. Of note, many surgeons advocate that a progressive stepwise compression of the pancreatic parenchyma before staple firing limits tissue crushing and trauma, thus reducing the likelihood of fistula occurrence [23]. Another option available to the surgeon includes the use of energy devices for pancreatic division, such as the electric scalpel and ultrasonic harmonic scalpels, in order to obtain tissue sealing by direct, coaptive coagulation, although superiority of such has not been ascertained thus far.

Moreover, many adjuncts have been proposed to optimize pancreatic stump closure, such as the employment of staplers reinforced with bioabsorbable materials, the application of fibrin sealant patches, glues, or meshes to cover the cut-surface, and the use of autologous tissue patch (e.g., omental or umbilical ligament flaps). Despite multiple randomized trials being conducted at this point, no technique has yet demonstrated substantial superiority over the others; therefore, the choice of employing such approaches is largely dependent on the surgeon's habits, intuition, background, availability of surgical devices, and considerations of cost-effectiveness.

As for pancreatoduodenectomy, routine drain placement following DP has been questioned for decades. Currently, drainless DP is considered an acceptable practice. In fact, a United States-based, multi-institutional RCT [24] demonstrated no differences in CR-POPF, postoperative percutaneous drain placement, reoperation, and mortality rates between patients who had and did not have intraperitoneal drain placed; the latter showed twice as high of an incidence of abdominal fluid collection (22 vs. 9%). Notably, in contrast to the Whipple procedure, no risk-based, data-driven protocol/algorithm exists yet to inform decision-making regarding drain placement after DP. Perhaps, that will change the given recent advent of the aforementioned risk scores for DP.

Management of Clinically Relevant Pancreatic Fistula

The first randomized clinical trial investigating optimal approaches for post-pancreatectomy management has been recently published. Conducted in the Netherlands between 2018 and 2019, the PORSCH trial [25] compared usual treatment (based on distinct institutional and physicians' practice habits) vs. the implementation of a standardized, multimodal algorithm for patient management. Specifically, such a protocol encompasses the assessment of vital signs, drain output, and serum markers of inflammation daily from POD3 to POD14, along with rigid criteria for performing CT scans, initiating antibiotic treatment, intraoperatively placed drain removal and placement of additional percutaneous drains (see Fig. 34.5). Despite not being specifically designed to reduce POPF-associated morbidity, the PORSCH trial demonstrated that the implementation of a structured, multilevel management protocol is capable of recognizing adverse events, allowing for a minimally invasive, step-up treatment approach when necessary. Undoubtedly, the proposed algorithm may constitute an effective, evidence-based paradigm in the

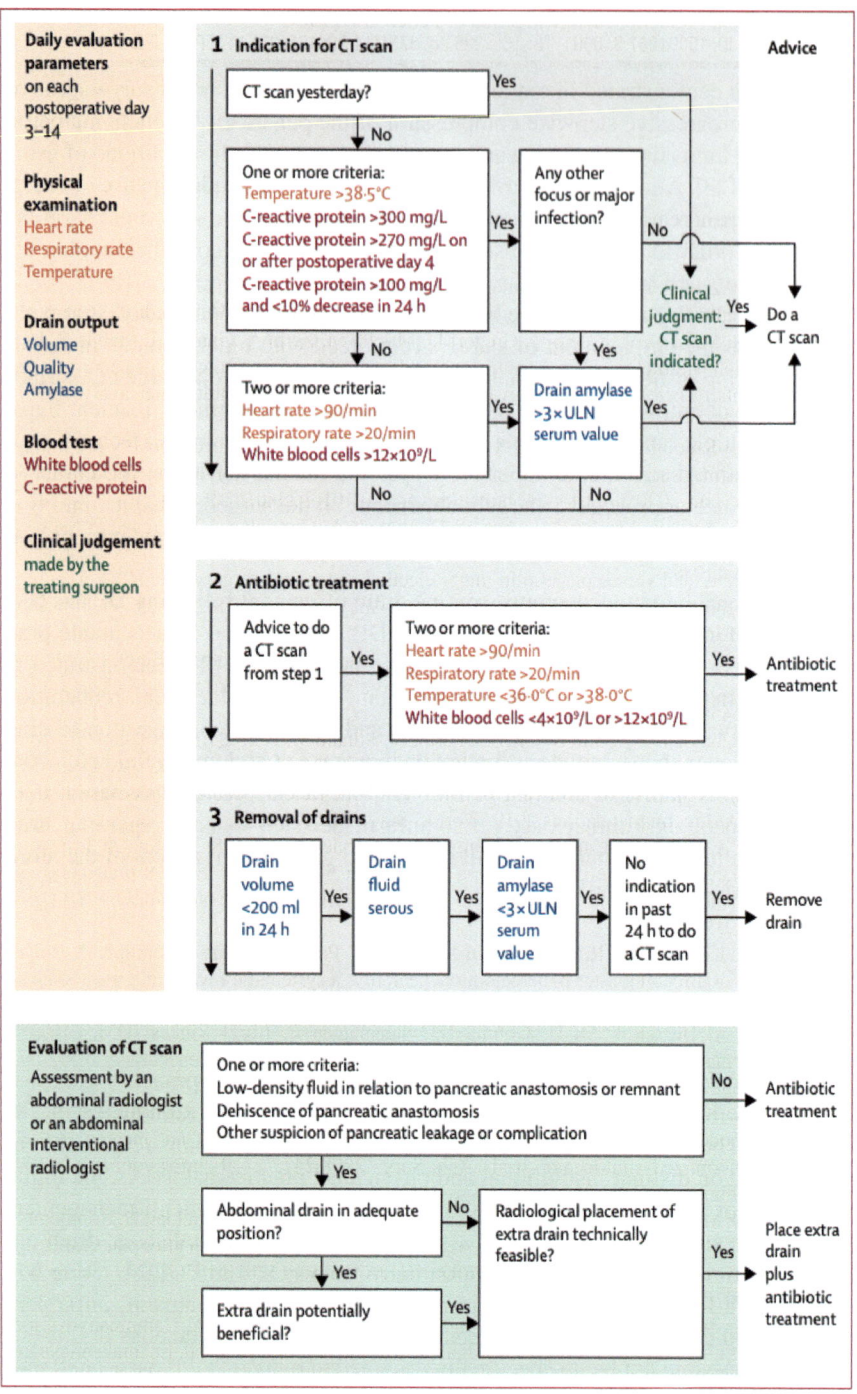

Fig. 34.5 Algorithm for the early recognition and management of complication following pancreatectomy employed in the PORSCHE trial. (Adapted from Smits FJ, Henry AC, Besselink MG, Busch OR, van Eijck CH, Arntz M, et al. Algorithm-based care vs. usual care for the early recognition and management of complications after pancreatic resection in the Netherlands: an open-label, nationwide, stepped-wedge cluster-randomized trial. Lancet. 2022;399(10338):1867–75)

management of pancreatic fistula. Notably, when employing such a tool, an overt reduction of organ failure and mortality rates was registered at both low-medium and high-volume institutions, indicating that a substantial outcome improvement can be achieved with standardization of practice and application of evidence-based patient management protocols irrespective of the surgeon/institution experience in pancreatic surgery.

An infected abdominal collection fed by pancreatic juice leakage can be reasonably suspected as soon as the patient presents some deviation from the normal clinical course. Therefore, continuous monitoring of patient status, vital signs, and drain output is paramount—as indicated in the PORSCH trial. Fever, chills, abdominal pain, nausea, and/or vomiting along with a purulent or creamy, malodorous drain effluent (so-called sinister effluent) are typical, early clinical manifestations of a pancreatic anastomotic leakage. An elevated C-reactive protein and leukocytosis often accompany such symptoms. In such a scenario, a contrast-enhanced CT scan will likely confirm the clinical suspect, revealing a pancreatico-enteric anastomosis disruption with surrounding free fluid (with or without gas), as well as peripancreatic collections (see Fig. 34.6). Most importantly, peripancreatic vessels should be carefully examined for wall irregularities, thrombosis, active bleeding, or pseudoaneurysm development. In addition, overt change of drain effluent to sanguineous nature is of immediate concern, reflecting the so-called sentinel bleed of a pseudoaneurysm, which can be approached through interventional radiology.

No well-established guidelines exist indicating the optimal treatment for pancreatic fistula, so that therapeutic approaches and algorithms employed vary across institutions. Following the lessons learned over time with acute pancreatitis, a step-up approach is recommended for the management of POPF. Requisites for optimal treatment are (1) intensive vital signs monitoring, either on the ward or transferring the patient to the intermediate/intensive care unit; (2) appropriate nutritional support; (3) extended-spectrum antibiotic treatment in the case of signs of infection/sepsis; and (4) when necessary, percutaneous catheter placement to externally drain

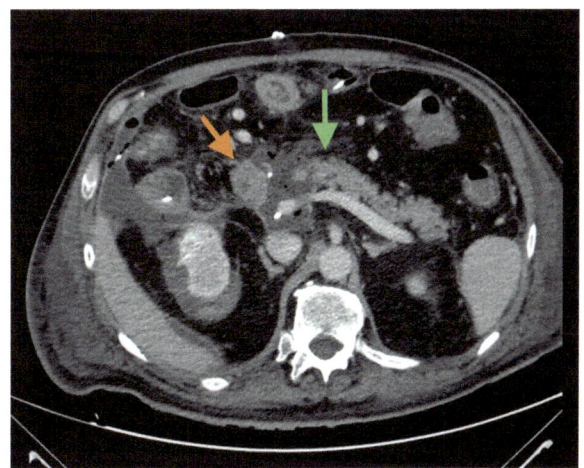

Fig. 34.6 Contrast-enhanced CT scan demonstrating pancreatico-jejunostomy dehiscence. A fluid collection with internal air bubbles is present between the jejunal loop (orange arrow) and the pancreatic stump (green arrow). Posteriorly, free fluid surrounds the superior mesenteric vein at the spleen vein confluence

purulent fluid, therefore obtaining source control. CT-guided procedures performed by dedicated interventional radiologists are preferred to prevent vascular and intestinal injuries, although US-guided catheter placement may be possible in the case of large, superficial collections. Moreover, endoscopic ultrasound-guided drainage procedures are also gaining consensus, in line with consolidated results obtained with the treatment of pancreatic pseudocysts/walled off pancreatic necrosis in the context of acute pancreatitis. This is especially useful for distal resection leaks. As indicated by a large retrospective study comparing primary non-operative and surgical management for CR-POPF [26] indicates that up to 77% of patients treated with primary catheter drainage display CR-POPF resolution without the need for surgery, with a significant advantage compared to those undergoing primary surgery in terms of mortality (14 vs. 36%), multiorgan failure (16 vs. 39%), new-onset diabetes (12 vs. 44%), as well as the need for additional laparotomies (22 vs. 45%), ICU admission (37 vs. 87%), and length of stay (median: 29 vs. 55 days).

Along with proper antimicrobial therapy and evacuation of intra-abdominal purulent fluid, nutritional support is also paramount to counterbalance a patient's increased catabolic demand. The preferred route of nutrition should be oral intake with standard diet, according to the results of recent randomized trials showing equivalent fistula closure rates with oral feeding when compared to total parenteral and enteral nutrition [27, 28]. It should be emphasized that total parenteral nutrition is associated with the risk of catheter contamination and fungal infection. Therefore, TPN should be administered only when both oral and enteral nutrition, either per a naso-jejunal tube or a feeding jejunostomy, are unable to guarantee adequate caloric and nutritional intake. Conversely, there is no concrete evidence supporting the efficacy of somatostatin-analogue administration in reducing fistula output and promoting fistula closure. Therefore, such drugs should not be employed as standard treatment.

As suggested by a long-time expert pancreatic surgeon: "[once a fistula occurs] keep cool and do not overreact, since 90% of fistulas will heal by just healing. The main problem of fistula is late bleeding; this is the primary reason for mortality. Thus, be prepared for dealing with bleeding" [2]. However, the decision to return to the operating room may ultimately be necessary. Reasons for proceeding with relaparotomy are the failure of previous interventions, a rapidly progressive impairment of patient status despite aggressive antimicrobial therapy and cardiocirculatory support, or when image-guided percutaneous catheter drainage of (infected) intra-abdominal fluid collections is not technically feasible. Unfortunately, neither solid clinical nor radiological parameters exists to guide decision-making, and resolution to undergo surgery needs to be made on a case-by-case basis. As previously ascertained for patients with necrotizing pancreatitis and secondary infection, reintervention is associated with mortality rates twice as high when compared to non-invasive approaches. Therefore, it is mandatory that the decision to commit to surgery would be shared with the anesthesiology and interventional radiology teams along with the patient (if capable to withdraw informed consent) and their family members, after ascertaining the infeasibility or ineffectiveness of non-invasive procedures (so-called step-up approach). In essence, reoperation represents the *last step* in this paradigm.

There is no consensus regarding the optimal strategy during relaparotomy. While committing to completion pancreatectomy might seem the most logical decision in order to remove the source of infection and inflammation, such an aggressive approach can lead to a rapid deterioration of organ failure, while being also burdened by the risk of damage of other organs/anastomoses and developing brittle pancreatic endocrine and exocrine insufficiency [29]. Mortality rates observed in patients who underwent salvage total pancreatectomy are significantly higher compared to those observed for pancreas-sparing procedures, being as high as 50–60%. Therefore, most expert pancreatic surgeons firmly discourage total pancreatectomy.

Similarly, redoing the anastomosis or conversion to an alternative anastomosis (i.e., from pancreatico-jejunostomy to pancreatico-gastrostomy, or vice versa) is usually discouraged, given the almost nil likelihood that a technically sound anastomosis could be fashioned in the face of local inflammatory changes and the innate glandular factors that undoubtedly led to the original anastomotic failure.

The most frequently employed approach consists of extended surgical drainage, encompassing the most accurate achievable removal of the peripancreatic necrotic/purulent tissue, followed by the application of multiple drains. Additional procedures include bridge-stenting techniques (namely the application of a stent inside the pancreatic duct that "bridges" it to the jejunal limb), direct external wirsungostomy or pancreatic duct occlusion with neoprene-based glue injection should be considered. Especially in the case of a highly contaminated surgical field and/or active bleeding, a savvy approach is to pursue a "damage control" management with open abdomen, in order to plan a surgical revision and, if possible, abdominal closure, within 24–48 h. If this is the case, we suggest leaving in place some rubber vascular loops that will help in the identification of peripancreatic vessels during second-look operations. This will be of utmost importance if vessel clamping or sutures were necessary in the first place, so that possible vascular injuries could be rapidly recognized and fixed thereafter. Additionally, the decision to place either a naso-jejunal feeding tube or, preferably, a nutritional jejunostomy should be kept in mind, as the critically ill patient might be unable to tolerate oral food for a long time thereafter.

References

1. Bassi C, Marchegiani G, Dervenis C, Sarr M, Abu Hilal M, Adham M, et al. The 2016 update of the international study group (ISGPS) definition and grading of postoperative pancreatic fistula: 11 years after. Surgery. 2017;161(3):584–91.
2. Casciani F, Bassi C, Vollmer C. Decision points in pancreatoduodenectomy: insights from the contemporary masters on prevention, mitigation and management of postoperative pancreatic fistula. Surgery. 2021;170(3):889–909.

3. Schuh F, Mihaljevic AL, Probst P, Trudeau MT, Muller PC, Marchegiani G, et al. A simple classification of pancreatic duct size and texture predicts postoperative pancreatic fistula: a classification of the international study group of pancreatic surgery (ISGPS). Ann Surg. 2021;277(3):e597–608.
4. Callery MP, Pratt WB, Kent TS, Chaikof EL, Vollmer CM Jr. A prospectively validated clinical risk score accurately predicts pancreatic fistula after pancreatoduodenectomy. J Am Coll Surg. 2013;216(1):1–14.
5. Trudeau MT, Casciani F, Ecker BL, Maggino L, Seykora TF, Puri P, et al. The fistula risk score catalog: toward precision medicine for pancreatic fistula after pancreatoduodenectomy. Ann Surg. 2020;275(2):e463–72.
6. McMillan MT, Malleo G, Bassi C, Allegrini V, Casetti L, Drebin J, et al. Multicenter, prospective trial of selective drain management for pancreatoduodenectomy using risk stratification. Ann Surg. 2017;265(6):1209–18.
7. Sachs T, Pratt W, Kent T, Callery M, Vollmer C. The pancreaticojejunal anastomotic stent: friend or foe? Surgery. 2013;153(5):651–62.
8. Ecker BL, McMillan MT, Asbun HJ, Ball CG, Bassi C, Beane JD, et al. Characterization and optimal management of high-risk pancreatic anastomoses during pancreatoduodenectomy. Ann Surg. 2018;267(4):608–16.
9. Andrianello S, Marchegiani G, Malleo G, Masini G, Balduzzi A, Paiella S, et al. Pancreaticojejunostomy with externalized stent vs pancreaticogastrostomy with externalized stent for patients with high-risk pancreatic anastomosis: a single-center, phase 3, randomized clinical trial. JAMA Surg. 2020;155(4):313–21.
10. Casciani F, Trudeau MT, Asbun H, Ball C, Bassi C, Behrman SW, et al. Surgeon experience contributes to improved outcomes in pancreatoduodenectomies at high risk for fistula development. Surgery. 2021;169(4):708–20.
11. Cannas S, Casciani F, Vollmer C. Extending quality improvement for pancreatoduodenectomy within the high-volume setting: the experience factor. Ann Surg. 2024;279(6):1036–45.
12. Mungroop TH, Klompmaker S, Wellner UF, Steyerberg EW, Coratti A, D'Hondt M, et al. Updated alternative fistula risk score (ua-FRS) to include minimally invasive pancreatoduodenectomy: Pan-European validation. Ann Surg. 2021;273(2):334–40.
13. Ecker BL, McMillan MT, Allegrini V, Bassi C, Beane JD, Beckman RM, et al. Risk factors and mitigation strategies for pancreatic fistula after distal pancreatectomy: analysis of 2026 resections from the international, multi-institutional distal pancreatectomy study group. Ann Surg. 2019;269(1):143–9.
14. Chong E, Ratnayake B, Lee S, French JJ, Wilson C, Roberts KJ, et al. Systematic review and meta-analysis of risk factors of postoperative pancreatic fistula after distal pancreatectomy in the era of 2016 international study group pancreatic fistula definition. HPB (Oxford). 2021;23(8):1139–51.
15. De Pastena M, van Bodengraven E, Mungroop T, Vissers F, Jones L, Marchegiani G, et al. Distal pancreatectomy fistula risk score (D-FRS): development and international validation. Ann Surg. 2023;227(5):e1099–3e1105.
16. Bonsdorff A, Ghorbani P, Helantera I, Tarvainen T, Kontio T, Belfrage H, et al. Development and external validation of DISPAIR fistula risk score for clinically relevant postoperative pancreatic fistula after distal pancreatectomy. Br J Surg. 2022;109(11):1131–9.
17. Marchegiani G, Perri G, Burelli A, Zoccatelli F, Andrianello S, Luchini C, et al. High-risk pancreatic anastomosis vs. total pancreatectomy after pancreatoduodenectomy: postoperative outcomes and quality of life analysis. Ann Surg. 2022;276(6):e905–13.
18. Balzano G, Zerbi A, Aleotti F, Capretti G, Melzi R, Pecorelli N, et al. Total pancreatectomy with islet transplantation as an alternative to high-risk pancreatojejunostomy after pancreatoduodenectomy: a prospective randomized trial. Ann Surg. 2023;277(6):894–903.
19. Andrianello S, Marchegiani G, Balduzzi A, Bastin A, Masini G, Esposito A. Pros and pitfalls of externalized, trans-anastomotic stent as a mitigation strategy for POPF: a prospective, risk-stratified observational series. HPB. 2021;23(7):1046–53.

20. Welsch T, Mussle B, Korn S, Sturm D, Bork U, Distler M, et al. Pancreatoduodenectomy with or without prophylactic falciform ligament wrap around the hepatic artery for prevention of postpancreatectomy haemorrhage: randomized controlled trial (PANDA trial). Br J Surg. 2021;109(1):37–45.

21. Seykora TF, Maggino L, Malleo G, Lee MK 4th, Roses R, Salvia R, et al. Evolving the paradigm of early drain removal following pancreatoduodenectomy. J Gastrointest Surg. 2019;23(1):135–44.

22. Diener MK, Seiler CM, Rossion I, Kleeff J, Glanemann M, Butturini G, et al. Efficacy of stapler versus hand-sewn closure after distal pancreatectomy (DISPACT): a randomised, controlled multicentre trial. Lancet. 2011;377(9776):1514–22.

23. Asbun HJ, Stauffer JA. Laparoscopic approach to distal and subtotal pancreatectomy: a clockwise technique. Surg Endosc. 2011;25(8):2643–9.

24. Van Buren G 2nd, Bloomston M, Schmidt CR, Behrman SW, Zyromski NJ, Ball CG, et al. A prospective randomized multicenter trial of distal pancreatectomy with and without routine intraperitoneal drainage. Ann Surg. 2017;266(3):421–31.

25. Smits FJ, Henry AC, Besselink MG, Busch OR, van Eijck CH, Arntz M, et al. Algorithm-based care versus usual care for the early recognition and management of complications after pancreatic resection in The Netherlands: an open-label, nationwide, stepped-wedge cluster-randomised trial. Lancet. 2022;399(10338):1867–75.

26. Smits FJ, van Santvoort HC, Besselink MG, Batenburg MCT, Slooff RAE, Boerma D, et al. Management of severe pancreatic fistula after pancreatoduodenectomy. JAMA Surg. 2017;152(6):540–8.

27. Wu J, Kuo T, Chen H, Wu C, Lai S, Yang C, et al. Randomized trial of oral versus enteral feeding for patients with postoperative pancreatic fistula after pancreatoduodenectomy. Br J Surg. 2019;106(3):190–8.

28. Fujii T, Nakao A, Murotani K, Okamura Y, Ishigure K, Hatsuno T, et al. Influence of food intake on the healing process of postoperative pancreatic fistula after pancreatoduodenectomy: a multi-institutional randomized controlled trial. Ann Surg Oncol. 2015;22(12):3905–12.

29. Groen JV, Smits FJ, Koole D, Besselink MG, Busch OR, den Dulk M, et al. Completion pancreatectomy or a pancreas-preserving procedure during relaparotomy for pancreatic fistula after pancreatoduodenectomy: a multicentre cohort study and meta-analysis. Br J Surg. 2021;108(11):1371–9.

Chapter 35
Post-Pancreatectomy Hemorrhage

Joshua P. Kronenfeld and Onur C. Kutlu

Introduction

Due to the often unpredictable environments and difficult to manage nature of its disease processes, the pancreas has a notorious reputation. Arguably the most famous of all rules in surgical residency is attributed to the pancreas: "Eat while you can, sleep while you can, and don't mess with the pancreas." [1] This rule is engraved into the minds of every young learner and will be recited from the beginning of clinical rotations until their retirement as physicians. Even as the experience of a surgeon increases, respect toward this challenging organ does not falter.

Despite much advancement in perioperative care and refinements in surgical technique, even in the hands of the most experienced surgeons and high-volume institutions, mortality and morbidity at 30 days after pancreatic surgery may reach 3% and 39%, respectively [2]. At 90 days, mortality has been reported to be double this rate [3]. Post-pancreatectomy hemorrhage (PPH) is a major contributor to "failure to rescue" and perioperative mortality, therefore should not be viewed as a simple post-surgical bleeding but as a severe and potentially devastating pancreatic surgery-specific complication.

Major causes of postoperative morbidity and mortality (e.g., pancreatic fistula, delayed gastric emptying, etc.) are outlined in their respective chapters in this manual and have been studied extensively. On the other hand, PPH has limited research with a lack of consensus in optimal medical and surgical management [4].

PPH is a potentially devastating complication with grave outcomes and arguably is the most feared of all events after pancreatectomy. The reported incidence rate is 3–29% with mortality rates reaching 7–31% [5, 6]. While most other adverse

J. P. Kronenfeld · O. C. Kutlu (✉)
DeWitt Daughtry Department of Surgery, University of Miami Miller School of Medicine, Miami, FL, USA
e-mail: okutlu@med.miami.edu

© The Author(s), under exclusive license to Springer Nature Switzerland AG 2025
E. P. Ceppa et al. (eds.), *The SAGES Manual of Evolving Techniques in Pancreatic Surgery*, https://doi.org/10.1007/978-3-031-78409-5_35

post-pancreatectomy events can be managed non-operatively or conservatively, early recognition and treatment of PPH are vital as operative or procedural management is often required [5]. The International Study Group of Pancreatic Surgery (ISGPS) classifies post-pancreatectomy hemorrhage based on time (e.g., early—less than 24 h vs. late—greater than 24 h), severity (e.g., mild vs. severe), and location (e.g., intraluminal vs. extraluminal) [7]. In this chapter, the source of bleeding vessel type (e.g., arterial vs. venous) will also be considered.

The pancreas is situated centrally in the retroperitoneum, and due to its embryological development, it is in an intimate relationship with the great abdominal vessels [8]. These include the first-order branches of the aorta: the celiac trunk and the superior mesenteric artery (SMA) and second-order branches: gastroduodenal artery (GDA) and common-proper hepatic artery. The arterial blood supply is provided by two rich arcades formed between branches of the SMA, GDA, and splenic artery including the superior and inferior pancreaticoduodenal arteries [9]. The venous anatomy, on the other hand, consists of low pressure systems with very high flow (e.g., inferior vena cava, renal veins, superior mesenteric vein, portal vein, inferior mesenteric vein, and splenic vein) [10].

The abundant blood supply, crowded vascular anatomy, and a difficult to access region of the abdomen contribute to the challenges of pancreatic surgery. Additionally, the pancreas produces proteolytic enzymes, which is a very important factor to the potential hemorrhagic complications of pancreatic surgery as these enzymes can potentially disrupt the hemostasis of vessels [11]. In addition to this, many patients who undergo pancreatectomy have a history of either acute or chronic pancreatitis, which complicates the issue even further due to chronic inflammation and weakening of the vasculature causing aneurysmal changes [12].

Current Classification and Definitions

PPH is a multifactorial complication and may originate from multiple sources due to the complex vascular anatomy and gastrointestinal reconstruction performed during the index operation. These sources can be summarized as injury to the arteries and veins, anastomotic suture or staple line dehiscence, bleeding from resection surfaces, pseudoaneurysms in surrounding arteries, bleeding from manipulation of the biliary structures, preexisting ulcer disease, and although rare, anatomical variances such as intrapancreatic arteries [13–15]. Bleeding can therefore be intraluminal or extraluminal depending on the source of hemorrhage.

The International Study Group of Pancreatic Surgery (ISGPS) classification published a consensus definition in 2007 categorizing the severity of PPH based on outcomes [7]. This guideline has been validated by many other studies, and it serves as the classification by which PPH is graded upon [6, 16, 17].

PPH Definitions According to ISGPS

Time of Onset

- Early hemorrhage ($\leq$24 h after the end of the index operation).
- Late hemorrhage (>24 h after the end of the index operation).

Location

- Intraluminal or intra-enteric (e.g., anastomotic suture line at stomach or duodenum, pancreatic surface at anastomosis, stress ulcer, pseudoaneurysm).
- Extraluminal or extra-enteric—into the abdominal cavity (e.g., arterial or venous vessels, diffuse bleeding from resection area, vascular anastomosis suture lines, and pseudoaneurysm).

Severity of Hemorrhage

Mild

- Small or medium volume blood loss (from drains, nasogastric tube, or identified on ultrasonography).
- Decrease in hemoglobin concentration < 3 g/dl.
- Mild clinical impairment of the patient, no therapeutic consequence.
- Possible need for noninvasive treatment with volume resuscitation or blood transfusions (2–3 units packed cells within 24 h of end of operation or 1–3 units if later than 24 h after operation).
- No need for reoperation or interventional angiographic embolization; endoscopic treatment of anastomotic bleeding may occur provided the other conditions apply.

Severe

- Large volume blood loss.
- Decrease in hemoglobin level by $\geq$3 g/dl.
- Clinically significant impairment of the patient (e.g., tachycardia, hypotension, oliguria, hypovolemic shock).
- Need for blood transfusion (>3 units packed cells).
- Need for invasive treatment (e.g., interventional angiographic embolization or additional surgical intervention).

ISGPS Grading of PPH

Grade	Onset/ severity	Clinical condition	Diagnosis	Treatment
A	Early/mild	Well	Close monitoring	None
			Hemoglobin checks	
			CT scan if necessary	
B	Early/severe	Often well-intermediate	Close monitoring	Transfusion of fluid/blood
	Late/mild	Rarely life threatening	Hemoglobin checks	Intermediate care unit or ICU
			CT scan	Relaparotomy for early PPH
			Angiogram	Embolization/stenting
			Endoscopy if intraluminal	Therapeutic endoscopy
C	Late/severe	Severely impaired	CT scan	ICU care
		Life threatening	Angiogram	Localization of bleeding
			Endoscopy if intraluminal	Angiography and embolization
				Relaparotomy
				Therapeutic endoscopy

Early PPH is often due to a technical error in intraoperative hemostasis or a coagulopathy (inherent or acquired) present in the patient. Late PPH is often related to a complication from the pancreatic resection such as a postoperative pancreatic, biliary or gastrointestinal anastomotic leak, or pseudoaneurysm, although inadequate surgical technique managing the gastroduodenal stump may also be an etiology [18, 19]. Due to the differences in underlying pathophysiology, early and late PPH should be considered as two distinct clinical entities.

Early Post-Pancreatectomy Hemorrhage

Early post-pancreatectomy hemorrhage, defined according to ISGPS guidelines as bleeding that occurs within 24 h of surgery, is most often due to one or a combination of a technical failure of appropriate hemostasis, failure of a suture or staple line at an anastomosis, bleeding from resection surfaces, or an acquired or inherent coagulopathy [13–15]. The location of early PPH may be intraluminal or extraluminal with each entity presenting its own clinical challenges.

Intraluminal PPH is defined as bleeding within a hollow-viscous organ such as the stomach, small intestine, or colon and can be identified as blood from a nasogastric tube, hematemesis, or melena. This type of bleeding represents about 11% of PPH and may be associated with ulcers at the anastomotic site or a fistula at an anastomosis [20]. Although some studies favor upper endoscopy in these cases, often times it is challenging to identify the source of bleeding during an acute bleed, and computed tomography (CT) angiography has been shown to be superior to endoscopy in diagnosis of significant intraluminal PPH [5, 21]. More importantly, even if a potential source can be identified via endoscopy, the bleeding may also originate outside the bowel and multiple sources of bleeding could be present. Thus, proceeding first with upper endoscopy in an intraluminal hemorrhage may delay diagnosis and treatment.

Extraluminal PPH, defined as bleeding that is freely into the abdominal cavity, is identified as blood egressing from a surgically placed drain or bleeding appreciated on postoperative cross-sectional imaging [15, 18, 20]. In rare circumstances, extraluminal blood can present as intraluminal bleeding and vice versa if breakdown of an anastomosis is present, so careful evaluation of any bleeding complication is imperative [15]. Early diagnosis and intervention are of paramount importance as mortality rates have been reported as high as 36% [18].

Once PPH is suspected, the initial step is to determine if the patient can tolerate diagnostic-therapeutic imaging [6]. For patients with obvious bleeding through the abdominal drains and hemodynamic instability, emergent surgical exploration should be considered [22]. This has been shown to result in definitive control of hemorrhage in up to 75% of the patients [6].

Late Post-Pancreatectomy Hemorrhage

Late or delayed PPH, defined to occur after 24 h from index operation, is the result of a multifactorial insult on the vasculature, in which the impact of post-operative pancreatic fistulae has been shown to be a significant contributor [11]. Although by definition late PPH presents 24 h after an operation, it may occur even weeks after the index procedure with a median presentation of 10–27 days and a range of 4–240 days, often after a patient has been discharged [5].

The effect of proteolytic enzymes on the vasculature is amplified by the intraoperative manipulation of the vessels, lymphadenectomy, subsequent vascular vulnerability, and the inflammation in the surgical bed [11]. This is even more profound in the presence of pseudoaneurysms due to the surgical intervention or due to previous episodes of acute or chronic pancreatitis in these patients [12].

Late or delayed PPH is often more common than early PPH and carries an incidence of 3.9% after pancreatic resection with a mortality of nearly 50% [5, 23]. Many delayed PPHs occur from arterial source such as the GDA stump, common hepatic artery, left hepatic artery, dorsal pancreatic artery, gastric arteries, or splenic artery [5, 13, 24]. Nearly 30% of patients with late PPH have a pseudoaneurysm present, which may be caused by proteolytic enzyme degradation from a pancreatic fistula, infection, or an intra-abdominal abscess [23]. Furthermore, the proportion of patients with late PPH increases to 65–80% of patients with either a pancreatic leak, intra-abdominal abscess, or both [23, 25, 26]. Presence of a pancreatic fistula was also an independent predictor of PPH and significantly increased the risk of mortality with an odds ratio of nearly 17 in one study [27]. The pathophysiology of PPH in these patients is hypothesized to be a pancreatic fistula or abscess that leads to weakening of vessel integrity, pseudoaneurysm formation, sentinel bleed, and ultimately catastrophic hemorrhage [13, 28].

Frequently, a sentinel bleed precedes massive hemorrhage. Sentinel bleeds are defined as small-volume blood loss through surgical drains, nasogastric tubes, hematemesis, or melena and are reported to occur in 30–100% of patients with PPH [7, 29]. It is, therefore, important to not overlook the changes in the characteristics of the drain output and have a high degree of suspicion for PPH if a drain suddenly becomes sanguineous, as this may imply the presence of a structural vascular defect that may precede a life-threatening hemorrhage [28]. As the blood loss becomes significant, the clinical signs will become apparent such as increased hemorrhagic output from tubes and drains, unexplained tachycardia and hypotension, clinical deterioration, alarming decreases in hemoglobin, hematemesis, and melena [30]. Once PPH is suspected, the patient should promptly be evaluated, as any delay in diagnosis would be detrimental and could negatively affect patient survival [6].

For the hemodynamically stable patients, emergent CT angiography or immediate percutaneous angiography should be performed [30]. Studies have shown contrast CT to have a 67% sensitivity in identifying the source of hemorrhage, similar to diagnostic invasive angiography, which has a mean sensitivity of 69% [31]. While CT angiography is noninvasive and effective alternative; however, invasive angiography has the advantage of being therapeutic in many cases of PPH [13].

Although emergent surgery should be considered for the hemodynamically unstable patient, for the patients that are stable enough, interventional radiologic management of these patients has been reported to have significantly lower rates of complications (36 vs. 70%) and mortality (17–21% vs. 36–42%) compared to open surgery [5].

Since late PPH is a relatively uncommon complication, it has not been feasible to formulate an algorithm or to create a predictive model to determine which treatment would be beneficial to each patient. Studies have shown that there is significant variability in the management of these patients even within the same institution [13, 25]. In a study by Jilesen et al., authors analyzed 1035 patients who underwent pancreaticoduodenectomy aiming to identify the predictors of which type of emergency intervention, surgical or radiological, a patient with late PPH should initially undergo [32]. However, no significant predictors were found that could be used to guide treatment in further episodes of late PPH.

While there is not an accepted algorithm for the treatment of a patient with late PPH, due to the aforementioned reasons, there is one generally accepted rule. Unstable patients with late PPH should immediately be transferred to an intensive care unit with aggressive resuscitation and the goal of achieving a level of stability that would allow for an endovascular intervention [7, 15]. In patients that cannot be resuscitated, immediate laparotomy should be considered even if unfavorable outcomes may frequently occur [33].

As in the case of early PPH, decisions are made based on the patient's hemodynamic stability. Although immediate laparotomy has been shown to control bleeding in 75% of the patients who present with massive hemorrhage after early PPH, late PPH inherently is a more challenging clinical scenario [6]. Contrary to early PPH, surgery for late PPH is more challenging due to inflammation, adhesions, and friable tissues [33]. Patients with delayed PPH are commonly critically ill, which contributes to the higher mortality rates seen in delayed PPH as should be expected from performing a long and challenging operation on a patient with hemodynamic instability [34].

In contrast, hemodynamically stable patients are typically better suited to undergo abdominal CT angiography at the first sign of bleeding [31]. CT angiography is a relatively quick diagnostic imaging modality, which can show the cause, nature, and site of bleeding and can guide treatment, especially when performed early before massive hemoperitoneum is present [15, 31]. However, some authors suggest directly performing an angiography as the sensitivity rate of identifying a bleeding source is 56–67%, compared with 69% for CT angiography [31]. Although more invasive, with a slight decrease in sensitivity, angiography has the advantage of not only identifying the source but also allowing for a successful therapeutic intervention in up to 87% of cases with an identifiable source of bleeding [15, 31]. In some situations, particularly when sentinel bleeding has occurred and since ceased, a clear bleeding site may be difficult or impossible to identify, further complicating the selection of ideal imaging and intervention modality [5, 15].

After the initial diagnostic workup, if the source of bleeding still cannot be identified, it is recommended to perform diagnostic angiography which could demonstrate contrast extravasation or vascular irregularities, although this may not be effective in case of diffuse or venous bleeding [13]. Historically, urgent surgical re-exploration was the procedure of choice, even for late PPH, as this would not only provide an opportunity to control hemorrhage but would also allow for drainage of collections and leaks which may have contributed to PPH [35]. Management of the pancreatic stump at the time of reoperation is also a major issue with little consensus. Wide drainage is one option mentioned previously; however, others advocate for removal of the pancreatic remnant to complete a total pancreatectomy. Others may choose to perform a new anastomosis with external and bridging drains. Furthermore, some surgeons have also proposed pancreatic duct occlusion with neoprene-based glue injection. Surgery has been associated with high rates of morbidity and mortality reaching 47% [35, 36]. Each situation is a case-by-case basis and in the era of interventional radiology is infrequently encountered. Therefore, unless the patient absolutely cannot tolerate interventional angiographic interventions and is not able to be resuscitated, percutaneous interventional radiology techniques should be prioritized [32].

Percutaneous angiographic interventions are recommended as a first-line approach by many authors. Systematic reviews and institutional case series report high rates of success in control of bleeding by interventional angiographic procedures (66–95%) [35]. Primarily coiling or gluing an arterial stump will most commonly be performed. It has also been described to cover the hepatic artery or a stump orifice off the SMA with a covered metal stent. The latter is more dangerous with downstream injury possible but are also performed in perilous situations for a complication with high fatality. Percutaneous interventional angiographic techniques have less complications rates (36 vs. 76%) and mortality (21 vs. 47%) when compared to open surgical interventions [35, 36]. Typically, rebleeding and need for multiple interventions are common.

While each clinical scenario of PPH may be different, clinical status will ultimately direct the optimal treatment modality offered to a patient. If clinically stable, it is clear that percutaneous interventional angiography is the treatment modality of choice, but more aggressive and invasive procedures, such as emergent laparotomy, may be required in unstable patients or in those where angiographic modalities are unsuccessful. Finally, institutional capabilities may also influence the intervention performed for a patient, as some institutions may not have the availability of advanced interventional specialists [32].

Conclusion

PPH is a dramatic complication of pancreatic surgery associated with high rates of mortality and morbidity. Although late PPH has a relatively lower incidence rate of 5%, the mortality rate is concerningly high at 14–41% [5]. A high index of suspicion, early recognition, and timely intervention are extremely important to minimizing adverse outcomes. Interventional procedures are advancing in the management of PPH with high rates of success in the management of bleeding with less mortality and morbidity compared to immediate relaparotomy, especially in case of late PPH. Despite the advances, PPH still has high rates of morbidity and mortality and contributes to failure to rescue after pancreatectomy. This still is the case even in high-volume centers with abundant resources. The data regarding PPH suggest that pancreatic surgery should be performed in high-volume centers where close collaboration with interventional specialties is capable of rescuing a patient from this relatively uncommon but lethal contributor to morbidity.

References

1. Biffl WL, Ball CG, Moore EE, et al. Don't mess with the pancreas! A multicenter analysis of the management of low-grade pancreatic injuries. J Trauma Acute Care Surg. 2021;91(5):820–8.
2. Hutchins RR, Kojodjojo P, Ho R, Bani-Hani A, Snooks SJ. Short and long-term outcome of pancreatic surgery in a district general hospital. J R Coll Surg Edinb. 2002;47(3):548–51.
3. Swanson RS, Pezzi CM, Mallin K, Loomis AM, Winchester DP. The 90-day mortality after pancreatectomy for cancer is double the 30-day mortality: more than 20,000 resections from the national cancer data base. Ann Surg Oncol. 2014;21(13):4059–67.
4. Ho CK, Kleeff J, Friess H, Buchler MW. Complications of pancreatic surgery. HPB (Oxford). 2005;7(2):99–108.

5. Biondetti P, Fumarola EM, Ierardi AM, Carrafiello G. Bleeding complications after pancreatic surgery: interventional radiology management. Gland Surg. 2019;8(2):150–63.
6. Ansari D, Tingstedt B, Lindell G, Keussen I, Ansari D, Andersson R. Hemorrhage after major pancreatic resection: incidence, risk factors, management, and outcome. Scand J Surg. 2017;106(1):47–53.
7. Wente MN, Veit JA, Bassi C, et al. Postpancreatectomy hemorrhage (PPH): an international study group of pancreatic surgery (ISGPS) definition. Surgery. 2007;142(1):20–5.
8. Ehrhardt JD, Gomez F. Embryology, pancreas. In: StatPearls. Treasure Island, FL: StatPearls Publishing; 2022.
9. Kulenovic A, Sarac-Hadzihalilovic A. Blood vessels distribution in body and tail of pancreas-a comparative study of age related variation. Bosn J Basic Med Sci. 2010;10(2):89–93.
10. Ibukuro K. Vascular anatomy of the pancreas and clinical applications. Int J Gastrointest Cancer. 2001;30(1–2):87–104.
11. Tien YW, Lee PH, Yang CY, Ho MC, Chiu YF. Risk factors of massive bleeding related to pancreatic leak after pancreaticoduodenectomy. J Am Coll Surg. 2005;201(4):554–9.
12. Vujasinovic M, Dugic A, Nouri A, et al. Vascular complications in patients with chronic pancreatitis. J Clin Med. 2021;10(16):3720.
13. Yekebas EF, Wolfram L, Cataldegirmen G, et al. Postpancreatectomy hemorrhage: diagnosis and treatment: an analysis in 1669 consecutive pancreatic resections. Ann Surg. 2007;246(2):269–80.
14. van Berge Henegouwen MI, Allema JH, van Gulik TM, Verbeek PC, Obertop H, Gouma DJ. Delayed massive haemorrhage after pancreatic and biliary surgery. Br J Surg. 1995;82(11):1527–31.
15. Puppala S, Patel J, McPherson S, Nicholson A, Kessel D. Hemorrhagic complications after Whipple surgery: imaging and radiologic intervention. AJR Am J Roentgenol. 2011;196(1):192–7.
16. Duarte Garces AA, Andrianello S, Marchegiani G, et al. Reappraisal of post-pancreatectomy hemorrhage (PPH) classifications: do we need to redefine grades a and B? HPB (Oxford). 2018;20(8):702–7.
17. Khuri S, Mansour S, Obeid A, Azzam A, Borzellino G, Kluger Y. Postpancreatoduodenectomy hemorrhage: association between the causes and the severity of the bleeding. Visc Med. 2021;37(3):171–9.
18. Wu X, Chen G, Wu W, et al. Management of late hemorrhage after pancreatic surgery: treatment strategy and prognosis. J Int Med Res. 2020;48(6):300060520929127.
19. Gao QX, Lee HY, Wu WH, et al. Factors associated with post-pancreaticoduodenectomy hemorrhage: 303 consecutive cases analysis. Chin Med J. 2012;125(9):1571–5.
20. Valcea S, Beuran M, Vartic M. Intraluminal postpancreatoduodenectomy hemorrhage—last 5 years experience. Chirurgia (Bucur). 2017;112(1):39–45.
21. Frattaroli FM, Casciani E, Spoletini D, et al. Prospective study comparing multi-detector row CT and endoscopy in acute gastrointestinal bleeding. World J Surg. 2009;33(10):2209–17.
22. Taghavi S, Nassar A, Askari R. Hypovolemic shock. In: StatPearls. Treasure Island, FL: StatPearls Publishing; 2022.
23. Limongelli P, Khorsandi SE, Pai M, et al. Management of delayed postoperative hemorrhage after pancreaticoduodenectomy: a meta-analysis. Arch Surg. 2008;143(10):1001–7. discussion 1007
24. Asai K, Zaydfudim V, Truty M, et al. Management of a delayed post-pancreatoduodenectomy haemorrhage using endovascular techniques. HPB (Oxford). 2015;17(10):902–8.
25. de Castro SM, Kuhlmann KF, Busch OR, et al. Delayed massive hemorrhage after pancreatic and biliary surgery: embolization or surgery? Ann Surg. 2005;241(1):85–91.
26. Manas-Gomez MJ, Rodriguez-Revuelto R, Balsells-Valls J, et al. Post-pancreaticoduodenectomy hemorrhage. Incidence, diagnosis, and treatment. World J Surg. 2011;35(11):2543–8.

27. Grutzmann R, Ruckert F, Hippe-Davies N, Distler M, Saeger HD. Evaluation of the international study group of pancreatic surgery definition of post-pancreatectomy hemorrhage in a high-volume center. Surgery. 2012;151(4):612–20.
28. Choi SH, Moon HJ, Heo JS, Joh JW, Kim YI. Delayed hemorrhage after pancreaticoduodenectomy. J Am Coll Surg. 2004;199(2):186–91.
29. Rajarathinam G, Kannan DG, Vimalraj V, et al. Post pancreaticoduodenectomy haemorrhage: outcome prediction based on new ISGPS clinical severity grading. HPB (Oxford). 2008;10(5):363–70.
30. Hooper N, Armstrong TJ. Hemorrhagic shock. In: StatPearls. Treasure Island, FL: StatPearls Publishing; 2022.
31. Floortje van Oosten A, Smits FJ, van den Heuvel DAF, van Santvoort HC, Molenaar IQ. Diagnosis and management of postpancreatectomy hemorrhage: a systematic review and meta-analysis. HPB (Oxford). 2019;21(8):953–61.
32. Jilesen AP, Tol JA, Busch OR, et al. Emergency management in patients with late hemorrhage after pancreatoduodenectomy for a periampullary tumor. World J Surg. 2014;38(9):2438–47.
33. Mimatsu K, Fukino N, Kano H, Kawasaki A, Oida T. Surgical laparotomy for repeated delayed arterial hemorrhage after pancreaticoduodenectomy. Case Rep Gastroenterol. 2019;13(1):50–7.
34. Lermite E, Sommacale D, Piardi T, et al. Complications after pancreatic resection: diagnosis, prevention and management. Clin Res Hepatol Gastroenterol. 2013;37(3):230–9.
35. Gaudon C, Soussan J, Louis G, Moutardier V, Gregoire E, Vidal V. Late postpancreatectomy hemorrhage: predictive factors of morbidity and mortality after percutaneous endovascular treatment. Diagn Interv Imaging. 2016;97(11):1071–7.
36. Das S, Ray S, Mangla V, et al. Post pancreaticoduodenectomy hemorrhage: a retrospective analysis of incidence, risk factors and outcome. Saudi J Gastroenterol. 2020;26:337–43.

Chapter 36
Delayed Gastric Emptying

Szu-Aun Long and Rebecca A. Snyder

Introduction

Despite advances in operative technique and improved perioperative care, postoperative morbidity following pancreatectomy remains high at 30–50% [1–4]. Delayed gastric emptying (DGE) is a common postoperative complication following pancreatic surgery affecting between 15 and 40% of patients following pancreatoduodenectomy (PD) [1, 5–7], 8–24% of patients following distal pancreatectomy (DP) [8, 9], and 36% of patients following total pancreatectomy (TP) [10]. Delayed gastric emptying is the inability to return to a standard diet due to symptoms of epigastric pain, early satiety, gastric fullness, and/or nausea and vomiting in the absence of mechanical obstruction. Although not fatal, it has been associated with increased hospital stay, higher readmission rates, need for transitional care upon discharge, and increased healthcare costs [11–14]. In a study conducted in California, the median length of stay for patients with DGE was 15 days compared to 8.5 days for patients without DGE. This resulted in an average additional cost of over $21,000 to the overall cost of hospitalization for those with DGE [12]. Additionally, patients with DGE report significantly worse quality of life outcomes 2 weeks after their operation [15], indicating that DGE contributes to the burden of additional healthcare costs and has profound effects on quality of life.

S.-A. Long
Department of Surgery, University of Cincinnati College of Medicine, Cincinnati, OH, USA

R. A. Snyder (✉)
Department of Surgical Oncology, The University of Texas MD Anderson Cancer Center, Houston, TX, USA
e-mail: rsnyder@mdanderson.org

© The Author(s), under exclusive license to Springer Nature Switzerland AG 2025
E. P. Ceppa et al. (eds.), *The SAGES Manual of Evolving Techniques in Pancreatic Surgery*, https://doi.org/10.1007/978-3-031-78409-5_36

Definitions of DGE

There have been several proposed definitions of DGE in the literature; most of these definitions have characterized DGE by the duration of nasogastric intubation and/or need for reinsertion of nasogastric tube (NGT), and the postoperative day when oral intake of regular food was tolerated [5]. Due to great variability in the definitions used by various surgical centers, the International Study Group of Pancreatic Surgery (ISGPS) suggested a standardized definition, with grades of DGE based on severity and clinical impact (Table 36.1), to facilitate the objective evaluation of various operative techniques and interventions.

The definition included three grades of DGE (A, B, C) based on increasing clinical severity. Grade A DGE is characterized by the patient requiring an NGT between postoperative day (POD) 4–7, if an NGT is reinserted after POD 3 for nausea or vomiting, or if a patient cannot tolerate a regular diet by POD 7 but can before POD 14. Grade B DGE is characterized by the patient requiring an NGT between POD 8 and 14, if an NGT is reinserted after POD 7 for symptoms, or if the patient is unable to tolerate a regular diet by POD 14 but can before POD 21. Grade C DGE is present if the NGT cannot be removed after POD 14, if the NGT has been replaced after POD 14, or if the patient is unable to tolerate a regular diet by POD 21. Typically, clinically relevant DGE (grade B/C) led to a greater length of time to resume diet and a greater need for prokinetic drugs, nutritional support, and diagnostic evaluations, leading to prolonged hospital stays. Grade B and C DGE were also associated with other postoperative complications such as pancreatic fistula [6]. The ISGPS definition has since been widely accepted and validated by several studies [16–19].

Pathophysiology of DGE

The mechanism behind DGE following pancreatectomy is not well understood. There have been several proposed mechanisms for primary DGE following PD and TP including vagal denervation and devascularization of the pylorus causing pylorospasm [20–22], decrease in plasma motilin levels following duodenectomy [23,

Table 36.1 The ISGPS definition of DGE after pancreatic surgery [5]

DGE grade	NGT required	Unable to tolerate solid oral intake by POD	Vomiting or gastric distension	Use of prokinetics
A	4–7 days or reinsertion > POD 3	7	±	±
B	8–14 days or reinsertion > POD 7	14	+	+
C	>14 days or reinsertion > POD 14	21	+	+

DGE delayed gastric emptying, *POD* postoperative day, *NGT* nasogastric tube

24], and reconstruction misalignment or angulation [23]. Risk factors contributing to the cause of DGE after PD do not apply to DP as there is minimal denervation of the duodenum or alimentary reconstruction. However, other postoperative complications such as pancreatic fistula, deep surgical infections, and peripancreatic fluid collections have been shown to increase the incidence of DGE in all three surgical operations [7, 9, 10, 25, 26].

Risk Factors of DGE

Patient Risk Factors

Several retrospective studies have used the ISGPS consensus definition of DGE to identify preoperative risk factors which may predispose a patient to develop DGE. In 2015, Eisenberg et al. retrospectively categorized over 700 patients from a single institution using the ISGPS definition and concluded that male sex (OR 1.92, $p = 0.007$) and prior smoking history (OR 1.75 $p = 0.033$) were positive predictors of DGE [13]. Other studies have utilized the large ACS-NSQIP database to identify predictive factors of DGE across all participating U.S. institutions. In a study conducted in 2019 of over 10,000 patients, Snyder et al. reported that age ≥65 years (OR 1.26, 95% confidence interval [CI] 1.13–1.41]), male sex (OR 1.54, 95% CI 1.38–1.72), body mass index (BMI) >30 (OR 1.22, 95% CI 1.06–1.40), and ASA class ≥3 (OR 1.24, 95% CI 1.08–1.42) were associated with increased rates of DGE [7]. Most recently, a large study analyzing over 15,000 patients reported age >70 (OR 1.23, 95%CI 0.98–1.54), coexisting chronic obstructive pulmonary disease (COPD) (OR 1.50, 95% CI 1.13–1.98), and ASA >2 (OR 1.17, 95% CI 1.05–1.32) to be positive predictors of DGE. Female sex (OR 0.74, 95% CI 0.66–0.84) and active smoking status (OR 0.78, CI 95% 0.66–0.93) were found to be protective factors [27].

Pylorus-Resecting Pancreatoduodenectomy (PrPD) Vs. Pylorus-Preserving Pancreatoduodenectomy (PpPD)

Both retrospective and prospective studies have investigated various operative techniques (Fig. 36.1) to explore associations between operative technique and DGE with conflicting reports. The classical pancreatoduodenectomy (cPD) as described by Kausch-Whipple in the 1930s included a distal hemigastrectomy [28]. In 1978, Traverso and Longmire introduced the pylorus-preserving pancreatoduodenectomy (PpPD) which aimed to prevent complications after gastrectomy such as dumping syndrome, reflux, or poor weight gain by preserving the pylorus [29]. However, early studies noted increased rates of DGE with PpPD compared to cPD

Fig. 36.1 Schematic illustration of the three types of PD: PrPD (cPD and SSPPD) and PpPD. In SSPPD, the stomach is resected at 2–3 cm proximal to the pyloric ring. (Borrowed from Hanna et al. 2015 [33] with permission from Springer)

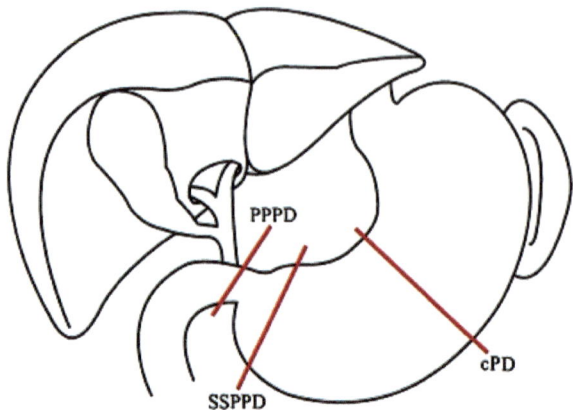

hypothesizing that pylorospasm may be contributing to the cause of DGE. Several techniques including pyloromyotomy [21] and pyloric dilatation [30, 31] were suggested to help mitigate DGE in PpPD. In Japan beginning in the 1990s, subtotal stomach-preserving pancreatoduodenectomy (SSPPD) was routinely performed in which only the pyloric ring is removed. This method was intended to maintain the pooling ability of the stomach while preserving the blood supply and innervation of the prepyloric region to help reduce the incidence of DGE [32]. Some studies noted a decrease in the incidence of DGE in SSPPD compared to PpPD. However, a recent meta-analysis analyzing three randomized-controlled trials and eight non-randomized studies with a total of 992 patients reported comparable rates of DGE between PrPD and PpPD suggesting no difference between the two procedures in regard to DGE [29].

Antecolic Reconstruction Vs. Retrocolic Reconstruction

Antecolic reconstruction of the gastrojejunostomy (GJ) during cPD or duodenojejunostomy (DJ) during PpPD has been preferred due to the theoretical advantage of the colon being between the gastroenteric reconstruction and the pancreatojejunostomy (PJ) to protect the anastomosis from pancreatic juices in the event of a postoperative pancreatic fistula [34, 35], less angulation or torsion of the GJ or DJ [35, 36], and a more mobile descending jejunal loop due to less venous congestion and bowel edema [37]. However, this remains controversial (Table 36.2). In 2006, Tani et al. retrospectively evaluated 159 patients and demonstrated that an antecolic route of reconstruction leads to a lower incidence of DGE compared to a retrocolic route in PpPD patients (5 vs. 50%) [38]. However, additional randomized-controlled trials conducted by Eshuis et al. and Tamandl et al. in 2014 later demonstrated that the route of gastroenteric reconstruction after PpPD does not influence the postoperative incidence of DGE [34, 39]. A recent meta-analysis published in 2019 analyzed

Table 36.2 Summary of comparative studies assessing DGE rates in antecolic vs. retrocolic reconstruction

| | | | Patient # | | DGE rates | | | |
References	Location	Study design	AC	RC	AC (%)	RC (%)	P- value	Study conclusion
[37]	Korea	Retro	46	104	6.5	31.7	0.0174	AC better
[42]	Japan	Retro	12	18	8	72	<0.001	AC better
[35]	Germany	Retro	100	100	5	24	<0.001	AC better
[43]	Japan	Retro	25	19	8	32	<0.0001	AC better
[38]	Japan	RCT	20	20	5	50	0.0014	AC better
[44]	Japan	Retro	78	54	10	81	<0.001	AC better
[45]	Japan	RCT	17	18	6	22	0.03	No difference
[46]	America	Retro	36	115	14	40	0.004	AC better
[47]	India	RCT	32	36	34.4	27.8	0.06	No difference
[48]	Japan	RCT	24	22	20.8	50.0	0.023	AC better
[49]	Netherlands	Retro	77	77	20	36	0.02	No difference
[34]	Netherlands	RCT	121	125	34	36	0.72	No difference
[50]	Japan	RCT	58	58	12.1	20.7	0.316	No difference
[39]	Australia	RCT	34	26	17.6	23.1	0.628	No difference
[51]	America	Retro	400	400	11	19	0.010	AC better
[41]	America	Retro	103	109	12.6	15.6	0.058	No difference

Retro retrospective cohort study, *RCT* randomized-controlled trial, *AC* antecolic, *RC* retrocolic

fifteen studies involving 2270 patients and found that antecolic reconstruction of the GJ or DJ was associated with a significantly lower rate of DGE (OR 0.29, 95% CI 0.16–0.50), shorter hospital stay, and faster recovery to a regular diet compared to retrocolic reconstruction [40]. Most recently, a randomized-controlled trial conducted in 2021 of 212 patients failed to determine non-inferiority of retrocolic to antecolic reconstruction in regard to DGE incidence following PD (15.6 vs. 12.6%, risk difference 2.97%, 95% CI −6.3–12.6%, $P = 0.058$) [41].

Billroth I Type Vs. Billroth II Type Vs. Roux-en-Y Reconstruction

The end-to-end duodenojejunostomy (Billroth I type) reconstruction has been proposed to be more physiologic in regard to regulation of pH and enzymatic digestion due to the resemblance of its anastomosis to normal anatomy in PpPD [52, 53]. This method of reconstruction has been favored in Japan [54] despite evidence of higher rates of DGE in patients with Billroth I type reconstruction compared to Billroth II type [36, 43, 55]. Randomized-controlled trials have compared rates of DGE with Billroth II type and Roux-en-Y reconstructions (Fig. 36.2) with conflicting reports. In 2013, Shimoda et al. reported significantly higher rates of DGE with Roux-en-Y reconstruction compared to Billroth II type reconstruction (20.4 vs. 5.7%) [56].

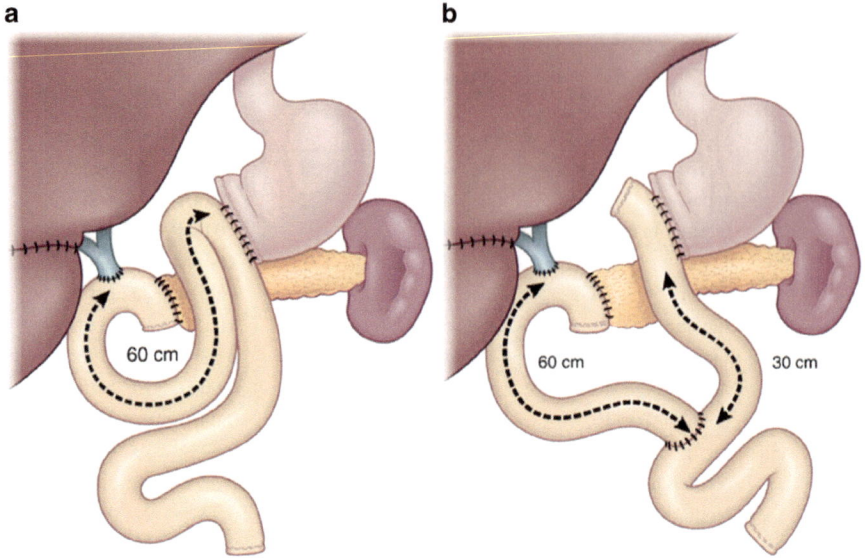

Fig. 36.2 Schematic illustration of Billroth II type reconstruction (**a**) and Roux-en-Y reconstruction (**b**). (Image adapted from Macutkiewicz 2021 [59] with permission from Springer)

Later in 2018, Busquets et al. published the randomized-controlled PAUDA trial which found equal rates of DGE in the Billroth II type and Roux-en-Y group (45 vs. 45%) [57]. A recent metanalysis published in 2021 examining 24 randomized-controlled trials and 2526 patients reported no difference in the rates of DGE in patients with a Billroth II type reconstruction vs. a Roux-en-Y [58].

Minimally Invasive Vs. Open Distal Pancreatectomy

Risk factors for DGE following DP have not been well studied compared to PD, likely due to the lower morbidity and incidence of DGE following DP. Studies have reported the incidence of DGE following elective DP to be 8–24% [8, 60, 61]. However, studies have demonstrated higher rates of DGE, up to three times, with open DP compared to laparoscopic and robot-assisted DP [8, 62]. In a randomized-controlled trial comparing minimally invasive vs. open DP, 20% patients who underwent open DP suffered from DGE compared to 6% in the minimally invasive group [62]. These studies suggest that a minimally invasive approach may limit the incidence of DGE and reduce hospital length of stay.

Assessment and Treatment of DGE

The ISGPS definition of DGE has been helpful in standardizing the reporting of DGE. However, there are no clear guidelines regarding the objective assessment of DGE. For secondary DGE, the treatment modality is determined according to the underlying etiology (i.e., drainage of the intra-abdominal abscess). For primary DGE, the management strategies are less clear. Some centers perform an upper endoscopy (Fig. 36.3) or obtain a contrast swallow study (Fig. 36.4) to confirm the patency of the gastroenteric anastomosis and to assess drainage of the afferent and efferent limbs [37, 63]. Other studies have shown that pyloric dilatation following PpPD decreases rates of DGE and facilitates earlier hospital discharge [64–66]. Gastric scintigraphy has been shown to be a non-invasive tool to objectively diagnose DGE and is considered the gold standard for measuring gastric motility [67, 68]. Therapeutic endoscopy in which recurrent intubations of the afferent and efferent limbs are performed with longer intubation times has been shown to be a possible treatment for primary DGE if medical treatments have failed [63].

Prevention and Therapeutic Strategies for DGE

Braun Enteroenterostomy

It has been proposed that bile reflux into the stomach from the gastroenterostomy is a possible etiology of DGE in cPD [69]. A Braun entero-enterostomy, first reported by Braun over 100 years ago in the context of gastric surgery, has been proposed as

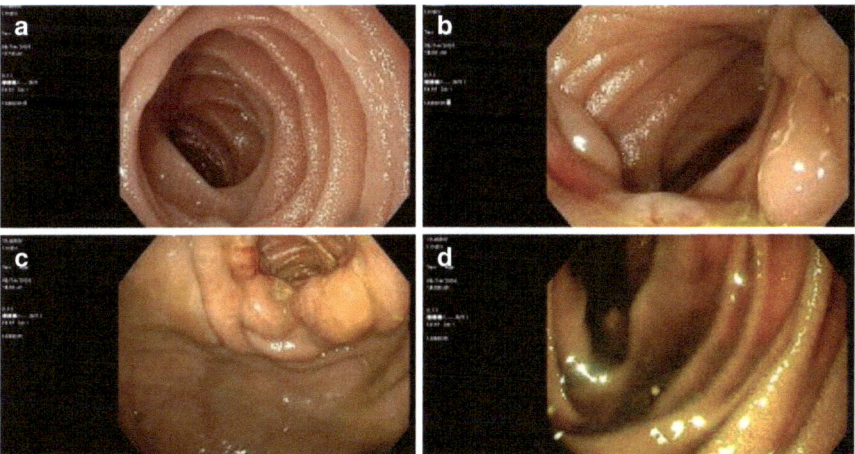

Fig. 36.3 Esophagogastroduodenoscopy demonstrating a patent afferent limb (**a**), gastrojejunostomy (**b**, **c**), and efferent limb (**d**) in a patient with DGE

Fig. 36.4 Upper GI study demonstrating contrast passage through the esophagus, stomach, and gastrojejunostomy in a patient with DGE

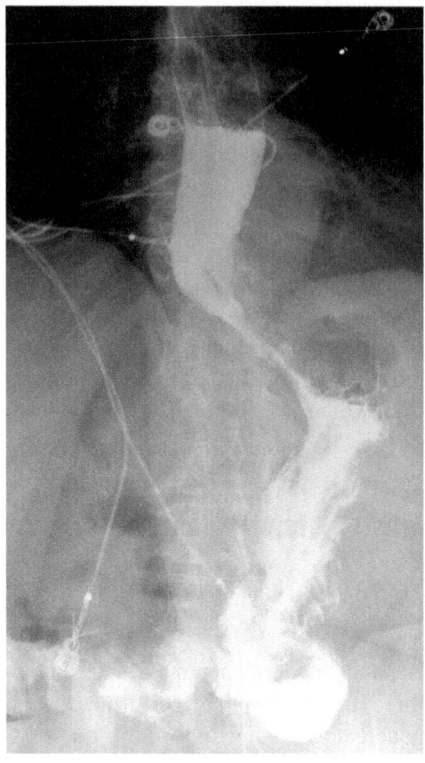

a mechanism to alleviate bile reflux and mitigate DGE. Here, an enteroenterostomy is made between the afferent and efferent limbs distal to the gastroenterostomy to divert bile and pancreatic secretions into the efferent limb to prevent reflux into the remnant stomach [70]. Additionally, it has been theorized that the Braun enteroenterostomy stabilizes the gastrojejunostomy and prevents twisting and angulation of the anastomosis which may contribute to DGE [46]. Meta-analyses on retrospective studies comparing DGE in patients with and without Braun entero-enterostomy have demonstrated that Braun entero-enterostomy can reduce the occurrence of DGE [71, 72]. However, recent randomized-controlled trials have shown no difference in rates of DGE between both groups [72, 73]. In 2018, Zhou et al. completed a meta-analysis of 11 studies (3 RCTs and 8 non-RCTs) and over 1600 patients and concluded that Braun entero-enterostomy decreases the incidence (OR 0.32, 95% CI 0.24–0.43) and severity (OR 0.27, 95% CI 0.15–0.51) of DGE following PD [74].

Nasogastric Tube

Current standards of fast-track surgery and enhanced recovery protocols recommend avoidance of nasogastric intubation following PD [75] to decrease postoperative morbidity. Data has shown that early removal of NGT following elective laparotomy is associated with an earlier return of bowel function and decrease in pulmonary complications [76]. Studies have demonstrated that elective liver, gastric, and colonic surgeries can be performed without nasogastric decompression [77]. Recently, retrospective studies have demonstrated that routine gastric decompression following PD can be safely avoided to minimize postoperative complications [77–79]. A randomized-controlled trial recently published in 2020 confirmed these findings and demonstrated that avoiding routine nasogastric intubation following PD is safe, although routine implementation into clinical practice has not yet been demonstrated [80].

Early Feeding

Surgeons have often been reluctant to introduce early postoperative oral feeding after PD due to concerns regarding pancreatic secretion stimulation, gastric distension, and anastomotic integrity. Distal enteral feeds by either nasojejunal feeding tube or jejunostomy tube have been shown to reduce complications and length of stay compared to total parenteral nutrition [81]. A recent randomized-controlled trial investigated whether early normal feeding following major upper gastrointestinal surgery (of which >22% of the operations were PD or DP) was safe compared to enteral tube feeding. This study concluded that initiating an early oral diet does not increase morbidity compared to enteral feeding [82]. Similarly, a study published in 2021 compared early oral feeding compared to early nasojejunal feeding following PpPD and found no association of feeding methods and DGE [83].

Prokinetic Drugs and Secretory Analogues

Metoclopramide has been shown as being an effective agent in treating delayed gastric emptying [84]. However, no randomized-controlled trial to date has studied metoclopramide in the setting of DGE following pancreatoduodenectomy. Yeo et al. studied erythromycin in a randomized-controlled trial in 1993. High-dose erythromycin (200 mg) administered on POD 3–10 was shown to significantly reduce the incidence of DGE by 37% [85]. However, erythromycin can cause adverse cardiac events due to QT-interval prolongation, so careful monitoring of drug interactions is warranted. Another study demonstrated that low doses of erythromycin (1 mg/kg) administered on POD 1–14 reduced the incidence of DGE by 75% after Billroth I type PpPD [86]. Somatostatin analogues result in an inhibition of gastrointestinal secretions and can be used to reduce output from postoperative pancreatic fistula. Although there have been concerns that octreotide could exacerbate DGE, studies to date have not demonstrated an impact of octreotide on gastric emptying following cPD or PpPD [87–89].

Chewing Gum

Gum chewing has been shown to restore gut activity following colorectal surgery [90]. In 2014, a small pilot study demonstrated lower rates of DGE and shorter length of stay following PD in patients who chewed gum for 30 min three times a day [91]. It is an easy, cheap, and safe agent that may have some beneficial effects on preventing DGE [92].

Indications for Nutritional Support

Following pancreatectomy, the nutritional status of the patient must be closely monitored. In the case of severe postoperative complications, DGE, or evidence of malnutrition [93], supplementary artificial nutrition should be started immediately. Enteral nutrition is preferred as its delivery to the stomach and small intestine stimulates the release of pancreatobiliary secretions to maintain gut contractility and blood flow as well as preserves the gut mucosal barrier to prevent bacterial translocation [94].

Enteral nutrition can be provided via a nasoenteric feeding tube or through more invasive options such as an endoscopic or percutaneous gastrostomy with jejunal extension or an operatively placed feeding jejunostomy tube [95]. Each technique has its own risk of complications which should be taken into consideration. Distal feeding is generally preferred to decrease risk of aspiration and to protect the anastamoses [93]. Although nasojejunal feeding tubes have been reported to dislodge in >30% of cases [96] and cause patients to experience more discomfort [97], they generally have less severe complications compared to jejunostomy tubes [96, 98]. Given the shift toward enhanced recovery pathway protocols, placement of nasojejunal feeding tubes for enteral nutrition appears to be the preferred approach [95]. It is recommended that nasojejunal feeding tubes be placed with the aid of endoscopic, fluoroscopic, or bedside electromagnetic guidance to reduce risk of complications from inadvertent placement of the tube into the bronchus [93, 99].

Mitigation Strategies for DGE

Feeding Jejunostomy Tube

Intraoperative placement of a feeding jejunostomy tube for postoperative nutrition was historically a routine practice at some institutions following PD. With increasing implementation of enhanced recovery after surgery pathway protocols, several studies have found that placement of a feeding jejunostomy tube is not associated with decreased morbidity following PD [100] and may in fact be associated with increased morbidity [101, 102]. A recent meta-analysis concluded that feeding jejunostomies are associated with increased rates of DGE and hospital length of stay without significant benefits [103]. However, to this date, no randomized-controlled trials have studied this specifically.

Risk-Stratified Perioperative Pathways

Perioperative care pathways and enhanced recovery pathway protocols have been designed to standardize care of all patients being treated for a specific surgical operation at an institution. Although clinical pathways have been designed and implemented for pancreatectomies, the results have been less dramatic compared to those observed with other operations [104–106]. In specific regard to DGE, initial studies showed that standardized clinical pathways may have no benefit on DGE rates [107, 108]. However, recent studies have now shown a benefit in preoperative individualized risk stratification to help reduce common complications following PD. In a recent study from MD Anderson Cancer Center, patients were assigned to one of three perioperative care pathways based on individual risk stratification for postoperative pancreatic fistula. After risk-stratified pathway implementation, median length of stay decreased from 10 to 6 days, and median costs of hospitalization were reduced by 22% [104]. Another study from MD Anderson Cancer Center specifically examined DGE rates after individual risk-stratification assignment to low- or high-risk care pathways and found that risk-stratified pathway implementation was the single most important factor in reducing DGE rates [109]. Recently, the *PrEDICT-DGE* score was developed to identify patients preoperatively who are at low-, intermediate-, and high-risk for DGE based on nine variables—age, gender, smoking status, COPD, ASA >2, preoperative blood transfusion, biliary stent, reconstruction technique (cPD, PpPD, invagination of PJ or PG), and concomitant procedures (adhesiolysis, feeding jejunostomy placement, vascular reconstruction) [27]. This tool or similar predictive models may be beneficial to identify patients who may warrant deviation from a standardized pathway.

Analgesia Modalities

Very few studies have examined the relationship of pain management following PD and DGE rates. A 2020 randomized trial evaluating gastrointestinal complications after pancreatoduodenectomy in patients with epidural vs. patient-controlled intravenous analgesia found no between-group difference in DGE [110]. A recent meta-analysis compared epidural analgesia and patient-controlled anesthesia following PD and DP and found no difference in DGE rates between groups [111].

Conclusion

Delayed gastric emptying is a common complication following pancreatic resection affecting 8–40% of patients based on the type of surgery. It is defined by a validated grading system based on severity and clinical impact. Risk factors associated with increased incidence include postoperative complications such as pancreatic fistula, deep surgical infections, and peripancreatic fluid collections. Additionally, various preoperative risk factors have been identified which may predispose a patient to develop DGE.

The association between surgical technique and DGE has been extensively studied in the literature with conflicting results. Current evidence suggests that surgical technique, specifically PpPD vs. PrPD, does not affect the incidence of DGE. The existing data suggest that antecolic reconstruction may be superior to retrocolic reconstruction in reducing DGE. Billroth II type and Roux-en-Y reconstruction have been shown to reduce rates of DGE compared to Billroth I type reconstruction for PpPD. Additionally, there is some data to suggest that Braun entero-enterostomy may be beneficial in reducing DGE, although the procedure has not been implemented routinely at most high-volume centers. Meticulous surgical technique to minimize the incidence of pancreatic fistula and avoid other postoperative complications is likely more important than the type of anastomosis or reconstruction technique performed.

With the use of enhanced recovery protocols gaining popularity following major abdominal operations, studies have recommended against routine use of nasogastric intubation and use of enteric feeding methods via nasojejunal feeding tubes or jejunostomy tubes. Based on a few recent studies, individualized risk-stratification pathways do appear to reduce DGE rates. In the postoperative period, prokinetic drugs such as metoclopramide and erythromycin and chewing gum may also be beneficial in reducing DGE.

References

1. Yeo CJ, Cameron JL, Sohn TA, Lillemoe KD, Pitt HA, Talamini MA, et al. Six hundred fifty consecutive pancreaticoduodenectomies in the 1990s: pathology, complications, and outcomes. Ann Surg. 1997;226(3):248.
2. Winter JM, Cameron JL, Campbell KA, Arnold MA, Chang DC, Coleman JA, et al. 1423 pancreaticoduodenectomies for pancreatic cancer: a single-institution experience. J Gastrointest Surg. 2006;10(9):1199–211.
3. Cameron JL, He J. Two thousand consecutive pancreaticoduodenectomies. J Am Coll Surg. 2015;220(4):530–6.
4. Trede M, Schwall G. The complications of pancreatectomy. Ann Surg. 1988;207(1):39.
5. Wente MN, Bassi C, Dervenis C, Fingerhut A, Gouma DJ, Izbicki JR, et al. Delayed gastric emptying (DGE) after pancreatic surgery: a suggested definition by the international study group of pancreatic surgery (ISGPS). Surgery. 2007;142(5):761–8.
6. Wente MN, Veit JA, Bassi C, Dervenis C, Fingerhut A, Gouma DJ, et al. Postpancreatectomy hemorrhage (PPH)-an international study group of pancreatic surgery (ISGPS) definition. Surgery. 2007;142(1):20–5.
7. Snyder RA, Ewing JA, Parikh AA. Delayed gastric emptying after pancreaticoduodenectomy: a study of the national surgical quality improvement program. Pancreatology. 2020;20(2):205–10.
8. Degisors S, Caiazzo R, Dokmak S, Truant S, Aussilhou B, Eveno C, et al. Delayed gastric emptying following distal pancreatectomy: incidence and predisposing factors. HPB. 2022;24(5):772–81.
9. Glowka TR, Webler M, Matthaei H, Schäfer N, Schmitz V, Kalff JC, et al. Delayed gastric emptying following pancreatoduodenectomy with alimentary reconstruction according to Roux-en-Y or Billroth-II. BMC Surg. 2017;17(1):24.
10. John GK, Singh VK, Pasricha PJ, Sinha A, Afghani E, Warren D, et al. Delayed gastric emptying (DGE) following total pancreatectomy with islet auto transplantation in patients with chronic pancreatitis. J Gastrointest Surg. 2015;19(7):1256–61.
11. Miedema BW, Sarr MG, Van Heerden JA, Nagorney DM, McIlrath DC, Ilstrup D. Complications following pancreaticoduodenectomy: current management. Arch Surg. 1992;127(8):945–50.
12. Grossi S, Lin A, Wong A, Namm J, Senthil M, Gomez N, et al. Costs and complications: delayed gastric emptying after pancreaticoduodenectomy. Am Surg. 2019;85(12):1423–8.
13. Eisenberg JD, Rosato EL, Lavu H, Yeo CJ, Winter JM. Delayed gastric emptying after pancreaticoduodenectomy: an analysis of risk factors and cost. J Gastrointest Surg. 2015;19(9):1572–80.
14. Robinson JR, Marincola P, Shelton J, Merchant NB, Idrees K, Parikh AA. Perioperative risk factors for delayed gastric emptying after a pancreaticoduodenectomy. HPB. 2015;17(6):495–501.
15. Eshuis WJ, De Bree K, Sprangers MAG, Bennink RJ, Van Gulik TM, ORC B, Gouma DJ. Gastric emptying and quality of life after pancreato-duodenectomy with retrocolic or antecolic gastroenteric anastomosis. Br J Surg. 2015;102:1123–32.
16. Malleo G, Crippa S, Butturini G, Salvia R, Partelli S, Rossini R, et al. Delayed gastric emptying after pylorus-preserving pancreaticoduodenectomy: validation of international study group of pancreatic surgery classification and analysis of risk factors. HPB. 2010;12:610–8.
17. Welsch T, Bonn M, Degrate L, Hinz U, Büchler MW, Wente MN. Evaluation of the international study group of pancreatic surgery definition of delayed gastric emptying after pancreatoduodenectomy in a high-volume centre. Br J Surg. 2010;97(7):1043–50.
18. Park JS, Hwang HK, Kim JK, Cho SI, Yoon DS, Lee WJ, Chi HS. Clinical validation and risk factors for delayed gastric emptying based on the international study group of pancreatic surgery (ISGPS) classification. Surgery. 2009;146(5):882–7.

19. Harnoss JC, Ulrich AB, Harnoss JM, Diener MK, Büchler MW, Welsch T. Use and results of consensus definitions in pancreatic surgery: a systematic review. Surgery. 2014;155(1):47–57.
20. Tanaka A, Ueno T, Oka M, Suzuki T. Effect of denervation of the pylorus and transection of the duodenum on acetaminophen absorption in rats; possible mechanism for early delayed gastric emptying after pylorus preserving pancreatoduodenectomy. Tohoku J Exp Med. 2000;192(4):239–47.
21. Kim DK, Hindenburg AA, Sharma SK, Suk CH, Gress FG, Staszewski H, et al. Is pyloro-spasm a cause of delayed gastric emptying after pylorus-preserving pancreaticoduodenec-tomy? Ann Surg Oncol. 2005;12(3):222–7.
22. Gauvin JM, Sarmiento JM, Sarr MG. Pylorus-preserving pancreaticoduodenectomy with complete preservation of the pyloroduodenal blood supply and innervation. Arch Surg. 2003;138(11):1261–3.
23. Tanaka M. Gastroparesis after a pylorus-preserving pancreatoduodenectomy. Surg Today. 2005;35:345–50.
24. Matsunaga H, Tanaka M, Naritomi G, Yokohata K, Yamaguchi K, Chijiiwa K. Effect of leu-cine 13-motilin (KW5139) on early gastric stasis after pylorus-preserving pancreatoduode-nectomy. Ann Surg. 1998;227(4):507–12.
25. Noorani A, Rangelova E, Del Chiaro M, Lundell LR, Ansorge C. Delayed gastric emptying after pancreatic surgery: analysis of factors determinant for the short-term outcome. Front Surg. 2016;3:25.
26. Ramanathan R, Mason T, Wolfe LG, Kaplan BJ. Predictors of short-term readmission after pancreaticoduodenectomy. J Gastrointest Surg. 2018;22(6):998–1006.
27. Werba G, Sparks AD, Lin PP, Johnson LB, Vaziri K. The PrEDICT-DGE score as a simple preoperative screening tool identifies patients at increased risk for delayed gastric emptying after pancreaticoduodenectomy. HPB. 2022;24(1):30–9.
28. Whipple AO. Present-day surgery of the pancreas. N Engl J Med. 2009;226(13):515–26.
29. Klaiber U, Probst P, Strobel O, Michalski CW, Dörr-Harim C, Diener MK, et al. Meta-analysis of delayed gastric emptying after pylorus-preserving versus pylorus-resecting pan-creatoduodenectomy. Br J Surg. 2018;105(4):339–49.
30. Balcom Iv JH, Rattner DW, Warshaw AL, Chang Y, Fernandez-Del Castillo C. Ten-year experience with 733 pancreatic resections: changing indications, older patients, and decreas-ing length of hospitalization. Arch Surg. 2001;136(4):391–8.
31. Uravić M, Zelić M, Petrošić N, Tokmadžić VS. Effect of pyloric dilatation on gastric emptying after pylorus-preserving pancreaticoduodenectomy. Hepato-Gastroenterology. 2011;58(112):2144–7.
32. Hayashibe A, Kameyama M, Shinbo M, Makimoto S. The surgical procedure and clinical results of subtotal stomach preserving pancreaticoduodenectomy (SSPPD) in comparison with pylorus preserving pancreaticoduodenectomy (PPPD). J Surg Oncol. 2007;95(2):106–9.
33. Hanna M, Gadde R, Tamariz L, Allen C, Meizoso J, Sleeman D, et al. Delayed gastric empty-ing after pancreaticoduodenectomy: is subtotal stomach preserving better or pylorus preserv-ing? J Gastrointest Surg. 2015;19(8):1542–52.
34. Eshuis WJ, Van Eijck CHJ, Gerhards MF, Coene PP, De Hingh IHJT, Karsten TM, et al. Antecolic versus retrocolic route of the gastroenteric anastomosis after pancreatoduodenec-tomy: a randomized controlled trial. Ann Surg. 2014;259(1):45–51.
35. Hartel M, Wente MN, Hinz U, Kleeff J, Wagner M, Müller MW, et al. Effect of antecolic reconstruction on delayed gastric emptying after the pylorus-preserving whipple procedure. Arch Surg. 2005;140(11):1094–9.
36. Ueno T, Takashima M, Iida M, Yoshida S, Suzuki N, Oka M. Improvement of early delayed gastric emptying in patients with Billroth I type of reconstruction after pylorus preserving pancreatoduodenectomy. J Hepato-Biliary-Pancreat Surg. 2009;16(3):300–4.
37. Park YC, Kim SW, Jang JY, Ahn YJ, Park YH. Factors influencing delayed gastric emptying after pylorus-preserving pancreatoduodenectomy. J Am Coll Surg. 2003;196(6):859–65.

38. Tani M, Terasawa H, Kawai M, Ina S, Hirono S, Uchiyama K, Yamaue H. Improvement of delayed gastric emptying in pylorus-preserving pancreaticoduodenectomy: results of a prospective, randomized, controlled trial. Ann Surg. 2006;243(3):316–20.
39. Tamandl D, Sahora K, Prucker J, Schmid R, Holst JJ, Miholic J, et al. Impact of the reconstruction method on delayed gastric emptying after pylorus-preserving pancreaticoduodenectomy: a prospective randomized study. World J Surg. 2014;38(2):465–75.
40. Qiu J, Li M, Du C, Koniaris LG. Antecolic reconstruction is associated with a lower incidence of delayed gastric emptying compared to retrocolic technique after Whipple or pylorus-preserving pancreaticoduodenectomy. Medicine. 2019;98(34):e16663.
41. Toyama H, Matsumoto I, Mizumoto T, Fujita H, Tsuchida S, Kanbara Y, et al. Influence of the retrocolic versus antecolic route for alimentary tract reconstruction on delayed gastric emptying after pancreatoduodenectomy: a multicenter, noninferiority randomized controlled trial. Ann Surg. 2021;274(6):935–44.
42. Sugiyama M, Abe N, Ueki H, Masaki T, Mori T, Atomi Y. A new reconstruction method for preventing delayed gastric emptying after pylorus-preserving pancreatoduodenectomy. Am J Surg. 2004;187(6):743–6.
43. Kurosaki I, Hatakeyama K. Clinical and surgical factors influencing delayed gastric emptying after pyloric-preserving pancreaticoduodenectomy. Hepato-Gastroenterology. 2005;52(61):143–8.
44. Murakami Y, Uemura K, Sudo T, Hayashidani Y, Hashimoto Y, Nakagawa N, et al. An antecolic roux-en y type reconstruction decreased delayed gastric emptying after pylorus-preserving pancreatoduodenectomy. J Gastrointest Surg. 2008;12(6):1081–6.
45. Chijiiwa K, Imamura N, Ohuchida J, Hiyoshi M, Nagano M, Otani K, et al. Prospective randomized controlled study of gastric emptying assessed by 13C-acetate breath test after pylorus-preserving pancreaticoduodenectomy: comparison between antecolic and vertical retrocolic duodenojejunostomy. J Hepato-Biliary-Pancreat Surg. 2009;16(1):49–55.
46. Nikfarjam M, Kimchi ET, Gusani NJ, Shah SM, Sehmbey M, Shereef S, Staveley-O'Carroll KF. A reduction in delayed gastric emptying by classic pancreaticoduodenectomy with an antecolic gastrojejunal anastomosis and a retrogastric omental patch. J Gastrointest Surg. 2009;13(9):1674–82.
47. Gangavatiker R, Pal S, Javed A, Dash NR, Sahni P, Chattopadhyay TK. Effect of antecolic or retrocolic reconstruction of the gastro/duodenojejunostomy on delayed gastric emptying after pancreaticoduodenectomy: a randomized controlled trial. J Gastrointest Surg. 2011;15(5):843–52.
48. Kurahara H, Shinchi H, Maemura K, Mataki Y, Iino S, Sakoda M, et al. Delayed gastric emptying after pancreatoduodenectomy. J Surg Res. 2011;171(2):e187–e92.
49. Eshuis WJ, Van Dalen JW, Busch ORC, Van Gulik TM, Gouma DJ. Route of gastroenteric reconstruction in pancreatoduodenectomy and delayed gastric emptying. HPB. 2012;14(1):54.
50. Imamura N, Chijiiwa K, Ohuchida J, Hiyoshi M, Nagano M, Otani K, Kondo K. Prospective randomized clinical trial of a change in gastric emptying and nutritional status after a pylorus-preserving pancreaticoduodenectomy: comparison between an antecolic and a vertical retrocolic duodenojejunostomy. HPB. 2014;16(4):384.
51. Sahora K, Morales-Oyarvide V, Thayer SP, Ferrone CR, Warshaw AL, Lillemoe KD, Fernández-Del CC. The effect of antecolic versus retrocolic reconstruction on delayed gastric emptying after classic non–pylorus-preserving pancreaticoduodenectomy. Am J Surg. 2015;209(6):1028–35.
52. Suzuki T, Imamura M, Kajiwara T, Kim HC, Miyashita T, Tobe T. A new method of reconstruction after pylorus-preserving pancreatoduodenectomy. World J Surg. 1988;12(5):645–50.
53. Takeda T, Yoshida J, Tanaka M, Matsunaga H, Yamaguchi K, Chijiiwa K. Delayed gastric emptying after Biliroth I pylorus-preserving pancreatoduodenectomy effect of postoperative time and cisapride. Ann Surg. 1999;229(2):223–9.

54. Watanabe Y, Ohtsuka T, Kimura H, Matsunaga T, Tamura K, Ideno N, et al. Braun entero-enterostomy reduces delayed gastric emptying after pylorus-preserving pancreatoduodenec-tomy: a retrospective review. Am J Surg. 2015;209(2):369–77.
55. Goei TH, Van Berge Henegouwen MI, Slooff MJH, Van Gulik TM, Gouma DJ, Eddes EH. Pylorus-preserving pancreatoduodenectomy: influence of a Billroth I versus a Billroth II type of reconstruction on gastric emptying. Dig Surg. 2001;18(5):376–80.
56. Shimoda M, Kubota K, Katoh M, Kita J. Effect of Billroth II or Roux-en-Y reconstruction for the gastrojejunostomy on delayed gastric emptying after pancreaticoduodenectomy: a randomized controlled study. Ann Surg. 2013;257(5):938–42.
57. Busquets J, Martin S, Secanella L, Peláez N, Ramos E, Fabregat J. Billroth II or Roux-en-Y reconstruction for gastrojejunostomy after pancreaticoduodenectomy. Randomized con-trolled trial (PAUDA TRIAL). Pancreatology. 2018;18(4):S6.
58. Varghese C, Bhat S, Wang THH, O'Grady G, Pandanaboyana S. Impact of gastric resection and enteric anastomotic configuration on delayed gastric emptying after pancreaticoduode-nectomy: a network meta-analysis of randomized trials. BJS Open. 2021;5(3):zrab035.
59. Macutkiewicz C. Delayed gastric emptying after pancreatic surgery. Textbook of pancreatic cancer. Cham: Springer International Publishing; 2021. p. 1069–82.
60. Paiella S, De Pastena M, Korrel M, Pan TL, Butturini G, Nessi C, et al. Long term outcome after minimally invasive and open Warshaw and Kimura techniques for spleen-preserving distal pancreatectomy: international multicenter retrospective study. Eur J Surg Oncol. 2019;45(9):1668–73.
61. Glowka TR, von Websky M, Pantelis D, Manekeller S, Standop J, Kalff JC, Schäfer N. Risk factors for delayed gastric emptying following distal pancreatectomy. Langenbeck's Arch Surg. 2016;401(2):161–7.
62. De Rooij T, Van Hilst J, Van Santvoort H, Boerma D, Van Den Boezem P, Daams F, et al. Minimally invasive versus open distal pancreatectomy (LEOPARD): a multicenter patient-blinded randomized controlled trial. Ann Surg. 2019;269(1):2–9.
63. Ozgun YM, Oter V, Piskin E, Colakoglu MK, Aydin O, Aksoy E, et al. Treatment modalities and the role of endoscopy for delayed gastric emptying after whipple operation: analysis of 53 patients. Am Surg. 2022;88(2):273–9.
64. Fischer CP, Hong JC. Method of pyloric reconstruction and impact upon delayed gastric emptying and hospital stay after pylorus-preserving pancreaticoduodenectomy. J Gastrointest Sur. 2006;10(2):215–9.
65. Manes K, Lytras D, Avgerinos C, Delis S, Dervenis C. Antecolic gastrointestinal recon-struction with pylorus dilatation. Does it improve delayed gastric emptying after pylorus-preserving pancreaticoduodenectomy? HPB. 2008;10(6):472.
66. Panwar R, Pal S. The international study group of pancreatic surgery definition of delayed gastric emptying and the effects of various surgical modifications on the occurrence of delayed gastric emptying after pancreatoduodenectomy. Hepatobiliary Pancreat Dis Int. 2017;16(4):353–63.
67. Van Samkar G, Eshuis WJ, Lemmers M, Gouma DJ, Bennink RJ, Hollmann MW, et al. Value of scintigraphy for assessing delayed gastric emptying after pancreatic surgery. World J Surg. 2013;37(12):2911–7.
68. Samaddar A, Kaman L, Dahiya D, Bhattacharyya A, Sinha SK. Objective assessment of delayed gastric emptying using gastric scintigraphy in post pancreaticoduodenectomy patients. ANZ J Surg. 2017;87(9):E80–E4.
69. Hochwald SN, Grobmyer SR, Hemming AW, Curran E, Bloom DA, Delano M, et al. Braun enteroenterostomy is associated with reduced delayed gastric emptying and early resumption of oral feeding following pancreaticoduodenectomy. J Surg Oncol. 2010;101(5):351–5.
70. Vogel SB, Drane WE, Woodward ER, Ritchie WP, Rutledge RH, Thompson JC. Clinical and radionuclide evaluation of bile diversion by Braun enteroenterostomy: prevention and treatment of alkaline reflux gastritis. An alternative to Roux-en-Y diversion. Ann Surg. 1994;219(5):458–66.

71. Xu B, Meng H, Qian M, Gu H, Zhou B, Song Z. Braun enteroenterostomy during pancreaticoduodenectomy decreases postoperative delayed gastric emptying. Am J Surg. 2015;209(6):1036–42.

72. Hwang HK, Lee SH, Han DH, Choi SH, Kang CM, Lee WJ. Impact of Braun anastomosis on reducing delayed gastric emptying following pancreaticoduodenectomy: a prospective, randomized controlled trial. J Hepatobiliary Pancreat Sci. 2016;23(6):364–72.

73. Fujieda H, Yokoyama Y, Hirata A, Usui H, Sakatoku Y, Fukaya M, Nagino M. Does Braun anastomosis have an impact on the incidence of delayed gastric emptying and the extent of intragastric bile reflux following pancreatoduodenectomy? A randomized controlled study. Dig Surg. 2017;34(6):462–8.

74. Zhou Y, Hu B, Wei K, Si X. Braun anastomosis lowers the incidence of delayed gastric emptying following pancreaticoduodenectomy: a meta-analysis. BMC Gastroenterol. 2018;18(1):176.

75. Lassen K, Kjæve J, Fetveit T, Tranø G, Sigurdsson HK, Horn A, Revhaug A. Allowing normal food at will after major upper gastrointestinal surgery does not increase morbidity: a randomized multicenter trial. Ann Surg. 2008;247(5):721–9.

76. Nelson R, Edwards S, Tse B. Prophylactic nasogastric decompression after abdominal surgery. Cochrane Database Syst Rev. 2004;3.

77. Gaignard E, Bergeat D, Courtin-Tanguy L, Rayar M, Merdrignac A, Robin F, et al. Is systematic nasogastric decompression after pancreaticoduodenectomy really necessary? Langenbeck's Arch Surg. 2018;403(5):573–80.

78. Flick KF, Soufi M, Yip-Schneider MT, Simpson RE, Colgate CL, Nguyen TK, et al. Routine gastric decompression after pancreatoduodenectomy: treating the surgeon? J Gastrointest Surg. 2021;25(11):2902–7.

79. Park JS, Kim JY, Kim JK, Yoon DS. Should gastric decompression be a routine procedure in patients who undergo pylorus-preserving pancreatoduodenectomy? World J Surg. 2016;40(11):2766–70.

80. Bergeat D, Merdrignac A, Robin F, Gaignard E, Rayar M, Meunier B, et al. Nasogastric decompression vs no decompression after pancreaticoduodenectomy: the randomized clinical IPOD trial. JAMA Surg. 2020;155(9):e202291.

81. Adiamah A, Ranat R, Gomez D. Enteral versus parenteral nutrition following pancreaticoduodenectomy: a systematic review and meta-analysis. HPB. 2019;21(7):793–801.

82. Lassen K, Kjæve J, Fetveit T, Tranø G, Sigurdsson HK, Horn A, Revhaug A. Allowing normal food at will after major upper gastrointestinal surgery does not increase morbidity. Ann Surg. 2008;247(5):721–9.

83. Liu X, Chen Q, Fu Y, Lu Z, Chen J, Guo F, et al. Early nasojejunal nutrition versus early oral feeding in patients after pancreaticoduodenectomy: a randomized controlled trial. Front Oncol. 2021;11:656332.

84. Perkel MS, Moore C, Hersh T, Davidson ED. Metoclopramide therapy in patients with delayed gastric emptying. Dig Dis Sci. 1979;24(9):662–6.

85. Yeo CJ, Barry MK, Sauter PK, Sostre S, Lillemoe KD, Pitt HA, et al. Erythromycin accelerates gastric emptying after pancreaticoduodenectomy. A prospective, randomized, placebo-controlled trial. Ann Surg. 1993;218(3):229.

86. Ohwada S, Satoh Y, Kawate S, Yamada T, Kawamura O, Koyama T, et al. Low-dose erythromycin reduces delayed gastric emptying and improves gastric motility after Billroth I pylorus-preserving pancreaticoduodenectomy. Ann Surg. 2001;234(5):668.

87. Kollmar O, Moussavian MR, Richter S, de Roi P, Maurer CA, Schilling MK. Prophylactic octreotide and delayed gastric emptying after pancreaticoduodenectomy: results of a prospective randomized double-blinded placebo-controlled trial. Eur J Surg Oncol. 2008;34(8):868–75.

88. El Nakeeb A, ElGawalby A, Ali M, Shehta A, Hamed H, El Refea M, et al. Efficacy of octreotide in the prevention of complications after pancreaticoduodenectomy in patients with

soft pancreas and non-dilated pancreatic duct: a prospective randomized trial. Hepatobiliary Pancreat Dis Int. 2018;17(1):59–63.

89. Adiamah A, Arif Z, Berti F, Singh S, Laskar N, Gomez D. The use of prophylactic somatostatin therapy following pancreaticoduodenectomy: a meta-analysis of randomised controlled trials. World J Surg. 2019;43(7):1788–801.

90. Vásquez W, Hernández AV, Garcia-Sabrido JL. Is gum chewing useful for ileus after elective colorectal surgery? A systematic review and meta-analysis of randomized clinical trials. J Gastrointest Surg. 2009;13(4):649–56.

91. Maheshwaran MU, Sathyanesan J, Perumal SK, Ramasamy R, Pitchaimuthu A, Rajendran K, et al. Impact of chewing gum protocol on delayed gastric emptying following pancreaticoduodenectomy. HPB. 2016;18:e763.

92. Lassen K, Coolsen MME, Slim K, Carli F, de Aguilar-Nascimento JE, Schäfer M, et al. Guidelines for perioperative care for pancreaticoduodenectomy: enhanced recovery after surgery (ERAS®) society recommendations. Clin Nutr. 2012;31(6):817–30.

93. Gianotti L, Besselink MG, Sandini M, Hackert T, Conlon K, Gerritsen A, et al. Nutritional support and therapy in pancreatic surgery: a position paper of the international study group on pancreatic surgery (ISGPS). Surgery. 2018;164(5):1035–48.

94. Schörghuber M, Fruhwald S. Effects of enteral nutrition on gastrointestinal function in patients who are critically ill. Lancet Gastroenterol Hepatol. 2018;3(4):281–7.

95. Robertson R, Russell K, Pandanaboyana S, Wu D, Windsor J. Postoperative nutritional support after pancreaticoduodenectomy in adults. Cochrane Database Syst Rev. 2022;2022(6):CD014792.

96. Gerritsen A, Besselink MG, Cieslak KP, Vriens MR, Steenhagen E, Van Hillegersberg R, et al. Efficacy and complications of nasojejunal, jejunostomy and parenteral feeding after pancreaticoduodenectomy. J Gastrointest Surg. 2012;16(6):1144–51.

97. Wang L, Tian Z, Liu Y. Nasoenteric tube versus jejunostomy for enteral nutrition feeding following major upper gastrointestinal operations: a meta-analysis. Asia Pac J Clin Nutr. 2017;26(1):20–6.

98. Abu-Hilal M, Hemandas AK, McPhail M, Jain G, Panagiotopoulou I, Scibelli T, et al. A comparative analysis of safety and efficacy of different methods of tube placement for enteral feeding following major pancreatic resection. A non-randomized study. Jop. 2010;11(1):8–13.

99. Gerritsen A, van der Poel MJ, de Rooij T, Molenaar IQ, Bergman JJ, Busch OR, et al. Systematic review on bedside electromagnetic-guided, endoscopic, and fluoroscopic placement of nasoenteral feeding tubes. Gastrointest Endosc. 2015;81(4):836–47.e2.

100. Li A, Shah R, Han X, Sood A, Steffes C, Kwon D. Pancreaticoduodenectomy and placement of operative enteral access: better or worse? Am J Surg. 2019;217(3):458–62.

101. Padussis JC, Zani S, Blazer DG, Tyler DS, Pappas TN, Scarborough JE. Feeding jejunostomy during Whipple is associated with increased morbidity. J Surg Res. 2014;187(2):361–6.

102. Waliye HE, Wright GP, McCarthy C, Johnson J, Scales A, Wolf A, Chung M. Utility of feeding jejunostomy tubes in pancreaticoduodenectomy. Am J Surg. 2017;213(3):530–3.

103. Vasavada B, Patel H. Routine use of feeding jejunostomy in pancreaticoduodenectomy: a metaanalysis. Surg Pract. 2021;25(2):104–13.

104. Denbo JW, Bruno M, Dewhurst W, Kim MP, Tzeng CW, Aloia TA, et al. Risk-stratified clinical pathways decrease the duration of hospitalization and costs of perioperative care after pancreatectomy. Surgery. 2018;164(3):424–31.

105. Hilal MA, Di Fabio F, Badran AA, Alsaati H, Clarke H, Fecher I, et al. Implementation of enhanced recovery programme after pancreatoduodenectomy: a single-centre UK pilot study. Pancreatology. 2013;13(1):58–62.

106. Kagedan DJ, Ahmed M, Devitt KS, Wei AC. Enhanced recovery after pancreatic surgery: a systematic review of the evidence. HPB. 2014;17:11–6.

107. Bai X, Zhang X, Lu F, Li G, Gao S, Lou J, et al. The implementation of an enhanced recovery after surgery (ERAS) program following pancreatic surgery in an academic medical center of China. Pancreatology. 2016;16(4):665–70.

108. Nussbaum DP, Penne K, Stinnett SS, Speicher PJ, Cocieru A, Blazer DG, et al. A standard-ized care plan is associated with shorter hospital length of stay in patients undergoing pancre-aticoduodenectomy. J Surg Res. 2015;193(1):237–45.
109. Arango NP, Prakash LR, Chiang YJ, Dewhurst WL, Bruno ML, Ikoma N, et al. Risk-stratified pancreatectomy clinical pathway implementation and delayed gastric emptying. J Gastrointest Surg. 2021;25(9):2221–30.
110. Klotz R, Larmann J, Klose C, Bruckner T, Benner L, Doerr-Harim C, et al. Gastrointestinal complications after pancreatoduodenectomy with epidural vs patient-controlled intravenous analgesia. JAMA Surg. 2020;155(7):e200794.
111. Akter N, Ratnayake B, Joh DB, Chan SJ, Bonner E, Pandanaboyana S. Postoperative pain relief after pancreatic resection: systematic review and meta-analysis of analgesic modalities. World J Surg. 2021;45(10):3165–73.

Chapter 37
Long-Term Sequelae: Pancreatic Exocrine and Endocrine Failure

Nicholas Caminiti and Robert Martin

Pancreatic Exocrine Insufficiency

Pancreatic exocrine insufficiency (PEI) is defined as the inability of the pancreas to secrete and/or deliver enough enzymes to the small intestine, resulting in impaired digestion and absorption of the contents of a meal [1, 2]. This results in multiple symptoms for patients including steatorrhea, weight loss, bloating, and nutrient deficiencies, especially fat-soluble vitamins (Table 37.1). Following pancreatic resection, PEI can develop if the remaining pancreas is unable to produce enough enzymes to adequately digest nutrients. Additionally, if the resection requires an anastomosis of the pancreas to the GI tract (i.e., pancreaticojejunostomy), an anastomotic stricture can impair adequate enzyme delivery. Finally, GI function is highly regulated and adequate digestion requires the release of pancreatic enzymes such that they are present in the duodenum when food leaves the stomach. If a pancreatic resection alters normal GI anatomy (i.e., pancreatoduodenectomy), PEI can develop when pancreatic enzymes are released but do not reach an alimentary limb while food is present.

The gold standard for diagnosis of PEI is the assessment of fecal elastase content (Table 37.1) [3]. Elastase is an enzyme released by the pancreas and passed in stool, thus low level of elastase in fecal material is a marker for inadequate production of pancreatic enzymes and PEI. The normal level of elastase is >200 µg elastase/g fecal material, with 100–200 µg elastase/g fecal material indicating moderate PEI, and < 100 µg elastase/g fecal material indicating severe PEI [4]. Unfortunately, fecal elastase testing is rather cumbersome, with samples rejected if stool is too watery or contains urine or plasma. The turnaround time for the test is 3–6 days and often requires that samples be sent to outside laboratories such that the average time

N. Caminiti · R. Martin (✉)
Department of Surgery, University of Louisville, Louisville, KY, USA
e-mail: nscami01@louisville.edu; Robert.martin@louisville.edu

Table 37.1 Pancreatic exocrine insufficiency (PEI)

Symptoms	Diagnosis	Treatment
Diarrhea Abdominal pain Steatorrhea Bloating Flatulence Unexpected weight loss	Fecal elastase testing considered the gold standard, often not necessary/ recommended in the correct clinical context	Pancreatic enzyme replacement therapy, at least 25,000 lipase units with snacks and 50,000 lipase units with meals

to diagnosis from sample collection is 10–14 days [1]. Furthermore, if adequate elastase is produced but does not reach a food bolus appropriately secondary to altered GI anatomy, fecal elastase levels may be normal in a patient with PEI symptoms. Given these difficulties, PEI following pancreatic resection is more often a clinical diagnosis based on the presence of typical symptoms after surgery.

The rate of PEI varies based on the type of pancreatic resection and the method of diagnosis, with fecal elastase testing generally showing a lower rate of PEI than a solely clinical diagnosis. Overall, 35–40% of patients appear to develop PEI following surgery although reported rates vary widely, with some studies reporting as low as 5% for parenchymal sparing resections and some reporting >80% PEI rates following pancreaticoduodenectomy [2, 5, 6]. In general, pancreatoduodenectomy appears to have a higher rate of PEI than distal pancreatectomy, with one study reporting PEI rates at 5 years of 58% and 29% respectively [7, 8]. The same study reported a 5-year PEI rate for atypical, parenchymal sparing (e.g., enucleation, central pancreatectomy) resections of 3%. Pylorus preservation versus resection during pancreatoduodenectomy does not seem to affect the occurrence of postoperative PEI [7].

The rate of PEI also seems to increase over time, especially in pancreatoduodenectomy patients. The previously discussed series found the rate of PEI 1 year following resection was 32%, 27%, and 3% for pancreaticoduodenectomy, distal pancreatectomy, and parenchymal sparing resections, respectively. These figures indicate a nearly two-fold increase of PEI in the pancreatoduodenectomy group, while distal pancreatectomy and parenchymal sparing resection remained similar over time [2]. Similarly, a large single institution review found that the mean time of PEI onset was 14 months following resection [9]. Other studies show high rates (80%) of PEI in the 30 days following resection, but persistent symptoms in only 49% of those undergoing pancreatoduodenectomy and 28% of those undergoing distal pancreatectomy [10]. A final study found that about half of all patients who develop PEI following pancreatic resection do so within 90 days of surgery and about half develop symptoms after 90 days [11]. Altogether these data seem to indicate that PEI is common following pancreatic head resection but has variable rates, also depending on the timing and method of diagnosis.

Multiple risk factors for postoperative PEI have been identified. Preoperative PEI is highly correlated with postoperative PEI requiring enzyme supplementation, although studies report that 15–20% of patients taking pancreatic enzymes preoperatively will no longer require them after resection [12]. Increasing age, history of tobacco use, a family history of diabetes, and malignancy as the indication for resection have all been shown to increase the risk of postoperative PEI [4]. Following resection, the development of steatorrhea or weight loss is highly correlated with the development of PEI requiring enzyme supplementation [2]. Malignancy specifically has been shown to dramatically increase the risk of PEI following resection, with PEI rates following benign tumor resection of 25% compared to 50% following resection for malignancy in some studies [13]. This can be related both to preoperative pancreatic duct obstruction by malignant neoplasms inducing parenchymal atrophy, and the need for additional therapies in the setting of malignancy. Both neoadjuvant and adjuvant chemotherapy, as well as adjuvant radiation therapy have been shown to increase the risk of PEI following pancreatic resection [11, 13].

The extent of resection has been extensively studied with regard to postoperative PEI rates. Preliminary evidence that the amount of remaining parenchyma is crucial for avoiding PEI can be seen in the lower rates of PEI following parenchymal sparing, atypical resections than in more traditional distal pancreatectomy and pancreaticoduodenectomy [2]. More formal assessments of pancreatic volume show that a radiographic thickness of less than 11.4 mm of the remaining parenchyma following resection predicts PEI [14]. Unfortunately, this measure is of limited predictive value, with a sensitivity of 88.9% and a specificity of 70%. Additionally, similar radiographic measures of pancreatic volume and thickness pre-resection have not been shown to predict PEI rates postoperatively [14]. Studies of distal pancreatectomy specifically have found no relationship between the extent of resection and the need for postoperative pancreatic enzyme supplementation [13].

The treatment of PEI consists of pancreatic enzyme supplementation, known as pancreatic enzyme replacement therapy (PERT) (Table 37.1). Commercially available pancrelipase consists of lipase, protease, and amylase coated with a capsule designed to maintain integrity through the stomach so that the enzymes are released in the intestine and not broken down by gastric acid. The enzymes are not absorbed, and it is generally recommended that they can be taken in the middle of a meal to ensure they reach the intestine with the food they are intended to help digest, although some patients report good results taking the capsules just prior to a meal. Studies show that as many as 33% of patients do not take their enzyme replacement appropriately, underscoring the importance of discussing this with them. Generic, uncoated pancrelipase is available at lower cost, but patients should be on some form of acid suppression to minimize degradation of the enzymes in the stomach [15]. Notably, all currently available forms of pancrelipase are porcine derived, a fact that should be discussed with patients prior to use. Pancrelipase is available in multiple dosages, which vary from country to country. Generally, a starting dose of at least 25,000 lipase units taken with snacks and 50,000 lipase units taken with meals is recommended [3]. A normal pancreas is estimated to release >700,000 lipase units of enzymes per meal, so increasing the dose is possible and recommended [15].

Given the prevalence of PEI following pancreatic resection and the limited side effect profile of pancrelipase, UK consensus guidelines now recommend therapy for all symptomatic patients without a confirmatory fecal elastase test, generally with a starting dose of one 36,000 unit pill with snacks and two 36,000 unit pills with meals (Table 37.1) [3]. Enzyme replacement in the setting of malignancy has been shown to prevent weight loss and malnutrition, and some studies have shown an improvement in overall survival. Similarly, an increase in overall survival was seen in patients following pancreatoduodenectomy for ampullary carcinoma when they received enzyme replacement in one recent retrospective series [16]. Therefore, a trial of pancrelipase following resection is warranted for any patient with signs or symptoms consistent with PEI. Although the quality of the available evidence is suboptimal, a 2018 position paper of the International Study Group on Pancreatic Surgery (ISGPS) on nutritional support and therapy in pancreatic surgery recommends initiating PERT routinely in patients who underwent pancreatoduodenectomy, continuing for at least 6 months after surgery [17]. In distal pancreatectomy patients, ISGPS recommends initiating PERT only in patients with PEI symptoms [17].

Endocrine Pancreatic Insufficiency

The pancreas plays a crucial role in glucose metabolism through the release of insulin and glucagon. These hormones are released from beta and alpha cells, respectively, which reside in nests in the pancreas called islets. These islets make up ~1–2% of the volume of the pancreas, found mostly in the body and tail, and loss of these cells can lead to derangements of glucose management and ultimately endocrine pancreatic insufficiency (EPI) following resection [18]. The failure of pancreatic endocrine function following resection manifests as new onset or worsening diabetes (Table 37.2). Although a specific definition is difficult to determine, EPI is identified by one of three clinical scenarios. A patient can progress from no evidence of diabetes to requiring either oral hypoglycemic agents or insulin, or a patient previously requiring oral hypoglycemic agents can progress to requiring insulin [7]. It is certainly plausible that a patient requiring insulin prior to surgery could see their insulin requirement increase following resection, but this is generally difficult to track and often excluded from research regarding EPI [7].

Table 37.2 Endocrine pancreatic insufficiency (EPI)

Symptoms	Diagnosis	Treatment
Traditional diabetes symptoms Large swings in glucose common	Hb A1c 6.5% or greater, routine testing following pancreatic resection is recommended	Subcutaneous insulin therapy, generally requiring similar insulin amounts to type I diabetics

Overall, the rate of EPI following pancreatic resection is reported to be 15–40%, based on the precise definition used and the length of follow-up, although persistent diabetes rates are roughly 20% in large cohorts [6]. In a large, single institution review over 15 years, the reported rate was found to be ~20%, with about 2/3 representing patients with new onset diabetes and 1/3 patients previously on oral hypoglycemic medications requiring a transition to insulin for adequate glucose control [18]. Distal pancreatectomy is reported to have a higher rate of EPI than pancreatoduodenectomy, although the overall difference is rather small in most studies. Atypical, parenchymal sparing resections clearly have a lower rate of EPI than either distal pancreatectomy or pancreaticoduodenectomy, with rates of <5% reported routinely depending on the extent of the atypical resection [7].

Post-resection EPI is not an immediate phenomenon. Patients often have deranged glucose in the immediate postoperative period as their diet is altered and they are placed on IV fluids with various glucose concentrations. However, a significant number of these patients will recover without evidence of new impaired glucose tolerance. In one study specifically examining the onset of EPI in patients who were not previously diabetic, 25% required new pharmacologic intervention within 30 days of resection while 40% did not require intervention until more than 90 days after their procedure [11]. A separate review found the mean time of EPI onset to be 20 months following resection [19].

Multiple risk factors for post-resection EPI have been identified. Increasing BMI, family history of diabetes or personal history of diabetes pre-resection, history of pancreatitis, and history of tobacco use have all been shown to increase the risk of postoperative EPI following pancreatic resection [2]. Resection for malignancy has been shown to increase the risk of EPI compared to resection for benign indications. This may partly be due to the use of adjuvant radiation following some resections for malignancy, which has been shown to increase the risk of EPI [11]. Additionally, DM is newly diagnosed with pancreatic adenocarcinoma in about 40% of cases. Despite loss of islets being the dominant explanation for postoperative EPI, extent of pancreatic resection and remnant pancreas volume are not predictive of EPI following distal pancreatectomy or pancreaticoduodenectomy [14].

Diabetes following pancreatic resection is often termed pancreatogenic diabetes or "brittle diabetes" and is characterized by labile blood glucose levels with abrupt transitions from hypo- to hyperglycemia (Table 37.2). This is likely secondary to the loss of glucagon producing alpha cells along with insulin producing beta cells during resection. As a result, patients with this form of diabetes experience hypoglycemic episodes in as many as 79% of cases [15]. Consensus guidelines now recommend routine monitoring of blood glucose and HbA1c levels following pancreatic resection to monitor for the development of diabetes (Table 37.2) [3, 15]. Once patients develop diabetes, management of their blood glucose often falls to primary care physicians or endocrinologists. However, the majority of these patients will require insulin therapy at dosages and intervals similar to type I diabetes patients (Table 37.2) [15]. Total pancreatectomy and autologous islet transplant will be discussed elsewhere in this text, but it should be noted that improved glucose control and insulin independence have been reported following such procedures. Unfortunately, malignancy precludes autologous islet transplantation and is now the most common indication for pancreatic resection. Similarly, parenchymal sparing resections reduce the rates of EPI but are not appropriate in oncologic settings and there are reports showing a higher rate of pancreatic fistula.

References

1. Moore JV, et al. Exocrine pancreatic insufficiency after pancreatectomy for malignancy: systematic review and optimal management recommendations. J Gastrointest Surg. 2021;25(9):2317–27.
2. Kusakabe J, et al. Long-term endocrine and exocrine insufficiency after pancreatectomy. J Gastrointest Surg. 2019;23(8):1604–13.
3. Phillips ME, et al. Consensus for the management of pancreatic exocrine insufficiency: UK practical guidelines. BMJ Open Gastroenterol. 2021;8(1):e000643.
4. Phillips ME. Pancreatic exocrine insufficiency following pancreatic resection. Pancreatology. 2015;15(5):449–55.
5. Falconi M, et al. Pancreatic insufficiency after different resections for benign tumours. Br J Surg. 2008;95(1):85–91.
6. Elliott IA, et al. Population-level incidence and predictors of surgically induced diabetes and exocrine insufficiency after partial pancreatic resection. Perm J. 2017;21:16–095.
7. Beger HG, et al. New onset of diabetes and pancreatic exocrine insufficiency after pancreaticoduodenectomy for benign and malignant tumors: a systematic review and meta-analysis of long-term results. Ann Surg. 2018;267(2):259–70.
8. Beger HG, Mayer B. Early postoperative and late metabolic morbidity after pancreatic resections: an old and new challenge for surgeons—a review. Am J Surg. 2018;216(1):131–4.
9. Pathanki AM, et al. Pancreatic exocrine insufficiency after pancreaticoduodenectomy: current evidence and management. World J Gastrointest Pathophysiol. 2020;11(2):20–31.
10. Goess R, Ceyhan GO, Friess H. Pancreatic exocrine insufficiency after pancreatic surgery. Panminerva Med. 2016;58(2):151–9.
11. Lim PW, et al. Thirty-day outcomes underestimate endocrine and exocrine insufficiency after pancreatic resection. HPB (Oxford). 2016;18(4):360–6.
12. Ghaneh P, Neoptolemos JP. Exocrine pancreatic function following pancreatectomy. Ann N Y Acad Sci. 1999;880:308–18.
13. Hallac A, et al. Exocrine pancreatic insufficiency in distal pancreatectomy: incidence and risk factors. HPB (Oxford). 2020;22(2):275–81.
14. Hartman V, et al. Prediction of exocrine and endocrine insufficiency after pancreaticoduodenectomy using volumetry. Acta Chir Belg. 2020;120(4):257–64.
15. Khatkov IE, et al. Russian consensus on exo- and endocrine pancreatic insufficiency after surgical treatment. Turk J Gastroenterol. 2021;32(3):225–39.
16. Roberts KJ, et al. Pancreas exocrine replacement therapy is associated with increased survival following pancreatoduodenectomy for periampullary malignancy. HPB (Oxford). 2017;19(10):859–67.
17. Gianotti L, et al. Nutritional support and therapy in pancreatic surgery: a position paper of the international study group on pancreatic surgery (ISGPS). Surgery. 2018 Nov;164(5):1035–48.
18. Berney T, et al. Long-term metabolic results after pancreatic resection for severe chronic pancreatitis. Arch Surg. 2000;135(9):1106–11.
19. Sikkens EC, et al. Prospective assessment of the influence of pancreatic cancer resection on exocrine pancreatic function. Br J Surg. 2014;101(2):109–13.

Chapter 38
How to Measure Postoperative Outcomes

Elizabeth L. Barbera, Alexandra M. Adams, and Timothy J. Vreeland

Introduction

Pancreas surgery was once considered to have a high, but acceptable, mortality rate of up to 30% in the 1970s and 1980s. With improvements in patient selection and surgical technique, pancreas surgery has become increasingly safe [1]. Recent series report extremely low mortality from distal pancreatectomy (<2.5%) and low rates even for pancreatoduodenectomy (2–6%) [1–3]. Despite such improvements, there remains a gap in outcomes between high and low volume centers, the latter in which mortality is considerably higher [4]. Efforts to close this gap must focus on both standardizing outcomes and assisting centers to reach these benchmarks. Additionally, with such dramatic improvements in morbidity and mortality, surgeons and patients have been able to shift the spotlight toward more patient-centered outcomes after pancreas surgery. The focus of these outcomes is not merely surviving the operation, but maintaining quality of life after surger as well.

This chapter will describe outcomes of pancreas surgery. We first discuss the clinical outcomes that have predominated the focus of these operations for many years but follow with a description of patient-centered outcomes that are increasingly recognized as distinct entities meriting further study.

E. L. Barbera · A. M. Adams · T. J. Vreeland (✉)
Brooke Army Medical Center, Fort Sam Houston, TX, USA

E. P. Ceppa et al. (eds.), *The SAGES Manual of Evolving Techniques in Pancreatic Surgery*, https://doi.org/10.1007/978-3-031-78409-5_38

Part I: Benchmarks in Pancreatic Surgery

Establishing Benchmarks

The standardization of benchmarks for complex surgical procedures with significant morbidity and mortality is a relatively new effort. Benchmarking establishes an opportunity to identify clinically relevant performance gaps in different patient cohorts or treatment centers and provide opportunities to implement specific quality improvement measures to improve outcomes [5, 6]. Benchmark methodology has also been used for other complex operations including liver transplantation, esophagectomy, and liver resection, but its application to pancreatic surgery has been much more recent [7–9].

The landmark paper in 2019 by Sanchez-Velazquez et al. used a large international patient cohort to establish 20 benchmarks for surgical and oncological outcomes after pancreatoduodenectomy (PD). Patients from 23 high-volume centers (defined as performing >50 complex pancreatic procedures per year) across three continents with a low preoperative risk profile were included to calculate a numeric benchmark cutoff for "best achievable" results. This was validated in two separate cohorts of patients with poorer preoperative risk profiles and those who underwent a minimally invasive approach. Strict selection criteria were used to identify low-risk benchmark patients, including those over 18 years old undergoing open PD, and excluding those undergoing extended or total pancreatectomy, resection of mesenteric artery or celiac trunk, with macroscopic positive margins, prior major abdominal surgery, extra-pancreatic metastases, of ASA class 3 or greater, BMI of greater than 35 or with other major comorbidities, or those on anticoagulants or two or more anti-diabetic drugs [10].

The benchmark cutoff was defined as the 75th percentile of the median value for each center. Twenty outcome indicators were selected, including intraoperative parameters, at discharge, and at 3, 6, and 12 months. Intraoperative outcomes included operative duration and blood transfusion, while outcomes at discharge included length of stay and in-hospital mortality. Outcomes measured at 3, 6, and 12 months included patients with at least one complication stratified by the Clavien-Dindo grading system, pancreatic fistula rate (including biochemical leak, grade B, and grade C), severe postoperative bleeding, failure-to-rescue rate, and readmission rate. Complications were also compiled and compared using the comprehensive complication index (CCI), which quantifies the cumulative comorbidity burden, adjusted for each complication's corresponding grade, for each patient over the first year. Oncologic outcomes included R1 resection rate, number of lymph nodes resected, and both 1-year and 3-year disease-free survival (DFS) [10].

An interesting secondary analysis in this study compared outcomes among the 23 high-volume centers, which found that outcomes were not associated with volume itself, but inversely related to the proportion of benchmark cases performed. Perhaps those centers performing more complex cases had better outcomes due to higher exposure to more complex cases, and robust multi-disciplinary approaches to

Table 38.1 Benchmark values for selected outcomes [10]

Outcome	Benchmark value
Operation duration	≤7.5 h
Length of stay	≤15 days
Readmission rate	≤21%
Postoperative 6-month morbidity[a]	≤73%
Pancreatic fistula rate	≤19%
Grade B	≤15%
Grade C	≤5%
In-hospital mortality	≤1.6%

[a] Patients with at least 1 complication (according to Clavien-Dindo scale definition)

complications. Regardless, their benchmark values for each of the 20 intra- and postoperative outcomes were validated among patients with more preoperative morbidity (ASA class 3 or greater) and among patients undergoing minimally invasive PD, with most outcomes among both cohorts remaining within the benchmark cutoffs [10]. These values can be used as a more objective measure of a center's performance and additionally can identify areas in need of quality improvement. Selected benchmark values for outcomes of interest from the work of Sánchez-Velázquez et al. are summarized in Table 38.1.

Textbook Outcomes

Another concept in standardization of high-quality pancreatic surgical care includes the definition of a "textbook outcome" (TBO). The TBO is a composite outcome which encompasses the ideal postoperative course of a patient receiving optimal care [11]. Achievement of a TBO relies on the all-or-none principle, and fulfilling a list of pre-specified outcomes [12]. The first study to examine TBO in hepatopancreatic surgery was among Medicare beneficiaries in 2018 by Merath et al. who defined TBO as no postoperative complications, no prolonged LOS, no 90-day readmission, and no 90-day postoperative mortality. Notably, TBO was achieved in 47.8% of patients undergoing minor pancreatic resection (distal pancreatectomy or other partial pancreatectomy) but only 24.7% undergoing major pancreatic resection (proximal pancreatectomy, PD, total pancreatectomy) in this study [13]. With less than a quarter of patients achieving an ideal short-term outcome, much room remains for quality improvement.

The use of TBOs provide a comprehensive composite measure of quality care for pancreatic surgery, but its primary criticism is a lack of consensus on its definition. As mentioned above, a more generalized TBO for hepatopancreatic surgery has been proposed as no postoperative complications, no prolonged LOS, no 90-day readmission, and no 90-day postoperative mortality [13]. Other papers utilize more pancreatic surgery-specific TBOs defined as absence of prolonged LOS, severe complications (Clavien-Dindo grade III or higher), postoperative pancreatic fistula (POPF, grade B/C), post-pancreatectomy hemorrhage (PPH, grade B/C), bile leakage (grade B/C), readmission, and in-hospital or 30-day mortality [12, 14].

The Dutch use this detailed definition within the nationwide prospective Dutch Pancreatic Cancer Audit (DPCA) to assess variation and compare quality between hospitals, with adjustments for case-mix. An analysis of the first 6 years of their nationwide audit demonstrated that TBOs remained stable (57–55%, $p = 0.283$), although there was a decrease in in-hospital mortality (4.1–2.4%, $p = 0.001$) and failure to rescue (13–7.4%, $p < 0.001$). The authors largely credit the improvements in outcomes to nationwide collaboration, transparency, and sharing of best practices [15]. The DPCA serves as a model for other healthcare systems to audit and share their outcomes, with the aim to collaborate and improve patient care.

Another benefit of a comprehensive metric such as TBO is to evaluate novel approaches to complex surgery, including new surgical techniques or perioperative processes. For example, Lof et al. utilized TBO to investigate the effectiveness of the Enhanced Recovery After Surgery (ERAS) protocol in a retrospective comparison of 250 patients undergoing this protocol and 125 patients undergoing standard perioperative management. A composite outcome such as TBO facilitated assessment of the multimodal nature of the ERAS protocol, demonstrating improvement in TBO from 44.0% to 56.4% ($p = 0.023$) with utilization of an ERAS protocol [14]. This composite TBO can also be used to evaluate implementation of new techniques within and/or between institutions, especially as minimally invasive approaches are more widely adopted.

Part II. Patient-Reported Outcome and Experience Measures

Introduction to Patient-Reported Outcome Measures and Patient-Reported Experience Measures

Patient-reported outcomes (PROs) are measures that represent the assessment of a patient's health or care experience from their own perspective, without interpretation by a clinician. These domains, which may include health-related quality of life (HRQOL), symptom burden, and sense of well-being, are particularly important considerations in pancreas surgery, given the morbidity of these operations for a potentially limited survival, particularly in the case of pancreatic adenocarcinoma [16, 17]. Consideration of these aspects may increase a patient's engagement in their treatment, foster a culture of shared decision-making, and facilitate patient-centered care [17–19].

Data surrounding these outcomes is inherently subjective and therefore a challenge to implement into practice. However, new means have been developed to translate this information into more objective forms. Patient-reported outcome measures (PROMs) and patient-reported experience measures (PREMs) are tools developed to provide a standardized determination of a patient's health and experience, respectively, from their own perspective [20]. The former focuses on aspects of a patient's care related to their health (e.g., a patient's view of their functional status after surgery) [21]. In contrast, the latter centers on a patient's experience with their health staff and provided services, such as wait times or overall humanity of care [21, 22]. For both PROMs and PREMs, measurements can be unidimensional (e.g., pain) or multidimensional (e.g., HRQOL) [23]. Varied methods have been developed to collect this information from patients, both at home and in the healthcare setting.

In the remainder of the chapter, we will discuss some of the available PROMs and PREMs within the discipline of pancreatic surgery, including specific examples both in research studies and clinical practice. Finally, we will cover barriers to implementation of these measures and methods by which these can be overcome.

PROMs and PREMs in Pancreatic Surgery

Numerous PROMs have been developed to capture the perspective of the patient with pancreatic disease. These instruments are most commonly identified in studies of patients with pancreatic cancer, with over 70 unique tools identified in one systematic review analyzing PROMs in this specific population, but other studies have investigated these measures in benign pancreatic disease as well. Notably, PROMs specific to recovery after pancreatic surgery are extremely limited, and more work is needed to fully represent the surgical recovery process.

The European Organization for Research and Treatment of Cancer (EORTC) pancreatic cancer disease-specific quality of life questionnaire (QLQ), the QLQ-PAN26, was recommended for patients with resectable disease in a systematic review of PROMS in pancreatic cancer [23]. This tool, published in 1999 by Fitzsimmons et al., was developed for use in combination with the EORTC core cancer module, the QLQ-C30, and aims to investigate important aspects of a patient's experience with pancreatic cancer in a 56-item questionnaire. Items queried include symptoms and side effects of treatments, such as loss of muscle strength and nighttime pain, but also the emotional burden of disease like fear of future health [24]. Importantly, this tool was later validated by Eaton et al. in a cohort of 300 patients who underwent pancreatic resection, noting acceptable reliability and validity of the scales with the caveat that the hepatic scale (encompassing two symptoms of pruritis and yellowing of the skin) had low internal consistency among postoperative patients [25, 26]. Multiple other studies have used the QLQ-PAN26 to investigate HRQOL outcomes in pancreas cancer, including the LEOPARD randomized controlled trial comparing outcomes for patients undergoing minimally invasive vs. open distal pancreatectomy [27–30].

For patients with unresectable cancer, Maharaj et al. recommend the Functional Assessment of Cancer Therapy-Hepatobiliary (FACT-HEP) [23]. This instrument is a 45-item questionnaire designed to measure quality of life in patients with hepatobiliary cancers. An initial series of questions are spread across physical, social, emotional, and functional domains, which are then followed by 16 hepatobiliary-specific symptom questions (e.g., appetite, dry mouth) [31]. While the original instrument was created to encompass patients with a broad spectrum of hepatobiliary cancers, to include primary and metastatic disease of the liver, it was later validated in patients with metastatic pancreatic adenocarcinoma alone [32]. This tool was subsequently applied in the setting of resectable disease by Cloyd et al. in a study investigating the impact of distal pancreatectomy vs. pancreatoduo-denectomy (PD) for pancreatic or periampullary tumors on long-term HRQOL and symptom burden. The authors found via the FACT-HEP that many survivors after pancreatectomy report generally positive health-related HRQOL at 6 months or later after surgery [33].

More generalized tools have been used in investigations of other pancreatic disease processes like acute pancreatitis, neuroendocrine tumors, and pancreatic cysts [23, 34–36]. For example, the Hospital Anxiety and Depression Scale (HADS) with its subscales for anxiety and depression was used to assess the psychological burden of surveillance for patients diagnosed with a pancreatic cyst. The majority of patients reported a positive attitude and low anxiety and/or depression scores via the HADS toward surveillance. Authors concluded that such a burden is low, a key finding when patients with pancreatic cysts may be followed with serial imaging for years to decades [34]. Information derived from PROMs in studies such as this one is therefore crucial to determine acceptability of such interventions from a patient's perspective.

Meanwhile, there are considerably fewer established PREMs for patients with pancreatic disease, particularly those undergoing surgery. Several research groups have identified this unmet need. A Belgian research team has recently published their protocol for the development of a PREM specific to patients with pancreatic cancer, with recruitment beginning in January 2022 [37]. In response to a systematic review by Apadula et al. revealing no specific PREMs for patients undergoing pancreatobiliary endoscopy, the authors are conducting a prospective observational cohort study to develop a PREM specific to endoscopic ultrasound [22, 38].

Otherwise, non-formalized surveys may currently provide the best quality information about patients with pancreatic disease and their experience with their health and the health system. In one study conducted over a 6-month period in 2018 in the United Kingdom, a cross-sectional questionnaire was administered to patients with pancreatic cancer, supplementing a PROM with questions regarding patient experience. While most patients responded positively to the care they received, this survey revealed otherwise important gaps in preoperative discussions. For example, approximately one-quarter of patients desired more information about their disease process at the time of diagnosis, and 10% of patients did not feel as though they were involved in treatment decision-making. Patients who underwent surgery vs. nonoperative management generally expressed a higher satisfaction with care and a better experience, though the authors acknowledged these results may be confounded with the generally poor prognosis of patients with unresectable disease. One important result of the study was the finding that while 83% were prescribed pancreatic enzyme replacement therapy (PERT), 33% of patients felt insufficiently educated about it [39]. Feelings of inadequate education about PERT, which addresses the malnutrition common in patients with pancreatic cancer and is associated with both improved HRQOL and survival, is an example of granular data to be gleaned from PREMs that may impact other clinical outcomes [40, 41].

In another study investigating patients' experience with surgery as management for pancreatic cystic lesions, the authors built a questionnaire that leaned heavily on surgeon experience, supplemented by research regarding shared decision-making and factors impacting patient satisfaction. This study had encouraging results regarding patient–surgeon interaction, with 84% reporting a "quite" or "extremely" detailed discussion with their surgeon and 91% agreeing that their surgeon took their personal beliefs into consideration during the visit. Almost 60% of patients reported fear of the cyst preoperatively, while relatively fewer (15%) reported negative emotions from postoperative changes in lifestyle. Studies such as these provide important insight into values of patients during preoperative discussions, and what may ultimately drive their decision to undergo surgery [42].

As can be seen in the above examples of PROMs and PREMs within the existing literature, these instruments are valuable tools for investigating the patients' perspective on aspects such as quality of life and experience with the healthcare system. While numerous PROMs have been published in the field of pancreatic disease, emphasis should be placed on including factors such as HRQOL more consistently as study outcomes. In comparison, relatively fewer PREMs are available, and research should focus on creating robust, validated tools for patients with pancreatic disease.

Use of PROMs and PREMs in Practice

These instruments are not only important tools in research but can also inform clinical decision-making and operative approach, as well as guide patient counseling.

Operative approach may not be associated with improved PROs in some disease processes, but other studies may demonstrate benefit. For example, pylorus-preserving PD vs. classic PD did not show any difference in patient-reported HRQOL as measured by the EORTC QLQ-C30 in one prospective study conducted over 2 years [43]. As discussed previously, the LEOPARD trial investigated the impact of minimally invasive vs. open distal pancreatectomy on long-term HRQOL using tools including the EORTC QLQ-C30, QLQ-PAN26, and a body image questionnaire. While there was no difference in quality-adjusted life years (primary outcome) or overall HRQOL, patients in the minimally invasive group did report a greater cosmetic satisfaction and reduced reduction of HRQOL at 30-days postoperatively compared to the open group [44]. These studies of how operative approach may or may not affect PROs for patients serve as important examples of how surgical technique may impact more than just clinical outcomes for patients.

Perhaps most importantly, studies investigating PROs provide information useful for patient counseling, especially of what to expect of symptoms pre- and postoperatively. As an example, Laitinen et al. conducted a study investigating HRQOL using the EORTC QLQ-C30 and QLQ-PAN26 for patients undergoing PD for pancreatic adenocarcinoma. The authors determined that global HRQOL was higher at 3 months postoperatively than prior to surgery, a finding which persisted for 2 years postoperatively for survivors. However, certain specific symptoms lasted up to 6 months after surgery, such as nausea and vomiting, before returning to preoperative levels. Physical functioning took 6 months before patients returned to baseline ability [45]. These findings are consistent with other reports that after a transient postoperative decline, most symptoms and physical function are improved by three to 6 months after surgery [46, 47]. Results of such studies are essential to share in combination with clinical outcomes with patients who are considering their treatment options.

Barriers to Implementation

Despite the clear benefits of incorporating PROs into routine outcomes measured for pancreatic disease, multiple barriers exist that hinder widespread inclusion and success of these tools in both research and practice.

Many instruments exist to measure patient outcomes, and the use of apps and other novel technologies has even further increased the total number of PROMs and PREMs. The challenge of such volume is that many tools may not be developed with the same rigor as those earlier discussed [23]. It is therefore essential that all tools be objectively assessed prior to inclusion in a trial or other intervention. As an example, Fitzpatrick et al. outlined a set of eight questions to be considered when evaluating a PROM for inclusion in a clinical trial, with the recommendation of close consideration of aspects of the instrument including validity, feasibility, and precision [48]. Furthermore, language and culture differences may affect test reliability, which must also be considered [49]. Selecting the right tool in the right context will maximize its success.

Additional obstacles to the implementation of PROs come from clinicians and other healthcare providers, who may believe they lack the training for use, fear their practice is judged on these scores alone, or resent lack of their input in selection of specific tools which may or may not apply to their patients. From an organization standpoint, there may be little support from higher administration for implementation, or lack of inclusion into existing clinical infrastructure. Mitigation strategies for these concerns include engaging clinicians in selection and implementation of instruments that are then incorporated into an existing clinical workflow, with high-quality training for all involved [50]. Ultimately, underscoring the importance of these tools as a means to incorporate the patient perspective, as well as emphasizing the underlying data behind their use, are additional strategies to achieve buy-in from stakeholders.

Conclusion

Pancreatic surgery can be morbid and the long-term outcomes can be limited, especially in the setting of pancreatic adenocarcinoma which has a low cure rate. Even in less ominous preoperative diagnoses such as pancreatic cysts or neuroendocrine tumors, the decision for pancreatectomy is complex and requires consideration of numerous factors, including individual patient factors and goals, surgeon and center experience, and many others. Communication of clinical outcomes is clearly necessary when counseling patients. However, discussions of other aspects of postoperative recovery, such as symptom burden and HRQOL, are equally important in the care of patients with pancreatic disease. Both recognition and benchmarking of clinical and patient-centered outcomes are an essential component of maintaining and improving both the safety of pancreas surgery and care of those undergoing these operations.

References

1. Narayanan S, Martin AN, Turrentine FE, Bauer TW, Adams RB, Zaydfudim VM. Mortality after pancreaticoduodenectomy: assessing early and late causes of patient death. J Surg Res. 2018;231:304–8.
2. Dominguez-Comesaña E, Gonzalez-Rodriguez FJ, Ulla-Rocha JL, Lede-Fernandez Á, Portela-Serra JL, Piñon-Cimadevila MÁ. Morbidity and mortality in pancreatic resection. Cirugía Española (English Edition). 2013;91(10):651–8.
3. Cardini B, Primavesi F, Maglione M, Oberschmied J, Guschlbauer L, Gasteiger S, et al. Outcomes following pancreatic resections—results and challenges of an Austrian university hospital compared to nationwide data and international centres. Eur Surg. 2019;51(3):81–9.
4. Ahola R, Sand J, Laukkarinen J. Centralization of pancreatic surgery improves results: review. Scand J Surg. 2020;109(1):4–10.
5. von Eiff W. International benchmarking and best practice management: in search of health care and hospital excellence. Adv Health Care Manag. 2015;17:223–52.
6. Staiger RD, Schwandt H, Puhan MA, Clavien PA. Improving surgical outcomes through benchmarking. Br J Surg. 2019;106(1):59–64.
7. Muller X, Marcon F, Sapisochin G, Marquez M, Dondero F, Rayar M, et al. Defining benchmarks in liver transplantation: a multicenter outcome analysis determining best achievable results. Ann Surg. 2018;267(3):419–25.
8. Rossler F, Sapisochin G, Song G, Lin YH, Simpson MA, Hasegawa K, et al. Defining benchmarks for major liver surgery: a multicenter analysis of 5202 living liver donors. Ann Surg. 2016;264(3):492–500.
9. Schmidt HM, Gisbertz SS, Moons J, Rouvelas I, Kauppi J, Brown A, et al. Defining benchmarks for transthoracic esophagectomy: a multicenter analysis of Total minimally invasive esophagectomy in low risk patients. Ann Surg. 2017;266(5):814–21.
10. Sanchez-Velazquez P, Muller X, Malleo G, Park JS, Hwang HK, Napoli N, et al. Benchmarks in pancreatic surgery: a novel tool for unbiased outcome comparisons. Ann Surg. 2019;270(2):211–8.
11. Tsilimigras DI, Pawlik TM, Moris D. Textbook outcomes in hepatobiliary and pancreatic surgery. World J Gastroenterol. 2021;27(15):1524–30.

12. van Roessel S, Mackay TM, van Dieren S, van der Schelling GP, Nieuwenhuijs VB, Bosscha K, et al. Textbook outcome: nationwide analysis of a novel quality measure in pancreatic surgery. Ann Surg. 2020;271(1):155–62.

13. Merath K, Chen Q, Bagante F, Beal E, Akgul O, Dillhoff M, et al. Textbook outcomes among medicare patients undergoing hepatopancreatic surgery. Ann Surg. 2020;271(6):1116–23.

14. Lof S, Benedetti Cacciaguerra A, Aljarrah R, Okorocha C, Jaber B, Shamali A, et al. Implementation of enhanced recovery after surgery for pancreatoduodenectomy increases the proportion of patients achieving textbook outcome: a retrospective cohort study. Pancreatology. 2020;20(5):976–83.

15. Suurmeijer JA, Henry AC, Bonsing BA, Bosscha K, van Dam RM, van Eijck CH, et al. Outcome of pancreatic surgery during the first six years of a mandatory audit within the Dutch pancreatic cancer group. Ann Surg. 2022;278:260–6.

16. Patient-Reported Outcomes. Washington, DC: National Quality Forum; https://www.quality-forum.org/Patient-Reported_Outcomes.aspx.

17. Liu JB, Pusic AL, Temple LK, Ko CY. Patient-reported outcomes in surgery: listening to patients improves quality of care. Bull Am Coll Surg. 2017;102(3):19–23.

18. Lavallee DC, Chenok KE, Love RM, Petersen C, Holve E, Segal CD, et al. Incorporating patient-reported outcomes into health care to engage patients and enhance care. Health Aff (Millwood). 2016;35(4):575–82.

19. Baumhauer JF, Bozic KJ. Value-based healthcare: patient-reported outcomes in clinical decision making. Clin Orthop Relat Res. 2016;474(6):1375–8.

20. Depla AL, Lamain-de Ruiter M, Laureij LT, Ernst-Smelt HE, Hazelzet JA, Franx A, et al. Patient reported outcome and experience measures in perinatal care to guide clinical practice: prospective observational study. J Med Internet Res. 2022;24(7):e37725.

21. Black N. Patient reported outcome measures could help transform healthcare. BMJ. 2013;346:f167.

22. Apadula L, Capurso G, Arcidiacono PG. Patient-reported experience measure in pancreatobiliary endoscopy: a systematic review to highlight areas for improvement. Eur J Gastroenterol Hepatol. 2021;33(6):832–8.

23. Maharaj AD, Samoborec S, Evans SM, Zalcberg J, Neale RE, Goldstein D, et al. Patient-reported outcome measures (PROMs) in pancreatic cancer: a systematic review. HPB (Oxford). 2020;22(2):187–203.

24. Fitzsimmons D, Johnson CD, George S, Payne S, Sandberg AA, Bassi C, et al. Development of a disease specific quality of life (QoL) questionnaire module to supplement the EORTC core cancer QoL questionnaire, the QLQ-C30 in patients with pancreatic cancer. Eur J Cancer. 1999;35(6):939–41.

25. Eaton AA, Karanicolas P, Bottomley A, Allen P, Gonen M. Psychometric validation of the EORTC QLQ-PAN26 pancreatic cancer module for assessing health related quality of life after pancreatic resection. J Pancreas. 2017;18(1):19–25.

26. Eaton AA, Gonen M, Karanicolas P, Jarnagin WR, D'Angelica MI, DeMatteo R, et al. Health-related quality of life after pancreatectomy: results from a randomized controlled trial. Ann Surg Oncol. 2016;23(7):2137–45.

27. Mackay TM, Latenstein AEJ, Sprangers MAG, van der Geest LG, Creemers GJ, van Dieren S, et al. Relationship between quality of life and survival in patients with pancreatic and periampullary cancer: a multicenter cohort analysis. J Natl Compr Cancer Netw. 2020;18(10):1354–63.

28. Heerkens HD, van Berkel L, Tseng DSJ, Monninkhof EM, van Santvoort HC, Hagendoorn J, et al. Long-term health-related quality of life after pancreatic resection for malignancy in patients with and without severe postoperative complications. HPB (Oxford). 2018;20(2):188–95.

29. Fong ZV, Sekigami Y, Qadan M, Fernandez-del Castillo C, Warshaw AL, Lillemoe KD, et al. Assessment of the long-term impact of pancreatoduodenectomy on health-related quality of life using the EORTC QLQ-PAN26 module. Ann Surg Oncol. 2021;28(8):4216–24.

30. de Rooij T, van Hilst J, Vogel JA, van Santvoort HC, de Boer MT, Boerma D, et al. Minimally invasive versus open distal pancreatectomy (LEOPARD): study protocol for a randomized controlled trial. Trials. 2017;18(1):166.
31. Heffernan N, Cella D, Webster K, Odom L, Martone M, Passik S, et al. Measuring health-related quality of life in patients with hepatobiliary cancers: the functional assessment of cancer therapy–hepatobiliary questionnaire. J Clin Oncol. 2002;20(9):2229–39.
32. Cella D, Butt Z, Kindler HL, Fuchs CS, Bray S, Barlev A, et al. Validity of the FACT hepatobiliary (FACT-Hep) questionnaire for assessing disease-related symptoms and health-related quality of life in patients with metastatic pancreatic cancer. Qual Life Res. 2013;22(5):1105–12.
33. Cloyd JM, Tran Cao HS, Petzel MQ, Denbo JW, Parker NH, Nogueras-González GM, et al. Impact of pancreatectomy on long-term patient-reported symptoms and quality of life in recurrence-free survivors of pancreatic and periampullary neoplasms. J Surg Oncol. 2017;115(2):144–50.
34. Overbeek KA, Kamps A, van Riet PA, Di Marco M, Zerboni G, van Hooft JE, et al. Pancreatic cyst surveillance imposes low psychological burden. Pancreatology. 2019;19(8):1061–6.
35. de-Madaria E, Sánchez-Marin C, Carrillo I, Vege SS, Chooklin S, Bilyak A, et al. Design and validation of a patient-reported outcome measure scale in acute pancreatitis: the PAN-PROMISE study. Gut. 2021;70(1):139–47.
36. Vinik A, Bottomley A, Korytowsky B, Bang YJ, Raoul JL, Valle JW, et al. Patient-reported outcomes and quality of life with sunitinib versus placebo for pancreatic neuroendocrine tumors: results from an international phase III trial. Target Oncol. 2016;11(6):815–24.
37. Moens K, Peeters M, Van den Bulcke M, Leys M, Horlait M. Development, testing, and implementation of the Belgian patient reported experience measure for pancreatic cancer care (PREPARE) project: protocol for a multi-method research project. JMIR Res Protoc. 2022;11(6):e29004.
38. Apadula L, Capurso G, Ambrosi A, Arcidiacono PG. Patient reported experience measure in endoscopic ultrasonography: the PREUS study protocol. Nurs Rep. 2022;12(1):59–64.
39. Watson EK, Brett J, Hay H, Witwicki C, Perris A, Poots AJ, et al. Experiences and supportive care needs of UK patients with pancreatic cancer: a cross-sectional questionnaire survey. BMJ Open. 2019;9(11):e032681.
40. Roberts KJ, Bannister CA, Schrem H. Enzyme replacement improves survival among patients with pancreatic cancer: results of a population based study. Pancreatology. 2019;19(1):114–21.
41. Pezzilli R, Caccialanza R, Capurso G, Brunetti O, Milella M, Falconi M. Pancreatic enzyme replacement therapy in pancreatic cancer. Cancers (Basel). 2020;12(2):275.
42. Puri PM, Watkins AA, Kent TS, Maggino L, Jeganathan JG, Callery MP, et al. Decision-making for the management of cystic lesions of the pancreas: how satisfied are patients with surgery? J Gastrointest Surg. 2018;22(1):88–97.
43. Schniewind B, Bestmann B, Henne-Bruns D, Faendrich F, Kremer B, Kuechler T. Quality of life after pancreaticoduodenectomy for ductal adenocarcinoma of the pancreatic head. Br J Surg. 2006;93(9):1099–107.
44. Korrel M, Roelofs A, van Hilst J, Busch OR, Daams F, Festen S, et al. Long-term quality of life after minimally invasive vs open distal pancreatectomy in the LEOPARD randomized trial. J Am Coll Surg. 2021;233(6):730–9.e9.
45. Laitinen I, Sand J, Peromaa P, Nordback I, Laukkarinen J. Quality of life in patients with pancreatic ductal adenocarcinoma undergoing pancreaticoduodenectomy. Pancreatology. 2017;17(3):445–50.
46. Rees JRE, Macefield RC, Blencowe NS, Alderson D, Finch-Jones MD, Blazeby JM. A prospective study of patient reported outcomes in pancreatic and peri-ampullary malignancy. World J Surg. 2013;37(10):2443–53.
47. Lewis AR, Pihlak R, McNamara MG. The importance of quality-of-life management in patients with advanced pancreatic ductal adenocarcinoma. Curr Probl Cancer. 2018;42(1):26–39.

48. Fitzpatrick R, Davey C, Buxton MJ, Jones DR. Evaluating patient-based outcome measures for use in clinical trials. Health Technol Assess. 1998;2(14):i–iv, 1–74

49. Saunders C, Carter DJ, Jordan A, Duffield C, Bichel-Findlay J. Cancer patient experience measures: an evidence review. J Psychosoc Oncol. 2016;34(3):200–22.

50. Foster A, Croot L, Brazier J, Harris J, O'Cathain A. The facilitators and barriers to implementing patient reported outcome measures in organisations delivering health related services: a systematic review of reviews. J Patient Rep Outcomes. 2018;2(1):46.

Chapter 39
SAGES University Master's Program: Pancreas Pathway

Hemasat Alkhatib, Voranaddha Vacharathit, and Kevin M. El-Hayek

The education of surgeons has evolved to become more structured during residency and fellowship [1]. However, the attending surgeon faces an ambiguous pathway to lifelong learning and skill advancement post-graduation. This disorganized continuance of education can lead to deficits that directly impact patient outcomes [2, 3]. Recognizing this, the Society of American Gastrointestinal and Endoscopic Surgeons (SAGES) sought to use its own vast educational content to create longitudinal, goal-directed education pathways within each clinical topics [4]. Their effort was termed the SAGES MASTERS Program (Fig. 39.1).

The SAGES MASTERS program is structured based on the Dreyfus Model for advanced stages of skill acquisition: competency, proficiency, and mastery [5]. Competency is what is expected of a graduating general surgery chief resident or Minimally Invasive Surgery (MIS) fellow; proficiency is what is expected from a surgeon approximately 3 years after completion of training; and mastery is what is expected of more experienced surgeons after several years of practice. The program currently has acute care surgery, biliary, bariatric, colorectal, foregut, hernia, flexible endoscopy, and leadership and professional development and robotic surgery modules. In this chapter, we describe the development of the pancreas pathway of the SAGES MASTERS program.

H. Alkhatib
Division of General Surgery, MetroHealth System, Cleveland, OH, USA

V. Vacharathit
Faculty of Medicine, Department of Surgery, Chulalongkorn University, Bangkok, Thailand

King Chulalongkorn Memorial Hospital, The Thai Red Cross Society, Bangkok, Thailand

K. M. El-Hayek (✉)
Division of General Surgery, MetroHealth System, Cleveland, OH, USA

Case Western Reserve University School of Medicine, Cleveland, OH, USA

Northeast Ohio Medical University, Rootstown, OH, USA

MASTERS PROGRAM

Welcome to the SAGES Masters Program. The goal is to organize all SAGES educational materials along three distinct curriculum pathways into blocks which can be achieved at the annual meeting or online. The program is currently in development. View our current educational resources.

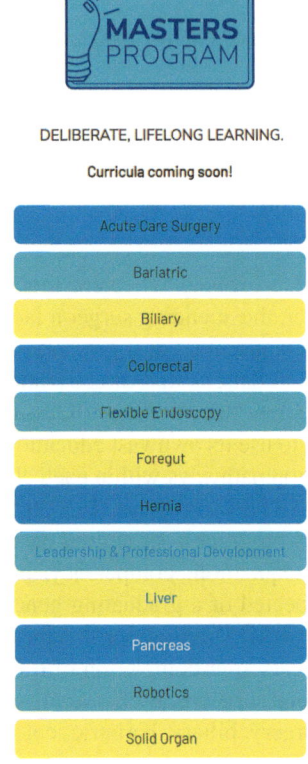

Fig. 39.1 SAGES MASTERS program. MASTERS PROGRAM https://www.sages.org/masters-program/ Accessed 2/26/2024

At each level of skill acquisition, the pancreas pathway aims to equip surgeons with level-appropriate knowledge of clinically relevant anatomy and patient considerations requisite to performing the anchoring procedures. To achieve this, the pathway provides resources derived from the SAGES library as well as seminal articles. Participants are evaluated by multiple choice questions, short-essay questions, and oral boards-style case scenarios. Finally, for each level of skill acquisition, surgeons can provide a video of an operation to be evaluated by an expert panel.

SAGES encourages an environment of collaborative teaching and peer-to-peer coaching through different online forums including membership only Facebook™ groups for each pathway. Figure 39.2 shows the Facebook™ group for the SAGES Hepatopancreatobiliary Surgery Master's Program Collaboration. Participants are

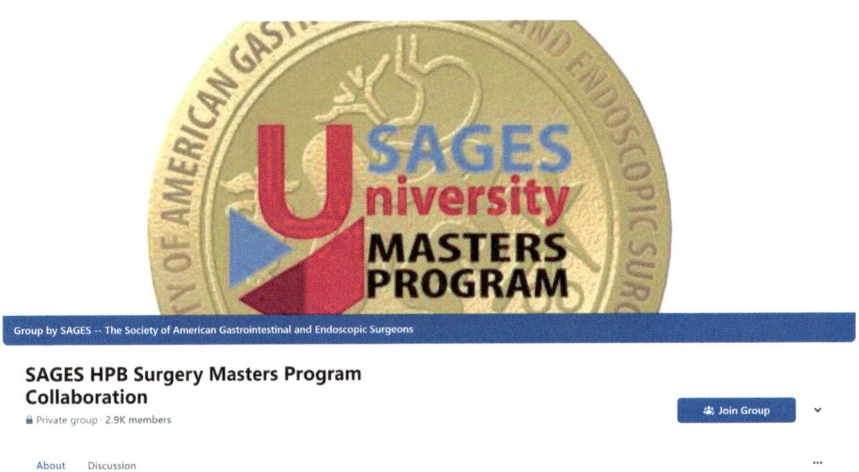

Fig. 39.2 The Facebook™ group for the SAGES Hepatopancreatobiliary Surgery Master's Program Collaboration. https://www.facebook.com/groups/900832470038666 Accessed 2/26/2024

encouraged to submit videos of critical steps of each procedure, while other members provide feedback and areas for improvement. These groups facilitate international participation, with sharing of unique experiences that the surgeon may otherwise not be exposed to. Collectively, these methods aim to improve comprehension, mastery, and collaboration on multiple levels: knowledge, practice, and technical skills.

Pancreas Curriculum

Currently in development, each level of the pancreas pathway is subdivided into three modules: preoperative, intraoperative, and postoperative modules. The preoperative module covers indications for surgery, including recognizing typical and atypical presentations, differential diagnoses, proper laboratory and radiographic work-up, results interpretation, and management options. The intraoperative module focuses on optimal patient and trocar setup, key anatomic landmarks, and critical operative steps, and exemplifying scenarios requiring further intraoperative modalities like intraoperative ultrasound. This module also covers possible intraoperative complications and bail-out maneuvers such as conversion to hand-assisted or open surgery. The postoperative module covers management in the immediate postoperative period including nutritional supplementation, medication titration, activity, and drain management. It also covers short- and long-term outcomes, as well as the work-up and management of postoperative complications.

Competency Level

The curriculum at the competency level focuses on the preoperative, intraoperative, and postoperative considerations for minimally invasive distal pancreatectomy with splenectomy. Table 39.1 lists all recommended educational resources for this module.

Table 39.1 Competency level: minimally invasive distal pancreatectomy with splenectomy

	Preoperative module
Videos	1. Minimally invasive distal pancreatectomy: To preserve or not preserve the spleen: https://www.sages.org/video/ minimally-invasive-distal-pancreatectomy-to-preserve-or-not-preserve-the-spleen/
Articles	1. Managing incidental pancreatic cysts (PMID: 29886564) [6]
	2. Surgical resection of lesions of the body and tail of the pancreas (UpToDate article) [7]
	3. Surgical management of pancreatic neuroendocrine tumors (PMID: 32151358) [8]
	4. The Miami international evidence-based guidelines on minimally invasive pancreas resection (PMID: 315675090) [9]
	5. Revisions of international consensus Fukuoka guidelines for the management of IPMN of the pancreas (PMID: 28735806) [10]
	Intraoperative module
Videos	1. Port placement for distal pancreatectomy: https://www.sages.org/video/ port-placement-for-distal-pancreatectomy/
	2. SAGES Top 21 Videos: Laparoscopic Distal Pancreatectomy: https://www.sages. org/video/sages-top-21-videos-laparoscopic-distal-pancreatectomy/
	3. Technique of minimal invasive distal pancreatectomy in the U.S.: https://www. sages.org/video/technique-of-minimal-invasive-distal-pancreatectomyin-the-u-s/
	4. Laparoscopic distal pancreatectomy: Clockwise (Asbun's) technique: https://www. sages.org/video/laparoscopic-distal-pancreatectomy-clockwise-asbuns-technique/
	5. Pancreatic transection techniques: https://www.sages.org/video/ pancreatic-transection-techniques/
	6. Pancreatic transection techniques 2: https://www.sages.org/video/ pancreatic-transection-techniques-2/
	7. Video face-off panel: Distal pancreatectomy panel discussion 2: https://www.sages. org/video/video-face-off-panel-distal-pancreatectomy-panel-discussion-2/
	8. Robotic approach to the distal pancreatectomy: Medial to lateral pancreatic exposure: https://www.sages.org/video/ robotic-approach-to-the-distal-pancreatectomy-medial-to-lateral-pancreatic-exposure/
Articles	1. Laparoscopic approach to distal and subtotal pancreatectomy: a clockwise technique (PMID: 21487886) [11]
	2. Technical aspects of laparoscopic distal pancreatectomy for benign and malignant disease: Review of the literature (PMID: 26240565) [12]

(continued)

Table 39.1 (continued)

	Postoperative module
Articles	1. Enhanced recovery pathways in pancreatic surgery: State of the art. (PMID: 27605881) [13]
	2. Enhanced recovery pathways in pancreatic surgery. (PMID: 27865279) [14]
	3. A prospective randomized multicenter trial of distal pancreatectomy with and without routine intraperitoneal drainage. (PMID: 28692468) [15]
	4. Drain management following distal pancreatectomy: Characterization of contemporary practice and impact of early removal. (PMID: 30943185) [16]
	5. Postpancreatectomy complications and management. (PMID: 27865280) [17]
	6. Postoperative management in patients undergoing major pancreatic resections. in: surgery for pancreatic and periampullary cancer. Springer, Singapore [18]
	7. Pancreatic exocrine insufficiency following pancreatic resection (PMID: 26145836) [19]
	8. New-onset diabetes after distal pancreatectomy: a systematic review. (PMID: 24983994) [20]
	9. Postoperative management in patients undergoing major pancreatic resections. In: Surgery for Pancreatic and Periampullary Cancer. Springer, Singapore [18] Complications in the adult asplenic patient: A review for the emergency clinician. (PMID: 32247651) [21]

Preoperative Module

Upon completion of the preoperative module, the learner should be able to:

1. Describe the typical presentation of patients with left-sided pancreatic lesions.
2. Distinguish between a solid mass vs. a cystic neoplasm.
3. Recall the work-up for cystic neoplasms based on current guidelines.
4. Recognize the utility of and indications for CT, MRI, and endoscopic ultrasound with fine needle aspiration biopsy.
5. Independently interpret fluid analyses from cystic neoplasms of the pancreas.
6. Identify patients who will benefit from distal pancreatectomy with splenectomy and incorporate the patient's comorbidities and work-up into procedure choice.
7. Recall the appropriate preoperative vaccinations for a patient with planned splenectomy.

Intraoperative Module

Upon completion of this module, the learner should be able to:

1. List possible patient positioning and trocar placements for distal pancreatectomy with splenectomy.
2. List several methods of mobilizing and retracting the greater curvature of the stomach and exposing the pancreatic tail.

3. Describe several techniques for verifying adequate parenchymal margin prior to transection.
4. Explain at least 3 methods of parenchymal transection.
5. Describe different methods of major peripancreatic vessel transection.
6. Describe the various factors that increase pancreatic fistula risk.
7. Describe the advantages and disadvantages of drain placement.
8. Describe strategies for managing intraoperative bleeding and demonstrate judgment as to when to convert to an open/hybrid approach.

Postoperative Module

Upon completion of this module, the learner should be able to:

1. Elaborate on the typical immediate postoperative pathway following a distal pancreatectomy and splenectomy (including nutrition, activity, medication changes, drain management, etc.).
2. List the typical expected outcomes of patients with curative surgery vs those who require ongoing surveillance (i.e., IPMN vs adenocarcinoma).
3. Identify the most common short-term postoperative complications, state their incidence, appropriate diagnostic work-up, and how to manage them. (i.e., post-pancreatectomy fistula/hemorrhage, deep vein thrombosis, and pulmonary embolism).
4. Identify the most common long-term postoperative complications, state their incidence, appropriate diagnostic work-up, and how to manage them (i.e., diabetes, post-splenectomy sepsis).

Proficiency Level

The proficiency level of the pancreas pathway covers MIS spleen-preserving distal pancreatectomy (MIS SPDP), with preoperative, intraoperative, and postoperative considerations. Table 39.2 lists the educational resources recommended for this module.

Table 39.2 Proficiency level: Minimally Invasive spleen preserving distal pancreatectomy

	Preoperative module
Videos	1. Minimally invasive distal pancreatectomy: To preserve or not preserve the spleen: https://www.sages.org/video/minimally-invasive-distal-pancreatectomy-to-preserve-or-not-preserve-the-spleen/ 2. Technical aspects of spleen preserving distal pancreatectomy: https://www.sages.org/video/technical-aspects-spleen-preserving-distal-pancreatectomy/ 3. Technique of minimal invasive distal pancreatectomy in Korea: https://www.sages.org/video/technique-of-minimal-invasive-distal-pancreatectomy-in-korea/
Articles	1. Laparoscopic spleen-preserving distal pancreatectomy with and without splenic vessel preservation—a comparative study [22] 2. Spleen-preserving pancreatic resections with preservation of splenic vessels: A cautionary note on the risk of vascular complications [23] 3. True learning curve of laparoscopic spleen-preserving distal pancreatectomy with splenic vessel preservation. (PMID: 29934868) [24] 4. Splenic preservation vs. splenectomy in laparoscopic distal pancreatectomy: a propensity score-matched study (PMID: 31236723) [25]
	Intraoperative module
Videos	1. Minimally invasive distal pancreatectomy: To preserve or not preserve the spleen: https://www.sages.org/video/minimally-invasive-distal-pancreatectomy-to-preserve-or-not-preserve-the-spleen/ 2. Sages distal pancreatectomy video faceoff: https://www.sages.org/video/sages-distal-pancreatectomy-video-faceoff/ 3. Laparoscopic splenic and vessel preserving distal pancreatectomy: https://www.sages.org/video/laparoscopic-splenic-and-vessel-preserving-distal-pancreatectomy/
Articles	1. Laparoscopic distal pancreatectomy combined with preservation of the spleen for cystic neoplasms of the pancreas (PMID: 15120376) [26] 2. Distal pancreatic resection: Technical differences between open and laparoscopic approaches (PMID: 18333239) [27] 3. Conservation of the spleen with distal pancreatectomy. (PMID: 3358679) [28] 4. Robotic distal pancreatectomy with or without preservation of spleen: a technical note (PMID: 25248464) [29]
	Postoperative module
Videos	1. Minimally invasive distal pancreatectomy: To preserve or not preserve the spleen: https://www.sages.org/video/minimally-invasive-distal-pancreatectomy-to-preserve-or-not-preserve-the-spleen/
Articles	1. Splenic preservation vs. splenectomy in laparoscopic distal pancreatectomy: a propensity score-matched study. (PMID: 31236723) [30] 2. Long-term outcome after minimally invasive and open Warshaw and Kimura techniques for spleen-preserving distal pancreatectomy: International multicenter retrospective study. (PMID: 31005470) [31] 3. ENETS Consensus Recommendations for the Standards of Care in Neuroendocrine Neoplasms: Follow-Up and Documentation. (PMID: 28222443) [32] 4. The North American Neuroendocrine Tumor Society Consensus Paper on the Surgical Management of Pancreatic Neuroendocrine Tumors. (PMID: 31856076) [33] 5. Revisions of international consensus Fukuoka guidelines for the management of IPMN of the pancreas. (PMID: 28735806) [10]

Preoperative Module

Upon completion of this module, the learner will be able to:

1. Describe the proper clinical and radiographic evaluation for a patient presenting with a pancreatic lesion who could be a candidate for spleen-preserving distal pancreatectomy.
2. Identify and describe the benefits of MIS SPDP based on clinical and radiographic findings.
3. Describe the recommended preoperative laboratory and radiographic work-up for pancreatic lesions amenable to MIS SPDP.
4. Use clinical and radiographic data to plan operations based on anatomic implications.
5. Propose and explain treatment strategies for a specific patient.
6. Describe the anticipated pre- and postoperative findings related to an oncologically safe and effective procedure.
7. Discuss indications and contraindications for spleen preservation during distal pancreatectomy.

Intraoperative Module

Upon completion of this module, the learner should be able to:

1. Describe different options for different key operative steps including vascular control, pancreatic dissection, achieving R0 margins, and node harvesting.
2. Describe differences between spleen-preserving distal pancreatectomy vs. the Warshaw technique.
3. Describe how the patient is to be positioned and secured for the procedure.
4. List the key operative steps including:

   - Access/incisions: How many ports, what sizes, location, energy devices, and stapling choices.
   - Key anatomic landmarks at, above, and below the pancreas, spleen, common anatomic variances, and need for en bloc resections.
   - Adequate resection margins and lymph node harvesting.

5. Describe final exploration: confirm hemostasis and closure (drain placement when applicable).
6. Identify reasons to convert to open surgery.

Postoperative Module

Upon completion of this module, the learner should be able to:

1. Describe the typical immediate postoperative pathway (including nutrition, activity, medication changes, vaccinations, drain management, etc.)
2. Describe the typical expected outcomes (i.e., margin status, incidence of conversion, incidence of fistula formation, wound infection, or other described complications) and expected postoperative signs and symptoms.
3. List the short-term postoperative complications following a MIS SPDP (such as pancreatic leak, wound infection, splenic vessel thrombosis, etc.), their incidence, work-up, and how to manage them in a timely and appropriate fashion.
4. List the long-term postoperative clinical outcomes (i.e., diabetes, local recurrence)—including their incidence, work-up, and management.

Mastery Level

The mastery level of the pancreas pathway covers MIS radical antegrade modular pancreatosplenectomy (RAMPS). Table 39.3 lists all recommended educational resources for this module.

Table 39.3 Mastery level: Minimally invasive radical antegrade modular pancreatosplenectomy

	Preoperative module
Articles	1. A systematic review of minimally invasive vs. open radical antegrade modular pancreatosplenectomy for pancreatic cancer (PMID: 35093863) [34]
	2. Radical antegrade modular pancreatosplenectomy procedure for adenocarcinoma of the body and tail of the pancreas: Ability to obtain negative tangential margins (PMID: 17254928) [35]
	3. Initial experience with laparoscopic radical antegrade modular pancreatosplenectomy for left-sided pancreatic cancer in a single institution: Technical aspects and oncological outcomes (PMID: 28061895) [36]
	Intraoperative module
Videos	1. Standard resection vs ramps: https://www.sages.org/video/standard-resection-vs-ramps/
	2. Standard resection vs ramps 2: https://www.sages.org/video/standard-resection-vs-ramps-2/
	3. Technique of minimal invasive distal pancreatectomy in Korea: https://www.sages.org/video/technique-of-minimal-invasive-distal-pancreatectomy-in-korea/
	4. Video face-off panel: Distal pancreatectomy conclusions: https://www.sages.org/video/video-face-off-panel-distal-pancreatectomy-conclusions/

(continued)

Table 39.3 (continued)

Articles	
	1. Robot-assisted radical antegrade modular pancreatosplenectomy including resection and reconstruction of the spleno-mesenteric junction (PMID: 31957748) [37]
	2. Radical antegrade modular pancreatosplenectomy procedure for adenocarcinoma of the body and tail of the pancreas: Ability to obtain negative tangential margins (PMID: 17254928) [35]
	3. Multimedia article. Laparoscopic modified anterior RAMPS in well-selected left-sided pancreatic cancer: Technical feasibility and interim results (PMID: 21298529) [38]
	4. Minimally invasive RAMPS in well-selected left-sided pancreatic cancer within Yonsei criteria: Long-term (>median 3 years) oncologic outcomes (PMID: 24853839) [39]
	5. Laparoscopic radical antegrade modular pancreatosplenectomy for left-sided pancreatic cancer using the ligament of Treitz approach (PMID: 28409377) [40]
	6. Initial experience with laparoscopic radical antegrade modular pancreatosplenectomy for left-sided pancreatic cancer in a single institution: Technical aspects and oncological outcomes (PMID: 28061895) [36]
	7. Robotic radical antegrade modular pancreatosplenectomy (RAMPS) vs. standard retrograde pancreatosplenectomy (SRPS): Study protocol for a randomized controlled trial (PMID: 32245518) [41]
	8. Outcomes and risk score for distal pancreatectomy with celiac axis resection (DP-CAR): An international multicenter analysis (PMID: 30610560) [42]
	9. Robotic and open distal pancreatectomy with celiac axis resection for locally advanced pancreatic body tumors: a single institutional assessment of perioperative outcomes and survival (PMID: 27506992) [43]
	10. A prospective randomized multicenter trial of distal pancreatectomy with and without routine intraperitoneal drainage (PMID: 28692468) [15]
	11. Enhanced recovery after pancreatic surgery: a systematic review of the evidence (PMID: 24750457) [44]
	12. Comprehensive comparative analysis of cost-effectiveness and perioperative outcomes between open, laparoscopic, and robotic distal pancreatectomy (PMID: 31217087) [45]
	13. Short-term surgical morbidity and mortality of distal pancreatectomy performed for benign vs. malignant diseases: a NSQIP analysis (PMID: 31598880) [46]
	14. Management of the pancreatic transection plane after left (distal) pancreatectomy: Expert consensus guidelines by the international study group of pancreatic surgery (ISGPS). (PMID: 32249092) [47]
	15. Risk Factors and Mitigation Strategies for Pancreatic Fistula After Distal Pancreatectomy: Analysis of 2026 Resections From the International, Multi-institutional Distal Pancreatectomy Study Group (PMID: 28857813) [48]

(continued)

Table 39.3 (continued)

	Postoperative module
Articles	1. Enhanced recovery pathways in pancreatic surgery: State of the art. (PMID: 27605881) [13]
	2. Enhanced recovery pathways in pancreatic surgery. (PMID: 27865279) [14]
	3. A prospective randomized multicenter trial of distal pancreatectomy with and without routine intraperitoneal drainage. (PMID: 28692468) [15]
	4. Drain management following distal pancreatectomy: Characterization of contemporary practice and impact of early removal. (PMID: 30943185) [16]
	5. Postpancreatectomy complications and management. (PMID: 27865280) [17]
	6. Postoperative management in patients undergoing major pancreatic resections. In: Surgery for pancreatic and periampullary cancer. Springer, Singapore [18]
	7. Pancreatic exocrine insufficiency following pancreatic resection. (PMID: 26145836) [19]
	8. New-onset diabetes after distal pancreatectomy: a systematic review. (PMID: 24983994) [20]
	9. Complications in the adult asplenic patient: A review for the emergency clinician. (PMID: 32247651) [21]
	10. NCCN guidelines for pancreatic adenocarcinoma [49]

Preoperative Module

Upon completion of this module, the learner should be able to:

1. Describe the typical and atypical presenting signs and symptoms of a patient with left-sided pancreatic adenocarcinoma.
2. Describe the oncologic rationale for RAMPS (complete regional lymph node harvest, negative tangential margins).
3. Recognize the utility of and indications for CT, MRI, and endoscopic ultrasound with fine needle aspiration biopsy.
4. Independently interpret CT/MRI images for vascular (portal vein, SMV, SMA, celiac axis) and adjacent organ involvement (left adrenal, stomach, transverse colon).
5. Discuss tumor characteristics on cross-sectional imaging that will be important in operative planning for RAMPS.
6. Identify patients who will benefit from RAMPS and decide on procedure choice while incorporating the patients' comorbidities and work-up into the decision-making.
7. Describe the appropriate usage of neoadjuvant chemotherapy for left-sided pancreatic adenocarcinoma. Discuss controversies and trends.

Intraoperative Module

Upon completion of this module, the learner should be able to:

1. Describe how to prepare patients for surgery (i.e., vaccinations, bowel prep, patient positioning).
2. Describe the key steps for RAMPS—techniques for exposure of the pancreatic body/tail, options for division of the pancreas, dissection along the SMV/PV, SMA and celiac axis, lymph node harvesting, and obtaining tangential resection margins.
3. Describe the difference between anterior and posterior RAMPS.
4. Discuss the options for drain placement.
5. Discuss the indications for multivisceral (adrenal, stomach, colon) and vascular resection (for instance, SMV-PV or celiac axis resection).
6. Describe the management of intraoperative complications and how to manage them.

Postoperative Module

Upon completion of this module, the learner should be able to:

1. Describe the typical immediate postoperative pathway following a distal pancreatectomy and splenectomy (including nutrition, activity, medication changes, drain management, etc.)
2. List the typical expected oncologic outcomes and describe the indications for adjuvant chemotherapy and radiation.
3. Identify the most common short-term postoperative complications (i.e., PE, DVT, hemorrhage, pancreatic fistula), state their incidence, appropriate diagnostic work-up, and how to manage them.
4. Identify the most common long-term post-op complications (i.e., diabetes, postsplenectomy sepsis), state their incidence, appropriate diagnostic work-up, and how to manage them.

References

1. Camison L, Brooker JE, Naran S, Potts JR III, Losee JE. The history of surgical education in the United States: past, present, and future. Ann Surg Open. 2022;3:e148.
2. Birkmeyer JD, Finks JF, O'Reilly A, Oerline M, Carlin AM, Nunn AR, Dimick J, Banerjee M, Birkmeyer NJ. Surgical skill and complication rates after bariatric surgery. N Engl J Med. 2013;369:1434–42.
3. Stulberg JJ, Huang R, Kreutzer L, Ban K, Champagne BJ, Steele SR, Johnson JK, Holl JL, Greenberg CC, Bilimoria KY. Association between surgeon technical skills and patient outcomes. JAMA Surg. 2020;155:960–8.

4. Jones DB, Stefanidis D, Korndorffer JR Jr, Dimick JB, Jacob BP, Schultz L, Scott DJ. SAGES University MASTERS program: a structured curriculum for deliberate, lifelong learning. Surg Endosc. 2017;31:3061–71.
5. Dreyfus SE. The five-stage model of adult skill acquisition. Bull Sci Technol Soc. 2004;24:177–81.
6. Phan J, Raman Muthusamy V. Managing incidental pancreatic cysts. Curr Gastroenterol Rep. 2018;20:32.
7. Donahue TR. Surgical resection of lesions of the body and tail of the pancreas. In: Stanley W, Ashley M, editors. UpToDate ; 2022.
8. Vaghaiwalla T, Keutgen XM. Surgical management of pancreatic neuroendocrine tumors. Surg Oncol Clin N Am. 2020;29:243–52.
9. Asbun HJ, Moekotte AL, Vissers FL, Kunzler F, Cipriani F, Alseidi A, D'Angelica MI, Balduzzi A, Bassi C, Björnsson B, Boggi U, Callery MP, Del Chiaro M, Coimbra FJ, Conrad C, Cook A, Coppola A, Dervenis C, Dokmak S, Edil BH, Edwin B, Giulianotti PC, Han HS, Hansen PD, van der Heijde N, van Hilst J, Hester CA, Hogg ME, Jarufe N, Jeyarajah DR, Keck T, Kim SC, Khatkov IE, Kokudo N, Kooby DA, Korrel M, de Leon FJ, Lluis N, Lof S, Machado MA, Demartines N, Martinie JB, Merchant NB, Molenaar IQ, Moravek C, Mou YP, Nakamura M, Nealon WH, Palanivelu C, Pessaux P, Pitt HA, Polanco PM, Primrose JN, Rawashdeh A, Sanford DE, Senthilnathan P, Shrikhande SV, Stauffer JA, Takaori K, Talamonti MS, Tang CN, Vollmer CM, Wakabayashi G, Walsh RM, Wang SE, Zinner MJ, Wolfgang CL, Zureikat AH, Zwart MJ, Conlon KC, Kendrick ML, Zeh HJ, Hilal MA, Besselink MG. The Miami international evidence-based guidelines on minimally invasive pancreas resection. Ann Surg. 2020;271:1–14.
10. Tanaka M, Fernández-Del Castillo C, Kamisawa T, Jang JY, Levy P, Ohtsuka T, Salvia R, Shimizu Y, Tada M, Wolfgang CL. Revisions of international consensus Fukuoka guidelines for the management of IPMN of the pancreas. Pancreatology. 2017;17:738–53.
11. Asbun HJ, Stauffer JA. Laparoscopic approach to distal and subtotal pancreatectomy: a clockwise technique. Surg Endosc. 2011;25:2643–9.
12. de Rooij T, Sitarz R, Busch OR, Besselink MG, Abu Hilal M. Technical aspects of laparoscopic distal pancreatectomy for benign and malignant disease: review of the literature. Gastroenterol Res Pract. 2015;2015:472906.
13. Pecorelli N, Nobile S, Partelli S, Cardinali L, Crippa S, Balzano G, Beretta L, Falconi M. Enhanced recovery pathways in pancreatic surgery: state of the art. World J Gastroenterol. 2016;22:6456–68.
14. Barton JG. Enhanced recovery pathways in pancreatic surgery. Surg Clin North Am. 2016;96:1301–12.
15. Van Buren G 2nd, Bloomston M, Schmidt CR, Behrman SW, Zyromski NJ, Ball CG, Morgan KA, Hughes SJ, Karanicolas PJ, Allendorf JD, Vollmer CM Jr, Ly Q, Brown KM, Velanovich V, Winter JM, McElhany AL, Muscarella P 2nd, Schmidt CM, House MG, Dixon E, Dillhoff ME, Trevino JG, Hallet J, NSG C, Nakeeb A, Behrns KE, Sasson AR, Ceppa EP, Abdel-Misih SRZ, Riall TS, Silberfein EJ, Ellison EC, Adams DB, Hsu C, Tran Cao HS, Mohammed S, Villafañe-Ferriol N, Barakat O, Massarweh NN, Chai C, Mendez-Reyes JE, Fang A, Jo E, Mo Q, Fisher WE. A prospective randomized multicenter trial of distal pancreatectomy with and without routine intraperitoneal drainage. Ann Surg. 2017;266:421–31.
16. Seykora TF, Liu JB, Maggino L, Pitt HA, Vollmer CM Jr. Drain management following distal pancreatectomy: characterization of contemporary practice and impact of early removal. Ann Surg. 2020;272:1110–7.
17. Malleo G, Vollmer CM Jr. Postpancreatectomy complications and management. Surg Clin North Am. 2016;96:1313–36.
18. Pulvirenti A, Pea A, De Pastena M, Marchegiani G, Salvia R, Bassi C. Postoperative management in patients undergoing major pancreatic resections. In: Tewari M, editor. Surgery for pancreatic and periampullary cancer: principles and practice. Singapore: Springer Singapore; 2018. p. 239–45.

19. Phillips ME. Pancreatic exocrine insufficiency following pancreatic resection. Pancreatology. 2015;15:449–55.
20. De Bruijn KM, van Eijck CH. New-onset diabetes after distal pancreatectomy: a systematic review. Ann Surg. 2015;261:854–61.
21. Long B, Koyfman A, Gottlieb M. Complications in the adult asplenic patient: a review for the emergency clinician. Am J Emerg Med. 2021;44:452–7.
22. Raveendran Nair S, Senadhipan B. Laparoscopic spleen-preserving distal pancreatectomy with and without splenic vessel preservation—a comparative study. HPB. 2016;18:e441.
23. Bissolati M, Muffatti F, Aleotti F, Nobile S, Salandini MC, Adamenko O, Crippa S, Partelli S, Falconi M, Balzano G. Spleen-preserving pancreatic resections with preservation of splenic vessels: a cautionary note on the risk of vascular complications. HPB. 2016;18:e772.
24. Kim HS, Park JS, Yoon DS. True learning curve of laparoscopic spleen-preserving distal pancreatectomy with splenic vessel preservation. Surg Endosc. 2019;33:88–93.
25. Moekotte AL, Lof S, White SA, Marudanayagam R, Al-Sarireh B, Rahman S, Soonawalla Z, Deakin M, Aroori S, Ammori B, Gomez D, Marangoni G, Abu Hilal M, For the Minimally Invasive l, Pancreatic Surgery Study Group UK. Splenic preservation versus splenectomy in laparoscopic distal pancreatectomy: a propensity score-matched study. Surg Endosc. 2020;34:1301–9.
26. Fernández-Cruz L, Martínez I, Gilabert R, Cesar-Borges G, Astudillo E, Navarro S. Laparoscopic distal pancreatectomy combined with preservation of the spleen for cystic neoplasms of the pancreas. J Gastrointest Surg. 2004;8:493–501.
27. Fernández-Cruz L. Distal pancreatic resection: technical differences between open and laparoscopic approaches. HPB. 2006;8:49–56.
28. Warshaw AL. Conservation of the spleen with distal pancreatectomy. Arch Surg (Chicago, Ill: 1960). 1988;123:550–3.
29. Parisi A, Coratti F, Cirocchi R, Grassi V, Desiderio J, Farinacci F, Ricci F, Adamenko O, Economou AI, Cacurri A, Trastulli S, Renzi C, Castellani E, Di Rocco G, Redler A, Santoro A, Coratti A. Robotic distal pancreatectomy with or without preservation of spleen: a technical note. World J Surg Oncol. 2014;12:295.
30. Moekotte AL, Lof S, White SA, Marudanayagam R, Al-Sarireh B, Rahman S, Soonawalla Z, Deakin M, Aroori S, Ammori B, Gomez D, Marangoni G, Abu Hilal M. Splenic preservation versus splenectomy in laparoscopic distal pancreatectomy: a propensity score-matched study. Surg Endosc. 2020;34:1301–9.
31. Paiella S, De Pastena M, Korrel M, Pan TL, Butturini G, Nessi C, De Robertis R, Landoni L, Casetti L, Giardino A, Busch O, Pea A, Esposito A, Besselink M, Bassi C, Salvia R. Long term outcome after minimally invasive and open Warshaw and Kimura techniques for spleen-preserving distal pancreatectomy: international multicenter retrospective study. Eur J Surg Oncol. 2019;45:1668–73.
32. Knigge U, Capdevila J, Bartsch DK, Baudin E, Falkerby J, Kianmanesh R, Kos-Kudla B, Niederle B, Nieveen van Dijkum E, O'Toole D, Pascher A, Reed N, Sundin A, Vullierme MP. ENETS consensus recommendations for the standards of care in neuroendocrine neoplasms: follow-up and documentation. Neuroendocrinology. 2017;105:310–9.
33. Howe JR, Merchant NB, Conrad C, Keutgen XM, Hallet J, Drebin JA, Minter RM, Lairmore TC, Tseng JF, Zeh HJ, Libutti SK, Singh G, Lee JE, Hope TA, Kim MK, Menda Y, Halfdanarson TR, Chan JA, Pommier RF. The North American neuroendocrine tumor society consensus paper on the surgical management of pancreatic neuroendocrine tumors. Pancreas. 2020;49:1–33.
34. Takagi K, Umeda Y, Yoshida R, Yagi T, Fujiwara T. A systematic review of minimally invasive versus open radical antegrade modular pancreatosplenectomy for pancreatic cancer. Anticancer Res. 2022;42:653–60.
35. Strasberg SM, Linehan DC, Hawkins WG. Radical antegrade modular pancreatosplenectomy procedure for adenocarcinoma of the body and tail of the pancreas: ability to obtain negative tangential margins. J Am Coll Surg. 2007;204:244–9.

36. Kim EY, Hong TH. Initial experience with laparoscopic radical antegrade modular pancreatosplenectomy for left-sided pancreatic cancer in a single institution: technical aspects and oncological outcomes. BMC Surg. 2017;17:2.
37. Napoli N, Kauffmann EF, Menonna F, Iacopi S, Cacace C, Boggi U. Robot-assisted radical antegrade modular pancreatosplenectomy including resection and reconstruction of the Spleno-mesenteric junction. J Vis Exp; 2020. https://doi.org/10.3791/60370.
38. Choi SH, Kang CM, Lee WJ, Chi HS. Multimedia article. Laparoscopic modified anterior RAMPS in well-selected left-sided pancreatic cancer: technical feasibility and interim results. Surg Endosc. 2011;25:2360–1.
39. Lee SH, Kang CM, Hwang HK, Choi SH, Lee WJ, Chi HS. Minimally invasive RAMPS in well-selected left-sided pancreatic cancer within Yonsei criteria: long-term (>median 3 years) oncologic outcomes. Surg Endosc. 2014;28:2848–55.
40. Ome Y, Hashida K, Yokota M, Nagahisa Y, Michio O, Kawamoto K. Laparoscopic radical antegrade modular pancreatosplenectomy for left-sided pancreatic cancer using the ligament of Treitz approach. Surg Endosc. 2017;31:4836–7.
41. Zhang G, Kang Y, Zhang H, Wang F, Liu R. Robotic radical antegrade modular pancreatosplenectomy (RAMPS) versus standard retrograde pancreatosplenectomy (SRPS): study protocol for a randomized controlled trial. Trials. 2020;21:306.
42. Klompmaker S, Peters NA, van Hilst J, Bassi C, Boggi U, Busch OR, Niesen W, Van Gulik TM, Javed AA, Kleeff J, Kawai M, Lesurtel M, Lombardo C, Moser AJ, Okada KI, Popescu I, Prasad R, Salvia R, Sauvanet A, Sturesson C, Weiss MJ, Zeh HJ, Zureikat AH, Yamaue H, Wolfgang CL, Hogg ME, Besselink MG. Outcomes and risk score for distal pancreatectomy with celiac axis resection (DP-CAR): an international multicenter analysis. Ann Surg Oncol. 2019;26:772–81.
43. Ocuin LM, Miller-Ocuin JL, Novak SM, Bartlett DL, Marsh JW, Tsung A, Lee KK, Hogg ME, Zeh HJ, Zureikat AH. Robotic and open distal pancreatectomy with celiac axis resection for locally advanced pancreatic body tumors: a single institutional assessment of perioperative outcomes and survival. HPB. 2016;18:835–42.
44. Kagedan DJ, Ahmed M, Devitt KS, Wei AC. Enhanced recovery after pancreatic surgery: a systematic review of the evidence. HPB. 2015;17:11–6.
45. Magge DR, Zenati MS, Hamad A, Rieser C, Zureikat AH, Zeh HJ, Hogg ME. Comprehensive comparative analysis of cost-effectiveness and perioperative outcomes between open, laparoscopic, and robotic distal pancreatectomy. HPB. 2018;20:1172–80.
46. Daniel FE, Tamim HM, Hosni MN, Mailhac AC, Khalife MJ, Jamali FR, Faraj W. Short-term surgical morbidity and mortality of distal pancreatectomy performed for benign versus malignant diseases: a NSQIP analysis. Surg Endosc. 2020;34:3927–35.
47. Miao Y, Lu Z, Yeo CJ, Vollmer CM Jr, Fernandez-Del Castillo C, Ghaneh P, Halloran CM, Kleeff J, de Rooij T, Werner J, Falconi M, Friess H, Zeh HJ, Izbicki JR, He J, Laukkarinen J, Dejong CH, Lillemoe KD, Conlon K, Takaori K, Gianotti L, Besselink MG, Del Chiaro M, Montorsi M, Tanaka M, Bockhorn M, Adham M, Oláh A, Salvia R, Shrikhande SV, Hackert T, Shimosegawa T, Zureikat AH, Ceyhan GO, Peng Y, Wang G, Huang X, Dervenis C, Bassi C, Neoptolemos JP, Büchler MW. Management of the pancreatic transection plane after left (distal) pancreatectomy: expert consensus guidelines by the international study group of pancreatic surgery (ISGPS). Surgery. 2020;168:72–84.
48. Ecker BL, McMillan MT, Allegrini V, Bassi C, Beane JD, Beckman RM, Behrman SW, Dickson EJ, Callery MP, Christein JD, Drebin JA, Hollis RH, House MG, Jamieson NB, Javed AA, Kent TS, Kluger MD, Kowalsky SJ, Maggino L, Malleo G, Valero V 3rd, Velu LKP, Watkins AA, Wolfgang CL, Zureikat AH, Vollmer CM Jr. Risk factors and mitigation strategies for pancreatic fistula after distal pancreatectomy: analysis of 2026 resections from the international, multi-institutional distal pancreatectomy study group. Ann Surg. 2019;269:143–9.
49. Network NCC NCCN guidelines for pancreatic adenocarcinoma.

Index